Nutrition for Brain Development

Nutrition for Brain Development

Editor

M. Hasan Mohajeri

MDPI • Basel • Beijing • Wuhan • Barcelona • Belgrade • Manchester • Tokyo • Cluj • Tianjin

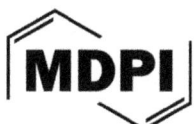

Editor
M. Hasan Mohajeri
Department of Human Medicine
University of Zurich
Zurich
Switzerland

Editorial Office
MDPI
St. Alban-Anlage 66
4052 Basel, Switzerland

This is a reprint of articles from the Special Issue published online in the open access journal *Nutrients* (ISSN 2072-6643) (available at: www.mdpi.com/journal/nutrients/special_issues/Nutrition_Brain_Development).

For citation purposes, cite each article independently as indicated on the article page online and as indicated below:

LastName, A.A.; LastName, B.B.; LastName, C.C. Article Title. *Journal Name* **Year**, *Volume Number*, Page Range.

ISBN 978-3-0365-3804-4 (Hbk)
ISBN 978-3-0365-3803-7 (PDF)

© 2022 by the authors. Articles in this book are Open Access and distributed under the Creative Commons Attribution (CC BY) license, which allows users to download, copy and build upon published articles, as long as the author and publisher are properly credited, which ensures maximum dissemination and a wider impact of our publications.

The book as a whole is distributed by MDPI under the terms and conditions of the Creative Commons license CC BY-NC-ND.

Contents

About the Editor . . . . **vii**

Preface to "Nutrition for Brain Development" . . . . **ix**

M. Hasan Mohajeri
Nutrition for Brain Development
Reprinted from: *Nutrients* 2022, 14, 1419, doi:10.3390/nu14071419 . . . . **1**

Federico Granziera, Maria Angela Guzzardi and Patricia Iozzo
Associations between the Mediterranean Diet Pattern and Weight Status and Cognitive Development in Preschool Children
Reprinted from: *Nutrients* 2021, 13, 3723, doi:10.3390/nu13113723 . . . . **5**

Saivageethi Nuthikattu, Dragan Milenkovic, Jennifer E. Norman, John Rutledge and Amparo Villablanca
Inhibition of Soluble Epoxide Hydrolase Is Protective against the Multiomic Effects of a High Glycemic Diet on Brain Microvascular Inflammation and Cognitive Dysfunction
Reprinted from: *Nutrients* 2021, 13, 3913, doi:10.3390/nu13113913 . . . . **17**

Kenjirou Ogawa, Ayumi Ishii, Aimi Shindo, Kunihiro Hongo, Tomohiro Mizobata and Tetsuya Sogon et al.
Spearmint Extract Containing Rosmarinic Acid Suppresses Amyloid Fibril Formation of Proteins Associated with Dementia
Reprinted from: *Nutrients* 2020, 12, 3480, doi:10.3390/nu12113480 . . . . **45**

Morgane Frapin, Simon Guignard, Dimitri Meistermann, Isabelle Grit, Valentine S. Moullé and Vincent Paillé et al.
Maternal Protein Restriction in Rats Alters the Expression of Genes Involved in Mitochondrial Metabolism and Epitranscriptomics in Fetal Hypothalamus
Reprinted from: *Nutrients* 2020, 12, 1464, doi:10.3390/nu12051464 . . . . **59**

Dawid Gawliński, Kinga Gawlińska, Małgorzata Frankowska and Małgorzata Filip
Maternal Diet Influences the Reinstatement of Cocaine-Seeking Behavior and the Expression of Melanocortin-4 Receptors in Female Offspring of Rats
Reprinted from: *Nutrients* 2020, 12, 1462, doi:10.3390/nu12051462 . . . . **83**

Zsolt Kovács, Brigitta Brunner and Csilla Ari
Beneficial Effects of Exogenous Ketogenic Supplements on Aging Processes and Age-Related Neurodegenerative Diseases
Reprinted from: *Nutrients* 2021, 13, 2197, doi:10.3390/nu13072197 . . . . **101**

Cristina Romani, Filippo Manti, Francesca Nardecchia, Federica Valentini, Nicoletta Fallarino and Claudia Carducci et al.
Cognitive Outcomes and Relationships with Phenylalanine in Phenylketonuria: A Comparison between Italian and English Adult Samples
Reprinted from: *Nutrients* 2020, 12, 3033, doi:10.3390/nu12103033 . . . . **137**

Shannon Morgan McCabe and Ningning Zhao
The Potential Roles of Blood–Brain Barrier and Blood–Cerebrospinal Fluid Barrier in Maintaining Brain Manganese Homeostasis
Reprinted from: *Nutrients* 2021, 13, 1833, doi:10.3390/nu13061833 . . . . **159**

Sylvia Docq, Marcia Spoelder, Wendan Wang and Judith R. Homberg
The Protective and Long-Lasting Effects of Human Milk Oligosaccharides on Cognition in Mammals
Reprinted from: *Nutrients* **2020**, *12*, 3572, doi:10.3390/nu12113572 . . . . **173**

Tom Knuesel and M. Hasan Mohajeri
The Role of the Gut Microbiota in the Development and Progression of Major Depressive and Bipolar Disorder
Reprinted from: *Nutrients* **2021**, *14*, 37, doi:10.3390/nu14010037 . . . . **189**

Shirley Mei-Sin Tran and M. Hasan Mohajeri
The Role of Gut Bacterial Metabolites in Brain Development, Aging and Disease
Reprinted from: *Nutrients* **2021**, *13*, 732, doi:10.3390/nu13030732 . . . . **211**

About the Editor

M. Hasan Mohajeri

Professor M. Hasan Mohajeri is a Lecturer at the Medical Faculty of the University of Zurich, Switzerland. He has a solid publication record, with more than 110 contributions in topics related to brain development and aging, as well as the interactions between the nervous system and the gut microbiota (https://scholar.google.co.uk/citations?hl=de&user=OWHRJzEAAAAJ).

He is the co-inventor of 25+ patents. He is also a member of the Editorial board of Several journals. Dr. Mohajeri studied Biochemistry at the University of Zurich, Switzerland, and achieved his Ph.D. in Neurosciences from the Swiss Federal Institute of Technology (ETH) in Zurich, Switzerland, in 1994. He has more than 20 years of scientific and managerial working experience in large international life sciences enterprises, as well as start-up companies in Europe and the United States.

Preface to "Nutrition for Brain Development"

This Special Issue focuses on factors that are implicated in the development of the brain, and thus have the potential to influence its functions. On the one hand, the brain depends on a steady and sufficient supply of oxygen and dietary ingredients for proper functioning. On the other hand, genetic predispositions and epigenetic and environmental factors may influence brain development and function. Imbalances in any of these factors may lead to the manifestation of developmental disorders at young ages, compromised daily capabilities, or age-associated brain disorders.

The goal of this Special Issue is to publish state-of-the-art contributions discussing the role of nutritional compounds, genetic factors, etc., on brain development, its functions, and aging. Mechanistic and epidemiological studies in vitro, in vivo, and in human subjects were considered for publication. The submission of original research articles, reviews, and meta-analyses was specifically encouraged. This book is of general interest to readership from medical and natural sciences interested in brain aging, the gut–brain axis, and nutrition.

M. Hasan Mohajeri
Editor

Editorial

Nutrition for Brain Development

M. Hasan Mohajeri

Department of Human Medicine, University of Zurich, Winterthurerstrasse 190, 8057 Zürich, Switzerland; mhasan.mohajeri@uzh.ch; Tel.: +41-79-938-1203

This Special Issue focuses on the fundamental role of nutrition in brain development. A steady and sufficient supply of oxygen and dietary ingredients are indispensable for proper brain functioning but genetic and environmental factors may influence brain development and function. Imbalance in any of these factors may lead to the manifestation of developmental disorders of young ages, compromised daily capabilities, or age-associated brain disorders. This editorial will focus on important topics discussed in individual reports included in this Special Issue.

Granziera et al. [1] studied the associations between habitual food consumption, body mass index (BMI), and cognitive outcomes in 54 preschool children born in 2011–2014 and living in Tuscany, Italy. These authors showed, by using the Griffiths Mental Development Scales-Extended Revised (GMDS-ER) test, that adherence to the Mediterranean diet was associated with higher cognitive scores. Importantly, a high body mass index negatively impacted cognition. All associations were independent of maternal IQ, socioeconomic status, breastfeeding, actual age at cognitive assessment, and gender.

Nuthikattu and colleagues [2] showed, using a multi-omic approach, that a high glycemic diet (HGD) leads to differential expression of 608 genes in vivo. HGD affected gene expression of brain microvessels in memory centers by up-regulating the protein-coding and non-coding genes involved in mitochondrial function, oxidation, inflammation, and microvascular functioning. This report showed that inhibition of soluble epoxide hydrolase protects against cognitive decline by down-regulating the above-mentioned differentially expressed genes up-regulated by HGD.

The effects of spearmint extract (SME) and rosmarinic acid (the major component of SME) were examined on the amyloid fibril formation of αSyn, Aβ, and Tau proteins in vitro [3]. Utilizing thioflavin T (ThioT) binding assays and transmission electron microscopy (TEM), it was concluded that rosmarinic acid could disassemble preformed fibrils of αSyn, Aβ, and Tau. Given the fact that a successful therapy for neurodegenerative disorders has not been developed despite decades of intensive research [4], rosmarinic acid may be a promising candidate to be tested in disease models of amyloidosis and supports the notion that dietary ingredients may exhibit a realistic potential to improve brain functions in vivo [5].

Dietary restriction is known to profoundly affect fetal brain development. The report by Frapin et al. asked the question as to which are the cellular and molecular systems underlying the effects of maternal protein restriction (MPR) during fetal development [6]. Transcriptomic analysis of the fetal rat hypothalamus revealed that some genes encoding proteins of the mitochondrial respiratory chain were overexpressed and the mitochondrial metabolic activity in the fetal hypothalamus was altered. Collectively, this report suggests that MPR leads to early alterations of neuronal development and subsequent impaired hypothalamus function in vivo.

In their study, Gawliński et al. evaluated how maternal diet determines the reinstatement of cocaine-seeking behavior and the expression of melanocortin-4 receptors in female rat offspring [7]. The authors showed that a maternal high-sugar diet is an important factor that triggers cocaine-seeking behavior in female offspring and the expression of melanocortin-4 (MC-4) receptors in the nucleus accumbens. Moreover, they suggested that an altered amount of macronutrients in the maternal diet disrupts the proper expression of MC-4 receptors in brain structures involved in cocaine relapse.

In their elaborated review, Kovacs et al. examined the potential beneficial effects of ketogenic supplements on the aging process and age-related neurodegenerative diseases. They concluded that exogenous ketogenic supplements (EKS), such as ketone salts and ketone esters, may mitigate aging processes, delay the onset of age-associated diseases and extend lifespan through ketosis. Consequently, the administration of EKS may be a potential therapeutic tool as an adjuvant therapeutics in combination with therapeutic drugs against age-related neurodegenerative diseases and increase the health span of the aging human population [8].

A collaborative effort of scientists in the United Kingdom and Italy [9] compared the test batteries, designed to monitor the effect of phenylketonuria (PKU) on cognitive performance. The parameter in the focus of this study included visual attention, visuomotor coordination, executive functions, sustained attention, verbal and visual memory, and learning. The results suggested that batteries with the same and/or matched tasks can be used to assess cognitive outcomes across countries allowing results to be compared and accrued.

Manganese (Mn) is a trace nutrient necessary for life but is toxic to the brain at high concentrations. McCabe and Zhao [10] provided an insight into the transport mechanisms of Mn through the blood–brain barrier (BBB) and the blood–CSF barrier (BCB) and its hemostasis in the brain by reviewing in vitro and in vivo models.

The potential effects of the human milk oligosaccharides (HMO) on cognitive functions were reviewed in mice, rats, and piglets [11]. The authors concluded that the administration of fucosylated (single or combined with Lacto-N-neoTetraose and other oligosaccharides) and sialylated HMOs results in marked age-dependent improvements in spatial memory and in an accelerated learning rate in operant tasks, which already become apparent during infancy. A combination of HMOs with other oligosaccharides yielded different effects on memory performance as opposed to single HMO administration, a topic that is being intensively researched.

Lastly, we evaluated in a systematic review [12] the available preclinical and clinical data on alterations of the gut microbiome, particularly on low taxonomic levels, and related them to the pathophysiology of major depressive (MDD) and bipolar disorder (BD). A discussion of diagnostic and treatment response parameters, their health-promoting potential, as well as novel adjunctive treatment options are also discussed. We also take on the task of systematically evaluating the role of the bacterial metabolites, beyond the short-chain fatty acids (SCFA), in brain development and different neurodegenerative diseases [13]. SCFA are extensively studied in various test systems, but the biology of other bacterial metabolites in health and disease is an overtly under-researched topic. Our data highlight the existence of altered bacterial metabolites in patients across various brain diseases and describe protective and detrimental effects of some bacterial metabolites in brain diseases such as autism spectrum disorder, affective disorders, multiple sclerosis, and Parkinson's disease. These findings could lead to further insights into the gut–brain axis and thus into potential diagnostic, therapeutic, or preventive strategies in brain diseases.

In conclusion, diet is of fundamental importance for the development of the brain. Given that diet directly or indirectly affects brain development and function, carefully planned and masterfully conducted basic and clinical research is needed to understand brain development better and to answer the question to which extent diet-related strategies can prevent brain disorders or be therapeutically exploited.

Funding: This research received no external funding.

Institutional Review Board Statement: Not applicable.

Informed Consent Statement: Not applicable.

Data Availability Statement: Not applicable.

Conflicts of Interest: The author declares no conflict of interest.

References

1. Granziera, F.; Guzzardi, M.A.; Iozzo, P. Associations between the mediterranean diet pattern and weight status and cognitive development in preschool children. *Nutrients* **2021**, *13*, 3723. [CrossRef] [PubMed]
2. Nuthikattu, S.; Milenkovic, D.; Norman, J.E.; Rutledge, J.; Villablanca, A. Inhibition of soluble epoxide hydrolase is protective against the multiomic effects of a high glycemic diet on brain microvascular inflammation and cognitive dysfunction. *Nutrients* **2021**, *13*, 3913. [CrossRef] [PubMed]
3. Ogawa, K.; Ishii, A.; Shindo, A.; Hongo, K.; Mizobata, T.; Sogon, T.; Kawata, Y. Spearmint extract containing rosmarinic acid suppresses amyloid fibril formation of proteins associated with dementia. *Nutrients* **2020**, *12*, 3480. [CrossRef] [PubMed]
4. Mohajeri, M.H.; Leuba, G. Prevention of age-associated dementia. *Brain Res. Bull.* **2009**, *80*, 315–325. [CrossRef] [PubMed]
5. Mechan, A.O.; Fowler, A.; Seifert, S.; Rieger, H.; Wohrle, T.; Etheve, S.; Wyss, A.; Schuler, G.; Colletto, B.; Kilpert, C.; et al. Monoamine reuptake inhibition and mood-enhancing potential of a specified oregano extract. *Br. J. Nutr.* **2011**, *105*, 1150–1163. [CrossRef] [PubMed]
6. Frapin, M.; Guignard, S.; Meistermann, D.; Grit, I.; Moulle, V.S.; Paille, V.; Parnet, P.; Amarger, V. Maternal protein restriction in rats alters the expression of genes involved in mitochondrial metabolism and epitranscriptomics in fetal hypothalamus. *Nutrients* **2020**, *12*, 1464. [CrossRef] [PubMed]
7. Gawlinski, D.; Gawlinska, K.; Frankowska, M.; Filip, M. Maternal diet influences the reinstatement of cocaine-seeking behavior and the expression of melanocortin-4 receptors in female offspring of rats. *Nutrients* **2020**, *12*, 1462. [CrossRef]
8. Kovacs, Z.; Brunner, B.; Ari, C. Beneficial effects of exogenous ketogenic supplements on aging processes and age-related neurodegenerative diseases. *Nutrients* **2021**, *13*, 2197. [CrossRef]
9. Romani, C.; Manti, F.; Nardecchia, F.; Valentini, F.; Fallarino, N.; Carducci, C.; De Leo, S.; Macdonald, A.; Palermo, L.; Leuzzi, V. Cognitive outcomes and relationships with phenylalanine in phenylketonuria: A comparison between Italian and English adult samples. *Nutrients* **2020**, *12*, 3033. [CrossRef]
10. McCabe, S.M.; Zhao, N. The potential roles of blood–Brain barrier and blood–Cerebrospinal fluid barrier in maintaining brain manganese homeostasis. *Nutrients* **2021**, *13*, 1833. [CrossRef] [PubMed]
11. Docq, S.; Spoelder, M.; Wang, W.; Homberg, J.R. The protective and long-lasting effects of human milk oligosaccharides on cognition in mammals. *Nutrients* **2020**, *12*, 3572. [CrossRef] [PubMed]
12. Knuesel, T.; Mohajeri, M.H. The role of the gut microbiota in the development and progression of major depressive and bipolar disorder. *Nutrients* **2021**, *14*, 37. [CrossRef] [PubMed]
13. Tran, S.M.-S.; Mohajeri, M.H. The role of gut bacterial metabolites in brain development, aging and disease. *Nutrients* **2021**, *13*, 732. [CrossRef] [PubMed]

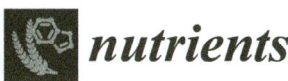

Article

Associations between the Mediterranean Diet Pattern and Weight Status and Cognitive Development in Preschool Children

Federico Granziera [1,2], Maria Angela Guzzardi [1,*] and Patricia Iozzo [1]

1. Institute of Clinical Physiology, National Research Council (CNR), 56124 Pisa, Italy; federico.granziera@santannapisa.it (F.G.); patricia.iozzo@ifc.cnr.it (P.I.)
2. Sant'Anna School of Advanced Studies, 56127 Pisa, Italy
* Correspondence: m.guzzardi@ifc.cnr.it; Tel.: +39-050-3152789

Abstract: Cognitive dysfunctions are a global health concern. Early-life diet and weight status may contribute to children's cognitive development. For this reason, we explored the associations between habitual food consumption, body mass index (BMI) and cognitive outcomes in 54 preschool children belonging to the Pisa birth Cohort (PISAC). We estimated groups of foods, nutrients and calorie intakes through a food frequency questionnaire (FFQ) and Italian national databases. Then, we adopted the Mediterranean diet (MD) score to assess relative MD adherence. Cognition was examined using the Griffiths Mental Development Scales-Extended Revised (GMDS-ER). We found that higher, compared to low and moderate, adherence to MD was associated with higher performance scores. Furthermore, white meat consumption was positively related to BMI, and BMI (age–gender specific, z-scores) categories were negatively related to practical reasoning scores. All associations were independent of maternal IQ estimates, parents' socioeconomic status, exclusive/non-exclusive breastfeeding, actual age at cognitive assessment and gender. In conclusion, in preschool children, very high adherence to MD seemed protective, whereas BMI (reinforced by the intake of white meat) was negatively associated with cognition.

Keywords: early childhood; nutrition; Mediterranean diet; body mass index; cognitive development

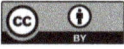

1. Introduction

Cognitive decline and impairment are globally increasing health concerns, associating with a growing prevalence of metabolic diseases [1] and with population aging [2]. Effective treatment is lacking, and early prevention targeting modifiable determinants is warranted [3]. Life-course studies have shown that a lower intelligence quotient (IQ) at 11 years is already predictive of dementia seven decades later [4], suggesting that the risk is partially settled at 11 years and preventive actions should focus on younger children.

Diet and body weight are accredited lifestyle determinants of cognitive (dys)function in adults and patients [5], but few studies have explored associations between nutrients or consumption of given foods or eating habits and cognitive outcomes in children from developed countries. Some have investigated the effects of individual micronutrients, such as vitamin B12, folic acid, zinc, iron, and iodine, but findings in non-IQ-deficient children are controversial [6]. In addition, studies investigating the association of plasma biomarkers of polyunsaturated fatty acids and cognition in children have provided inconsistent results [7]. For example, a study observed a direct relationship between the proportion of docosahexaenoic acid (DHA) and eicosapentaenoic acid (EPA) in blood and working memory in children [8]; instead, Boucher et al. found no associations between the proportions of DHA, EPA, or other omega-3 fatty acids in blood and working memory in children [9]. Several other studies have focused on macronutrients and whole foods [10]. For example, an observational study in 586 European children aged 7–9 years documented that consumption of two fish (including one fatty fish) meals per week reduced social, attention, and behavioural problems [11]. Another study in 5200 Canadian children aged 10–11 showed that lower fat and higher fruit and vegetable intakes were associated with better reading and writing achievements [12]. Sugar intake did not emerge as a factor affecting behaviour or cognitive performance in children in meta-analysis studies [13], but consumption of sugar-sweetened beverages was recently reported as negative predictor of higher verbal scores in 3-year-old American children [14]. Other studies found that low-glycaemic index (GI) breakfasts predicted better attention and memory, and declarative-verbal memory and high-GI breakfasts were associated with better vigilance in 6–11 and 11–14-year-old children [15,16]. Taki et al. showed that brain grey and white matter volumes were greater in children eating rice than bread at breakfast, speculating that this may depend on the lower glycaemic index of rice [17]. However, a recent systematic review concluded that there is a lack of research comparing breakfast types, precluding recommendations for the size and composition of an optimal breakfast for children's cognitive function [18].

Dietary patterns and diet quality indices have been suggested to better reflect a real-life diet, where foods are the combination of various nutrients that act synergistically and are interrelated [19,20]. These diet quality indices mostly describe a diet high in vegetables, fruit and berries, non-refined cereals products and fish and low in meats and saturated fat. Among whole-diet scores, the Healthy Eating Index (HEI-2005), Dietary Approaches to Stop Hypertension (DASH) score, Baltic Sea Diet Score (BSDS) and the Finnish Children Healthy Eating Index (FCHEI) were linked to better reading skills or cognition among 6–9-year-old children [7].

This overview highlights that the current understanding of the diet–cognitive development relationship is limited, and a great majority of studies have been focused on children who have entered school, in whom the influence of academic education may represent a relevant confounder, whereas very sparse knowledge has been produced in preschool children.

The aim of this study was to explore, comparatively, the impact of food habits, amount of ingested daily calories, macro- and micronutrient intakes, and Mediterranean diet (MD) adherence in preschool children on cognitive outcomes while taking into account the most important known confounders, i.e., maternal IQ estimate, parental socio-economic status, exclusive or non-exclusive breastfeeding, actual age at cognitive assessment and children's gender.

2. Materials and Methods
2.1. Study Population

The study was conducted in a subgroup of n = 54, 5-year-old preschool children of the Pisa birth Cohort (PISAC). Overall, the PISAC cohort includes 90 families—father, mother and infants born in 2011–2014 and living in Tuscany, Italy—enrolled during pregnancy to investigate the effects of maternal obesity on offspring cardiometabolic and cognitive health. The cohort was intended to represent the general population and, therefore, the inclusion criteria were broad, namely, (1) mothers within the first trimester of pregnancy at the first visit or at delivery; (2) any parents' age; (3) any BMI; (4) willingness of mothers and fathers to participate and to actively collect questionnaires and samples; (5) capacity of mothers and fathers to understand the study and its implications; (6) signature of the informed consent by mothers and fathers; (7) absence of major diseases (mothers and fathers) and perinatal complications. Exclusion criteria were (1) history of major diseases in the mother and in the father (kidney failure, liver failure, cardiac failure, major lung disease, autoimmune disease, cancer, psychiatric illness, also including anorexia–bulimia nervosa and substance abuse); (2) major health complications during the perinatal period; (3) failure to understand the study's implications, comply with the study's schedule or sign the consent form. Follow-up visits were carried out from birth to the children's age of five years and consisted of anthropometric, echocardiographic and cognitive assessments and collection of biological samples (cord–blood, faeces and saliva) and of FFQs (at 5 years). Families were given the option to participate in all or only part of the assessment visits

(0, 12, 18, 24, 36 and 60 months of life); therefore, the sample size varied across age points and measurements. In particular, families not included in this analysis did not have time to attend all 60 months' visits and chose to have cardiac or anthropometric evaluations rather than cognitive assessments or no evaluation at all. At 60 months, children's body weight (in kg to the nearest 0.1 kg) and length (in cm to the nearest 0.5 cm) were measured by weight scale and stadiometer, with children wearing light clothes and standing straight without shoes and with heels close together [21]. Then, the children's BMI (kg/m^2) was calculated, and BMI-for-age (gender-specific, z-scores) categories were defined as follows: moderately underweight (>−3 to <−2 standard deviations), normal weight (>−2 to <+1 standard deviations), overweight (>+1 to <+2 standard deviations), obesity (>+2 standard deviations) [22]. Data on parents' jobs were transformed in socioeconomic classes using the European Socio-economic Classification (ESeC) [23].

The study was conducted in accordance with the Declaration of Helsinki and approved by the Ethics Committee of Massa and Carrara and the latest amendments by the Ethical Committee of the Area Vasta Nord-Ovest (CEAVNO), Pisa, Italy (Study ID 394, approval decree/document n. 75 and 71512). Parents gave their written informed consent before inclusion.

2.2. Food Frequency Questionnaire (FFQ)

Dietary assessment was conducted for 65 children throughout a validated, self-administered, semi-quantitative FFQ, with minor modifications [24]. However, the current analyses pertained to the 54 children who also underwent the cognitive visit. The FFQ consisted of 53 commonly used food items (including 124 foods) classified into 22 groups (bread, pizza, crackers and breadsticks, pasta or rice, minestrone soup with pasta or rice, barley and spelled, polenta, couscous, potatoes, eggs, fresh and processed meats, fish, cheeses, milk, yogurt, vegetables, olives, fruit and nuts, legumes, cakes and snacks, sugar and honey teaspoons added to milk and drinks and beverages). Vegetable drinks, milk-shakes, wine and beer were included in the FFQ but were not consumed in our population. The type of fat (extra virgin olive (EVO) oil, olive oil, seed oil, butter, margarine, cooking cream, bacon and lard) used for preparing, cooking and dressing food was also addressed.

Frequency response categories for foods items were the following: never, less than once a month, 1–3 times a month, once a week, 2–4 and 5–6 times a week, once a day and 2–3 and 4–5 times a day. Frequency response categories for cooking and dressing fats included: always (2–3 times per day), sometimes (twice per month) and never. The parents filled in the FFQ on the child's behalf. Data were checked for completeness and consistency, considering incompleteness in >25% items as grounds for a priori exclusion [25]. All FFQs were valid to be submitted into data processing and analysis. A total of 23 specific food groups were further grouped into 13 broader categories (cereals, potatoes, eggs, red and processed meats, white meat, fish, dairy products, legumes, vegetables, fruit and nuts, cakes and snacks, sugar-sweetened drinks and cooking–dressing fats ratio) based on their nutritional content. To estimate the weekly grams consumed for each food category, we first calculated the consumptions of the 53 food items, multiplying the frequency of consumption by the age-appropriate standard portion [26], and we summed the amounts consumed of each food item belonging to the specific category, thus obtaining relative consumption. To estimate daily nutrients and calories intakes, we started by obtaining the nutritional values of the original 124 foods using the Food Composition Tables for Epidemiological Studies in Italy (BDA) [27] or the Food Composition Tables (Council for Agricultural Research and Analysis of the Agricultural Economy, CREA) [28]. The nutritional content of each food was used to calculate the mean amount/portion for each nutrient in the 53 food items. Then, we obtained the daily intake of each nutrient through the weighted sum of the consumption frequency of each food item by its amount/portion. Furthermore, the daily caloric intake was estimated through the weighted sum of each macronutrient intake by its calories. Among the 65 children, eight participants had food allergies or intolerances (i.e., to gluten, milk or lactose, tomato, chickpeas, sesame, shellfish and egg-white), and eighteen had taken food supplements (i.e., prebiotics, probiotics, vitamins and minerals) in the last month. None of the parents declared any other major food-related illnesses affecting their children.

2.3. Mediterranean Diet (MD) Score

The degree of children's adherence to the traditional Mediterranean diet was estimated according to the score proposed by Trichopoulou et al., with a minor modification [29]. Briefly, based on median consumption values, a score of 0 or 1 was assigned to each of the following 9 food categories: vegetables, legumes, fruits and nuts, cereals, fish, red and processed meats, white meat, dairy products and the ratio of unsaturated fatty acids to saturated fatty acids (cooking–dressing fats). For dietary components that are considered protective in the MD (vegetables, legumes, fruits and nuts, cereal, fish and a high ratio of unsaturated/saturated fatty acids), a score of 0 was attributed if consumption was below the median value of the population, and 1 point was given if it was equal or above the median value. The opposite was done for the other components (i.e., red/processed and white meats and dairy products). Thus, the total MD score ranged from 0 (reflecting no adherence at all) to 9 points (maximal adherence to the traditional MD). Finally, adherence to the MD score was categorised into 4 categories: low (score 0–2), moderate (score 3–4), high (score 5–6), and very high (score 7–9).

2.4. Neuropsychological Assessment

The children's cognitive development was evaluated by a trained psychologist in a dedicated hospital room using the GMDS-ER version [30–32] in $n = 54$ of the children, addressing the following 6 cognitive domains: locomotor, personal–social, hearing and language, hand–eye coordination, performance and practical reasoning. Maternal IQ was estimated in $n = 52$ women by the Raven's progressive matrices.

2.5. Statistical Analysis

SPSS for Windows (version 26, Chicago, IL, USA) was used for statistical analysis. Regression models, such as bivariate correlation analysis, were performed to assess associations between continuous variables, and partial correlation analyses to adjust for covariates (i.e., mothers' IQ estimate, parents' ESeC, exclusive or non-exclusive breastfeeding, actual age at cognitive assessment and gender). To avoid chance findings, p-values were corrected for multiple comparison, using the Benjamini–Hochberg false discovery rate ($Q = 0.20$). General linear models and t-tests or two-way ANOVAs (analysis of variance) were performed for two or more than two group comparisons, and ANCOVA (analysis of covariance) was used to incorporate covariates). The results are presented as the mean $\pm$ standard deviation (SD) or standard error (SEM), and p-values ≤ 0.05 were established as the threshold for rejecting the null hypothesis.

3. Results

3.1. Description of the Study Population

The characteristics of the study's population are reported in Table 1. The number of boys slightly prevailed over that of girls, and nearly half of the children were exclusively breastfed in the first 6 months of life [21]. According to WHO's child growth standards [22], half of the children were modestly underweight and <20% were overweight. The parents' mean age was 39.1 ± 4.2 years for mothers and 41.7 ± 4.6 years for fathers. With reference to the ESeC 3-class model [23], parents were well distributed between working and intermediate classes, and were less represented in the salariat class. Finally, children's mean age at cognitive assessment was 5.2 ± 0.1 and all children were cognitively healthy, like their mothers [31].

Table 1. Characteristics of the study population.

Variable	N	Descriptive Results
Boys/girls, N (%)	54	30 (55.6)/24 (44.4)
Breastfeeding (exclusively/non-exclusively), N (%)	54	25 (46.3)/29 (53.7)
Weight at 5 years (kg), mean ± SD	54	20.6 ± 3.7
BMI at 5 years (kg/m^2), mean ± SD	54	17.1 ± 2.4
BMI UW/NW/OW/OB at 5 years, N (%)	54	27 (50)/18 (33.3)/9 (16.7)/0
BMI UW/NW/OW/OB at 5 years (kg/m^2), mean ± SD	54	15.3 ± 0.9/17.6 ± 0.5/21.1 ± 0.5/0
Mothers' BMI in pregnancy	51	29.4 ± 4.9
Mother's age (years), mean ± SD	54	39.1 ± 4.2
Father's age (years), mean ± SD	54	41.7 ± 4.6
Mothers' ESeC WK/IN/SA, N (%)	53	18 (33.3)/21 (38.9)/14 (25.9)
Fathers' ESeC WK/IN/SA, N (%)	48	19 (35.2)/19 (35.2)/10 (18.5)
Mothers' IQ estimate, mean ± SD	48	114.9 ± 9.5
Actual age at cognitive assessment	54	5.2 ± 0.1
Locomotor score, mean ± SD	54	103.8 ± 7.3
Personal–social score, mean ± SD	54	104.8 ± 8.6
Hearing and speech score, mean ± SD	54	101.6 ± 10.0
Hand–eye coordination score, mean ± SD	54	99.2 ± 10.0
Performance score, mean ± SD	54	112.0 ± 7.1
Practical reasoning score, mean ± Practical SD	54	95.7 ± 9.2
MD scores, mean ± SD	54	4.3 ± 1.6
MD score 0–2/3–4/5–6/7–9 categories, N (%)	54	8 (14.8)/20 (37)/20 (37)/6 (11.1)

Population characteristics are given as the mean ± SD or number and (%), as appropriate. UW = moderately underweight, NW = normal weight, OW = overweight, OB = obesity, WK = working class, IN = intermediate class, SA = salariat class and MD = Mediterranean diet.

3.2. Children's Food, Calories and Nutrients Intake

The consumption of the 13 food categories and nutritional and caloric intake are reported in Table 2. We found no difference between boys and girls, and the average weekly food consumption was mostly in line with the Guidelines for Healthy Italian Food Habits, with the exception of a lower consumption of eggs (<100 g/week) [26]. The estimated calories and (micro-)nutrients amounts were in accordance with the Nutrient and Energy Reference Intake Levels for the Italian population aged 4–6, except for vitamin D, the consumption of which was almost 90% below the recommended amount (10 µg/day) [33]. Among cooking and dressing fats, the intake of unsaturated (over saturated) fats prevailed, reflecting a predominant use of EVO, olive and seed oils.

Table 2. Children's weekly food groups and daily energy and nutrients intakes.

Dietary Variable	N	Children's Intake
Cereals (g/week)	53	1110.8 ± 484.0
Potatoes (g/week)	53	173.1 ± 124.9
Legumes (g/week)	53	41.5 ± 38.9
Eggs (g/week)	53	49.5 ± 47.4
Red and processed meats (g/week)	54	140.6 ± 96.6
White meat (g/week)	54	120.8 ± 70.1
Fish (g/week)	54	137.5 ± 104.0
Dairy products (g/week)	54	582.3 ± 486.5
Vegetables (g/week)	54	492.5 ± 447.1
Fruit and nuts (g/week)	54	1152.5 ± 868.8
Cakes and snacks (g/week)	54	406.8 ± 358.7
Sugar-sweetened drinks	53	865.5 ± 644.3
Unsaturated/saturated fats ratio	54	4.7/1 ± 1.1
Daily calorie (kcal/day)	54	1569.0 ± 394.7

Table 2. Cont.

Dietary Variable	N	Children's Intake
Proteins (g/day)	54	48.3 ± 13.4
Lipids (g/day)	54	60.4 ± 13.9
Carbohydrates (g/day)	54	202.4 ± 61.5
Fibres (g/day)	54	11.0 ± 3.7
Retinol (mg/day)	54	414.1 ± 163.6
Vitamin B1 (mg/day)	54	0.5 ± 0.1
Vitamin B6 (mg/day)	54	0.9 ± 0.2
Folate (μg/day)	54	144.4 ± 48.2
Vitamin C (mg/day)	54	75.5 ± 48.7
Vitamin D (μg/day)	54	0.6 ± 0.3
Vitamin E (mg/day)	54	7.9 ± 1.6
Iron (mg/day)	54	5.2 ± 1.5
Calcium (mg/day)	54	649.1 ± 245.0
Sodium (mg/day)	54	1264.0 ± 468.6
Potassium (mg/day)	54	1728.2 ± 481.7
Phosphorous (mg/day)	54	797.8 ± 241.4
Zinc (mg/day)	54	5.4 ± 1.5

Continuous data are reported as the mean ± SD.

3.3. Correlations between Food Categories and BMI and Cognitive Outcomes

Relevant associations between weekly consumption of foods included in the MD score and children's BMI or cognitive outcomes are reported in Table 3. Bivariate analysis showed that the consumption of white meat was related to BMI ($p = 0.005$), unsaturated/saturated fats ratio (cooking–dressing) was related to hand–eye coordination ($p = 0.005$), dairy products were related to performance scores and vegetable consumption was associated with personal–social scores ($p = 0.015$). In addition, BMI categories were negatively related to practical reasoning score ($p = 0.010$) (Table 3). The other variables in Table 2 did not show associations with cognitive scores or BMI.

Table 3. Correlations between MD food categories and BMI (including BMI categories) and cognitive outcomes.

Variables	Regression Model	BMI	Locomotor	Personal–Social	Hearing and Language	Hand–Eye Coordination	Performance	Practical Reasoning
Cereals (g/week)	Bivariate	−0.188	0.029	0.208	−0.010	0.032	−0.030	0.137
	Adjusted	−0.042	0.004	0.274	0.109	0.035	−0.055	0.227
Potatoes (g/week)	Bivariate	−0.077	0.078	−0.012	−0.021	0.037	−0.057	0.116
	Adjusted	−0.307	0.114	−0.049	−0.210	0.008	−0.010	0.158
Legumes (g/week)	Bivariate	0.096	0.011	0.061	0.002	−0.093	0.103	−0.105
	Adjusted	0.113	0.079	0.104	−0.009	−0.044	0.188	−0.146
Eggs (g/week)	Bivariate	−0.162	−0.085	0.068	−0.130	0.229	0.188	−0.028
	Adjusted	−0.059	−0.089	−0.049	−0.213	0.380	0.199	−0.113
Red and processed meats (g/week)	Bivariate	0.237	0.033	0.097	0.121	0.012	−0.007	−0.006
	Adjusted	0.319	0.185	0.217	0.188	0.059	0.057	0.056
White meat (g/week)	Bivariate	0.377 **	0.081	0.084	0.054	0.009	−0.111	−0.080
	Adjusted	0.440 **	0.267	0.303	0.067	0.089	0.023	−0.015
Vegetables (g/week)	Bivariate	−0.067	0.242	0.295 *	0.067	0.037	0.101	0.030
	Adjusted	0.073	0.285	0.315	−0.009	0.051	0.005	−0.006
Fruit and nuts (g/week)	Bivariate	−0.030	0.059	0.044	−0.168	0.018	−0.124	−0.032
	Adjusted	0.085	0.053	0.046	−0.088	0.199	−0.102	0.181
Dairy products (g/week)	Bivariate	−0.232	0.030	−0.015	0.053	0.101	0.275 *	0.233
	Adjusted	−0.177	−0.021	−0.093	0.024	0.027	0.272	0.233
Unsaturated/saturated fats ratio	Bivariate	−0.023	−0.078	−0.018	−0.037	0.369 **	0.254	0.212
	Adjusted	−0.009	−0.282	−0.224	−0.086	0.295	0.222	−0.002
BMI categories	Bivariate	0.792 **	−0.131	−0.083	−0.115	−0.005	−0.100	−0.358 **
	Adjusted	0.811 **	−0.122	0.084	−0.126	0.101	0.063	−0.329 *

The table provides the results of the regression analysis for both the bivariate and adjusted models. Bivariate analyses were performed in $n = 53$ (list-wise deletion) and partial correlation analyses were performed in $n = 43$ (list-wise deletion); p-values were corrected for the false discovery rate using the Benjamini–Hochberg (Q = 0.20). * $p < 0.05$, ** $p < 0.01$. Adjustment for confounders in multivariate analyses includes mothers' IQ estimate, parents' ESeC, exclusive/non-exclusive breastfeeding, actual age at cognitive assessment and gender.

Among potential confounders, we found that some intakes in children were correlated with maternal IQ and parents' ESeC or exclusive/non-exclusive breastfeeding in the first 6 months of life. In particular, maternal IQ estimate was related to children's unsaturated/saturated fats ratio intake (r = 0.367, p = 0.007), to hand–eye coordination scores (r = 0.305, p = 0.035) and practical reasoning scores (r = 0.376, p = 0.008); parents' ESeC was related to children's cereals intake (r = 0.320, p = 0.014) and to unsaturated/saturated fats ratio intake (r = 0.437, p = 0.001). Moreover, exclusively breastfed children consumed more potatoes than non-exclusively breastfed children (t-test, p = 0.017). In addition, the actual age (in months) at cognitive assessment was negatively related with all but two cognitive domains, hearing and language and hand–eye coordination (r = −0.326, p = 0.016 locomotor; r = −0.441, p = 0.001 personal–social; r = −0.327, p = 0.016 performance; r = −0.498, p < 0.001 practical reasoning domains). For this reason, the above correlative analyses were adjusted for these variables and for children's gender. Instead, mothers' BMI during pregnancy was not related to any dietary or cognitive outcome.

After adjustment, partial correlation analyses showed that white meat consumption was significantly related to BMI, and BMI categories remained negatively related to practical reasoning scores. Instead, associations between food categories and cognitive outcomes did not remain significant (Table 3).

3.4. Adherence to MD and Cognitive Outcomes

Continuous data did not show significance. Children were further stratified into tertiles of cognitive scores (gender-specific high, medium and low tertiles), and univariate and adjusted analyses were performed. In the unadjusted model, children with maximum adherence to the MD had higher performance scores than those with low and moderate adherence to the MD (p = 0.003, p = 0.014, respectively; p trend = 0.008). In the other five cognitive domains, no difference was seen between the four MD categories (data not shown). Adjustment for the relevant covariates confirmed the above results, as shown by significance levels given in Figure 1. According to Ivens et al. [31], children in the second tertile were within the average range of performance scores, and children in the third tertile were above average to the very high range. The grouping in tertiles reduced the interindividual variability effects and resulted in the detection of very high MD adherence as a significant thresholding range.

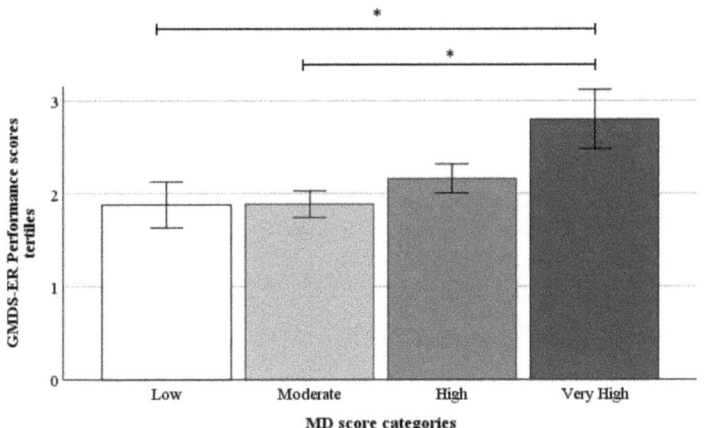

Figure 1. The children's performance in tertiles (low = 1<; medium = >1 to 2<; high = >2) stratified by the Mediterranean diet score categories (n = 44). Data are shown as mean ± SEM. * p < 0.05.

4. Discussion

In the present study, we found that stricter MD adherence was positively related with scores in the performance domain in preschool children. Furthermore, children's BMI was associated with white meat consumption (positively) and with practical reasoning scores (inversely).

Among cognitively healthy school children, two cohort studies have shown that a higher quality diet was associated with better cognitive tasks. Khan et al. explored the association between inhibitory control (Kaufman Brief Intelligence Test or the Woodcock-Johnson Tests of Cognitive Abilities) and overall diet quality (HEI-2005 score) among 65 American 7–9-year-old children using three-day dietary records. They found that the HEI-2005 scores were negatively associated with response accuracy interference, suggesting greater cognitive flexibility [34]. Haapala et al. suggested that diet quality favours precocious non-verbal fluid intelligence and abstract reasoning in 428 Finnish children aged 6–8 years, in whom DASH and BSDS scores, calculated by a four-day food record, were directly associated with Raven's Coloured Progressive Matrices scores (i.e., higher cognitive performance) [35]. In the present study, we evaluated diet quality through the use of the MD score. To our knowledge, these findings are the first evidence for the associations of adherence to the MD and cognition in preschool children, even if limited to a small population. The expectation when adopting this score was to reinforce the impact of the single components by their pooling and establish the level of MD adherence that would result into a clinically significant difference. Interestingly, a two-point MD adherence score difference has been shown to lower overall and cardiovascular mortality, and the incidence of Parkinson's and Alzheimer's diseases in the general population [29]. Though neural mechanisms underlying cognitive benefits of the MD have not been clarified [36], there is evidence that circulating levels of glucose, choline, tyrosine and tryptophan, polyunsaturated fatty acids, vitamins/minerals, antioxidants and the gut microbiota affect neurochemistry, neurotransmission and neuroprotection in the human brain [37–39].

In addition, due to the sample size's limitation, the ability to control for confounders was limited. Other important confounders may include cognitive stimulation, parental educational attainment, etc.

We aimed to dissect single food categories or macro- and micronutrients that could contribute to explaining cognitive scores in children. However, it may be difficult to separate the specific effects of single nutrients/foods because of the interactive/synergistic nature of nutrients, high intercorrelation among nutrients and foods, potential small effect of a single food or nutrient and the residual confounding by dietary patterns [8]. We applied false discovery rate corrections to our analyses and then adjusted for confounders, maximising rigor and minimising chances for significant findings. Therefore, we consider that bivariate associations surviving false discovery rate corrections retain the value of hypothesis generating observations. They suggest positive effects of high intakes of vegetables (vs. personal–social scores), dairy products (vs. performance scores) and unsaturated/saturated fats ratios (vs. hand–eye coordination scores). These correlations were not significant after introducing parental and children's confounders, which may be due to the inter-correlation, limited sample and/or lack of a direct relationship and, overall, the correlations must be interpreted in light of the risk of type II error (i.e., false negative).

We noted that the intake of vitamin D in children seemed very low. Though food is not the main source and indicator of circulating vitamin D, there are recommended daily vitamin D intake ranges, and the observation of a 90% reduction below this range in our children is consistent with the estimated 80% prevalence of vitamin D deficiency in children living in developed countries, including countries with ample sunrays [40].

As a secondary study outcome, we found an inverse association between weight status and practical reasoning scores. Childhood overweight and obesity rates have risen dramatically over the past few decades. Although obesity has been linked to poorer neurocognitive functioning in adults, much less is known about this relationship in children and adolescents [41,42]. Our finding is in line with a recent meta-analysis showing a negative relationship between BMI and various aspects of neurocognitive function such as executive function, attention, visuo-spatial performance and motor skills in healthy children [43]. Our results strongly support these authors' statement, that longitudinal studies are urgently needed to determine the directionality of such relationships and identify the critical intervention time periods in order to develop effective treatment programs [43].

The present findings should be interpreted within the context of the study's strengths and limitations. Strengths of the present study include the assessment of children's diet with a validated dietary questionnaire, well-established outcome measures and control for several family, maternal and children's characteristics. We opted for the FFQ to reflect usual eating habits rather than short-lasting dietary exposures [44], and cognitive development was objectively measured by a trained psychologist by using the GMDS-ER test. Dietary estimations were based on a total of 124 foods using validated Italian food databases; however, given the FFQ format, we recognise that adopting standard portion sizes may be less accurate than actually measuring portions. Another important limitation is the small sample size. Therefore, our findings should be interpreted as hypothesis generating observations. We also acknowledge that there are possibly more comprehensive tests to assess cognition at the age of 5 years, but our children were followed from the age of 6 months, and we chose to preserve the same (though age-adapted) test longitudinally. We recognise that comparison with other studies is rather complex, mainly because of different methodological approaches, including dietary records, type of dietary scores/indices, control of confounding factors, type of cognitive subtests, age range of children, with very few studies addressing preschool children. Although our results incorporated information on the most known relevant confounders, we acknowledge that the ability to control for confounders could be reduced because of the sample size, and that residual confounding effects related to other unmeasured variables, such as cognitive stimulation, parental educational attainment and physical activity, may still occur. Moreover, the age at cognitive assessment had a negative association with cognitive outcomes, but we can only speculate that other unaccounted factors could be involved. Finally, the cross-sectional design cannot establish causal relationships.

5. Conclusions

The present study provides limited but novel evidence linking children's diet, weight status and cognition, suggesting potentially positive impacts of the Mediterranean diet and negative impacts of a high BMI. Our data are compatible with the hypothesis that an optimal intake of key foods, acting in synergy with the MD, may confer protection. Our hypothesis-generating findings on single foods support the conduct of larger prospective and mechanistic studies to confirm the positive relationship observed between intake of dairy products, vegetables or unsaturated (vs saturated) fats and cognitive outcomes.

Author Contributions: Formal analysis, writing—original draft, F.G.; data collection, supervision of analyses, writing—review and editing of the manuscript, M.A.G.; conceptualisation, funding acquisition, writing—review and editing of the manuscript, P.I. All authors have read and agreed to the published version of the manuscript.

Funding: This study was partly supported by the EU-FP7-HEALTH DORIAN Project: Development Origins of Healthy and Unhealthy Aging: The Role of Maternal Obesity (grant agreement No. 278603), the JPI-HDHL-INTIMIC Knowledge Platform of Food, Diet, Intestinal Microbiomics, and Human Health (sub-project No. KP-778 MISVILUPPO, Italian Ministry of Agricultural, Food, and Forestry Policies, Ministry Decree 23092/7303/19), and the JPI-HDHL-INTIMIC Joint Transnational Research program (project No. INTIMIC-085 GUTMOM, Italian Ministry of Education, University and Research, Ministry Decree No. 946/2019). Projects supported by the Joint Action "European Joint Programming Initiative: A Healthy Diet for a Healthy Life" (JPI HDHL) were funded by the respective national/regional funding organisations: Fund for Scientific Research (FRS–FNRS, Belgium); Research Foundation—Flanders (FWO, Belgium); INSERM Institut National de la Santé et de la Recherche Médicale (France); Federal Ministry of Food and Agriculture (BMEL) represented by the Federal Office for Agriculture and Food (BLE, Germany); Ministry of Education, University and Research (MIUR), Ministry of Agricultural, Food, and Forestry Policies (MiPAAF), National Institute of Health (ISS) on behalf of the Ministry of Health (Italy); National Institute of Health Carlos III (Spain); The Netherlands Organisation for Health Research and Development (ZonMw, The Netherlands); Austrian Research Promotion Agency (FFG) on behalf of the Austrian Federal Ministry for Education, Science, and Research (BMBWF); the Ministry of Science and Technology (Israel); Formas (Sweden). The funders had no role in the study's design, data collection and analysis or preparation of the manuscript.

Institutional Review Board Statement: The study was conducted in accordance with the Declaration of Helsinki and approved by the Ethics Committee of Massa and Carrara and the latest amendments by the Ethical Committee of the Area Vasta Nord-Ovest (CEAVNO), Pisa, Italy (study ID 394, approval decree/document n. 75 and 71512). Parents gave their written informed consent before inclusion.

Informed Consent Statement: Informed consent was obtained from all parents involved in the study.

Data Availability Statement: The data presented in this study are available on request from the corresponding author.

Acknowledgments: We wish to acknowledge the families participating in the study.

Conflicts of Interest: The authors declare no conflict of interest.

References

1. Luchsinger, J.A.; Ryan, C.; Lenore, J.; Cowie, L.C.C.; Casagrande, S.S.; Menke, A.; Cissell, M.A.; Eberhardt, M.S.; Meigs, J.B.; Gregg, E.W.; et al. (Eds.) Diabetes and Cognitive Impairment. In *Diabetes in America*, 3rd ed.; National Institute of Diabetes and Digestive and Kidney Diseases: Bethesda, MD, USA, 2018.
2. Glisky, E.L.; Riddle, D.R. (Eds.) Changes in Cognitive Function in Human Aging. In *Brain Aging: Models, Methods, and Mechanisms*; CRC Press/Taylor & Francis: Boca Raton, FL, USA, 2007.
3. Ligia, J.; Dominguez, L.J.; Mario Barbagallo, M. Nutritional prevention of cognitive decline and dementia. *Acta Biomed.* **2018**, *89*, 276–290.
4. Russ, T.C.; Hannah, J.; Batty, G.D.; Booth, C.C.; Deary, I.J.; Starr, J.M. Childhood Cognitive Ability and Incident Dementia: The 1932 Scottish Mental Survey Cohort into their 10th Decade. *Epidemiology* **2017**, *28*, 361–364. [CrossRef]
5. Bhat, Z.F.; Morton, J.D.; Mason, S.; Bekhit, A.E.-D.A.; Bhat, H.F. Obesity and neurological disorders: Dietary perspective of a global menace. *Crit. Rev. Food. Sci. Nutr.* **2019**, *59*, 1294–1310. [CrossRef]
6. Lam, L.F.; Lawlis, T.R. Feeding the brain—The effects of micronutrient interventions on cognitive performance among school-aged children: A systematic review of randomized controlled trials. *Clin. Nutr.* **2017**, *36*, 1007–1014. [CrossRef] [PubMed]
7. Naveed, S.; Lakka, T.; Haapala, E.A. An Overview on the Associations between Health Behaviors and Brain Health in Children and Adolescents with Special Reference to Diet Quality. *Int. J. Environ. Res. Public Health* **2020**, *17*, 953.
8. Montgomery, P.; Burton, J.R.; Sewell, R.P.; Spreckelsen, T.F.; Richardson, A.J. Low blood long chain omega-3 fatty acids in UK children are associated with poor cognitive performance and behavior: A cross-sectional analysis from the DOLAB study. *PLoS ONE* **2013**, *8*, e66697. [CrossRef]
9. Boucher, O.; Burden, M.J.; Muckle, G.; Saint-Amour, D.; Ayotte, P.; Dewailly, E.; Nelson, C.A.; Jacobson, S.W.; Jacobson, J.L. Neurophysiologic and neurobehavioral evidence of beneficial effects of prenatal omega-3 fatty acid intake on memory function at school age. *Am. J. Clin. Nutr.* **2011**, *93*, 1025–1037. [CrossRef] [PubMed]
10. Nyaradi, A.; Li, J.; Hickling, S.; Foster, J.; Oddy, W.H. The role of nutrition in children's neurocognitive development, from pregnancy through childhood. *Front. Hum. Neurosci.* **2013**, *26*, 97. [CrossRef] [PubMed]
11. Gispert-Llaurado, M.; Perez-Garcia, M.; Escribano, J.; Closa-Monasterolo, R.; Luque, V.; Grote, V.; Weber, M.; Torres-Espínola, F.J.; Czech-Kowalska, J.; Verduci, E.; et al. Fish consumption in mid-childhood and its relationship to neuropsychological outcomes measured in 7–9 year old children using a NUTRIMENTHE neuropsychological battery. *Clin. Nutr.* **2016**, *35*, 1301–1307. [CrossRef] [PubMed]
12. Florence, M.D.; Asbridge, M.; Veugelers, P.J. Diet quality and academic performance. *J. Sch. Health* **2008**, *78*, 209–215, quiz 239. [CrossRef]
13. Wolraich, M.L.; Wilson, D.B.; White, J.W. The effect of sugar on behavior or cognition in children. A meta-analysis. *JAMA* **1995**, *274*, 1617–1621. [CrossRef]
14. Cohen, J.F.W.; Rifas-Shiman, S.L.; Young, J.; Oken, E. Associations of Prenatal and Child Sugar Intake with Child Cognition. *Am. J. Prev. Med.* **2018**, *54*, 727–735. [CrossRef]
15. Ingwersen, J.; Defeyter, M.A.; O Kennedy, D.; Wesnes, K.A.; Scholey, A.B. A low glycaemic index breakfast cereal preferentially prevents children's cognitive performance from declining throughout the morning. *Appetite* **2007**, *49*, 240–244. [CrossRef]
16. Micha, R.; Rogers, P.J.; Nelson, M. Glycaemic index and glycaemic load of breakfast predict cognitive function and mood in school children: A randomised controlled trial. *Br. J. Nutr.* **2011**, *106*, 1552–1561. [CrossRef] [PubMed]

17. Taki, Y.; Hashizume, H.; Sassa, Y.; Takeuchi, H.; Asano, M.; Asano, K. Breakfast staple types affect brain gray matter volume and cognitive function in healthy children. *PLoS ONE* **2010**, *5*, e15213. [CrossRef]
18. Hoyland, A. A systematic review of the effect of breakfast on the cognitive performance of children and adolescents. *Nut. Res. Rev.* **2009**, *22*, 220–243. [CrossRef]
19. Allès, B.; Samieri, C.; Féart, C.; Jutand, M.A.; Laurin, D.; Barberger-Gateau, P. Dietary patterns: A novel approach to examine the link between nutrition and cognitive function in older individuals. *Nutr. Res. Rev.* **2012**, *25*, 207–222. [CrossRef] [PubMed]
20. Vassiloudis, I.; Yiannakouris, N.; Panagiotakos, D.B.; Apostolopoulos, K.; Costarelli, V. Academic performance in relation to adherence to the Mediterranean diet and energy balance behaviors in Greek primary schoolchildren. *J. Nutr. Educ. Behav.* **2014**, *46*, 164–170. [CrossRef] [PubMed]
21. Guzzardi, M.A.; Granziera, F.; Sanguinetti, E.; Ditaranto, F.; Muratori, F.; Iozzo, P. Exclusive Breastfeeding Predicts Higher Hearing-Language Development in Girls of Preschool Age. *Nutrients* **2020**, *12*, 2320. [CrossRef]
22. World Health Organization. Available online: https://www.who.int/toolkits/child-growth-standards/standards/body-mass-index-for-age-bmi-for-age (accessed on 29 July 2021).
23. Institute for Social and Economic Research, University of Essex. Available online: https://www.iser.essex.ac.uk/files/esec/guide/docs/UserGuide.pdf (accessed on 29 July 2021).
24. The ZOOM8 Study: Nutrition and Physical Activity of Primary School Children. Reports ISTISAN. Available online: https://www.ncbi.nlm.nih.gov/nlmcatalog/101602341 (accessed on 29 July 2021). (In Italian)
25. Saravia, L.; Miguel-Berges, M.L.; Iglesia, I.; Nascimento-Ferreira, M.V.; Perdomo, G.; Bove, I.; Slater, B.; Moreno, L.A. Relative validity of FFQ to assess food items, energy, macronutrient and micronutrient intake in children and adolescents: A systematic review with meta-analysis. *Br. J. Nutr.* **2020**, *125*, 792–818. [CrossRef] [PubMed]
26. Guidelines for a Healthy Diet, Scientific Dossier 2017, Chapter 10. Available online: https://www.crea.gov.it/documents/59764/0/Dossier+LG+2017_CAP10.pdf/627ccb4d-4f80-cc82-bd3a7156c27ddd4a?t=1575530729812 (accessed on 29 July 2021). (In Italian)
27. Food Composition Database for Epidemiological Studies in Italy (BDA). Available online: http://www.bda-ieo.it/wordpress/en/?page_id=31 (accessed on 29 July 2021). (In Italian)
28. Council for Agricultural Research and Agricultural Economics Analysis (CREA). Available online: https://www.crea.gov.it/-/tabella-di-composizione-degli-alimenti (accessed on 29 July 2021). (In Italian)
29. Francesco Sofi, F.; Francesca Cesari, F.; Rosanna Abbate, R.; Gian Franco Gensini, G.F.; Alessandro Casini, A. Adherence to Mediterranean diet and health status: Meta-analysis. *BMJ* **2008**, *337*, a1344. [CrossRef] [PubMed]
30. Luiz, D.M.; Foxcroft, C.D.; Stewart, R. The construct validity of the Griffiths Scales of Mental Development. *Child Care Health Dev.* **2001**, *27*, 73–83. [CrossRef] [PubMed]
31. Ivens, J.; Martin, N. A common metric for the Griffiths Scales. *Arch. Dis. Child.* **2002**, *87*, 109–110. [CrossRef] [PubMed]
32. Luiz, D.M.; Faragher, B.; Barnard, A.; Knoesen, N.; Kotras, N.; Burns, L.E.; Challis, D. *GMDS-ER: Griffiths Mental Development Scales—Extended Revised Analysis Manual*; Hogrefe—The Test Agency Ltd.: Oxford, UK, 2006.
33. Tables LARN 2014. Available online: https://sinu.it/tabelle-larn-2014/ (accessed on 29 July 2021). (In Italian).
34. Khan, N.A.; Raine, L.B.; Drollette, E.S.; Scudder, M.R.; Kramer, A.F.; Hillman, C.H. Dietary fiber is positively associated with cognitive control among prepubertal children. *J. Nutr.* **2015**, *145*, 143–149. [CrossRef] [PubMed]
35. Haapala, E.A.; Eloranta, A.E.; Venäläinen, T.; Jalkanen, H.; Poikkeus, A.M.; Ahonen, T.; Lindi, V.; Lakka, T.A. Diet quality and academic achievement: A prospective study among primary school children. *Eur. J. Nutr.* **2017**, *56*, 2299–2308. [CrossRef] [PubMed]
36. Dauncey, M.J.; Bicknell, R.J. Nutrition and neurodevelopment: Mechanisms of developmental dysfunction and disease in later life. *Nutr. Res. Rev.* **1999**, *12*, 231–253. [CrossRef]
37. Martínez García, R.M.; Jiménez Ortega, A.I.; López Sobaler, A.M.; Ortega, R.M. Nutrition strategies that improve cognitive function. *Nutr. Hosp.* **2018**, *35*, 16–19.
38. Zeisel, S.H. Dietary influences on neurotransmission. *Adv. Pediatr.* **1986**, *33*, 23–47.
39. Ceppa, F.; Mancini, A.; Tuohy, K. Current evidence linking diet to gut microbiota and brain development and function. *Int. J. Food Sci. Nutr.* **2019**, *70*, 1–19. [CrossRef]
40. Holick, M.F. Vitamin D deficiency. *N. Engl. J. Med.* **2007**, *357*, 266–281. [CrossRef]
41. Pearce, A.L.; Leonhardt, C.A.; Vaidya, C.J. Executive and Reward-Related Function in Pediatric Obesity: A Meta-Analysis. *Child Obes.* **2018**, *14*, 265–279. [CrossRef]
42. Reinert, K.R.S.; Po'e, E.K.; Barkin, S.L. The relationship between executive function and obesity in children and adolescents: A systematic literature review. *J. Obes.* **2013**, *2013*, 820956. [CrossRef] [PubMed]
43. Liang, J.; Matheson, B.E.; Kaye, W.H.; Boutelle, K.N. Neurocognitive correlates of obesity and obesity-related behaviors in chil-dren and adolescents. *Int. J. Obes.* **2014**, *38*, 494–506. [CrossRef]
44. Thompson, F.E.; Byers, T. Dietary assessment resource manual. *J. Nutr.* **1994**, *124* (Suppl. 11), 2245S–2317S. [PubMed]

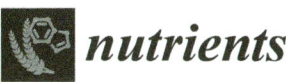

Article

Inhibition of Soluble Epoxide Hydrolase Is Protective against the Multiomic Effects of a High Glycemic Diet on Brain Microvascular Inflammation and Cognitive Dysfunction

Saivageethi Nuthikattu [1], Dragan Milenkovic [1,2,3], Jennifer E. Norman [1], John Rutledge [1] and Amparo Villablanca [1,*]

1. Division of Cardiovascular Medicine, University of California, Davis, CA 95616, USA; snuthikattu@ucdavis.edu (S.N.); dragan.milenkovic@inra.fr (D.M.); jenorman@ucdavis.edu (J.E.N.); jcrutledge@ucdavis.edu (J.R.)
2. Department of Nutrition, University of California, Davis, CA 95616, USA
3. Unité de Nutrition Humaine, INRA, Université Clermont Auvergne, CRNH Auvergne, F-63000 Clermont-Ferrand, France
* Correspondence: avillablanca@ucdavis.edu; Tel.: 530-752-0718; Fax: 530-752-3264

Abstract: Diet is a modifiable risk factor for cardiovascular disease (CVD) and dementia, yet relatively little is known about the effect of a high glycemic diet (HGD) on the brain's microvasculature. The objective of our study was to determine the molecular effects of an HGD on hippocampal microvessels and cognitive function and determine if a soluble epoxide hydrolase (sEH) inhibitor (sEHI), known to be vasculoprotective and anti-inflammatory, modulates these effects. Wild type male mice were fed a low glycemic diet (LGD, 12% sucrose/weight) or an HGD (34% sucrose/weight) with/without the sEHI, trans-4-[4-(3-adamantan-1-yl-ureido)-cyclohexyloxy]-benzoic acid (t-AUCB), for 12 weeks. Brain hippocampal microvascular gene expression was assessed by microarray and data analyzed using a multi-omic approach for differential expression of protein and non-protein-coding genes, gene networks, functional pathways, and transcription factors. Global hippocampal microvascular gene expression was fundamentally different for mice fed the HGD vs. the LGD. The HGD response was characterized by differential expression of 608 genes involved in cell signaling, neurodegeneration, metabolism, and cell adhesion/inflammation/oxidation effects reversible by t-AUCB and hence sEH inhibitor correlated with protection against Alzheimer's dementia. Ours is the first study to demonstrate that high dietary glycemia contributes to brain hippocampal microvascular inflammation through sEH.

Keywords: multi-omics; microvascular; brain; dementia; high glycemic diet; soluble epoxide hydrolase inhibitor; maless

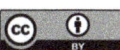

1. Introduction

Dementias are the seventh leading cause of death globally and contribute significantly to health care costs [1]. Several studies suggest that a high-fat diet or Western diet (high fat and high glycemic content) can lead to reduced cognitive function [2–6]. It has also become increasingly recognized that vasculature plays an important role in the development of dementias [7]. Our group has previously demonstrated the multi-omic and lipotoxic effect of a Western diet on the brain microvasculature and its negative consequences on cognitive function in male and female mice [8–11]. While there have been numerous mechanistic studies focusing on cognitive function with high-fat diets, few studies have explored the impact of high glycemia in the absence of high levels of dietary fat.

There is compelling epidemiological data to suggest that the effects of a high glycemic diet (HGD) on cognitive function and the brain are an important area of study. High blood glucose and high dietary glycemic load were both found to be related to poorer performance in perceptual speed and spatial ability [12]. An HGD has also been associated with a greater cerebral amyloid burden [13]. Further, consumption of a high glycemic index afternoon snack was associated with cognitive decline in apolipoprotein E4 allele carriers [14]. However, there is relatively sparse animal data on the effects of an HGD on the brain and cognitive function. In rats, an HGD had detrimental effects on memory [15,16], disrupted hypothalamic redox homeostasis [17], and increased hippocampal endoplasmic reticulum stress [18]. In a mouse model of Alzheimer's disease, an HGD was found to increase neuroinflammation and cortical levels of Amyloid-β [19]. These studies suggest that an HGD is associated with cognitive impairment in animal models.

The impact of high glycemia on cognition may be reversible. One study in rats found that a high sucrose diet increased brain unesterified arachidonic acid and the activity of enzymes facilitating the release of arachidonic acid from phospholipids [20]. Arachidonic acid is metabolized by cytochrome P450 enzymes to epoxyeicosatrienoic acid isomers (EETs), which are short-lasting and locally active neuroprotective, vasodilatory, and anti-inflammatory [21] signaling molecules. Soluble epoxide hydrolase (sEH) is an enzyme that converts EETs into dihydroxyeicosatrienoic acids (DHETs), which have less biological activity [21,22]. Inhibiting sEH activity thus increases the amount of beneficial EETs [22]. Studies have implicated soluble epoxide hydrolase (sEH) in many disorders of the central nervous system, including Parkinson's disease, white matter hyperintensities, vascular cognitive decline/impairment, and Alzheimer's disease [22–26]. Inhibitors of sEH (sEHI) have been shown to be protective in animal models of stroke [27,28]. Inhibition of sEH is of great clinical interest as it has also been shown to reduce neuroinflammation and cognitive impairment in animal models of cerebral hypoperfusion and type 1 and type 2 diabetes mellitus [29–33]. Further, the use of sEHI and genetic knockout of the sEH gene reduces cognitive impairment in animal models of age-related cognitive decline and Alzheimer's disease [26,34,35].

The hippocampus is central to the formation of memory [36], and dysfunction of the microvasculature can contribute to the development of dementia [37]. To our knowledge, no studies have been published to date examining the effects of an HGD on brain hippocampal microvascular gene expression. The objectives of this study were to use a male murine model to comprehensively characterize the effect of an HGD on neurovascular function through hippocampal microvascular multi-omics and to assess the impact of an HGD on cognitive function. We hypothesized that an HGD would result in injurious differential gene expression changes characterized by brain hippocampal microvascular oxidation, inflammation, and blood–brain barrier disruption. Further, we aimed to determine whether the deleterious genomic effects of an HGD could be mitigated by inhibiting sEH.

2. Materials and Methods

2.1. Experimental Animals and Soluble Epoxide Hydrolase Inhibitor (sEHI) Treatment

19-week-old C57BL/6J wild type (WT) male mice (Jackson Laboratories, stock 000664) were fed a standard chow diet (catalog no 0915 from Envigo Teklad Diets, Madison, WI, USA) and allowed to acclimate for one week prior to beginning the study procedures. Mice were then fed for 12 weeks either a Low Glycemic Index diet (LGD, catalog no TD.08485 from Envigo Teklad Diets, Madison, WI, USA) composed of 13% fat, 19.1% protein, 67.9% carbohydrate, as percent kcal, containing 12% sucrose by weight, or a High Glycemic Index diet (HGD, catalog no. TD.05230, Envigo Teklad Diets, Madison, WI, USA) composed of 12.6% fat, 18.7% protein, 68.7% carbohydrate, as percent kcal, containing 34% sucrose by weight. Mice receiving each diet were given 10mg/L of soluble epoxide hydrolase inhibitor (sEHI), trans-4-[4-(3-adamantan-1-yl-ureido)-cyclohexyloxy]-benzoic acid (t-AUCB) (Cayman Chemical, Ann Arbor, MI, USA) containing 1% v/v polyethylene glycol 400 (PEG400) (Millipore, Burlington, MA, USA) in the drinking water for 12 weeks at which point mice were 32 weeks of age and sacrificed. Mice consumed approximately 7 to 7.5 mL of water each day, consistent with previously published work [38], and 2.5 to 3 mg of t-AUCB (sEHI) per kg per day. There were a total of four experimental treatment groups (n = 7 mice/gp): LGD alone, LGD with sEHI (LGD+sEHI), HGD alone, and HGD with sEHI (HGD+sEHI). Mice were randomly assigned to the dietary groups.

Animals were housed one mouse per cage in a temperature- and humidity-controlled environment with a 12 h light/dark cycle in the University of California, Davis Mouse Biology Program. Body weight was measured at baseline and at the completion of the dietary intervention period, and activity, water, and food intake were monitored daily by vivarium staff. The research was conducted in conformity with the Public Health Service Policy on Humane Care and Use of Laboratory Animals and all protocols approved by the Institutional Animal Care and Use Committee of the University of California, Davis.

2.2. Serum Lipid, Glucose, and Insulin Assays

Mice were fasted overnight for 8 hours, and blood obtained by submandibular nick blood draw for the pre diet samples, and by ventricular puncture at the time of sacrifice following completion of the dietary feeding period for the post diet samples. Blood samples were stored at $-80\ °C$. Lipid, glucose and insulin levels were measured in fasted serum samples. Total cholesterol (TC), high-density lipoprotein cholesterol (HDL), and low-density lipoprotein cholesterol (LDL) were measured using enzymatic assays from Fisher Diagnostics (Middleton, VA, USA), and precipitation separation from AbCam (Cambridge, MA, USA) adapted to a microplate format. Glucose was measured using enzymatic assays from Fisher Diagnostics (Middleton, VA, USA), and insulin was determined by electrochemiluminescence from Meso Scale Discovery (Rockville, MD, USA) according to the manufacturer's instructions. All serum assays were performed by the UC Davis Mouse Metabolic Phenotyping Center (MMPC) on non-pooled serum samples.

2.3. Isolation and Cryosection of Murine Brain Hippocampus

Following completion of the 12 week dietary feeding period, mice were anesthetized by intraperitoneal xylazine/ketamine and euthanized by exsanguination during the light phase of their light/dark cycle. Intact brains were rapidly removed under RNAse free conditions, cut into regions including the temporal lobe segment containing the hippocampus, and embedded using HistoPrep Frozen Tissue Embedding Media (Fisher Scientific, Pittsburgh, PA, USA). To identify the hippocampus and hippocampal neurons, brain sections in the medial aspect of the temporal lobe were stained with hematoxylin and visualized with microscopy as previously described [8]. The hippocampus was then coronally cryosectioned (8 μm, Leica Frigocut 2800n Cryostat, Leica Biosystems, Buffalo Grove, IL, USA) and placed on charged RNA-free PEN Membrane Glass slides, treated with RNAlater®-ICE (Life Technologies, Grand Island, NY, USA) to prevent RNA degradation, and stored at $-80\ °C$ until use. When ready for use, cryosections from the hippocampal segments were submerged in nuclease-free water and dehydrated in desiccant.

2.4. Laser Capture Microdissection (LCM) of Hippocampal Microvessels

For analysis of gene transcriptome of hippocampal brain microvessels, endothelial microvessels (<20um) were first identified in the hippocampal brain cryosections by alkaline phosphatase staining utilizing 5-bromo-4-chloro-3-indolyl phosphate/nitro blue tetrazolium chloride (BCIP/NBT) substrate as previously described [39]. Laser capture microdissection (LCM) was then used to isolate the microvascular endothelium in hippocampal cryosections by capture of the entire vessel wall under direct microscopic visualization using a Leica LMD6000 Laser Microdissection Microscope (Leica Microsystems, Wetzlar, Germany). Microvessels were not categorized by hippocampal region or subregion, although they primarily corresponded to endothelial enriched sections in hippocampus dorsal segments that would have included CA1 and CA3 regions.

2.5. RNA Extraction from Laser Captured Brain Microvessels

Total RNA was extracted from the laser-captured hippocampal brain microvessels (300 per mice, 3 mice per experimental group) using an Arcturus PicoPure™ RNA Isolation

Kit (Thermo Fisher Scientific, Santa Clara, CA, USA) according to the manufacturer's instructions. The quality of the RNA from the LCM-derived vessels was assessed by Nanodrop. RNA quantification was performed according to Affymetrix RNA quantification kit with SYBR Green I and ROX™ Passive Reference Dye protocol (Affymetrix, Santa Clara, CA, USA).

2.6. Microarray Hybridization and Transcriptome Analysis

For transcriptomics analysis, we used Clariom D Mouse Array (one array per mouse), containing more than 7 million probes for protein-coding and protein non-coding genes such as micro RNAs (miRNAs), small nucleolar RNAs (snoRNAs), and long non-coding RNAs (LncRNAs) (Thermo Fisher, Santa Clara, CA, USA). RNA (122.3 pg) was used to prepare cRNA and sscDNA using GeneChip®WT Pico Kit (Thermo Fisher, Santa Clara, CA, USA). SscDNA (5.5 µg) was fragmented by uracil-DNA glycosylase (UDG) and apurinic/apyrimidinic endonuclease 1 (APE 1) and labeled by terminal deoxynucleotidyl transferase (TdT) using the DNA Labeling Reagent that is covalently linked to biotin. Fragmented and labeled sscDNA samples were then submitted to the UC Davis Genome Center shared resource core for hybridization, staining, and scanning using Thermo Fisher Scientific WT array hybridization protocol following the manufacturer's protocol. Hybridization of fragmented and labeled sscDNA samples was performed using GeneChip™Hybridization Oven 645, and samples were then washed and stained using GeneChip™ Fluidics Station 450. The arrays were scanned using GeneChip™ Scanner 3000 7G (Thermo Fisher Scientific, Santa Clara, CA, USA). Quality control of the microarrays and data analysis was performed using Thermo Fisher Scientific Transcriptome Analysis Console software version 4.0.2. We have deposited the microarray data in GEO, and the accession number is GSE185057.

2.7. Bioinformatic Analysis

Bioinformatics analysis of differentially expressed genes was performed by two of the study investigators (SN and DM) using multiple software tools. We compared the following study groups: (A) HGD to LGD (to determine the effect of the HGD diet) and (B) HGD+sEHI to HGD (to determine the effect of the inhibitor on the HGD diet) as shown in the flow chart in Figure 1.

The Principal Component Analysis (PCA) plot of identified differentially expressed genes (DEG) was obtained through ClustVis [40]. miRNA targets of DEG were identified using Mienturnet [41]. LncRNAs of DEG were identified using LncRRIsearch [42] and Rtools CBRC [43]. Canonical pathway analysis was conducted using GeneTrial2 online database [44,45]. Networks were constructed and visualized using Cytoscape software (version 3.7.1) [46–49]. Data preparation was performed with the use of several R packages including splitstackshape [50], data.table [51], dplyr [52,53] and string [54,55]. Pathway networks were built for pathways enriched from a global pathway analysis, considering all omic layers components together.

Transcription factor analyses were performed using Enrichr [56–58]. Hierarchical clustering and heat map representations of differentially expressed genes (DEG) were performed using PermutMatrix software [59,60].

We performed Pearson's correlation analysis between the genes differentially expressed by the HGD vs. LGD and the HGD+sEHI vs. HGD. We used the ggpubr package in R [61] to obtain the correlation coefficient and the significance level, as well as the scatter plot with regression line and confidence interval. We then performed prediction of neurodegenerative disease trait by performing correlation analysis between the obtained changes in the expression of genes following the HGD vs. LGD or the HGD+sEHI vs. HGD and the gene expression profiles observed in patients with Alzheimer's disease or cognitive disorders. The human genome data were extracted from the gene expression profile database, which was deposited in the GEO (gene expression omnibus) database. The identification of differentially expressed genes between patients and healthy volunteers was performed using GEO2R [62], an NCBI web tool that allows comparisons between two or more groups of samples in the GEO series to identify differentially expressed genes across the experimental conditions. The differentially expressed genes were screened according to *p*-values < 0.05. Pearson's correlation analysis between the genes identified as differentially expressed, following the HGD vs. LGD or the HGD + sEHI vs. HGD, and patients with neurogenerative diseases was performed using ggpubr package in R [61].

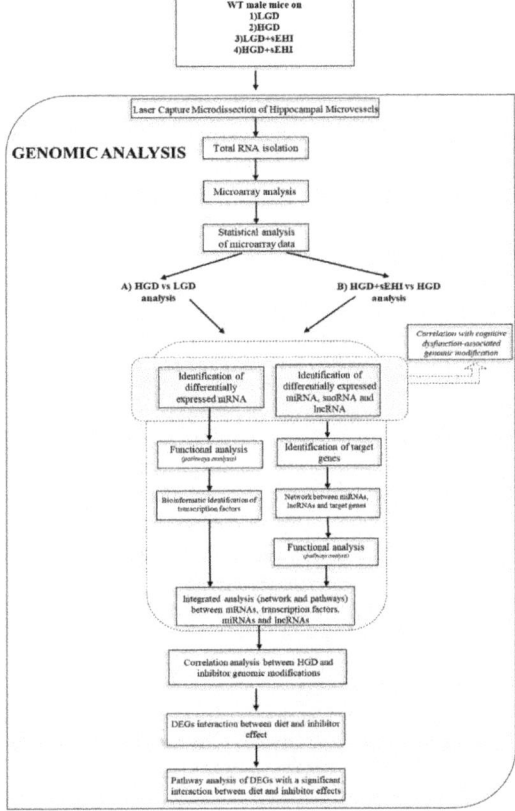

Figure 1. Research methodology flow chart. The flow chart shows the steps in the genomic analysis for: (A) the high glycemic diet compared to the low glycemic diet (HGD vs LGD), and (B) the high glycemic diet with the soluble epoxide hydrolase inhibitor (sEHI) compared to without the sEHI (HGD + sEHI vs HGD).

Interaction of diet and inhibitor effects was performed using Thermo Fisher Scientific Transcriptome Analysis Console software version 4.0.2. Interaction was defined by a ≥ 2 or ≤ -2 delta fold change and a *p*-value < 0.05 when comparing HGD+sEHI vs. LGD+sEHI to HGD vs. LGD.

2.8. Statistical Methods

For microarray, ANOVA ebayes (Thermo Fisher Scientific Transcriptome Analysis Console software, Santa Clara, CA, USA) were used for statistical analysis of microvessel transcriptomes. All genes from the microarray with $p < 0.05$ and ± 2.0-fold change were considered as differentially expressed. Mean body weight and plasma lipid levels were expressed as means $\pm$ standard error of the mean (SEM), and significance was determined at $p \leq 0.05$ using unpaired Student's *t*-tests (GraphPad software, La Jolla, CA, USA).

3. Results

The dietary treatment resulted in the expected weight gain in the study mice as follows: The mean weight for male mice at 20 weeks of age, on the chow diet, prior to initiation of the study diets, was 30 g and increased significantly ($p < 0.05$) after 12 weeks in both diet groups (LGD mean 36 g, HGD mean 34g). The soluble epoxide hydrolase inhibitor (sEHI) had no effect on body weight.

Total cholesterol (TC) levels at the end of the feeding period increased significantly ($p < 0.05$) in all the groups when compared to the baseline measurement at 20 weeks of age and did not statistically differ between the LGD (154.9 mg/dL) and HGD (146.2 mg/dL). The sEHI had no significant effect on total cholesterol levels.

Glucose and insulin levels also increased significantly ($p < 0.05$) in both the LGD (416.1 mg/dL) and HGD (374.7 mg/dL) treatment groups but did not statistically differ between them. The sEHI had no significant effect on glucose and insulin levels.

3.1. Effect of the High Glycemic Diet on the Hippocampal Microvascular Genome

3.1.1. Global Gene Expression and Hierarchical Clustering

To define the molecular mechanisms in brain hippocampal microvessels in response to the HGD, we began by assessing global gene expression using principal component analysis (PCA), a genetic distance visualization tool that shows relatedness between populations. PCA plot analysis showed that the global gene expression profiles of mice on the HDG and LGD were distinctly different from each other (Figure 2A). Using loading plot analysis, we further defined that the genes relevant to the separation of the PCA had opposite expression patterns with the HGD vs the LGD diet. Plots for a few genes (*Higd2a*, *Gm24400*, *Snora30*, *Cox5b*, *Mir5125*, *Acta2*, and *Map3k7cl*) that contributed to separation of the two dietary groups are provided as examples in Figure 2B.

We then performed hierarchical clustering of global gene expression profiles. Hierarchical clustering groups similar data points together and then organizes the clusters into a hierarchy. Using this strategy, we further confirmed that genes with higher levels of expression with the HGD had lower levels of expression with the LGD, and vice versa (Figure 3). Thus, the effect of the HGD on global hippocampal microvascular gene expression was fundamentally opposite compared to the LGD.

3.1.2. Differential Gene Expression

To study the effect of the HGD on gene expression, we compared the HGD to the LGD (flow chart Figure 1A). Statistical analysis of microarray data revealed 608 differentially expressed genes (DEGs) in hippocampal microvessels following the HGD, with the majority of the DEGs being up-regulated by the HGD (468 genes up-regulated vs. 140 genes down-regulated) when compared to the LGD, Supplemental Figure S1. The fold-change varied from 2.0 to 25.94 for up-regulated genes and from -16.65 to -2.01 for down-regulated genes (see Supplemental Table S1 for a complete listing of the DEGs). To our knowledge, we also show for the first time that the HGD regulates the expression of protein-coding genes (221) and non-coding genes (78) in male murine hippocampal microvessels (Supplemental Figure S2), including 32 long non-coding RNAs (lncRNAs), 25 microRNAs (miRNAs), and 21 small nucleolar RNAs (snoRNAs). The remaining 309 DEGs were other genes (pseudogenes, ribosomal RNAs (rRNAs), unassigned genes, and multiple-complex genes).

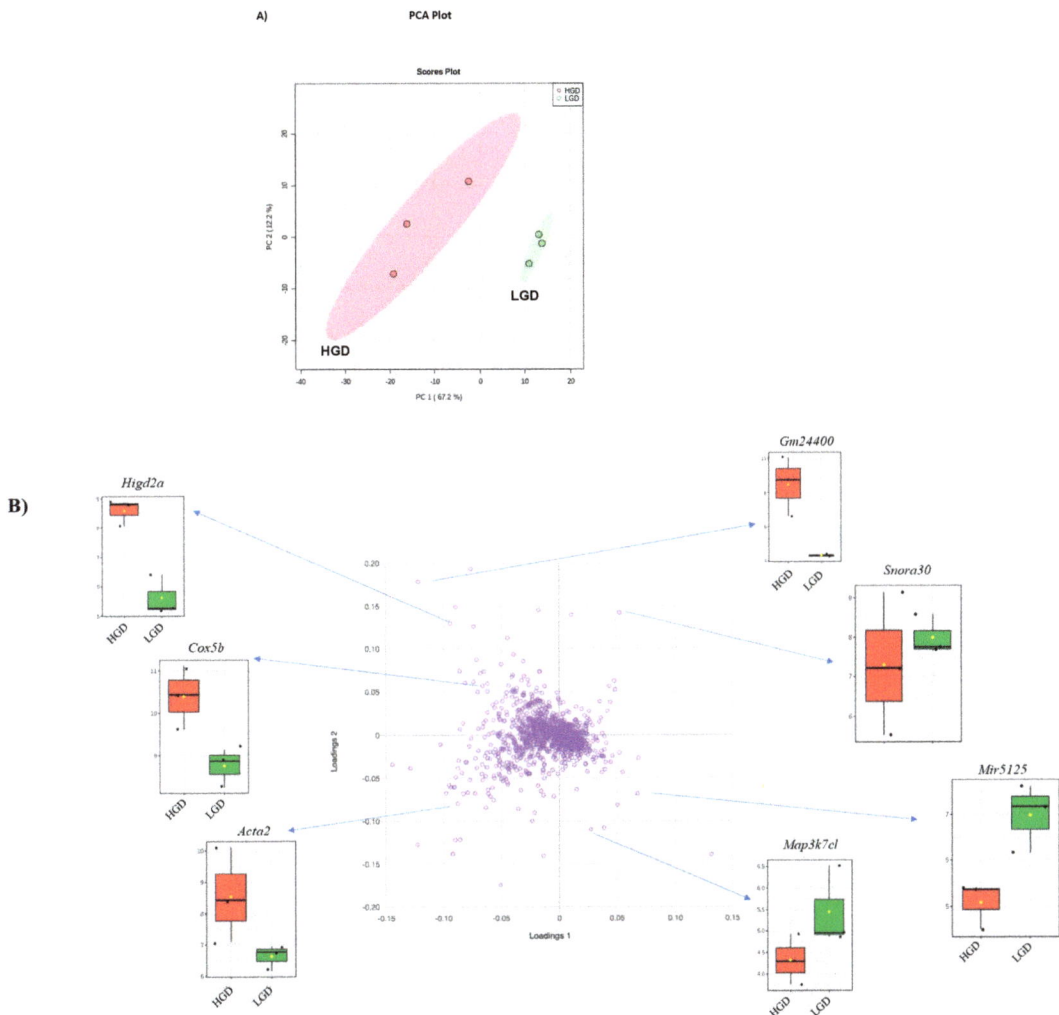

Figure 2. Principal Component Analysis (PCA) and loading plot of genes expressed in hippocampal microvessels of the high glycemic diet (HGD) and the low glycemic diet (LGD). (**A**) PCA scatter plot of the microarray data shows the trends of the expression profiles of the hippocampal microvasculature in the high glycemic diet (HGD, red circles) and low glycemic diet (LGD, green circles), respectively. The PCA plot captures the variance in a dataset in terms of principal components and displays the most significant of these on the x and y axes. The percentages of the total variation that are accounted for by the 1st and 2nd principal components are shown on the x- and y-axes labels. The data are shown for three biological replicates for each dietary group. (**B**) Loading plot of genes (violet circles) relevant to the separation of PCA. Blue arrows show box plots with expression levels of a few genes (*Higd2a, Gm24400, Snora30, Cox5b, Mir5125, Acta2, Map3k7cl, Snora30* and *Map3k7cl*) that contribute to separation of the two dietary groups (HGD, LGD). In the box plots, the black dots represent gene expression levels, the notch indicates 95% confidence interval around the median of each group, and yellow diamond indicates the average gene expression of each group.

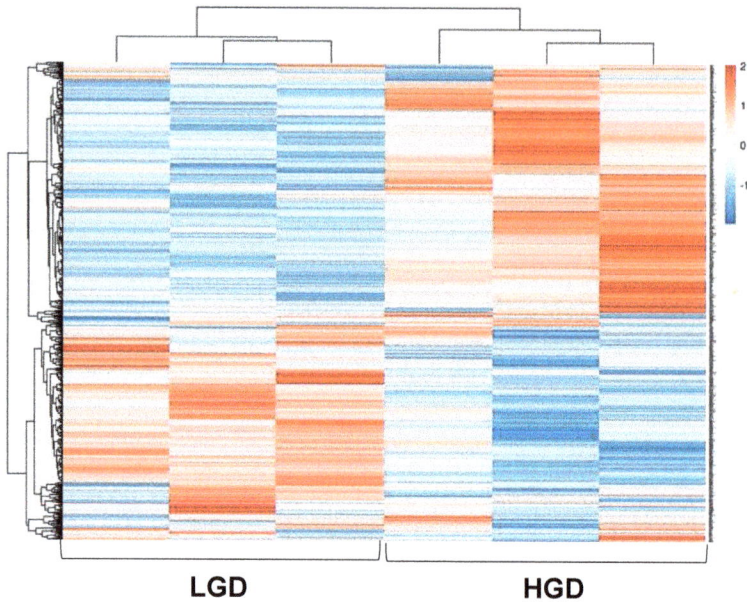

Figure 3. Hierarchical clustering of differentially expressed genes in hippocampal microvessels of the low glycemic diet (LGD) and the high glycemic diet (HGD). Upregulated genes are in red and downregulated genes are in blue. The data are shown for three biological replicates for each dietary group.

3.1.3. Pathways and Networks for Coding and Non-Coding Differentially Expressed Genes

Next, we performed bioinformatic analysis to find cellular pathways involving differentially expressed (DE) protein-coding genes. Among the 56 cellular pathways we identified were those involved in the regulation of neurodegenerative diseases (e.g., Alzheimer's disease), pathways involved in the regulation of cellular energy pathways (e.g., oxidative phosphorylation), and cellular metabolism (e.g., fatty acid metabolism). We also observed several cellular signaling pathways, cell adhesion pathways, as well as other pathways such as cell cycle or protein processing in endoplasmic reticulum (Supplemental Figure S3). Therefore, the HGD led to genomic modification in brain microvasculature pathways primarily by modulating the expression of genes involved in neurodegeneration, metabolism, and cell signaling. We also performed bioinformatics analyses of DEGs to identify potential transcription factors (TFs) whose activity could be modulated by the HGD and result in the observed genomic effects. Enrichr database analysis of the top 25 TFs and the DEGs regulated by them is shown in Supplemental Figure S4. The most statistically significant transcription factors were STAT3 (Signal Transducer and Activator of Transcription 3) involved in focal adhesion, DNMT1 (DNA Methyl Transferase 1), and PPARA (Peroxisome Proliferator-Activated Receptor Alpha) involved in Alzheimer's disease (Supplemental Table S2).

Microarray analysis also revealed that the HGD could induce differential expression of non-coding RNAs (miRNAs, lncRNAs, and snoRNAs). Of the 25 DE miRNAs in HGD vs. LGD (Supplemental Table S3), 12 were down-regulated (fold change −5.81 to −2.01) and 13 up-regulated (fold change 2.01 to 25.94). Using MIENTURNET software and database interrogation, we identified 442 potential target genes for 17 of the 25 miRNAs. The network of interactions between these miRNAs and their target genes is presented in Supplemental Figure S5. While most genes were the target of a single miRNA, we showed redundancy in that some genes were targets of two or three different miRNAs. Pathway analyses of miRNA target genes revealed they were involved in pathways regulating cell transduction, cell–cell adhesion, permeability, and neurofunction (Supplemental Figure S6). Eleven of the miRNA target genes pathways were in common with the protein-coding DEG pathways, such as Hypoxia-inducible factor 1 (HIF-1) signaling involved in endothelial cell function. Pathways unique to miRNA targets were primarily related to inflammation and cell signaling, whereas protein-coding DEGs specific pathways were primarily involved in cellular metabolism.

Together with miRNAs, our analysis also revealed 32 DE lncRNAs (Supplemental Table S4) following the HGD. Among these, 4 were down-regulated (fold-change -16.65 to -2.02), and 28 were up-regulated (fold-change 2.02 to 5.34). Using LncRRIsearch and Rtools CBRC databases, we were able to identify 458 potential target genes for 5 of the 32 lncRNAs (Supplemental Figure S7). Pathway analysis of these target genes showed that they were involved in pathways such as nitric oxide signaling, N-cadherin that regulate vascular endothelial function, as well as Alzheimer's disease (Supplemental Figure S8), which was also one of the 7 pathways in common with the miRNA targets pathways.

We also studied the expression of snoRNAs in the HGD compared to LGD. Among the 21 DE snoRNAs, 9 were up-regulated (fold change 2.36 to 19.44), and 12 were down-regulated (fold change -10.37 to -2.07) (Supplemental Table S5). A literature review did not identify any known target genes for the DE snoRNAs.

3.1.4. Integrated Analysis of Differentially Expressed Genes, Key Pathways and Networks

Following the individual omic analysis, we performed integrated analysis of all the identified DEGs including mRNAs, miRNAs and their targets, lncRNAs and their targets, and the identified potential transcription factors. This analysis allowed us to obtain networks of interactions (Figure 4A), and showed that in comparison to the LGD, the HGD significantly impacted the expression levels of different RNA types which interact and form a large molecular network. This molecular network can have a significant effect on cellular functions. Therefore, in order to determine if there was a pattern of functional coordination in the molecular differential expression pattern of the HGD on brain microvessels, we performed integrated pathway and network analysis using DE mRNAs, miRNAs and lncRNAs targets for the HGD compared to LGD. This analysis indeed revealed differential regulation of 5 key cellular pathways including for neurodegenerative diseases (such as Alzheimer's disease), cell signaling pathways (such as PPAR signaling and phosphoinositide-3-kinase-protein kinase B (PI3K-Akt) signaling), cell adhesion and mobility (including focal adhesion), cellular metabolism (including oxidative phosphorylation and electron transport chain), and other cellular pathways (such as mRNA processing and oxidative damage) (Figure 4B and 4C). Integrated pathways for DEGs, transcription factors, miRNAs and their targets, and lncRNAs and their targets are shown for the focal adhesion pathway (Figure 4D) and the Alzheimer's disease pathway (Figure 4E). Pathways are discussed in further detail in the Discussion section.

3.2. Effect of the Soluble Epoxide Hydrolase Inhibitor (sEHI) on the Hippocampal Microvascular Genome of Mice fed the High Glycemic Diet

In order to determine whether the soluble epoxide hydrolase inhibitor (sEHI) could inhibit the seemingly deleterious molecular effects of the HGD on hippocampal microvessels (upregulation of genes in pathways such as PPAR signaling, PI3K-Akt signaling that play an important role in oxidative stress, inflammation and Alzheimer's disease), we again performed hierarchical clustering of global gene expression profiles for the LGD and the HGD in the presence of the inhibitor (Figure 5). Since the gene expression profile of the LGD group did not substantially differ from the LGD with the inhibitor (Figure 5), the effect of the inhibitor was primarily analyzed in reference to the HGD in our analytic comparisons. Interestingly, in the presence of the sEHI, the gene expression profile of the HGD on hippocampal microvessels was nearly completely reversed and similar to that on the LGD.

Using PCA analysis, we were further able to show that the gene expression profile of hippocampal microvessels following the HGD was distinctly different from that of the

HGD+sEHI (Figure 6A). We used loading plot to identify genes important to the separation of PCA (Figure 6B). Genes such as *Gm24400, Resp18, Rheb, Brms1l, Ndufa13,* and *Ighv5-12-4* showed opposite expression in the HGD with inhibitor when compared to the HGD alone.

Statistical analysis of microarray data showed that there were a larger number of DEGs (1701) for the comparison of the HGD+sEHI vs. HGD (Supplemental Table S6) than there were for the HGD vs. LGD comparison. The sEHI primarily down-regulated both protein-coding and non-coding DEGs in the HGD (Figure 7A, and Supplemental Figures S9 and S10). We then performed correlation analysis between the DEGs of the HGD+sEHI vs. HGD and the HGD vs. LGD and identified a highly significant negative correlation with the sEHI (Figure 7B). This suggests that the inhibitor counteracts the effects of the HGD on differential gene expression.

A)

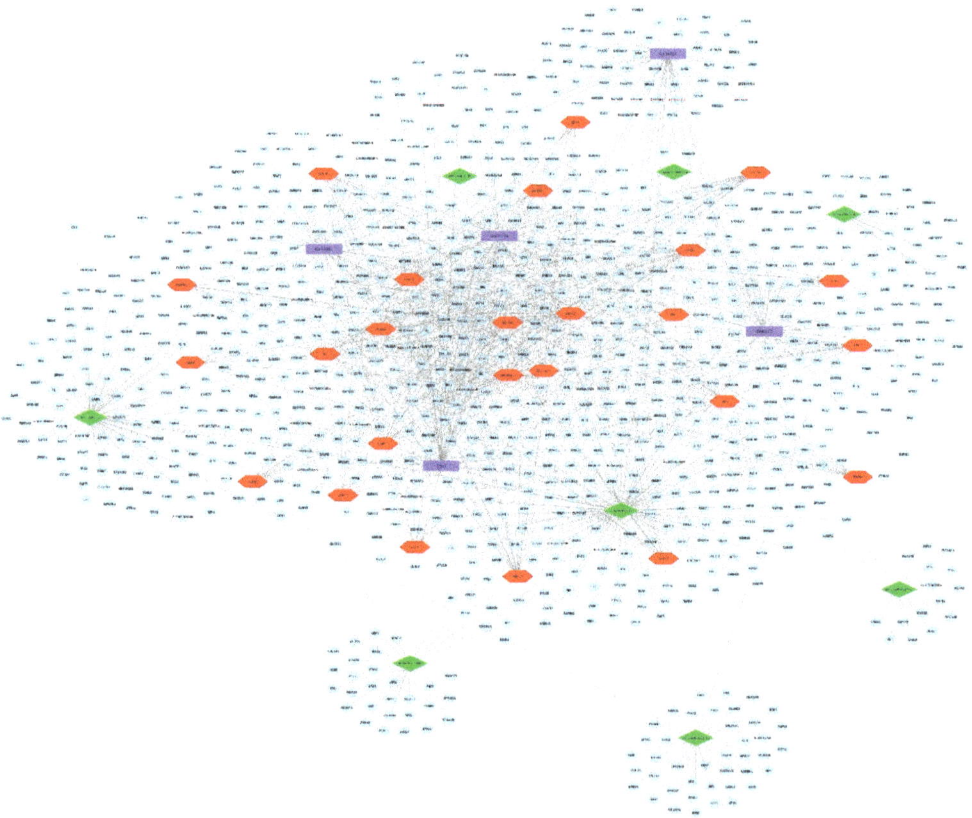

Figure 4. *Cont.*

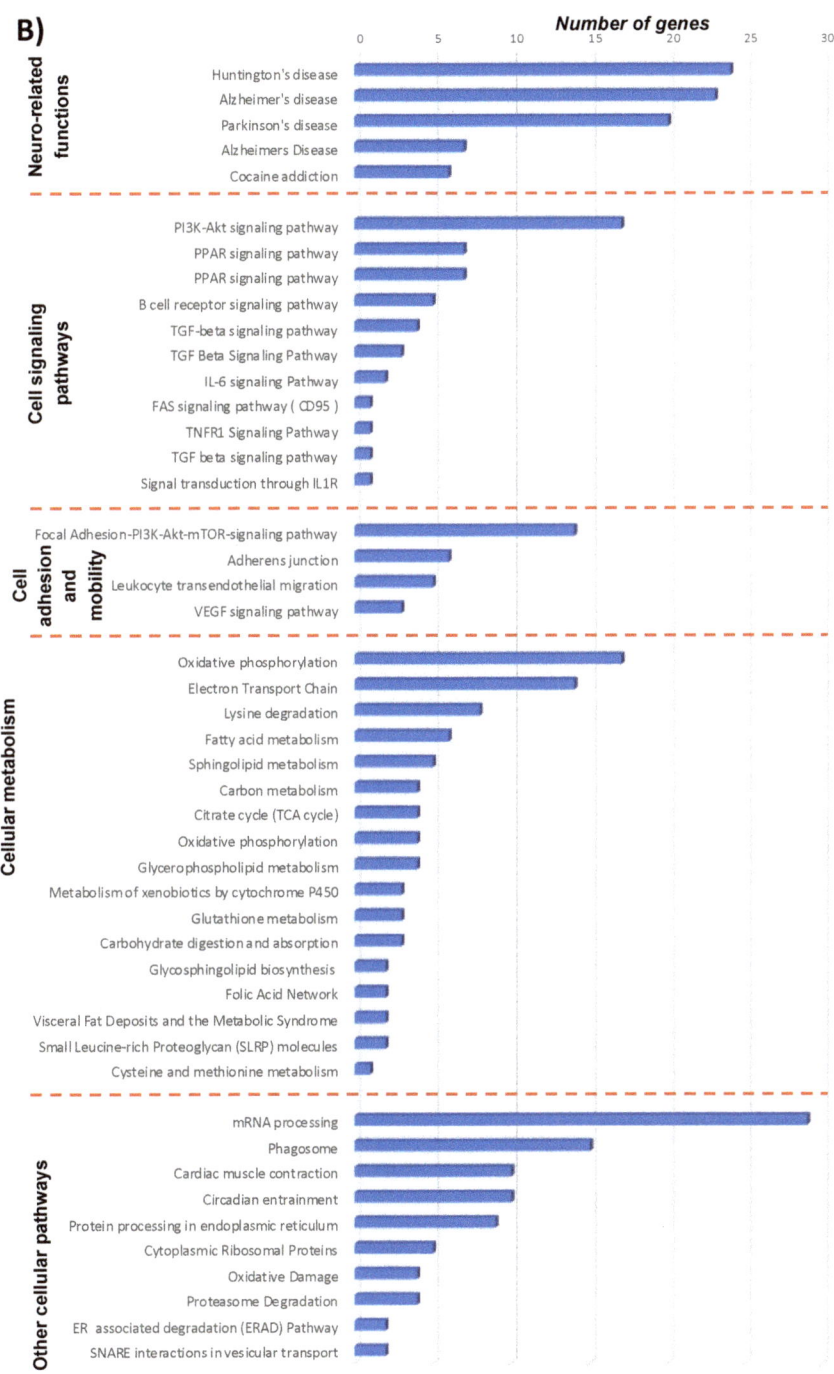

Figure 4. *Cont.*

C)

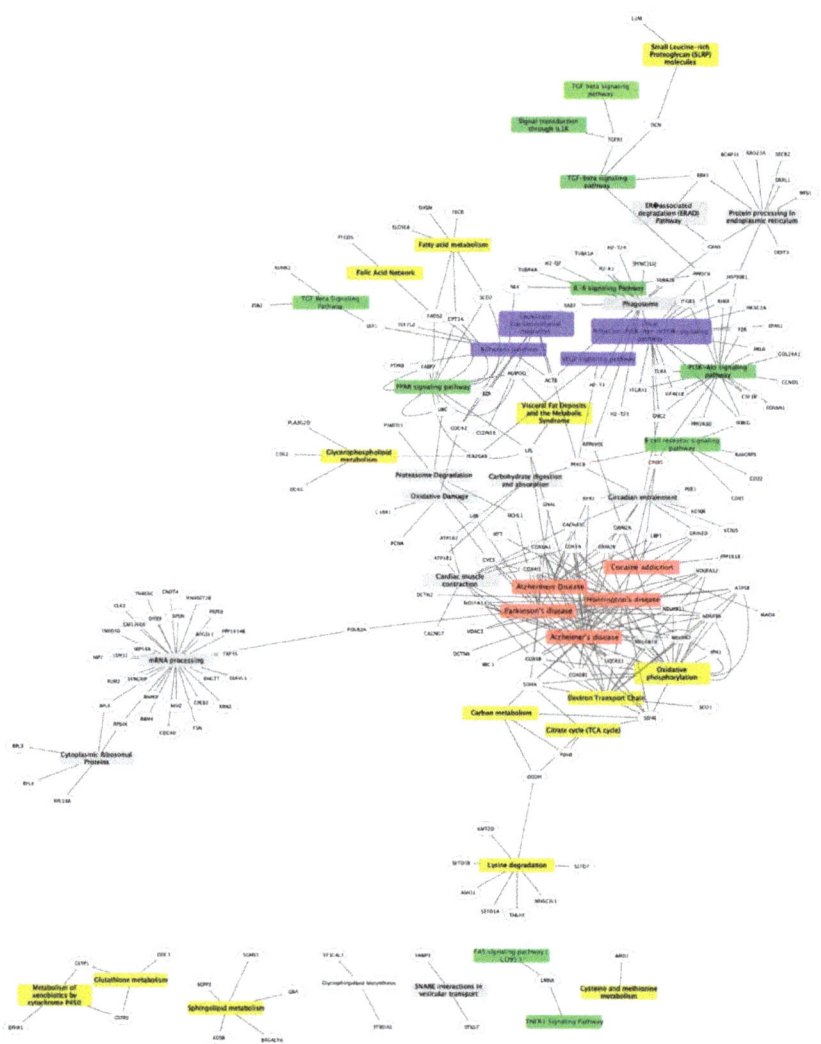

Figure 4. *Cont.*

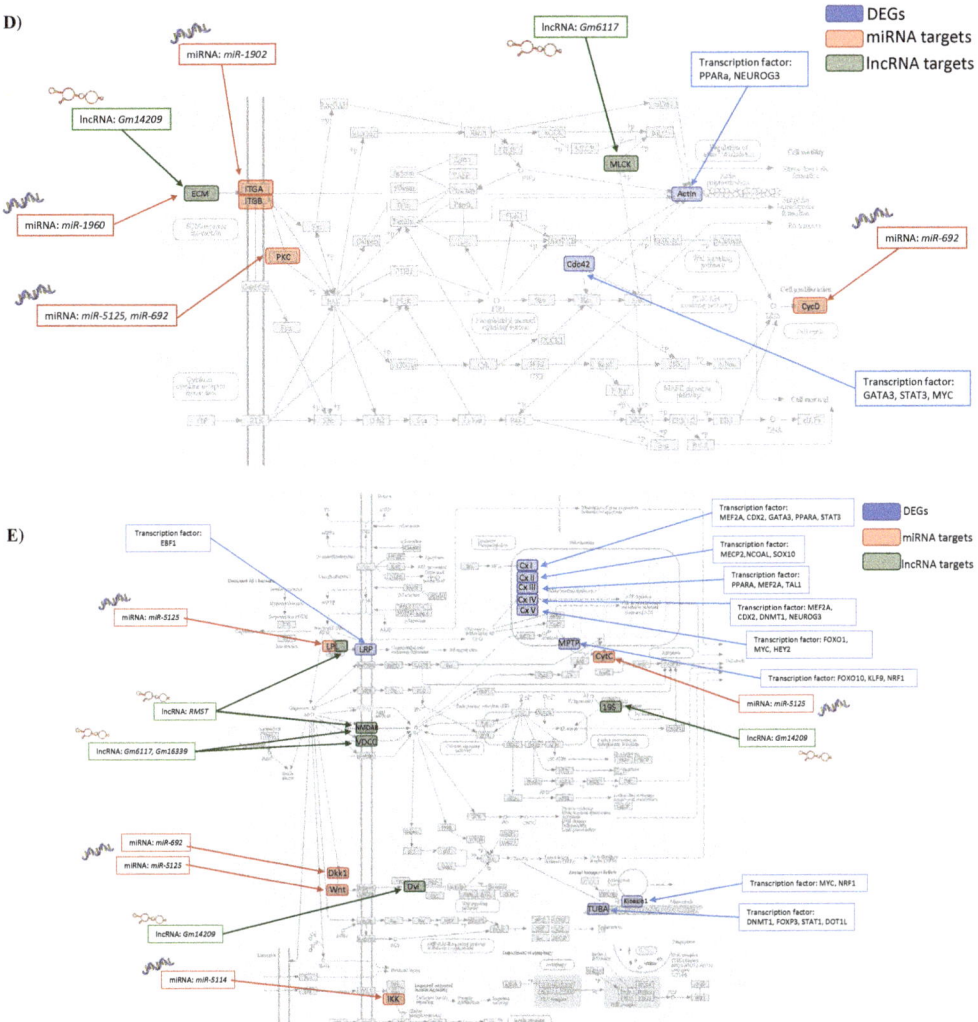

Figure 4. Effect of the high glycemic diet (HGD) on cellular pathways of differentially expressed protein-coding genes, miRNA targets, and LncRNA targets in the hippocampal microvasculature. (**A**) Network of differentially expressed protein-coding genes (grey circles), transcription factors (red hexagons), miRNAs (green diamonds) and their targets (blue circles), LncRNAs (purple rectangles) and their targets (blue circles) in the hippocampal microvessels for the high glycemic diet (HGD) compared to the low glycemic diet (LGD). (**B**) Histogram of a subset of the relevant pathways of differentially expressed protein-coding genes, miRNA targets, and LncRNA targets in the hippocampal microvasculature for the HGD vs LGD. The data are shown for three biological replicates for each dietary group. Statistically significant pathways ($p < 0.05$) were identified using Genetrial2 online database and grouped by cellular function. (**C**) Network of important cellular pathways shown in (**B**) and their genes. Pathways are shown in boxes and color coded based on cellular function such as neuro-related (red), cell signaling (green), cell adhesion and mobility (purple), cellular metabolism (yellow), and other cellular pathways (grey). White circles are differentially expressed genes (DEGs) or target genes of miRNAs and lncRNAs. Integrated analysis of (**D**) Focal adhesion and (**E**) Alzheimer's disease pathways. Blue=DEGs with potential transcription factors (TFs); Red= differentially expressed miRNAs and their targets; Green= differentially expressed lncRNAs and their targets.

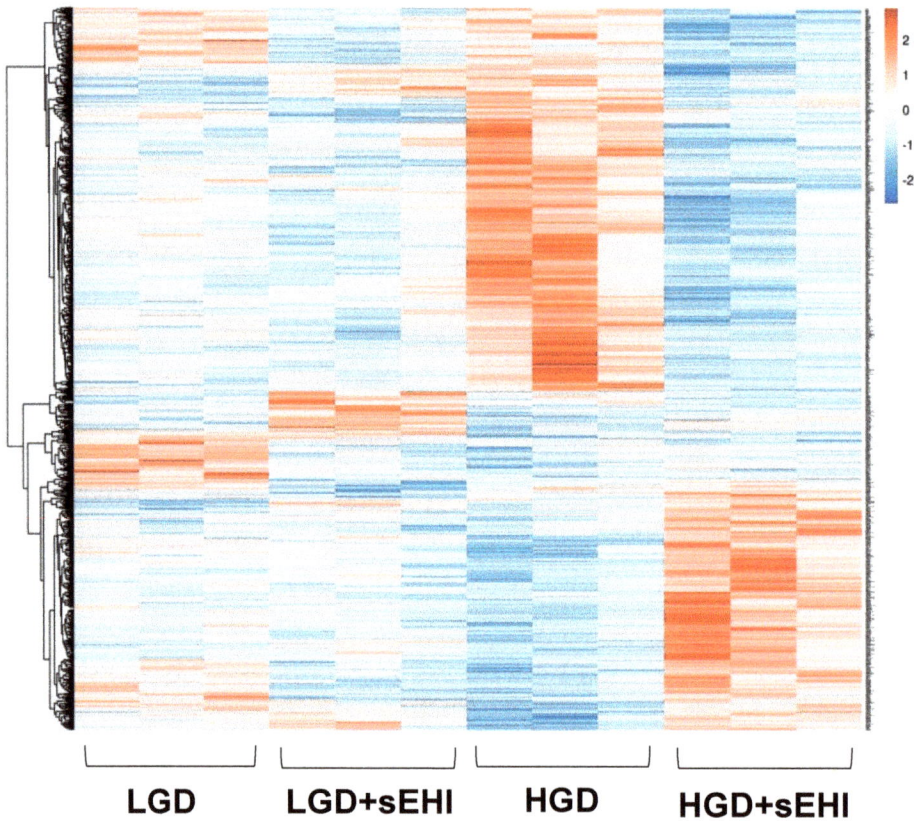

Figure 5. Hierarchical clustering of differentially expressed genes in hippocampal microvessels for the low glycemic diet (LGD) and the high glycemic diet (HGD) with and without soluble epoxide hydrolase inhibitor (sEHI). Hierarchical clustering of differentially expressed gene profiles in hippocampal microvessels of four experimental treatment groups: low glycemic diet (LGD), LGD with soluble epoxide hydrolase inhibitor (LGD+sEHI), high glycemic diet (HGD), and HGD with sEHI (HGD+sEHI). The data are shown for three biological replicates for each dietary group. Up-regulated genes are in red, and down-regulated genes are in blue. In the presence or absence of inhibitor, LGD groups had similar gene expression profiles while HGD groups had opposite gene expression profiles.

Most of the protein-coding genes down-regulated by the sEHI were involved in similar pathways (such as Alzheimer's disease, oxidative phosphorylation, and fatty acid metabolism) activated by the HGD alone (Supplemental Figure S11), suggesting that the inhibitor may offset the effect of the HGD on differential gene expression by targeting similar pathways. We also found 17 TFs in common between the HGD with and without inhibitors such as NEUROG3 (Neurogenin 3), MECP2 (Methyl-CpG Binding Protein 2), KLF9 (Kruppel Like Factor 9), and PPARA (Supplemental Table S2). Target genes of these TFs were up-regulated by the HGD but down-regulated by the inhibitor (Supplemental Figure S12). These target genes were involved in neurological disease pathways (e.g., Alzheimer's disease), oxidative phosphorylation (e.g., electron transport chain), apoptosis-related pathways (e.g., proteasome degradation), and cell signaling pathways (e.g., HF-1 signaling).

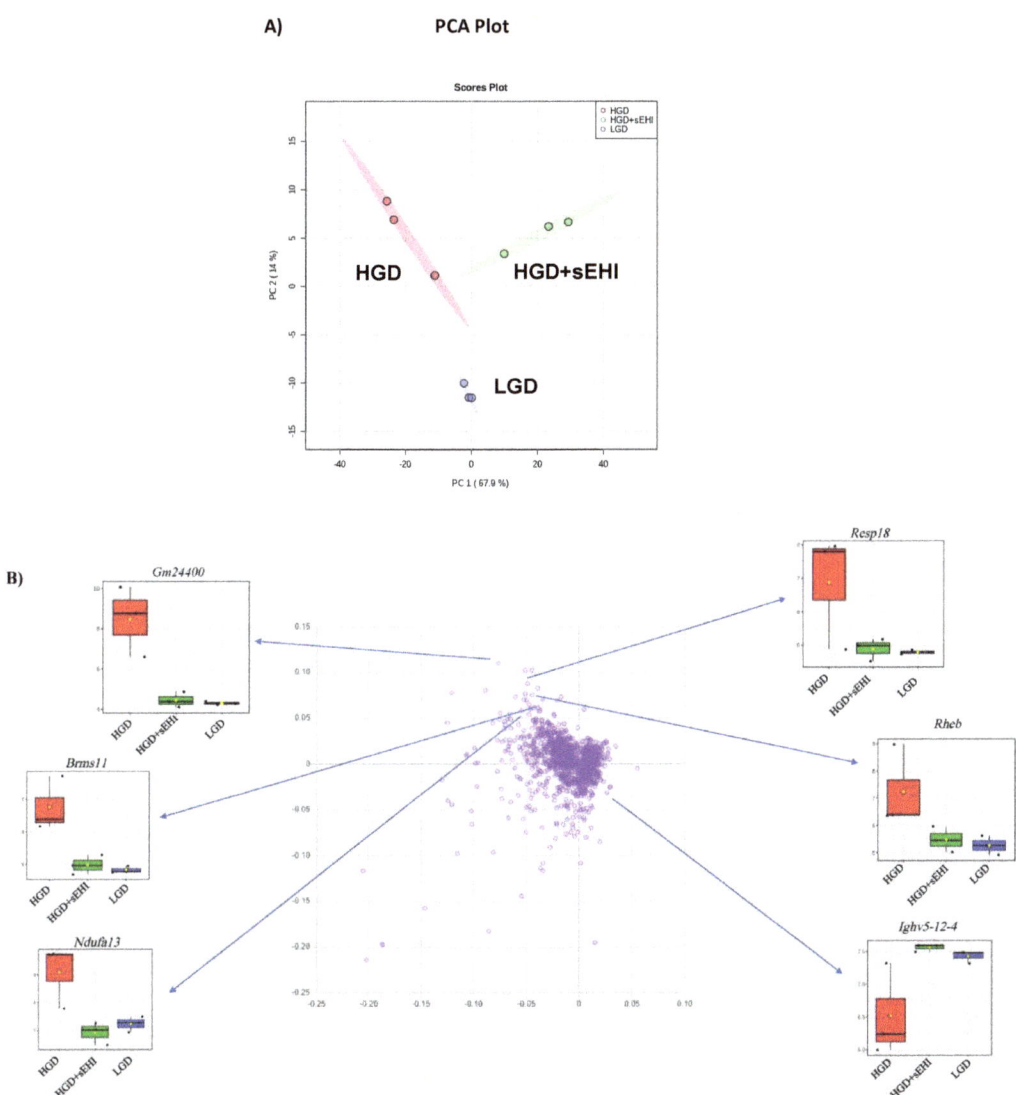

Figure 6. Principal Component Analysis (PCA) and loading plot of genes expressed in hippocampal microvessels for the high glycemic diet (HGD) with and without soluble epoxide hydrolase inhibitor (sEHI). (**A**) PCA scatter plot of the microarray data shows the trends of the expression profiles of the hippocampal microvasculature of the high glycemic diet with (HGD+sEHI, green circles) and without (HGD, red circles) the soluble epoxide hydrolase inhibitor compared to the low glycemic diet (LGD, blue circles). The PCA plot captures the variance in a dataset in terms of principal components and displays the most significant of these on the x and y axes. The percentages of the total variation that are accounted for by the 1st and 2nd principal components are shown on the x- and y-axes labels. The data are shown for three biological replicates for each dietary group. (**B**) Loading plot of genes (violet circles) relevant to the separation of PCA. Blue arrows show box plots with the expression levels of a few genes (*Gm24400, Resp18, Rheb, Brms1l, Ndufa13, Ighv5-12-4*) that contribute to separation of the three dietary groups (HGD, HGD+sEHI, LGD). In the box plots, the black dots represent gene expression levels, the notch indicates 95% confidence interval around the median of each group, and the yellow diamond indicates the average gene expression of each group.

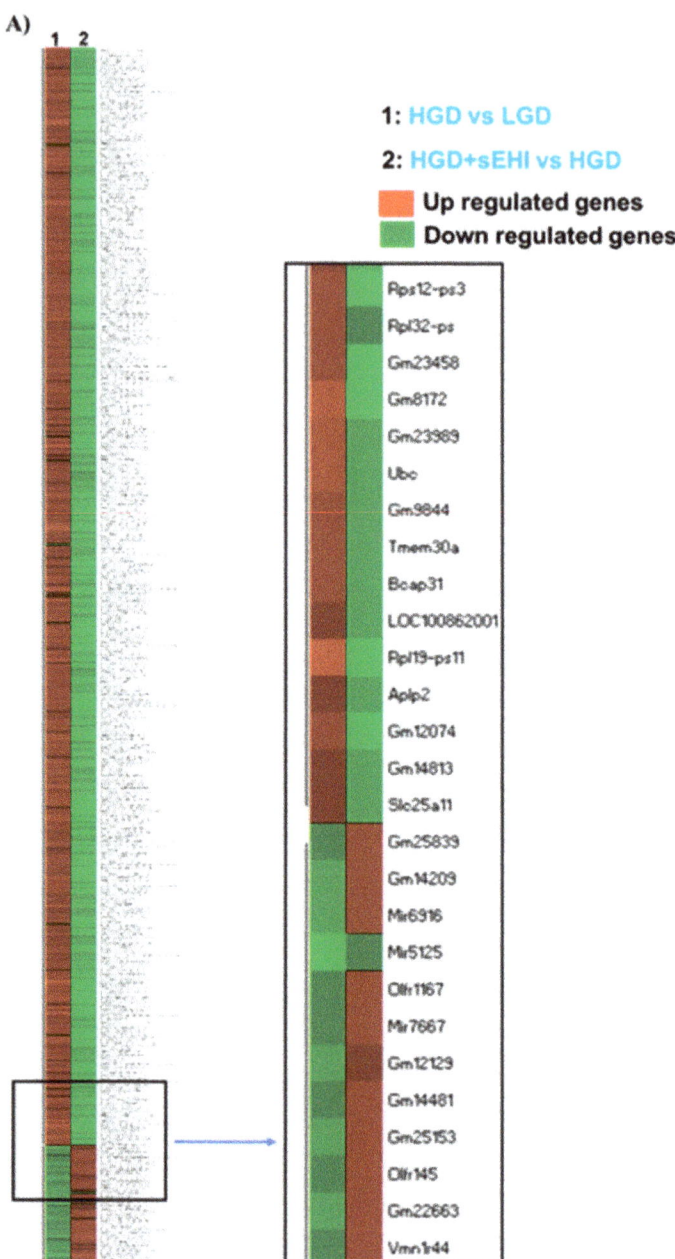

Figure 7. Cont.

B)

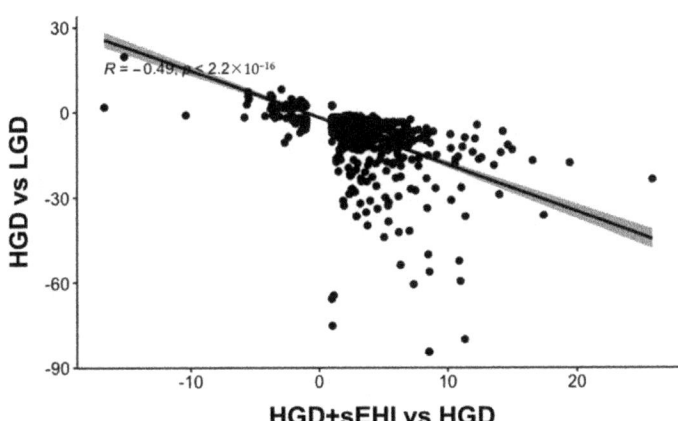

Figure 7. The effect of the high glycemic diet with and without soluble epoxide hydrolase inhibitor (sEHI) on differential gene expression in the hippocampal microvasculature. (**A**) Heat map showing individual differentially expressed genes (DEGs) in rows, and the two different experimental dietary comparison groups in columns, as follows: column 1: high glycemic diet compared to low glycemic diet (HGD vs LGD); column 2: HGD with soluble epoxide hydrolase inhibitor compared to without inhibitor (HGD+sEHI vs HGD). The data are shown for three biological replicates for each dietary group. Up-regulated genes are shown in red, and down-regulated genes in green. The rectangular box insert shows the list of genes with opposite gene expression patterns in the two comparisons (HGD vs. LGD compared to HGD+sEHI vs. HGD). (**B**) Pearson's correlation analysis of the DEGs between the comparisons, HGD vs. LGD and HGD+sEHI vs. HGD.

A higher number of DE non-coding RNAs (171 miRNAs, 127 snoRNAs, and 80 lncRNAs) were modulated by the sEHI (Supplemental Tables S3, S4, and S5, respectively) than the HGD alone. Most of the DE miRNAs that were up-regulated by the HGD were down-regulated by the inhibitor by targeting 300 genes (Supplemental Figure S13) that were involved in apoptosis-related pathways (such as PTEN dependent cell cycle arrest and Ubiquitin mediated proteolysis) (Supplemental Figure S14) and pathways related to cell degradation and death. The majority of DE lncRNAs that were up-regulated by the HGD were down-regulated by the inhibitor and again targeted a greater number of genes (785) compared to the HGD alone (Supplemental Figure S15) and were mainly involved in cell signaling (Supplemental Figure S16).

We then performed an integrated analysis of all the identified DEGs, including mRNAs, miRNAs and their targets, lncRNAs and their targets, and the potential TFs. We obtained a large molecular network of interactions of the different types of RNAs modulated by the inhibitor (Figure 8A). Integrated pathway analysis of this molecular network (Figure 8B) revealed that the inhibitor regulated similar pathways as the HGD, namely neuro-related pathways (such as Alzheimer's disease), cell signaling, cell adhesion (such as focal adhesion), and cellular metabolism, but once again, in opposite directions to the HGD. In toto, these data suggest that the inhibitor may counteract the effect of an HGD by robustly reversing the deleterious pattern of differential gene expression on cellular function and on the operative TFs, particularly by down-regulating the protein-coding and non-protein-coding DEGs that are up-regulated by the HGD.

3.3. Correlation of Genomics with Human Alzheimer's Disease Data

To evaluate the genomic modifications induced by the HGD on the development of neurodegenerative diseases, we analyzed the correlations between the genes modulated by the HGD and the genes associated with Alzheimer's disease. We analyzed the available GEO datasets with GEO2R and differentially expressed mRNAs were correlated with those extracted from the analyzed publications using the R program. These analyses showed that the gene expression profile in the brain of patients with Alzheimer's disease (GSE118553) was correlated, with high statistical significance, to the gene expression profile identified in our mice after the consumption of the HGD (Figure 9A). The gene expression profile of mice on the HGD in our study was also correlated with the gene expression profile obtained in another study (GSE132903) of brains of patients presenting with Alzheimer's disease (Figure 9B). This analysis suggests that consumption of the HGD induces changes in the expression of genes in murine hippocampus that correlates with the development of Alzheimer's disease in humans. Using the same approach, we also tested correlations between the genes modulated in our study by the HGD in the presence of the sEHI and the gene expression profiles obtained in both of the above noted genomic studies using the brains of patients with Alzheimer's disease. Interestingly, we observed a negative correlation between the human AD data and the gene expression profile of our brain microvasculature for animals on the HGD with the sEHI (Figure 9C,D). These results suggest that the inhibitor can prevent, at least partially, changes in the expression of genes induced by the HGD that are associated with the development of Alzheimer's disease in humans and can therefore exert a potentially protective effect against this neurological disorder.

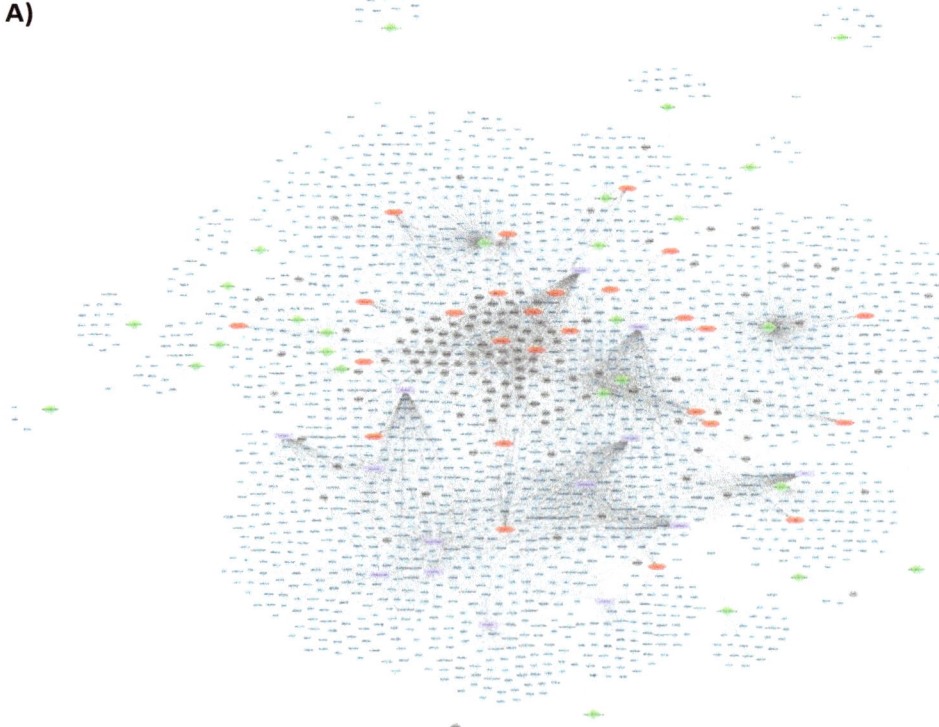

Figure 8. *Cont.*

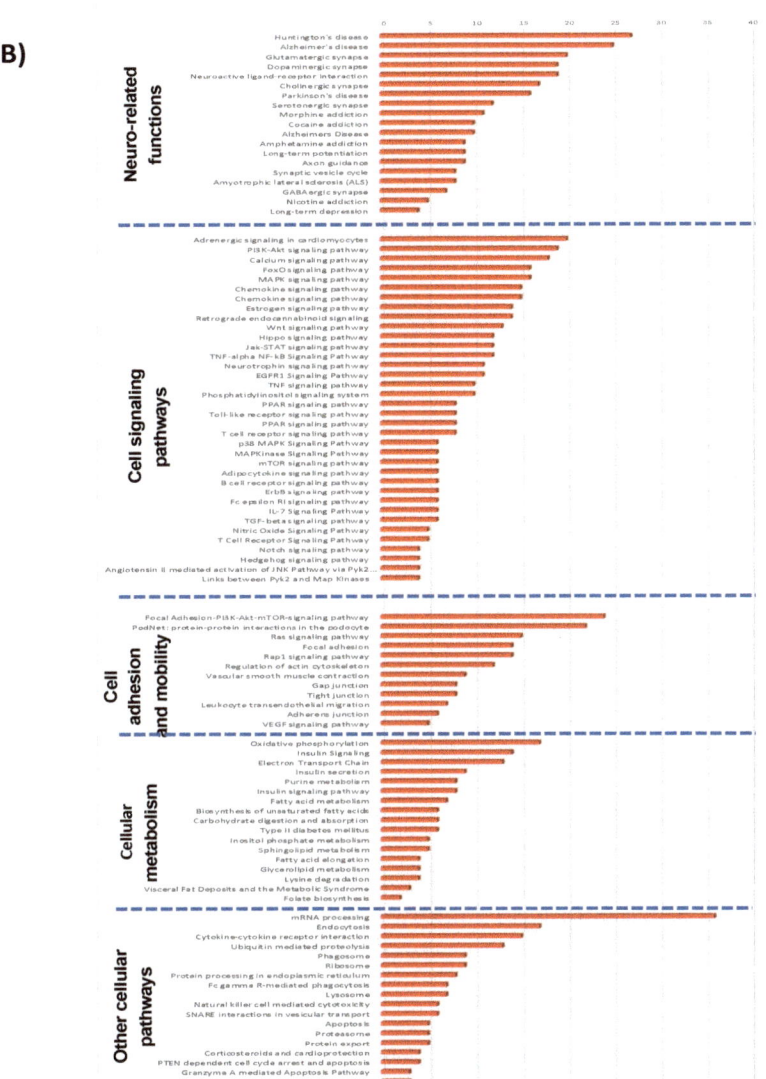

Figure 8. Effect of the high glycemic diet (HGD) with soluble epoxide hydrolase inhibitor (sEHI) on cellular pathways of differentially expressed protein-coding genes, miRNA targets, and LncRNA targets in the hippocampal microvasculature. (**A**) Network of differentially expressed protein-coding genes (grey circles), transcription factors (red hexagons), miRNAs (green diamonds) and their targets (blue circles), LncRNAs (purple rectangles) and their targets (blue circles) in the hippocampal microvessels for the high glycemic diet (HGD) with soluble epoxide hydrolase inhibitor (sEHI) when compared to HGD without sEHI. (**B**) Histogram of subset of relevant pathways of differentially expressed protein-coding genes, miRNA targets, and LncRNA targets in the hippocampal microvasculature for the HGD+sEHI vs HGD. The data are shown for three biological replicates for each dietary group. Statistically significant pathways ($p < 0.05$) were identified using Genetrial2 online database and are grouped by cellular function such as neuro-related, cell signaling, cell adhesion and mobility, cellular metabolism, and other.

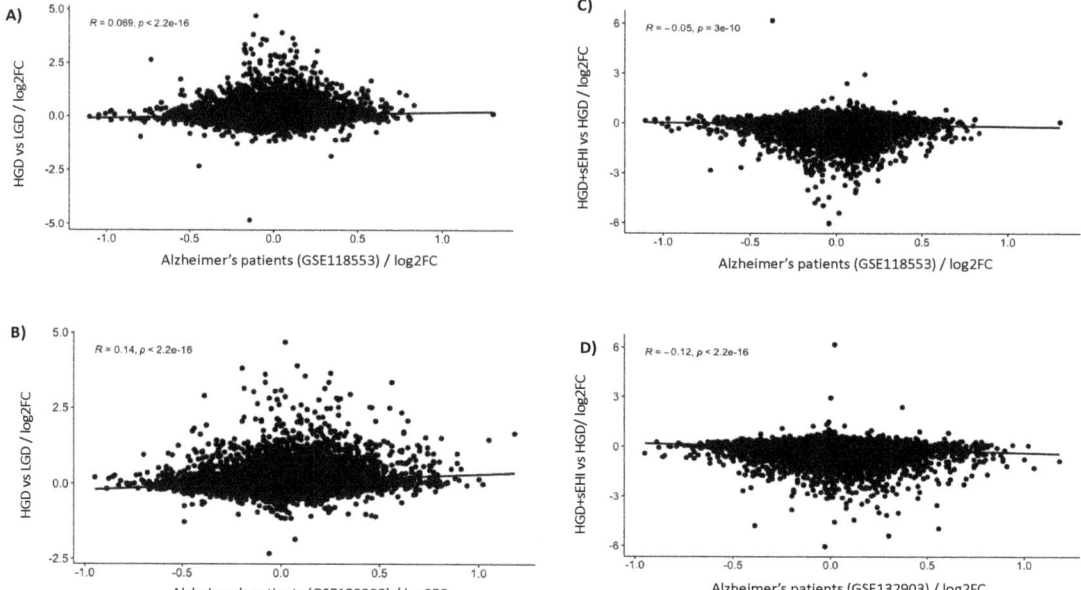

Figure 9. Correlation of the high glycemic diet (HGD) with and without inhibitor to Alzheimer's disease. Pearson correlation analysis between the genes modulated by the HGD vs LGD and the gene expression profiles observed in patients with Alzheimer's disease extracted from GEO database number (**A**) *GSE118553* and (**B**) *GSE132903*. Correlation between genes modulated by the HGD+sEHI vs LGD and patients with Alzheimer's disease extracted from GEO database number (**C**) *GSE118553* and (**D**) *GSE132903*.

3.4. Interaction of Effects of the Glycemic Diet and the Soluble Epoxide Hydrolase Inhibitor

In order to more clearly define how the sEHI modulated the response of hippocampal microvessels to an HGD, we used two-factor analysis to identify the DEGs with a significant interaction between the effects of the diet and the effects of the inhibitor. For this analysis, the LGD+sEHI group was included as it was necessary to use this additional control group for the two-factor analysis and to determine the delta fold change [(HGD+sEHI vs. LGD+sEHI) vs. (HGD vs. LGD)]. A positive delta fold change indicates a gene that is "more up-regulated" or "less down-regulated" by HGD in sEHI treated mice (compared to those with no inhibitor). A negative delta fold change indicates a gene that is "more down-regulated" or "less up-regulated" by an HGD in sEHI treated mice (compared to those with no inhibitor). We identified a total of 1543 DEGs (Supplemental Table S7) that had a significant interaction between diet and inhibitor, the majority of which had a negative delta fold change. In many cases, the direction of the regulation of the DEGs by the HGD was opposite in direction in the presence of the inhibitor when compared to the effects of the HGD on that same gene in the absence of the inhibitor. The DEGs with a negative delta fold change were diversified between RNA types, including coding, non-coding, multiple complex, and pseudogenes. The 583 DEGs with a positive delta fold change were primarily non-coding genes. Pathway analyses using the KEGG and WikiPathway databases for all of the coding DEGs (positive and negative delta fold change) demonstrated that the sEHI modulated the effects of the HGD for pathways involved in the electron transport chain, oxidative phosphorylation, focal adhesion, HIF-1 signaling pathway, and pathways active in neurological diseases (Alzheimer's pathway) (Figure 10A).

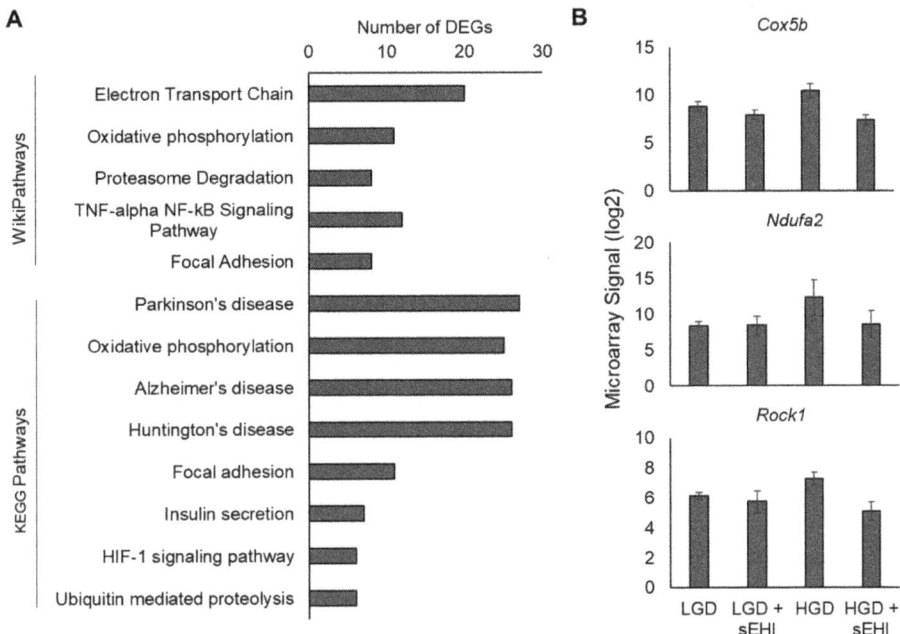

Figure 10. Analysis of DEGs with a significant interaction of diet and inhibitor. (**A**) Relevant enriched WikiPathways and KEGG Pathways for DEGs with an interaction between diet and inhibitor effects. (**B**) Signal plots of selected DEGs with an interaction between diet and inhibitor effects. Data shown are from three biological replicates (mean +/− standard deviation). The DEGs displayed are cytochrome c oxidase subunit Vb (Cox5b), NADH dehydrogenase (ubiquinone) 1 alpha subcomplex 2 (Ndufa2), and Rho-associated coiled-coil containing protein kinase 1 (Rock1).

An additional finding of the two-factor analysis was that when the individual DEGs of the relevant pathways shown in Figure 10A (77 DEGs) were examined, it again became apparent that the sEHI reverted the gene expression profile of brain hippocampal microvascular endothelium of mice on the HGD to a profile similar to that of the LGD. Examples of three genes (*Rock1, Ndufa2, and Cox5b*) are shown in Figure 10B. These DEGs were selected because they were each represented in multiple relevant pathways including focal adhesion (*Rock1*), electron transport chain (*Ndufa2* and *Cox5b*), and oxidative phosphorylation (*Ndufa2* and *Cox5b*).

4. Discussion

In this study, we characterized the effect of a high glycemic diet (HGD) on murine neurovascular function and cognition using hippocampal microvascular multiomics of mice exposed to high or low glycemic index diets. Utilizing similar techniques of large-scale transcriptome gene profiling, we have previously shown the effect of lipid stress and a Western diet (WD) on hippocampal microvascular injury and cognitive decline in male and female mice ApoE-/- and LDL-R-/- mice [8–11]. However, the molecular footprint of the glycemic component of the WD on the brain microvasculature, and whether and how the HGD may contribute to microvascular injury, was up to now unknown. A HGD is a risk factor for dementia [14] and is associated with poor cognitive performance [15,16], but whether the effect can be reversed has also been unknown. Given that in murine models of diabetes, soluble epoxide hydrolase inhibitors (sEHI) reduce neuroinflammation and cognitive decline [32–34], we also aimed to examine their role in our model.

We used a relevant model of glycemic index and demonstrated the expected significant differences in weight, cholesterol, glucose, and insulin levels consistent with what has been published previously for these experimental models [19,63–65]. To our knowledge, the present study shows for the first time that the HGD has distinct differential effects on gene expression that are different from the LGD and characterized by up-regulation of differentially expressed protein-coding genes, transcription factors, as well as non-protein-coding genes (miRNAs, snoRNAs, and lncRNAs), that are involved in five major cellular pathways: neurodegenerative diseases (Alzheimer's disease), endothelial cell function (focal adhesion), cell signaling (PPAR signaling, PI3K-Akt signaling), cellular metabolism (oxidative phosphorylation, electron transport chain), and other cellular pathways (mRNA processing, oxidative damage). Below we discuss our multi-omics integrative analysis for the focal adhesion and Alzheimer's disease pathways to illustrate the complexity and characterize the molecular regulation in response to the HGD.

Integrative analyses allowed us to identify the protein-coding genes, TFs, and the non-coding genes modulated by the HGD in the focal adhesion pathway. *Cdc42* (Cell Division Control Protein Homolog 42) is a protein-coding DEG up-regulated by the HGD and targeted by STAT3 (Signal Transducer and Activator of Transcription 3) transcription factor. *Cdc42* is up-regulated in aging endothelial cells via the focal adhesion pathway [66,67] and mediates the activation of proinflammatory genes [68]. STAT3 transcription factor is activated by oxidative stress [69,70] and is associated with neurovascular inflammation and Alzheimer's disease [71]. The HGD also up-regulated differentially expressed miRNA *miR-1902* that targets *ITGB* (Integrin β). Activation of ITGB induces a reduction in endothelial barrier function by destabilizing intercellular junctions and abnormal remodeling of extracellular matrix (ECM) [72]. Another example of differentially expressed miRNAs up-regulated by the HGD is *miR-5125* and *miR-692* which target *PKC* (Protein Kinase C). PKC is associated with endothelial dysfunction, insulin resistance [73], and neuroinflammation [74]. The HGD also up-regulated differential expression of LncRNA *Gm6117* that targets *MLCK* (Myosin Light Chain Kinase). Activation of MLCK induces endothelial vascular hyperpermeability, microvascular barrier dysfunction, and inflammation [75]. Another interesting pathway activated by the HGD was the vascular endothelial growth factor (VEGF) signaling pathway. VEGF is associated with an increase in microvascular permeability by activating PKC [76], which then signals the activation of MLCK [75]. Taken together, this molecular cascade suggests that an HGD may promote endothelial cell dysfunction by microvascular hyper permeability and activating proinflammatory TFs, protein, and non-protein-coding genes.

We also performed an integrated analysis of the Alzheimer's disease pathway and identified TFs, protein-coding, and non-coding RNAs modulated by the HGD. Mitochondrial *complex IV* protein-coding DEG was up-regulated by the HGD and targeted by DNMT1 (DNA Methyl Transferase 1) transcription factor. Increased expression of *complex IV* has been observed in the hippocampus of AD patients [77], and DNMT1 expression is up-regulated in late-onset AD [78]. Alterations in mitochondrial function are also associated with diabetes [79]. Another example of a DEG up-regulated by the HGD was *LRP1* (LDLR-related protein). Expression of *LRP1* is increased in the hippocampus of AD patients [80], particularly in the microvasculature close to amyloid plaques in AD brains [81,82]. DE miRNA, *miR-5125* was activated by the HGD and is known to target *DKK1* (Dickkopf-1). Increased expression of *DKK1* has been detected in the plasma and brain of AD patients and AD transgenic mice [83,84]. Another target of *miR-5125* was *LPL* (Lipoprotein lipase). LPL accumulates in senile plaques [85], and its expression has been shown to be increased in the hippocampus of AD mice [86]. LncRNAs *Gm6117* and *Gm16339* were also up-regulated by the HGD and target *NMDAR* (N-methyl-D-aspartate receptor). An increase in NMDAR activity induces apoptosis and neurodegeneration in AD [87]. Yet another interesting pathway modulated by the HGD was the PI3K-Akt signaling pathway. Activation of the PI3K/Akt pathway promotes oxidative stress-mediated cell death [88]. Thus, our findings suggest that an HGD may be involved in previously defined Alzheimer's disease-related pathways via deleterious effects on the brain microvasculature by promoting mitochondrial dysfunction, apoptosis, and neurodegeneration, and similar to the focal adhesion pathway, via up-regulation of pathway-associated TFs, protein-coding, and non-coding genes.

Our work with the soluble epoxide hydrolase inhibitor (sEHI) trans-4-[4-(3-adamantan-1-yl-ureido)-cyclohexyloxy]-benzoic acid (t-AUCB) showed several novel findings. sEH enzyme degrades anti-inflammatory and neuroprotective fatty acid epoxides (EETs) to biologically less active diols (DHETs) which are known to be involved in vascular cognitive impairment and Alzheimer's disease [24,25]. In animal models of stroke, sEH inhibitors have been shown to be neuroprotective [27,28]. In our study, we show for the first time that the sEHI reversed the deleterious phenotype of the HGD by down-regulating the differentially expressed genes up-regulated by the HGD and their TFs, and also by differential expression of non-coding RNAs (miRNA, snoRNA, and lncRNA) and that this proceeds by targeting the same pathways up-regulated by the HGD. When looking at specific DEGs targeted by the inhibitor, we identified interesting DEGs. For example, the presence of the sEHI down-regulated the expression of *Cdc42*, and the deletion of *Cdc42* is known to have protective effects against chronic inflammation in endothelial cells [67]. The sEHI also down-regulated the expression of the genes targeted by the PPAR (Peroxisome Proliferator-Activated Receptor) transcription factor, which is known to play a protective role against neuroinflammation in AD [89]. Furthermore, the sEHI down-regulated DE miRNAs, *miR-5125*, and *miR-692*, and their targets, *DKK1* and *PKC*, respectively. Inhibition of DKK1 has been shown to improve cognitive impairment [90] and protect against neurotoxicity [91]. PKC inhibition also protects against vascular injury of the blood–brain barrier [74]. Additionally, the sEHI also down-regulated DE lncRNA *Gm6117* and its target, *MLCK*. MLCK inhibitors play a protective role against vascular hyperpermeability and microvascular dysfunction [75]. These findings indicate that the sEHI served to protect against the neurotoxicity, endothelial- and neuro-inflammation, and blood– brain barrier permeability injury associated with the HGD.

Furthermore, our correlation analysis of the DEGs modulated by the HGD and inhibitor with the gene expression profiles obtained from the brains of Alzheimer's disease patients showed that the HGD is positively correlated, and the inhibitor is negatively correlated with the genes associated with Alzheimer's disease.

Our 2-factor interactive analysis served to further identify DEGs having a significant interaction between diet and the soluble epoxide hydrolase inhibitor. These DEGs were involved in Alzheimer's disease, electron transport chain, oxidative phosphorylation, and focal adhesion. The sEHI also was shown to restore the gene expression profile of hippocampal microvessels of mice on the HGD to a profile similar to that of the LGD, including for genes such as *Rock1* (Rho-associated protein kinase 1), which was increased by an HGD and decreased by the sEHI. *ROCK1* is activated in Alzheimer's disease, and reduction of *ROCK1* protects against AD by depleting amyloid-β levels in the brain [92]. In vitro exposure of brain microvascular endothelial cells to EETs, which generally increase after inhibition of sEH, has been shown to inhibit rho kinase (ROCK) activity [93]. Taken together, our molecular results suggest that the soluble epoxide hydrolase inhibitor may offset the effect of an HGD by robustly reversing the deleterious pattern of differential gene expression to that similar to an LGD and likely thereby protecting against vascular injury, neuroinflammation, and neurodegeneration. Furthermore, the sEHI was associated with improved cognition by down-regulating the TFs, protein-coding, and non-protein-coding DEGs that were up-regulated by the HGD.

5. Conclusions and Clinical Implications

In alignment with our hypothesis, our results show that an HGD has deleterious effects on differential gene expression of brain microvessels in memory centers in the brain by up-regulating the protein-coding and non-coding genes involved in alterations of mitochondrial function, oxidation, inflammation, and microvascular dysfunction. These processes play an important role in the pathophysiology of dementia. We also showed that inhibition of sEH protects against neuroinflammation, apoptosis, vascular injury, and cognitive decline by down-regulating the DEGs up-regulated by an HGD. The clinical role of sEHIs has been reviewed [22]. In clinical trials, sEHIs play a protective role in hypertension [94], and in animal models, they demonstrate neuroprotection in stroke [27,28], cerebral hypoperfusion, and in diabetes type 1 and type 2 [29–33]. Our studies show that sEHIs may also be promising therapeutic targets in the microvascular endothelial dysfunction that accompanies Alzheimer's and vascular dementias.

Supplementary Materials: The following are available online at https://www.mdpi.com/article/10.3390/nu13113913/s1, Figure S1: Volcano plot of differential gene expression changes in hippocampal microvessels for the high glycemic diet (HGD) compared to the low glycemic diet (LGD), Figure S2: Distribution of differentially expressed RNAs in hippocampal microvessels for the high glycemic diet (HGD) when compared to the low glycemic diet (LGD), Figure S3: Histogram of differentially expressed protein coding genes pathways in hippocampal microvessels for the high glycemic diet (HGD) when compared to the low glycemic diet (LGD), Figure S4. Target gene networks of differentially expressed transcription factors (TFs) in hippocampal microvessels for the high glycemic diet (HGD) compared to the low glycemic diet (LGD), Figure S5. Target gene networks of differentially expressed miRNAs in hippocampal microvessels with the high glycemic diet (HGD) compared to the low glycemic diet (LGD), Figure S6: Histogram of differentially expressed miRNA targets pathways in hippocampal microvessels with the high glycemic diet (HGD) when compared to the low glycemic diet (LGD), Figure S7. Target gene networks of differentially expressed LncRNAs in hippocampal microvessels with the high glycemic diet (HGD) compared to the low glycemic diet (LGD), Figure S8: Histogram of differentially expressed lncRNA targets pathways in hippocampal microvessels with the high glycemic diet (HGD) when compared to the low glycemic diet (LGD), Figure S9: Volcano plot of differential gene expression changes in hippocampal microvessels for the high glycemic diet (HGD) with soluble epoxide hydrolase inhibitor (sEHI) compared to without sEHI treatment, Figure S10: Distribution of differentially expressed RNAs in hippocampal microvessels from the high glycemic diet (HGD) with soluble epoxide hydrolase inhibitor (sEHI) compared to without sEHI treatment, Figure S11: Histogram of protein coding differentially expressed genes pathways in hippocampal microvessels for the high glycemic diet (HGD) with soluble epoxide hydrolase inhibitor (sEHI) compared to without sEHI treatment, Figure S12: Target gene networks of differentially expressed transcription factors (TFs) in hippocampal microvessels for the high glycemic diet (HGD) with and without soluble epoxide hydrolase inhibitor (sEHI), Figure S13: Target gene networks of differentially expressed miRNAs in hippocampal microvessels for the high glycemic diet (HGD) with and without soluble epoxide hydrolase inhibitor (sEHI), Figure S14: Histogram of differentially expressed miRNA targets pathways in hippocampal microvessels for the HGD with soluble epoxide hydrolase inhibitor (sEHI) compared to without sEHI treatment, Figure S15: Target gene networks of differentially expressed LncRNAs in hippocampal microvessels for the high glycemic diet (HGD) with and without soluble epoxide hydrolase inhibitor (sEHI), Figure S16: Histogram of differentially expressed lncRNA targets pathways in hippocampal microvessels for the high glycemic diet (HGD) with soluble epoxide hydrolase inhibitor (sEHI) compared to without the sEHI; Table S1: Differentially expressed genes for the high glycemic diet (HGD) compared to the low glycemic diet (LGD), Table S2: Top 30 transcription factors (TFs) differentially expressed by a high glycemic diet (HGD) with and without soluble epoxide hydrolase inhibitor (sEHI) in hippocampal microvascular endothelium, Table S3: Effect of the high glycemic diet (HGD) with and without soluble epoxide hydrolase inhibitor (sEHI) on the expression of microRNAs (miRNAs) in hippocampal microvessels, Table S4: Effect of the high glycemic diet (HGD) with and without soluble epoxide hydrolase inhibitor (sEHI) on the expression of long non-coding RNAs (lncRNAs) in hippocampal microvessels, Table S5: Effect of the high glycemic diet (HGD) with and without soluble epoxide hydrolase inhibitor (sEHI) on the expression of small nucleolar RNAs (snoRNAs) in hippocampal microvessels, Table S6: Differentially expressed genes for the high glycemic diet (HGD) with soluble epoxide hydrolase inhibitor (sEHI) compared to without sEHI, Table S7: Differentially expressed genes with a significant interaction of diet and inhibitor.

Author Contributions: Individual contributions of the authors were as follows. Conceptualization, A.V. and J.R.; methodology, S.N., A.V.; software, S.N., A.V., D.M., J.E.N.; validation, A.V., S.N., D.M. and J.E.N.; formal analysis, S.N., D.M., A.V., J.E.N.; investigation, S.N.; resources, A.V. and J.R.; data curation, A.V., D.M., S.N., J.E.N.; writing—original draft preparation, A.V. and S.N.; writing—review and editing, A.V., S.N., D.M., J.E.N.; visualization, A.V., S.N., D.M., J.E.N.; supervision, A.V., J.R., D.M.; project administration, S.N.; funding acquisition, A.V. and J.R. All authors have read and agreed to the published version of the manuscript.

Funding: This work was supported by an award from the Richard A. and Nora Eccles Foundation (A20-0111), the Richard A. and Nora Eccles Harrison Endowed Chair in Diabetes Research (J.C.R.), and the Frances Lazda Endowed Chair in Women's Cardiovascular Medicine (A.C.V). Laser Capture Microdissection and Cryo-Sectioning were conducted at the Cellular and Molecular Imaging core facility at the University of California Davis (UC Davis) Center for Health and the Environment. The laser capture microscope was funded by NIHS10RR-023555. Microarray Scanning and Hybridization was done by the Genomics Shared Resource at the UC Davis Medical Center. We are also grateful for the technical support and/or services provided to our research by the UC Davis Mouse Metabolic Phenotyping Center which assisted with the metabolic assays supported by U24 DK092993.

Institutional Review Board Statement: The institutional review board of the University of California, Davis, the Institutional Animal Care and Use Committee (IACUC) approved this project protocol number 20943 on 18 April 2019.

Informed Consent Statement: Not applicable.

Data Availability Statement: We have deposited the microarray data in GEO and the accession number is GSE185057.

Acknowledgments: We thank Nikita Patel, Anthony Pham, Taarini Hariharan, Nejma Wais, Ryan Vinh, and Corey Buckley for technical assistance in this project.

Conflicts of Interest: The authors declare no conflict of interest.

References

1. Duplantier, S.C.; Gardner, C.D. A Critical Review of the Study of Neuroprotective Diets to Reduce Cognitive Decline. *Nutrients* **2021**, *13*, 2264. [CrossRef]
2. Więckowska-Gacek, A.; Mietelska-Porowska, A.; Chutorański, D.; Wydrych, M.; Długosz, J.; Wojda, U. Western Diet Induces Impairment of Liver-Brain Axis Accelerating Neuroinflammation and Amyloid Pathology in Alzheimer's Disease. *Front. Aging Neurosci.* **2021**, *13*, 654509. [CrossRef]
3. Leigh, S.J.; Morris, M.J. Diet, Inflammation and the gut microbiome: Mechanisms for obesity-associated cognitive impairment. *Biochim. Biophys. Acta Mol. Basis Dis.* **2020**, *1866*, 165767. [CrossRef]
4. Buie, J.J.; Watson, L.S.; Smith, C.J.; Sims-Robinson, C. Obesity-related cognitive impairment: The role of endothelial dysfunction. *Neurobiol. Dis.* **2019**, *132*, 104580. [CrossRef]
5. Rutkowsky, J.M.; Lee, L.L.; Puchowicz, M.; Golub, M.S.; Befroy, D.E.; Wilson, D.W.; Anderson, S.; Cline, G.; Bini, J.; Borkowski, K.; et al. Reduced cognitive function, increased blood-brain-barrier transport and inflammatory responses, and altered brain metabolites in LDLr -/- and C57BL/6 mice fed a western diet. *PLoS ONE* **2018**, *13*, e0191909. [CrossRef]
6. Nguyen, J.C.; Killcross, A.S.; Jenkins, T.A. Obesity and cognitive decline: Role of inflammation and vascular changes. *Front. Neurosci.* **2014**, *8*, 375. [CrossRef] [PubMed]
7. Gorelick, P.B.; Counts, S.E.; Nyenhuis, D. Vascular cognitive impairment and dementia. *Biochim. Biophys. Acta (BBA)—Mol. Basis Dis.* **2016**, *1862*, 860–868. [CrossRef]
8. Aung, H.H.; Altman, R.; Nyunt, T.; Kim, J.; Nuthikattu, S.; Budamagunta, M.; Voss, J.C.; Wilson, D.; Rutledge, J.C.; Villablanca, A.C. Lipotoxic brain microvascular injury is mediated by activating transcription factor 3-dependent inflammatory and oxidative stress pathways. *J. Lipid Res.* **2016**, *57*, 955–968. [CrossRef] [PubMed]
9. Nuthikattu, S.; Milenkovic, D.; Rutledge, J.; Villablanca, A. The Western Diet Regulates Hippocampal Microvascular Gene Expression: An Integrated Genomic Analyses in Female Mice. *Sci Rep.* **2019**, *9*, 19058. [CrossRef] [PubMed]
10. Nuthikattu, S.; Milenkovic, D.; Rutledge, J.C.; Villablanca, A.C. Lipotoxic Injury Differentially Regulates Brain Microvascular Gene Expression in Male Mice. *Nutrients* **2020**, *12*, 1771. [CrossRef]
11. Nuthikattu, S.; Milenkovic, D.; Rutledge, J.C.; Villablanca, A.C. Sex-Dependent Molecular Mechanisms of Lipotoxic Injury in Brain Microvasculature: Implications for Dementia. *Int. J. Mol. Sci.* **2020**, *21*, 8146. [CrossRef] [PubMed]
12. Seetharaman, S.; Andel, R.; McEvoy, C.; Dahl Aslan, A.K.; Finkel, D.; Pedersen, N.L. Blood glucose, Diet-based glycemic load and cognitive aging among dementia-free older adults. *J. Gerontol. A Biol. Sci. Med. Sci.* **2015**, *70*, 471–479. [CrossRef]
13. Taylor, M.K.; Sullivan, D.K.; Swerdlow, R.H.; Vidoni, E.D.; Morris, J.K.; Mahnken, J.D.; Burns, J.M. A high-glycemic diet is associated with cerebral amyloid burden in cognitively normal older adults. *Am. J. Clin. Nutr.* **2017**, *106*, 1463–1470. [CrossRef]
14. Gentreau, M.; Raymond, M.; Chuy, V.; Samieri, C.; Féart, C.; Berticat, C.; Artero, S. High Glycemic Load Is Associated with Cognitive Decline in Apolipoprotein E ε4 Allele Carriers. *Nutrients* **2020**, *12*, 3619. [CrossRef]

15. Saikrishna, K.; Kumari, R.; Chaitanya, K.; Biswas, S.; Nayak, P.G.; Mudgal, J.; Kishore, A.; Nandakumar, K. Combined Administration of Monosodium Glutamate and High Sucrose Diet Accelerates the Induction of Type 2 Diabetes, Vascular Dysfunction, and Memory Impairment in Rats. *J. Environ. Pathol. Toxicol. Oncol.* **2018**, *37*, 63–80. [CrossRef] [PubMed]
16. Wong, A.; Dogra, V.R.; Reichelt, A.C. High-sucrose diets in male rats disrupt aspects of decision making tasks, motivation and spatial memory, but not impulsivity measured by operant delay-discounting. *Behav. Brain Res.* **2017**, *327*, 144–154. [CrossRef]
17. Żebrowska, E.; Chabowski, A.; Zalewska, A.; Maciejczyk, M. High-Sugar Diet Disrupts Hypothalamic but Not Cerebral Cortex Redox Homeostasis. *Nutrients* **2020**, *12*, 3181. [CrossRef]
18. Pinto, B.A.; Melo, T.M.; Flister, K.F.; França, L.M.; Kajihara, D.; Tanaka, L.Y.; Laurindo, F.R.; Paes, A.M. Early and sustained exposure to high-sucrose diet triggers hippocampal ER stress in young rats. *Metab. Brain Dis.* **2016**, *31*, 917–927. [CrossRef]
19. Yeh, S.H.; Shie, F.S.; Liu, H.K.; Yao, H.H.; Kao, P.C.; Lee, Y.H.; Chen, L.M.; Hsu, S.M.; Chao, L.J.; Wu, K.W.; et al. A high-sucrose diet aggravates Alzheimer's disease pathology, attenuates hypothalamic leptin signaling, and impairs food-anticipatory activity in APPswe/PS1dE9 mice. *Neurobiol. Aging* **2020**, *90*, 60–74. [CrossRef] [PubMed]
20. Taha, A.Y.; Gao, F.; Ramadan, E.; Cheon, Y.; Rapoport, S.I.; Kim, H.W. Upregulated expression of brain enzymatic markers of arachidonic and docosahexaenoic acid metabolism in a rat model of the metabolic syndrome. *BMC Neurosci.* **2012**, *13*, 131. [CrossRef]
21. Wang, L.; Luo, G.; Zhang, L.F.; Geng, H.X. Neuroprotective effects of epoxyeicosatrienoic acids. *Prostaglandins Other Lipid Mediat.* **2018**, *138*, 9–14. [CrossRef]
22. Zarriello, S.; Tuazon, J.P.; Corey, S.; Schimmel, S.; Rajani, M.; Gorsky, A.; Incontri, D.; Hammock, B.D.; Borlongan, C.V. Humble beginnings with big goals: Small molecule soluble epoxide hydrolase inhibitors for treating CNS disorders. *Prog. Neurobiol.* **2019**, *172*, 23–39. [CrossRef]
23. Ren, Q.; Ma, M.; Yang, J.; Nonaka, R.; Yamaguchi, A.; Ishikawa, K.I.; Kobayashi, K.; Murayama, S.; Hwang, S.H.; Saiki, S.; et al. Soluble epoxide hydrolase plays a key role in the pathogenesis of Parkinson's disease. *Proc. Natl. Acad. Sci. USA* **2018**, *115*, E5815–E5823. [CrossRef]
24. Nelson, J.W.; Young, J.M.; Borkar, R.N.; Woltjer, R.L.; Quinn, J.F.; Silbert, L.C.; Grafe, M.R.; Alkayed, N.J. Role of soluble epoxide hydrolase in age-related vascular cognitive decline. *Prostaglandins Other Lipid Mediat.* **2014**, *113–115*, 30–37. [CrossRef] [PubMed]
25. Yu, D.; Hennebelle, M.; Sahlas, D.J.; Ramirez, J.; Gao, F.; Masellis, M.; Cogo-Moreira, H.; Swartz, R.H.; Herrmann, N.; Chan, P.C.; et al. Soluble Epoxide Hydrolase-Derived Linoleic Acid Oxylipins in Serum Are Associated with Periventricular White Matter Hyperintensities and Vascular Cognitive Impairment. *Transl. Stroke Res.* **2019**, *10*, 522–533. [CrossRef] [PubMed]
26. Griñán-Ferré, C.; Codony, S.; Pujol, E.; Yang, J.; Leiva, R.; Escolano, C.; Puigoriol-Illamola, D.; Companys-Alemany, J.; Corpas, R.; Sanfeliu, C.; et al. Pharmacological Inhibition of Soluble Epoxide Hydrolase as a New Therapy for Alzheimer's Disease. *Neurotherapeutics* **2020**, *17*, 1825–1835. [CrossRef]
27. Simpkins, A.N.; Rudic, R.D.; Schreihofer, D.A.; Roy, S.; Manhiani, M.; Tsai, H.J.; Hammock, B.D.; Imig, J.D. Soluble epoxide inhibition is protective against cerebral ischemia via vascular and neural protection. *Am. J. Pathol.* **2009**, *174*, 2086–2095. [CrossRef] [PubMed]
28. Shaik, J.S.; Ahmad, M.; Li, W.; Rose, M.E.; Foley, L.M.; Hitchens, T.K.; Graham, S.H.; Hwang, S.H.; Hammock, B.D.; Poloyac, S.M. Soluble epoxide hydrolase inhibitor trans-4-[4-(3-adamantan-1-yl-ureido)-cyclohexyloxy]-benzoic acid is neuroprotective in rat model of ischemic stroke. *Am. J. Physiol. Heart Circ. Physiol.* **2013**, *305*, H1605–H1613. [CrossRef]
29. Chen, Y.; Tian, H.; Yao, E.; Tian, Y.; Zhang, H.; Xu, L.; Yu, Z.; Fang, Y.; Wang, W.; Du, P.; et al. Soluble epoxide hydrolase inhibition Promotes White Matter Integrity and Long-Term Functional Recovery after chronic hypoperfusion in mice. *Sci. Rep.* **2017**, *7*, 7758. [CrossRef]
30. Hao, J.; Chen, Y.; Yao, E.; Liu, X. Soluble epoxide hydrolase inhibition alleviated cognitive impairments via NRG1/ErbB4 signaling after chronic cerebral hypoperfusion induced by bilateral carotid artery stenosis in mice. *Brain Res.* **2018**, *1699*, 89–99. [CrossRef]
31. Matin, N.; Fisher, C.; Lansdell, T.A.; Hammock, B.D.; Yang, J.; Jackson, W.F.; Dorrance, A.M. Soluble epoxide hydrolase inhibition improves cognitive function and parenchymal artery dilation in a hypertensive model of chronic cerebral hypoperfusion. *Microcirculation* **2021**, *28*, e12653. [CrossRef] [PubMed]
32. Minaz, N.; Razdan, R.; Hammock, B.D.; Goswami, S.K. An inhibitor of soluble epoxide hydrolase ameliorates diabetes-induced learning and memory impairment in rats. *Prostaglandins Other Lipid Mediat.* **2018**, *136*, 84–89. [CrossRef]
33. Wu, J.; Fan, Z.; Zhao, Y.; Chen, Q.; Xiao, Q. Inhibition of soluble epoxide hydrolase (sEH) protects hippocampal neurons and reduces cognitive decline in type 2 diabetic mice. *Eur. J. Neurosci.* **2021**, *53*, 2532–2540. [CrossRef] [PubMed]
34. Ghosh, A.; Comerota, M.M.; Wan, D.; Chen, F.; Propson, N.E.; Hwang, S.H.; Hammock, B.D.; Zheng, H. An epoxide hydrolase inhibitor reduces neuroinflammation in a mouse model of Alzheimer's disease. *Sci. Transl. Med.* **2020**, *12*. [CrossRef]
35. Lee, H.T.; Lee, K.I.; Chen, C.H.; Lee, T.S. Genetic deletion of soluble epoxide hydrolase delays the progression of Alzheimer's disease. *J. Neuroinflamm.* **2019**, *16*, 267. [CrossRef]
36. Knierim, J.J. The hippocampus. *Curr. Biol.* **2015**, *25*, R1116–R1121. [CrossRef]
37. Han, F. Cerebral microvascular dysfunction and neurodegeneration in dementia. *Stroke Vasc. Neurol.* **2019**, *4*, 105–107. [CrossRef]
38. Gui, Y.J.; Yang, T.; Liu, Q.; Liao, C.X.; Chen, J.Y.; Wang, Y.T.; Hu, J.H.; Xu, D.Y. Soluble epoxide hydrolase inhibitors, t-AUCB, regulated microRNA-1 and its target genes in myocardial infarction mice. *Oncotarget* **2017**, *8*, 94635–94649. [CrossRef] [PubMed]
39. Ball, H.J.; McParland, B.; Driussi, C.; Hunt, N.H. Isolating vessels from the mouse brain for gene expression analysis using laser capture microdissection. *Brain Res. Brain Res. Protoc.* **2002**, *9*, 206–213. [CrossRef]

40. Metsalu, T.; Vilo, J. ClustVis: A web tool for visualizing clustering of multivariate data using Principal Component Analysis and heatmap. *Nucleic Acids Res.* **2015**, *43*, W566–W570. [CrossRef]
41. Licursi, V.; Conte, F.; Fiscon, G.; Paci, P. MIENTURNET: An interactive web tool for microRNA-target enrichment and network-based analysis. *BMC Bioinform.* **2019**, *20*, 545. [CrossRef]
42. Fukunaga, T.; Iwakiri, J.; Ono, Y.; Hamada, M. LncRRIsearch: A Web Server for lncRNA-RNA Interaction Prediction Integrated With Tissue-Specific Expression and Subcellular Localization Data. *Front. Genet.* **2019**, *10*, 462. [CrossRef] [PubMed]
43. Rtools CBRC. Available online: http://rtools.cbrc.jp/cgi-bin/RNARNA/index.pl (accessed on 25 April 2021).
44. GeneTrail2. Available online: https://genetrail2.bioinf.uni-sb.de (accessed on 2 June 2019).
45. Stockel, D.; Kehl, T.; Trampert, P.; Schneider, L.; Backes, C.; Ludwig, N.; Gerasch, A.; Kaufmann, M.; Gessler, M.; Graf, N.; et al. Multi-omics enrichment analysis using the GeneTrail2 web service. *Bioinformatics* **2016**, *32*, 1502–1508. [CrossRef]
46. Cytoscape. Available online: https://cytoscape.org/ (accessed on 2 June 2019).
47. Cytoscape Network Analyzer Application. Available online: http://apps.cytoscape.org/apps/networkanalyzer (accessed on 2 March 2020).
48. Shannon, P.; Markiel, A.; Ozier, O.; Baliga, N.S.; Wang, J.T.; Ramage, D.; Amin, N.; Schwikowski, B.; Ideker, T. Cytoscape: A software environment for integrated models of biomolecular interaction networks. *Genome Res.* **2003**, *13*, 2498–2504. [CrossRef]
49. Su, G.; Morris, J.H.; Demchak, B.; Bader, G.D. Biological network exploration with Cytoscape 3. *Curr. Protoc. Bioinform.* **2014**, *47*, 8–13. [CrossRef]
50. Splitstackshape. Available online: https://github.com/mrdwab/splitstackshape (accessed on 2 March 2020).
51. Rdata.table. Available online: https://github.com/Rdatatable/data.table (accessed on 2 March 2020).
52. Dplyr Tidyverse. Available online: http://dplyr.tidyverse.org (accessed on 2 March 2020).
53. Dplyr Tidyverse Github. Available online: https://github.com/tidyverse/dplyr (accessed on 2 March 2020).
54. String Tidyverse. Available online: http://stringr.tidyverse.org (accessed on 2 March 2020).
55. String Tidyverse Github. Available online: https://github.com/tidyverse/stringr (accessed on 2 March 2020).
56. Chen, E.Y.; Tan, C.M.; Kou, Y.; Duan, Q.; Wang, Z.; Meirelles, G.V.; Clark, N.R.; Ma'ayan, A. Enrichr: Interactive and collaborative HTML5 gene list enrichment analysis tool. *BMC Bioinform.* **2013**, *14*, 128. [CrossRef]
57. Kuleshov, M.V.; Jones, M.R.; Rouillard, A.D.; Fernandez, N.F.; Duan, Q.; Wang, Z.; Koplev, S.; Jenkins, S.L.; Jagodnik, K.M.; Lachmann, A.; et al. Enrichr: A comprehensive gene set enrichment analysis web server 2016 update. *Nucleic Acids Res.* **2016**, *44*, W90–W97. [CrossRef] [PubMed]
58. Xie, Z.; Bailey, A.; Kuleshov, M.V.; Clarke, D.J.B.; Evangelista, J.E.; Jenkins, S.L.; Lachmann, A.; Wojciechowicz, M.L.; Kropiwnicki, E.; Jagodnik, K.M.; et al. Gene Set Knowledge Discovery with Enrichr. *Curr. Protoc.* **2021**, *1*, e90. [CrossRef] [PubMed]
59. PermutMatrix. Available online: http://www.atgc-montpellier.fr/permutmatrix/ (accessed on 2 June 2019).
60. Caraux, G.; Pinloche, S. PermutMatrix: A graphical environment to arrange gene expression profiles in optimal linear order. *Bioinformatics* **2005**, *21*, 1280–1281. [CrossRef]
61. ggpubr R package. Available online: http://www.sthda.com/english/articles/24-ggpubr-publication-ready-plots/78-perfect-scatter-plots-with-correlation-and-marginal-histograms/ (accessed on 25 July 2021).
62. NCBI GEO2R. Available online: https://www.ncbi.nlm.nih.gov/geo/info/geo2r.html (accessed on 25 July 2021).
63. Van Schothorst, E.M.; Bunschoten, A.; Schrauwen, P.; Mensink, R.P.; Keijer, J. Effects of a high-fat, low-versus high-glycemic index diet: Retardation of insulin resistance involves adipose tissue modulation. *FASEB J.* **2009**, *23*, 1092–1101. [CrossRef]
64. Zhu, Y.; Smith, K.; Rowan, S.; Greenberg, A. The Short-Term Effect of a High-Glycemic Diet on Mouse Obesity and Intestinal Microbiota Composition. *Curr. Dev. Nutr.* **2020**, *4* (Suppl. 2), 1602. [CrossRef]
65. Sousa, L.G.O.d.; Marshall, A.G.; Norman, J.E.; Fuqua, J.D.; Lira, V.A.; Rutledge, J.C.; Bodine, S.C. The effects of diet composition and chronic obesity on muscle growth and function. *J. Appl. Physiol.* **2021**, *130*, 124–138. [CrossRef]
66. Cho, K.A.; Ryu, S.J.; Oh, Y.S.; Park, J.H.; Lee, J.W.; Kim, H.P.; Kim, K.T.; Jang, I.S.; Park, S.C. Morphological adjustment of senescent cells by modulating caveolin-1 status. *J. Biol. Chem.* **2004**, *279*, 42270–42278. [CrossRef] [PubMed]
67. Flentje, A.; Kalsi, R.; Monahan, T.S. Small GTPases and Their Role in Vascular Disease. *Int. J. Mol. Sci.* **2019**, *20*, 917. [CrossRef]
68. Ito, T.K.; Yokoyama, M.; Yoshida, Y.; Nojima, A.; Kassai, H.; Oishi, K.; Okada, S.; Kinoshita, D.; Kobayashi, Y.; Fruttiger, M.; et al. A crucial role for CDC42 in senescence-associated inflammation and atherosclerosis. *PLoS ONE* **2014**, *9*, e102186. [CrossRef]
69. Zouein, F.A.; Booz, G.W.; Altara, R. STAT3 and Endothelial Cell-Cardiomyocyte Dialog in Cardiac Remodeling. *Front. Cardiovasc. Med.* **2019**, *6*, 50. [CrossRef]
70. Bourgeais, J.; Gouilleux-Gruart, V.; Gouilleux, F. Oxidative metabolism in cancer: A STAT affair? *Jak-Stat* **2013**, *2*, e25764. [CrossRef]
71. Millot, P.; San, C.; Bennana, E.; Porte, B.; Vignal, N.; Hugon, J.; Paquet, C.; Hosten, B.; Mouton-Liger, F. STAT3 inhibition protects against neuroinflammation and BACE1 upregulation induced by systemic inflammation. *Immunol. Lett.* **2020**, *228*, 129–134. [CrossRef] [PubMed]
72. Faurobert, E.; Rome, C.; Lisowska, J.; Manet-Dupé, S.; Boulday, G.; Malbouyres, M.; Balland, M.; Bouin, A.P.; Kéramidas, M.; Bouvard, D.; et al. CCM1-ICAP-1 complex controls β1 integrin-dependent endothelial contractility and fibronectin remodeling. *J. Cell Biol.* **2013**, *202*, 545–561. [CrossRef]

73. Naruse, K.; Rask-Madsen, C.; Takahara, N.; Ha, S.W.; Suzuma, K.; Way, K.J.; Jacobs, J.R.; Clermont, A.C.; Ueki, K.; Ohshiro, Y.; et al. Activation of vascular protein kinase C-beta inhibits Akt-dependent endothelial nitric oxide synthase function in obesity-associated insulin resistance. *Diabetes* **2006**, *55*, 691–698. [CrossRef] [PubMed]
74. Tang, Y.; Soroush, F.; Sun, S.; Liverani, E.; Langston, J.C.; Yang, Q.; Kilpatrick, L.E.; Kiani, M.F. Protein kinase C-delta inhibition protects blood-brain barrier from sepsis-induced vascular damage. *J. Neuroinflamm.* **2018**, *15*, 309. [CrossRef]
75. Shen, Q.; Rigor, R.R.; Pivetti, C.D.; Wu, M.H.; Yuan, S.Y. Myosin light chain kinase in microvascular endothelial barrier function. *Cardiovasc. Res.* **2010**, *87*, 272–280. [CrossRef]
76. Wu, H.M.; Huang, Q.; Yuan, Y.; Granger, H.J. VEGF induces NO-dependent hyperpermeability in coronary venules. *Am. J. Physiol.* **1996**, *271*, H2735–H2739. [CrossRef]
77. Manczak, M.; Park, B.S.; Jung, Y.; Reddy, P.H. Differential expression of oxidative phosphorylation genes in patients with Alzheimer's disease: Implications for early mitochondrial dysfunction and oxidative damage. *Neuromol. Med.* **2004**, *5*, 147–162. [CrossRef]
78. Di Francesco, A.; Arosio, B.; Falconi, A.; Micioni Di Bonaventura, M.V.; Karimi, M.; Mari, D.; Casati, M.; Maccarrone, M.; D'Addario, C. Global changes in DNA methylation in Alzheimer's disease peripheral blood mononuclear cells. *Brain Behav. Immun.* **2015**, *45*, 139–144. [CrossRef] [PubMed]
79. Potenza, M.A.; Sgarra, L.; Desantis, V.; Nacci, C.; Montagnani, M. Diabetes and Alzheimer's Disease: Might Mitochondrial Dysfunction Help Deciphering the Common Path? *Antioxidants* **2021**, *10*, 1257. [CrossRef] [PubMed]
80. Akram, A.; Schmeidler, J.; Katsel, P.; Hof, P.R.; Haroutunian, V. Association of ApoE and LRP mRNA levels with dementia and AD neuropathology. *Neurobiol. Aging* **2012**, *33*, 628.e1–628.e14. [CrossRef] [PubMed]
81. Ruzali, W.A.; Kehoe, P.G.; Love, S. LRP1 expression in cerebral cortex, choroid plexus and meningeal blood vessels: Relationship to cerebral amyloid angiopathy and APOE status. *Neurosci. Lett.* **2012**, *525*, 123–128. [CrossRef]
82. Donahue, J.E.; Flaherty, S.L.; Johanson, C.E.; Duncan, J.A., 3rd; Silverberg, G.D.; Miller, M.C.; Tavares, R.; Yang, W.; Wu, Q.; Sabo, E.; et al. RAGE, LRP-1, and amyloid-beta protein in Alzheimer's disease. *Acta Neuropathol.* **2006**, *112*, 405–415. [CrossRef]
83. Caricasole, A.; Copani, A.; Caraci, F.; Aronica, E.; Rozemuller, A.J.; Caruso, A.; Storto, M.; Gaviraghi, G.; Terstappen, G.C.; Nicoletti, F. Induction of Dickkopf-1, a negative modulator of the Wnt pathway, is associated with neuronal degeneration in Alzheimer's brain. *J. Neurosci.* **2004**, *24*, 6021–6027. [CrossRef]
84. Rosi, M.C.; Luccarini, I.; Grossi, C.; Fiorentini, A.; Spillantini, M.G.; Prisco, A.; Scali, C.; Gianfriddo, M.; Caricasole, A.; Terstappen, G.C.; et al. Increased Dickkopf-1 expression in transgenic mouse models of neurodegenerative disease. *J. Neurochem.* **2010**, *112*, 1539–1551. [CrossRef] [PubMed]
85. Rebeck, G.W.; Harr, S.D.; Strickland, D.K.; Hyman, B.T. Multiple, Diverse senile plaque-associated proteins are ligands of an apolipoprotein E receptor, the alpha 2-macroglobulin receptor/low-density-lipoprotein receptor-related protein. *Ann. Neurol.* **1995**, *37*, 211–217. [CrossRef]
86. Blain, J.F.; Poirier, J. Could lipoprotein lipase play a role in Alzheimer's disease? *Sci. World J.* **2004**, *4*, 531–535. [CrossRef]
87. Wang, R.; Reddy, P.H. Role of Glutamate and NMDA Receptors in Alzheimer's Disease. *J. Alzheimer's Dis.* **2017**, *57*, 1041–1048. [CrossRef]
88. Nogueira, V.; Park, Y.; Chen, C.C.; Xu, P.Z.; Chen, M.L.; Tonic, I.; Unterman, T.; Hay, N. Akt determines replicative senescence and oxidative or oncogenic premature senescence and sensitizes cells to oxidative apoptosis. *Cancer Cell* **2008**, *14*, 458–470. [CrossRef]
89. Heneka, M.T.; Reyes-Irisarri, E.; Hüll, M.; Kummer, M.P. Impact and Therapeutic Potential of PPARs in Alzheimer's Disease. *Curr. Neuropharmacol.* **2011**, *9*, 643–650. [CrossRef]
90. Ortiz-Matamoros, A.; Arias, C. Chronic infusion of Wnt7a, Wnt5a and Dkk-1 in the adult hippocampus induces structural synaptic changes and modifies anxiety and memory performance. *Brain Res. Bull.* **2018**, *139*, 243–255. [CrossRef]
91. Fortress, A.M.; Frick, K.M. Hippocampal Wnt Signaling: Memory Regulation and Hormone Interactions. *Neuroscientist* **2016**, *22*, 278–294. [CrossRef] [PubMed]
92. Henderson, B.W.; Gentry, E.G.; Rush, T.; Troncoso, J.C.; Thambisetty, M.; Montine, T.J.; Herskowitz, J.H. Rho-associated protein kinase 1 (ROCK1) is increased in Alzheimer's disease and ROCK1 depletion reduces amyloid-β levels in brain. *J. Neurochem.* **2016**, *138*, 525–531. [CrossRef] [PubMed]
93. Gupta, N.C.; Davis, C.M.; Nelson, J.W.; Young, J.M.; Alkayed, N.J. Soluble epoxide hydrolase: Sex differences and role in endothelial cell survival. *Arterioscler. Thromb. Vasc. Biol.* **2012**, *32*, 1936–1942. [CrossRef] [PubMed]
94. Chen, D.; Whitcomb, R.; MacIntyre, E.; Tran, V.; Do, Z.N.; Sabry, J.; Patel, D.V.; Anandan, S.K.; Gless, R.; Webb, H.K. Pharmacokinetics and pharmacodynamics of AR9281, an inhibitor of soluble epoxide hydrolase, in single- and multiple-dose studies in healthy human subjects. *J. Clin. Pharmacol.* **2012**, *52*, 319–328. [CrossRef] [PubMed]

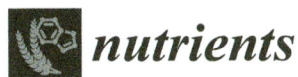

Article

Spearmint Extract Containing Rosmarinic Acid Suppresses Amyloid Fibril Formation of Proteins Associated with Dementia

Kenjirou Ogawa [1], Ayumi Ishii [2], Aimi Shindo [3], Kunihiro Hongo [2,3,4], Tomohiro Mizobata [2,3,4], Tetsuya Sogon [5] and Yasushi Kawata [2,3,4,*]

1. Organization for Promotion of Tenure Track, University of Miyazaki, Miyazaki 889-2192, Japan; ogawa.kenjirou.u2@cc.miyazaki-u.ac.jp
2. Department of Chemistry and Biotechnology, Graduate School of Engineering, Tottori University, Tottori 680-8552, Japan; bshijing80@gmail.com (A.I.); hongo@tottori-u.ac.jp (K.H.); mizobata@tottori-u.ac.jp (T.M.)
3. Department of Biomedical Science, Institute of Regenerative Medicine and Biofunction, Graduate School of Medical Science, Tottori University, Tottori 680-8552, Japan; a.3kmt10@gmail.com
4. Center for Research on Green Sustainable Chemistry, Tottori University, Tottori 680-8552, Japan
5. R&D Department, Wakasa Seikatsu Co. Ltd., 22 Naginataboko-cho, Shijo-Karasuma, Shimogyo-ku, Kyoto 600-8008, Japan; sogon@blueberryeye.co.jp
* Correspondence: kawata@tottori-u.ac.jp; Tel.: +81-857-31-5787

Received: 7 October 2020; Accepted: 11 November 2020; Published: 13 November 2020

Abstract: Neurological dementias such as Alzheimer's disease and Lewy body dementia are thought to be caused in part by the formation and deposition of characteristic insoluble fibrils of polypeptides such as amyloid beta (Aβ), Tau, and/or α-synuclein (αSyn). In this context, it is critical to suppress and remove such aggregates in order to prevent and/or delay the progression of dementia in these ailments. In this report, we investigated the effects of spearmint extract (SME) and rosmarinic acid (RA; the major component of SME) on the amyloid fibril formation reactions of αSyn, Aβ, and Tau proteins in vitro. SME or RA was added to soluble samples of each protein and the formation of fibrils was monitored by thioflavin T (ThioT) binding assays and transmission electron microscopy (TEM). We also evaluated whether preformed amyloid fibrils could be dissolved by the addition of RA. Our results reveal for the first time that SME and RA both suppress amyloid fibril formation, and that RA could disassemble preformed fibrils of αSyn, Aβ, and Tau into non-toxic species. Our results suggest that SME and RA may potentially suppress amyloid fibrils implicated in the progression of Alzheimer's disease and Lewy body dementia in vivo, as well.

Keywords: spearmint; rosmarinic acid; polyphenol; amyloid fibril; amyloid beta; alpha-synuclein; Tau; dementia

1. Introduction

Alzheimer's disease, Lewy body dementia, and Parkinson's disease are often caused by the formation of fibrillar aggregated proteins (amyloid fibrils) of amyloid beta (Aβ), Tau (identified in Alzheimer's disease patients), and α-synuclein (αSyn; identified in cases of Lewy body dementia and Parkinson's disease) [1–6]. During the formation of these protein fibrils, various soluble cyto-toxic oligomeric species are formed prior to the maturation of insoluble fibrils [7]. The deposition of Aβ, Tau and αSyn plaques, both inside and outside vital nerve cells, affects synaptic function and is associated with symptoms of dementia, which include onset of cognitive defects such as the impairment of learning and memorizing capabilities in the mouse and human brain [8], as well as various biological and neurochemical symptoms such as astrogliosis, neuronal dystrophy, and decline in acetylcholine levels [9]. Accordingly, it is important to suppress the aggregation of these proteins associated with dementia to prevent these symptoms.

Spearmint (*Mentha spicata*) is a prominent member of the *Labiatae* family, which is noted for its high rosmarinic acid (RA) content [10] (the chemical structure of (R)-(+)-rosmarinic acid is shown in Figure 1A. A significant increase in RA content was achieved in cultivars produced in breeding experiments performed in Indiana, USA [11], and spearmint extracts (SME) used in food supplements are prepared from such specially cultivated species (shown in Figure 1B). In addition to a high concentration of RA, smaller amounts of 65 additional phenolic compounds may also be found in SME [12]. Administration of SME has been shown to prevent the degradation of cognitive functions such as learning and memory, and also to suppress the oxidation of brain tissue in senescence accelerated mouse-prone 8 (SAMP8) mice, a naturally occurring mouse line with an accelerated aging phenotype [13]. In addition, in human clinical trials, intake of SME by healthy elderly patients resulted in improvements in cognitive function, for example, attention span, concentration span, language comprehension abilities, and working memory [14,15].

Biochemically, RA has been shown to promote numerous biological activities, including antioxidative, anti-inflammatory, antiangiogenic, neuroprotective, antimicrobial, and immunomodulatory activities [16–22]. Previously, it was reported that RA displays the ability to prevent the oligomerization of αSyn, reduce the deposition of Aβ in mouse brains and suppress synaptic toxicity [20,23,24]. However, there are no reports regarding the in vitro effects of SME and RA upon the amyloid fibril formation/aggregation reactions of proteins such as Aβ peptide, Tau, and αSyn.

In the present study, we demonstrate that SME and RA are capable of directly suppressing the amyloid fibril formation of αSyn, Aβ, and Tau in vitro, by diverting molecules of these proteins toward a non-aggregated form. Furthermore, we show that RA is also capable of destabilizing and disassembling pre-formed amyloid fibrils of αSyn, Aβ, and Tau proteins. From these interesting results, we suggest that it may be feasible to achieve an effective suppression of the formation and the accumulation of amyloid fibrils related to dementia using SMA and RA.

A

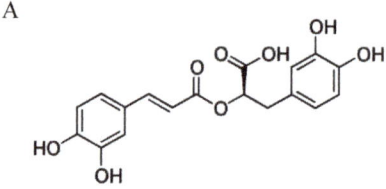

Rosmarinic acid

B

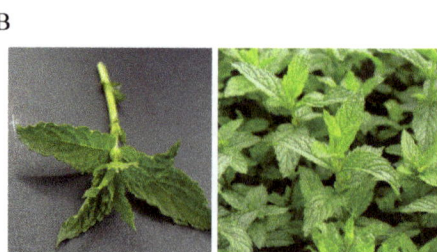

Figure 1. Chemical structure of rosmarinic acid and spearmint leaves: (**A**) chemical structure of rosmarinic acid; (**B**) spearmint (*Mentha spicata* L.) cultivated in Indiana, USA contains more rosmarinic acid and phenolic compounds than conventional spearmint due to selective breeding.

2. Materials and Methods

2.1. Materials

SME samples were purchased from Kemin Japan Co. Ltd. (Tokyo, Japan), and the composition of compounds in the extracts was confirmed by high performance liquid chromatography (HPLC). Analysis showed that SME preparations typically consisted of mainly RA (12.0%), with trace amounts of various other phenolic components. Pure RA was purchased from FUJIFILM Wako Pure Chemical Co. Ltd (Osaka, Japan). Human A$\beta_{1\text{-}42}$ peptide was purchased from Peptide Institute, Inc. (Osaka, Japan). Thioflavin T (ThioT) was obtained from Wako (Osaka).

2.2. Expression and Purification of αSyn and Tau Proteins

Human αSyn was over-expressed in *Escherichia coli* (*E. coli*) and purified according to methods reported previously [25]. For preparation of αSyn samples, lyophilized purified αSyn was dissolved in 4 M guanidine hydrochloride and then desalted with a PD-10 column (GE Healthcare, Tokyo, Japan). The concentration of αSyn in the samples was determined by using a molar absorption coefficient of ε 280 nm = 0.354 [26].

A pET23a-hTau40 gene was constructed by ligation of a synthesized hTau40 gene optimized for *E. coli* expression (Thermo Fisher, Waltham, MA, USA) with a DNA fragment obtained from the expression vector pET-23a(+). Both fragments were digested with the restriction enzymes *Nde*I and *Hind*III prior to ligation. After validation through DNA sequencing, the resultant pET23a-hTau40 expression vector was introduced into *E. coli* BLR(DE3) (Novagen) to establish an over-expression system for the human Tau protein (*E. coli* BLR(DE3)/pET23a-hTau40). The cultured cells were suspended in purification buffer (50 mM Tris-HCl, pH 7.8, containing 2 mM EDTA•2Na, 2 mM dithiothreitol (DTT), 0.2 mM phenylmethylsulfonyl fluoride (PMSF)) and incubated on ice before disruption using a combination of lysozyme chloride and sonication. After this process, the supernatant was recovered by centrifugation of the sample at 10,000 rpm, at 4 °C for 20 min. Sodium chloride was then added to the supernatant to a final concentration of 0.5 M, after which samples were heated to 80 °C for 10 min. Immediately afterwards, samples were cooled on ice, and then centrifuged to remove insoluble matter. Streptomycin sulfate (final concentration was 2.5%) was added to this clarified supernatant and the sample was stirred on ice for 30 min to precipitate nucleic acids. After removal of precipitated nucleic acids by centrifugation, the supernatant was dialyzed overnight against purification buffer. The dialysate containing Tau was centrifuged to remove debris and applied to an SP-Sepharose cation exchange column equilibrated with purification buffer. Bound samples were eluted by applying a linear gradient of 0–0.5 M NaCl. Eluted fractions containing Tau were recovered and dialyzed against 1 mM ammonium bicarbonate, and then lyophilized to obtain the final purified sample. Protein concentrations of purified Tau were determined by using a protein dye assay (Protein Assay Kit, Bio-Rad Laboratories) with bovine serum albumin (Sigma-Aldrich Japan, Tokyo, Japan) as a standard.

2.3. Amyloid Fibril Formation and ThioT Binding Assay

αSyn: αSyn (1 mg/mL) was incubated in 50 mM Tris-HCl buffer, pH 7.0, containing 150 mM NaCl, and 20 µM ThioT (Wako) with or without various concentrations of SME and RA added, in 96-well plates (Greiner, Kremsmuenster, Austria). Sample plates were incubated and monitored for changes in ThioT-derived fluorescence at 37 °C using an ARVO X (PerkinElmer Japan Co., Ltd., Yokohama, Japan) fluorescent plate reader with continuous agitation. ThioT fluorescence intensities were monitored by using an emission cutoff filter at >486 nm, with the excitation wavelength set to 450 nm.

Aβ: amyloid fibril formation of Aβ by using ThioT binding assay was performed according to methods reported previously, with some modifications [27]. Lyophilized human A$\beta_{1\text{-}42}$ was dissolved in aqueous 0.02% ammonia to prepare a 500 µM Aβ stock solution. Samples of 16.65 µM Aβ were prepared from this stock in 5 mM phosphate buffered saline (PBS) buffer, pH 7.4, containing 150 mM NaCl, 20 µM ThioT, and various concentrations of SME or RA dissolved in DMSO. Fluorescence changes were monitored using 96-well plates at 37 °C using a SpectraMax M2e multi-mode fluorescence plate reader (Molecular Devices, Tokyo, Japan) without agitation. ThioT fluorescence was monitored at 480 nm with an excitation wavelength of 440 nm.

Tau: hTau40 (0.5 mg/mL) was incubated in 25 mM Tris-HCl buffer, pH 7.4, 150 mM NaCl, 2 mM DTT, 5 μM heparin, 20 μM ThioT and containing various concentrations of SME or RA. ThioT fluorescence of samples in 96-well plates was monitored at 37 °C using an ARVO X (Perkin Elmer) fluorescence plate reader with continuous agitation. Fluorescence intensities at >486 nm were monitored by using an emission cutoff filter, with the excitation wavelength set to at 450 nm. Alternatively, emission measurements were taken at more precise wavelengths using the SpectraMax M2e multi-mode fluorescence plate reader (Molecular Devices, USA) with the emission wavelength set to 480 nm and the excitation wavelength set to 440 nm.

2.4. Transmission Electron Microscopy (TEM) Measurements of Fibril Samples

TEM measurements were performed on a JEOL-1400plus transmission electron microscope operating at 80 kV, as previously described [25]. Samples of αSyn, Aβ, or Tau protein incubated with or without SME or RA were diluted five-fold with water and applied to collodion-covered carbon mesh disks for 90 sec. Excess samples were blotted off and the sample disks were briefly rinsed by applying 5 μL of Milli-Q water followed by immediate blotting. Samples were stained by the application of a ten-fold diluted solution of EM Stainer (Nisshin EM Co., Ltd., Tokyo, Japan) to these washed samples for 30 sec followed by the blotting and air-drying of the completed sample.

2.5. Measurement of Cell Viability

The cell viability measurements were performed according to previous studies on the mouse neuroblastoma cell line Neuro2a (N2a), using a Tali™ Image-Based Cytometer (Thermo Fisher Scientific, Waltham, MA, USA) [28]. N2a cells were obtained from Public Health England. Cells were grown in Minimum Essential Medium (MEM, Thermo Fisher Scientific, Waltham, MA, USA) containing 10% fetal bovine serum, MEM non-essential amino acid solution (FUJIFILM Wako Pure Chemical Corporation, Osaka, Japan), 100 μM sodium pyruvate solution (FUJIFILM Wako Pure Chemical Corporation, Osaka, Japan), and 100 U/mL penicillin-streptomycin (Thermo Fisher Scientific, Waltham, MA, USA). Cell stock was seeded into 48 well plates and cultured at 37 °C with 5% CO_2 until the cells in the wells reached 80–90% confluence. N2a cells were then incubated with samples of amyloid fibril (either 1 mg/mL αSyn, 500 μM Aβ, or 0.5 mg/mL Tau) that had been pretreated with or without RA for differing intervals (40 h for αSyn, 12 h for Aβ, and 48 h for Tau). The specific times of incubation for amyloid proteins with RA were adjusted to correspond to the time required for fibril disassembly, detected by the decrease in ThioT fluorescence intensity for each protein (30 h and 40 h for αSyn, 7.5 h and 12 h for Aβ, and 36 h and 48 h for Tau). After incubation, fibril samples were collected for assays. Furthermore, 70% ethanol was used as a positive toxicity control. After incubating the cells for 24 h with each fibril sample, the cells were washed with PBS, collected to form cell suspensions, and then incubated with 1 μM 3′,6′-di(O-acetyl)-2′,7′-bis[N,N-bis(carboxymethyl)aminomethyl] fluorescein tetra-acetoxymethyl ester (Calcein AM) and 400 nM ethidium homodimer-1 (EthD-1) (LIVE/DEAD™ Viability/Cytotoxicity Kit for mammalian cells, Thermo Fisher Scientific, Waltham, MA, USA) for 30 min in the dark. Subsequently, 25 μL of the N2a cell suspension was injected into Tali™ Cellular Analysis Slides (Thermo Fisher Scientific, Waltham, MA, USA), after which changes in EthD-1 fluorescence were monitored with the Tali™ Image-Based Cytometer to estimate the number of dead cells in the sample.

2.6. Statistical Analysis

Data are presented as means ± SEM. Statistical comparisons were made using one-way analysis of variance followed by Student's *t*-test, Dunnett's multiple comparison test, or Tukey–Kramer multiple comparison test. A value of $p < 0.05$ was considered statistically significant.

3. Results

3.1. Suppression of the αSyn, Aβ and Tau Amyloid Fibril Formations by SME

First, we examined the effects of direct SME addition to the fibril formation reactions of αSyn, Aβ, and Tau, in individual assays. The formation of amyloid fibrils of αSyn, Aβ, and Tau were monitored for 40 h, 12 h, and 25 h, respectively, by utilizing the specific fluorescence that is emitted by fibril bound ThioT. The concentrations of SME added to each sample were calculated to correspond to 0.5, 1, 2, and 5 molar equivalents of RA relative to αSyn (Figure 2A), 0.05, 0.1, and 0.5 molar equivalents of RA relative to Aβ (Figure 2B), and 0.5, 1, and 2 molar equivalents of RA relative to Tau (Figure 2C), respectively. In the absence of SME (shown as control), an increase in ThioT fluorescence intensity over time for each protein was observed, which reflected a typical fibrillation reaction time course of each protein. In the presence of SME, however, fibrillation was either completely suppressed or reduced significantly. Fibrillation of αSyn and Aβ was almost completely inhibited by the addition of SME at concentrations that corresponded to a five-fold molar equivalent of RA relative to the protein monomer. A prolongation of the lag-phase interval was also observed for αSyn (Figure 2A). In the case of Aβ samples containing SME, the ThioT fluorescence was seen to increase initially to a maximum value, and subsequently this intensity decreased gradually to almost the original values at the beginning of each experiment (Figure 2B). We plotted the ratio of maximum to minimum ThioT fluorescence intensities for each sample, as shown in Figure 2A–C, to gauge the concentration-dependent effects of SME on the fibril reaction of each sample. As shown in Figure 2D–F, significant decreases in the maximum/minimum ratio were observed in samples containing substoichiometric concentrations of RA (0.5 molar equivalent for αSyn, 0.05 molar equivalent for Aβ), and a more moderate but significant suppressive effect was seen when two-molar equivalents of RA were added to Tau, respectively.

3.2. Suppression of the αSyn, Aβ and Tau Amyloid Fibril Formations by RA

Next, we evaluated the effects of pure RA on αSyn, Aβ, and Tau amyloid fibril formation. The concentrations of RA tested corresponded to 0.5, 1, 2, and 5 molar equivalents for αSyn, 0.5, 1, 2, and 3 molar equivalents for Aβ, and 3, 10, 20, and 30 molar equivalents for Tau, respectively. As shown in Figure 3, similar to the effects seen for SME, the addition of RA suppressed the increase in ThioT fluorescence over time for all three proteins relative to the control sample. The fibril suppression effects on αSyn (Figure 3A,D), Aβ (Figure 3B,E), and Tau (Figure 3C,F) were similar to the effects seen for SME (Figure 2), although the effective concentrations were different. Experiments for Tau using concentrations of RA that were comparable to those used for the other two targets (0.5, 1, 2 molar equivalents) failed to elicit a measurable effect on Tau fibrillation (data not shown), suggesting that the concentrations of pure RA required to alter Tau fibrillation were higher than the concentrations of SME needed to trigger a similar response. This unexpected result suggests that there may be an additional component present in SME that complements or enhances the effects of RA, which is relevant only to Tau fibrillation.

3.3. Suppression of Amyloid Fibril Formations of αSyn, Aβ, and Tau Detected by TEM

From the results that we show in Figures 2 and 3, we observe that both SME and RA have the ability to suppress amyloid fibril formation of αSyn, Aβ, and Tau. In order to determine the specific effects of SME and RA on aggregate morphology, we next observed samples of αSyn, Aβ, and Tau incubated in the presence and absence of SME and RA using TEM. Samples were taken from the end point of each fibrillation experiment shown in Figures 2 and 3. As shown in Figure 4, the structure of amyloid fibrils formed by αSyn, Aβ, and Tau in the absence of SME or RA may be described as bundles of linear fibril structures (shown as control). In contrast, in samples of the three amyloidogenic proteins incubated with SME (five-fold molar equivalent to αSyn, 0.5-fold molar equivalent to Aβ, and two-fold molar equivalent to Tau) or RA (five-fold molar equivalent to αSyn, three-fold molar equivalent to Aβ, and 30-fold molar equivalent to Tau), visible fibrillar structures were markedly reduced. Additionally, extremely short fibril structures and amorphous, non-linear aggregates were both detected in samples incubated with SME or RA. In the case of the Tau protein, we could observe long fibrillar structures even in samples containing SME or RA, although the relative abundance of these structures in the samples was low. The fibrillar structures of Tau in the presence of RA also tended toward more twisted and curved structures, although we were unable to quantify these morphological differences. These results clearly show that SME and RA altered the morphologies of αSyn, Aβ, and Tau protein aggregates in a specific manner.

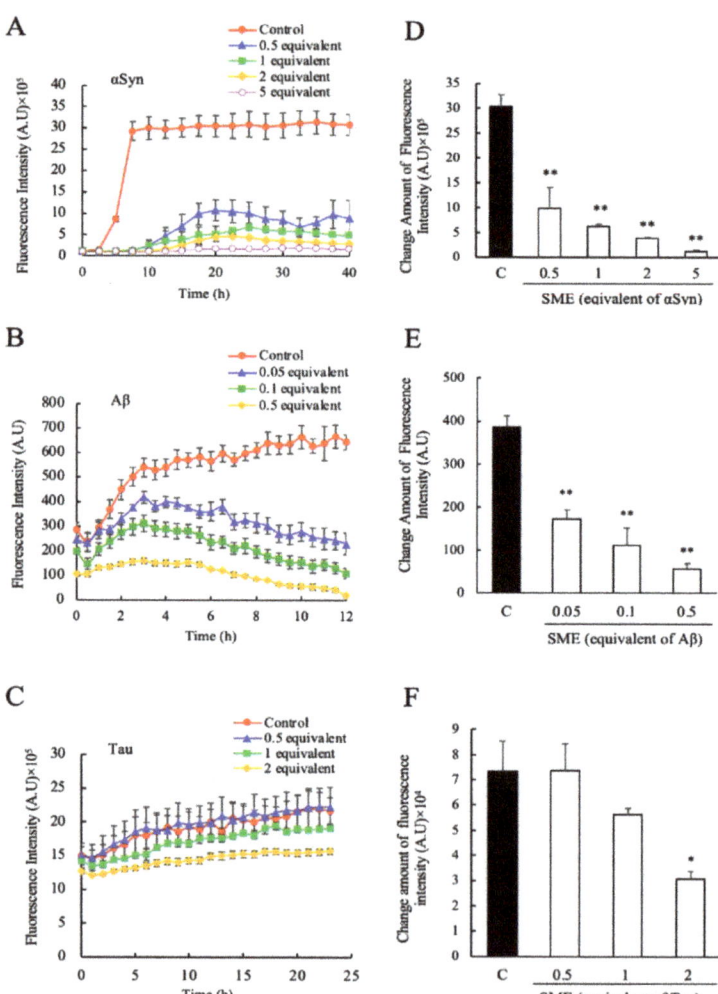

Figure 2. Inhibitory effects of spearmint extract (SME) against α-synuclein (αSyn), amyloid beta (Aβ), and Tau amyloid fibril formation. The degree of amyloid fibril formation was detected over time by measuring the specific fluorescence of fibril-bound thioflavin T (ThioT) in the presence and absence of SME; (**A**) αSyn (0.5–5 equivalents rosmarinic acid (RA)), (**B**) Aβ (0.05–0.5 equivalents RA), (**C**) Tau (0.5–2 equivalents RA). The net amount of fluorescence intensity change was estimated by the ratio between the maximum value and initial measurement value of its intensity; (**D**) αSyn, (**E**) Aβ, (**F**) Tau. Data are means ± SEM (n = 3). C, control. * $p < 0.05$, ** $p < 0.01$ vs. the control group (Dunnett's multiple comparison test).

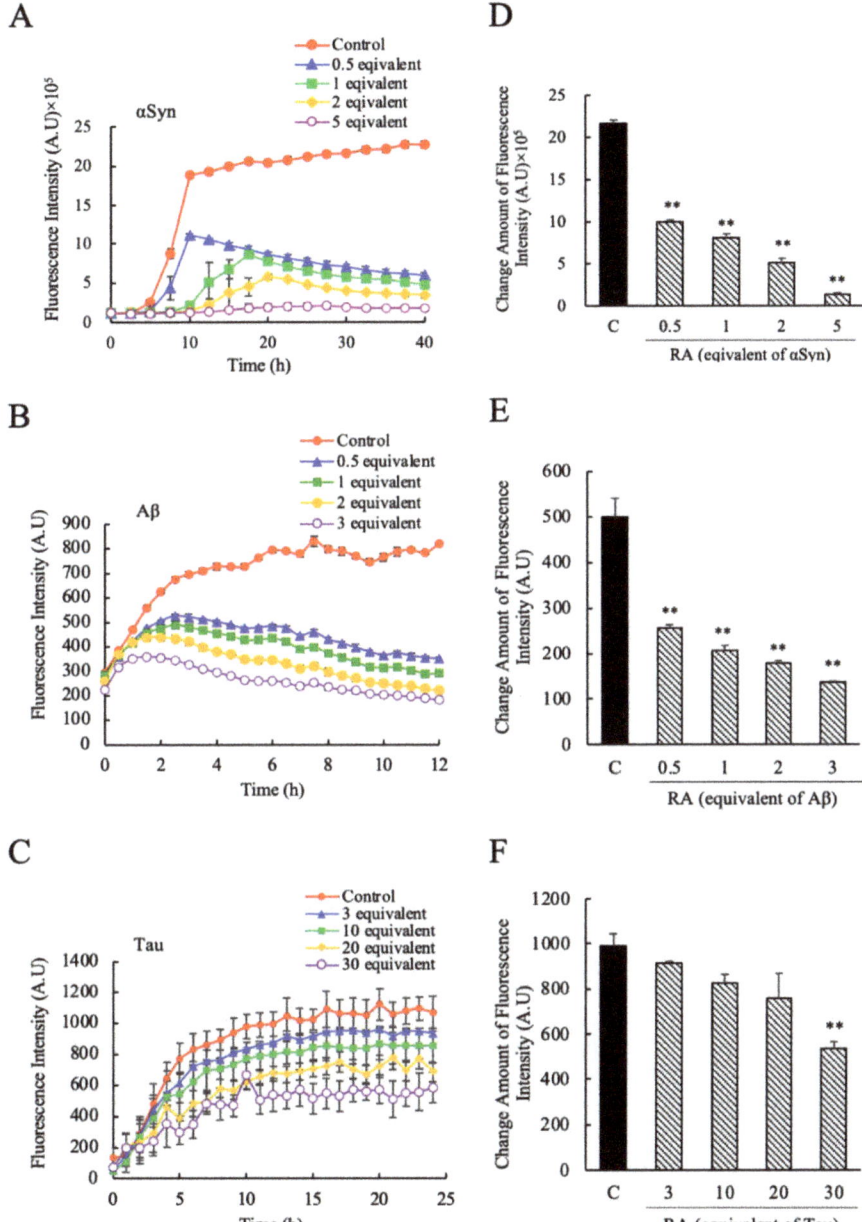

Figure 3. The inhibitory effects of pure rosmarinic acid (RA) against α-synuclein (αSyn), amyloid beta (Aβ), and Tau amyloid fibril formation. The degree of amyloid fibril formation was detected over time by measuring ThioT fluorescence in the presence and absence of pure RA; (**A**) αSyn (0.5–5 equivalent-mol RA), (**B**) Aβ (0.5–3 equivalent-mol RA), (**C**) Tau (3–30 equivalent-mol RA). The net amount of fluorescence intensity change was estimated by the ratio between the maximum value and initial measurement value of its intensity; (**D**) αSyn, (**E**) Aβ, (**F**) Tau. Data are means ± SEM ($n = 3$). C, control. ** $p < 0.01$ vs. the control group (Dunnett's multiple comparison test).

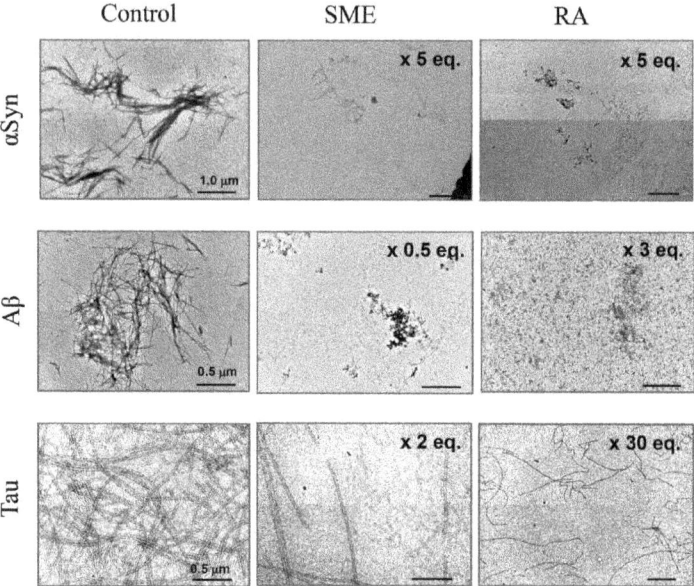

Figure 4. Transmission electron microscopy (TEM) measurements of amyloid fibrils of α-synuclein (αSyn), amyloid beta (Aβ), and Tau incubated with spearmint extract (SME) or pure rosmarinic acid (RA). αSyn, Aβ, and Tau amyloid fibril peptides were incubated with SME (5, 0.5, or 2 equivalent molar RA to each peptide) or pure RA (5, 3, 30 equivalent molar to each peptide) for the respective intervals (40 h for αSyn, 12 h for Aβ, and 25 h for Tau), after which samples were treated for observation with TEM. Scale bars, 1.0 μm on αSyn images, 0.5 μm on Aβ and Tau images.

3.4. Disassembly of Pre-Formed Amyloid Fibrils of αSyn, Aβ, and Tau by Addition of RA and Toxicity Evaluation

In the time course experiments shown in Figure 3A,B, we observed that for αSyn and Aβ, the ThioT fluorescence intensities in the presence of RA decreased after initially attaining a maximum value that was dependent on the concentration of added RA. From this result, we hypothesized that RA might possess the ability to disaggregate amyloid fibrils that had been formed. Therefore, in order to confirm this hypothesis, we studied the effects of adding RA to samples of preformed αSyn, Aβ, and Tau fibrils. As shown in Figure 5A, we observed that upon addition of RA to samples containing amyloid fibrils (as determined by the ThioT fluorescence intensities) a decrease in ThioT fluorescence was immediately triggered in each case. This fluorescence decrease seemed to be initiated regardless of the type of protein, and the effects of RA addition were independent of the specific stage at which RA was added to the reaction (for example, RA was able to trigger a fluorescence decrease during the extension phase of fibrillation of Aβ). TEM measurements confirmed that this decrease in ThioT fluorescence was accompanied by a loss of observable fibrillar aggregates (Figure 5B). These results clearly demonstrate that the RA can disassemble amyloid fibrils.

In the final experiment, we have evaluated the cytotoxicity of the disassembled species formed in the presence of RA using the Tali™ Image-Based Cytometer and the mouse N2a cell model. As shown in Figure 5C, we found that the disaggregated molecular samples that formed as a result of RA addition were completely inert against N2a cells, regardless of the type of fibrillogenic protein studied, or the time frame where RA addition was initiated. The result demonstrates rather clearly that RA disassembled amyloid fibrils of αSyn, Aβ, and Tau to a non-toxic, soluble form. In particular for Tau protein, this is the first instance of an isolated and characterized compound that shows such potent effects on fibril morphology and cytotoxicity.

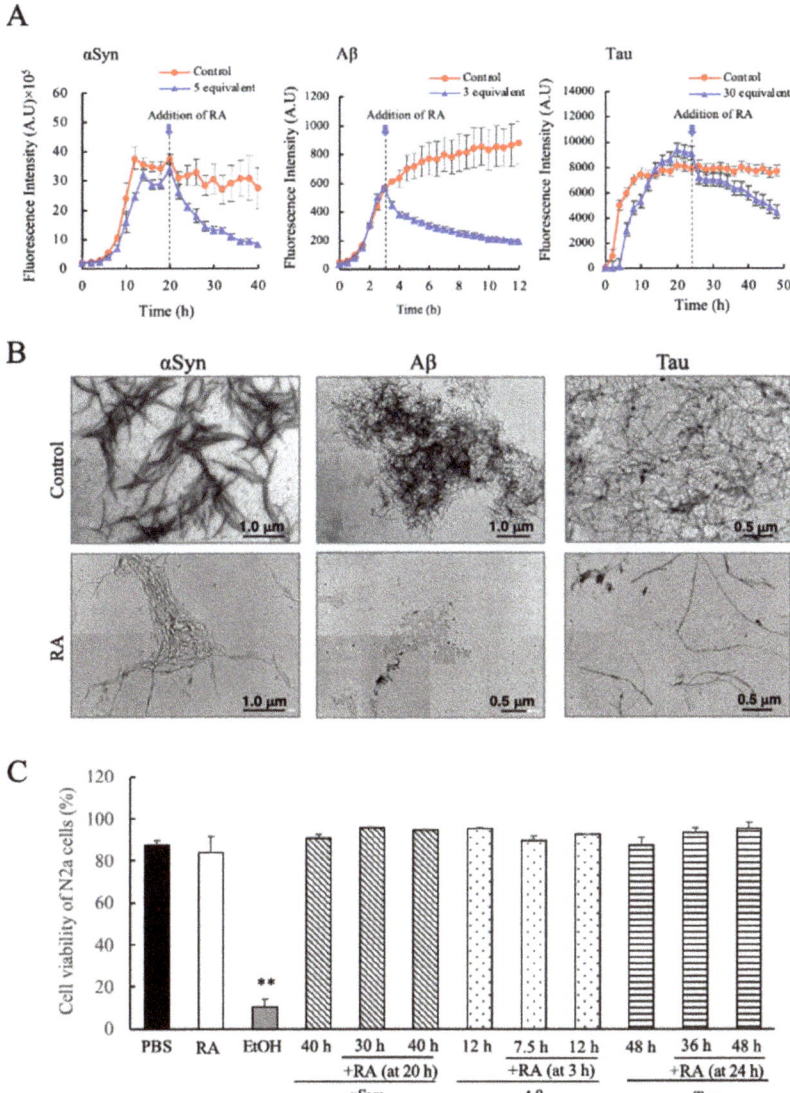

Figure 5. Evaluation of the fibril dissociative abilities of rosmarinic acid (RA) on preformed amyloid fibrils of α-synuclein (αSyn), amyloid beta (Aβ), and Tau. (**A**) RA was added to experiments where each fibrillogenic protein was allowed to form fibrils for a designated interval (20 h for αSyn, 3 h for Aβ, and 24 h for Tau). The specific instance that RA was added to each sample is denoted within each figure by the dotted lines and arrows. (**B**) TEM images of αSyn (at 40 h), Aβ (at 12 h), and Tau (at 48 h) samples after the addition of RA according to the protocol described in (**A**). (**C**) Determination of the cytotoxicity of RA-containing fibril samples, measured by Tali™ Cytometer analysis on Neuro2a (N2a) cells. Each fibril sample (either treated or not treated with RA) was collected at the indicated times (at 30 h and 40 h for αSyn, 12 h and 7.5 h for Aβ, 36 h and 48 h for Tau) and assayed for cytotoxicity. Data are means ± SEM ($n = 3$). PBS, phosphate buffered saline; EtOH, 70% ethanol solution. There are no significant differences in toxicity between RA-treated and non-treated fibril samples. ** $p < 0.01$ vs. the PBS groups (Tukey–Kramer multiple comparison test).

4. Discussion

In the present paper, we describe our efforts to characterize the suppressive effects of SME and its main component RA on the fibrillation of αSyn, Aβ, and Tau. SME is the water-soluble extract from a specially cultivated spearmint grown in Indiana, USA containing an enriched concentration of RA compared to other common cultivars. We demonstrated through our experiments that SME suppressed the in vitro amyloid fibril formation of αSyn, Aβ and also, for the first time, Tau protein (Figures 2 and 4). We further determined that pure RA could also effectively suppress fibrillation (Figures 3 and 4). This latter result strongly suggests that RA was the active component in SME that prevented the formation of characteristic amyloid fibrils of αSyn, Aβ, and Tau. Various polyphenolic compounds, including an antioxidative polyphenol RA [29], have been shown in previous studies to inhibit the formation of amyloid fibrils of proteins such as αSyn and Aβ [30,31]. Although RA has been shown to suppress the accumulation and aggregation of Aβ in vitro and in vivo [24,32], studies to determine whether SME (which contains a rich amount of RA) has the capability to directly suppress the fibrillation of proteins such as αSyn and Tau have not been performed to date.

From a detailed analysis of our data regarding the effects of SME and RA on fibril formation, we determined that the nature of the suppressive effects shown by these two chemical preparations was slightly different for each protein target. For instance, with respect to αSyn, SME and RA affected not only the rate of ThioT fluorescence increase (which reflects the rate at which fibrils are formed), but also affected the lag phase of fibrillation, which was prolonged (Figures 2A and 3A). This suggested that SME and RA inhibited both initial fibril nucleus formation as well as fibril extension of αSyn. In contrast, an increase in the lag interval was not observed in experiments using Aβ and Tau. Interestingly, when we compared the concentration dependence of the suppressive effects of SME and RA on the three targets studied, we identified another subtle difference. In the case of αSyn, the concentration range in which the effect was observed was similar (was roughly the same order) for both SME and RA (0.5–5 equivalent molar; Figure 2A,D and Figure 3A,D). In contrast, with regard to Aβ and Tau, the effective concentration of SME that was required to bring about a suppressive effect was roughly 10-fold lower for SME compared to pure RA (Figure 2B,E and Figure 3B,E for Aβ; Figure 2C,F and Figure 3C,F for Tau). This interesting discrepancy suggests that SME is more potent in suppressing Aβ and Tau fibrillation compared to pure RA, and indicates that additional active compounds may be present in SME, and that we are observing in our experiments a differential effect of such additional compounds for αSyn versus the other two targets. The SME used in our experiments typically contains 65 additional minor components other than RA and its derivative, such as quinic acid, citric acid, caftaric acid, coumaric acid, salvianolic acid, coumaric acid, caffeic acid, ferulic acid, rutin (quercetin-rutinoside), luteolin, narirutin (naringnin-7-O-rutinoside), sagerinic acid, acacetin, apigenin, danshensu (dihydroxyphenyllactic acid), and their derivative hydroxylated forms [12]. These additional compounds may potentially bind to the proteins susceptible to forming amyloid fibrils and elicit an effect similar to that seen for RA [33–35]. It would be necessary to identify the effects derived from each phenolic composition included in SME, especially against Aβ and Tau, in future experiments to clarify this.

One of the more intriguing results seen in our experiments was that SME displayed suppressive effects against Tau fibrillation in vitro (Figure 2C,F). Fibrillated Tau protein has been linked strongly to neurodegeneration, explained as the cause of disrupted axonal transport in Alzheimer's disease and related tauopathies [36]. Thus, we consider it significant that a naturally derived extract (SME) could suppress Tau fibrillation and aggregation so strongly. Another intriguing finding was the ability shown by RA to disassemble previously formed amyloid fibrils of αSyn and Tau (Figure 5A,B). Additionally, we found out that the molecular intermediates formed during the disassembly of preformed fibrils showed no cytotoxicity to N2a (Figure 5C). Although similar reports using a variety of polyphenols including RA were performed to find compounds that could destabilize preformed αSyn fibrils [30,37–39], as far as we know, this is the first case where an evaluation of cell toxicity regarding the disassembled samples that were formed as a result have also been reported.

Finally, we would like to discuss potential molecular mechanisms by which SME and RA suppress and disassemble amyloid fibrils. Previous studies have suggested that the addition of certain compounds results in the chemical modification of proteins through interactions between polyphenol and certain amino acid side chains [40]. Chemical modification of Lys residues (at εNH_2), by oxidized flavonoids derived from taxifolin or quercetin, was demonstrated to occur in experiments involving Aβ [41], and the significance of a non-covalent binding event of (-)-epigallocatechin gallate (EGCG) to the C-terminal region of αSyn was probed by NMR [42]. Although it was unknown whether covalent modification or non-covalent interaction occurs for Tau, it was reported that polyphenols, including catechol and flavonoids that have two adjacent phenolic hydroxyl groups, could effectively inhibit Tau filament formation [43]. These direct modification and non-covalent binding events of polyphenols to amyloidogenic proteins may result in the stabilization of the soluble monomer form of each protein, which would effectively stop the development of higher-order oligomers that eventually lead to the fibril form. Thus, it may be postulated that RA and SME (rich in RA) may function to suppress and to disassemble the fibrillation of αSyn, Aβ, and Tau proteins in a similar manner. It remains to be determined if a common molecular mechanism exists that explains the broadly applicable effects of RA and other potential polyphenols on protein fibrillation. Additionally, oral administration of SME to an experimental neurodegenerative disease animal model would be worthwhile in the future, since prevention of Alzheimer's pathological Aβ aggregation and deposition in Tg2576 mice brain has been reported by oral administration of RA [44].

5. Conclusions

In conclusion, the present study suggests that water soluble SME and RA have the ability to suppress the amyloid fibril formation of αSyn, Aβ, and Tau, which is related to Lewy body dementia and Alzheimer's disease. Furthermore, RA is able to disassemble preformed aggregated fibrils of these molecular targets into non-toxic species. In the future, we expect that functional research of SME will progress to clinical trials to elucidate the potential of spearmint to prevent dementia-related ailments.

Author Contributions: Conceptualization, Y.K. and K.O.; methodology, Y.K.; validation, K.O., T.M., and Y.K.; formal analysis, K.O., A.I., A.S., K.H., T.M.; investigation, K.O., A.I., A.S., and Y.K.; resources, T.S.; data curation, K.O., T.S., T.M., and Y.K.; writing manuscript, K.O., T.M., and Y.K.; visualization, K.O., A.I., A.S., K.H., T.M., and Y.K.; supervision, T.M. and Y.K.; project administration, T.S.; funding acquisition, Y.K. All authors have read and agreed to the published version of the manuscript.

Funding: This work was supported in part by grant-in-aid for Scientific Research (C) (no.25440027 to Y.K.) from the Japan Society for the Promotion of Science (JSPS) and grant-in-aid for Scientific Research on Innovative Areas (no.24113716 and no.18H04557 to Y.K.) from the Ministry of Education, Culture, Sports, Science and Technology of Japan (MEXT). This study has also been partially supported by financial aid from WAKASA SEIKATSU Co., Ltd., Japan.

Acknowledgments: We thank Y. Ashisada of Tottori University for technical assistance in measurements of electron microscopy.

Conflicts of Interest: This study was performed in cooperation with WAKASA SEIKATSU Co., Ltd., Japan, which markets dietary supplements commercially to the domestic market in Japan. One of the coauthors (T.S.) is an employee of WAKASA SEIKATSU Co., Ltd. This affiliation does not affect the role of this author in the following activities relevant to this study: Data curation; Project administration; Final decision regarding manuscript publication.

References

1. Stéphan, A.; Laroche, S.; Davis, S. Generation of aggregated beta-amyloid in the rat hippocampus impairs synaptic transmission and plasticity and causes memory deficits. *J. Neurosci.* **2001**, *21*, 5703–5714. [CrossRef] [PubMed]
2. Wischik, C.M.; Harrington, C.R.; Storey, J.M. Tau-aggregation inhibitor therapy for Alzheimer's disease. *Biochem. Pharmacol.* **2014**, *88*, 529–539. [CrossRef] [PubMed]
3. Guo, J.L.; Lee, V.M. Seeding of normal Tau by pathological Tau conformers drives pathogenesis of Alzheimer-like tangles. *J. Biol. Chem.* **2011**, *286*, 15317–15331. [CrossRef] [PubMed]

4. Holmes, B.B.; Furman, J.L.; Mahan, T.E.; Yamasaki, T.R.; Mirbaha, H.; Eades, W.C.; Belaygorod, L.; Cairns, N.J.; Holtzman, D.M.; Diamond, M.I. Proteopathic tau seeding predicts tauopathy in vivo. *Proc. Natl. Acad. Sci. USA* **2014**, *111*, E4376–E4385. [CrossRef] [PubMed]
5. Baba, M.; Nakajo, S.; Tu, P.-H.; Tomita, T.; Nakaya, K.; Lee, V.M.-Y.; Trojanowsk, J.Q.; Iwatsubo, T. Aggregation of α-Synuclein in Lewy Bodies of Sporadic Parkinson's Disease and Dementia with Lewy Bodies. *Am. J. Pathol.* **1998**, *152*, 879–884.
6. Kramer, M.L.; Schulz-Schaeffer, W.J. Presynaptic alpha-synuclein aggregates, not Lewy bodies, cause neurodegeneration in dementia with Lewy bodies. *J. Neurosci.* **2007**, *27*, 1405–1410. [CrossRef]
7. Gadad, B.S.; Britton, G.B.; Rao, K.S. Targeting Oligomers in Neurodegenerative Disorders: Lessons from α-Synuclein, Tau, and Amyloid-β Peptide. *J. Alzheimer's Dis.* **2011**, *24*, 223–232. [CrossRef]
8. Clinton, L.K.; Blurton-Jones, M.; Myczek, K.; Trojanowski, J.Q.; LaFerla, F.M. Synergistic Interactions between Aβ, Tau, and α-Synuclein: Acceleration of Neuropathology and Cognitive Decline. *J. Neurosci.* **2010**, *30*, 7281. [CrossRef]
9. Sharma, P.; Srivastava, P.; Seth, A.; Tripathi, P.N.; Banerjee, A.G.; Shrivastava, S.K. Comprehensive review of mechanisms of pathogenesis involved in Alzheimer's disease and potential therapeutic strategies. *Prog. Neurobiol.* **2019**, *174*, 53–89. [CrossRef]
10. Shekarchi, M.; Hajimehdipoor, H.; Saeidnia, S.; Gohari, A.R.; Hamedani, M.P. Comparative study of rosmarinic acid content in some plants of Labiatae family. *Pharmacogn. Mag.* **2012**, *8*, 37–41.
11. Narasimhamoorthy, B.; Zhao, L.Q.; Liu, X.; Yang, W.; Greaves, J.A. Differences in the chemotype of two native spearmint clonal lines selected for rosmarinic acid accumulation in comparison to commercially grown native spearmint. *Ind. Crops Prod.* **2015**, *63*, 87–91. [CrossRef]
12. Cirlini, M.; Mena, P.; Tassotti, M.; Herrlinger, K.A.; Nieman, K.M.; Dall'Asta, C.; del Rio, D. Phenolic and Volatile Composition of a Dry Spearmint (Mentha spicata L.). Extract. *Mol.* **2016**, *21*, 1007. [CrossRef] [PubMed]
13. Farr, S.A.; Niehoff, M.L.; Ceddia, M.A.; Herrlinger, K.A.; Lewis, B.J.; Feng, S.; Welleford, A.; Butterfield, D.A.; Morley, J.E. Effect of botanical extracts containing carnosic acid or rosmarinic acid on learning and memory in SAMP8 mice. *Physiol. Behav.* **2016**, *165*, 328–338. [CrossRef] [PubMed]
14. Nieman, K.M.; Sanoshy, K.D.; Bresciani, L.; Schild, A.L.; Kelley, K.M.; Lawless, A.L.; Ceddia, M.A.; Maki, K.C.; Rio, D.D.; Herrlinger, K.A. Tolerance, bioavailability, and potential cognitive health implications of a distinct aqueous spearmint extract. *Funct. Foods Health Dis.* **2015**, *5*, 165–187. [CrossRef]
15. Herrlinger, K.A.; Nieman, K.M.; Sanoshy, K.D.; Fonseca, B.A.; Lasrado, J.A.; Schild, A.L.; Maki, K.C.; Wesnes, K.A.; Ceddia, M.A. Spearmint Extract Improves Working Memory in Men and Women with Age-Associated Memory Impairment. *J. Altern. Complement. Med.* **2018**, *24*, 37–47. [CrossRef]
16. del Baño, M.J.; Lorente, J.; Castillo, J.; Benavente-García, O.; del Río, J.A.; Ortuño, A.; Quirin, K.-W.; Gerard, D. Phenolic Diterpenes, Flavones, and Rosmarinic Acid Distribution during the Development of Leaves, Flowers, Stems, and Roots of Rosmarinus officinalis. Antioxidant Activity. *J. Agric. Food Chem.* **2003**, *51*, 4247–4253. [CrossRef]
17. Osakabe, N.; Takano, H.; Sanbongi, C.; Yasuda, A.; Yanagisawa, R.; Inoue, K.-I.; Yoshikawa, T. Anti-inflammatory and anti-allergic effect of rosmarinic acid (RA); inhibition of seasonal allergic rhinoconjunctivitis (SAR) and its mechanism. *BioFactors* **2004**, *21*, 127–131. [CrossRef]
18. Rocha, J.; Eduardo-Figueira, M.; Barateiro, A.; Fernandes, A.; Brites, D.; Bronze, R.; Duarte, C.M.M.; Serra, A.T.; Pinto, R.; Freitas, M.; et al. Anti-inflammatory effect of rosmarinic acid and an extract of *rosmarinus officinalis* in rat models of local and systemic inflammation. *Basic Clin. Pharmacol. Toxicol.* **2015**, *116*, 398–413. [CrossRef]
19. Huang, S.; Zheng, R. Rosmarinic acid inhibits angiogenesis and its mechanism of action in vitro. *Cancer Lett.* **2006**, *239*, 271–280. [CrossRef]
20. Iuvone, T.; De Filippis, D.; Esposito, G.; D'Amico, A.; Izzo, A.A. The spice sage and its active ingredient rosmarinic acid protect PC12 cells from amyloid-beta peptide-induced neurotoxicity. *J. Pharmacol. Exp. Ther.* **2006**, *317*, 1143–1149. [CrossRef]
21. Moreno, S.; Scheyer, T.; Romano, C.S.; Vojnov, A.A. Antioxidant and antimicrobial activities of rosemary extracts linked to their polyphenol composition. *Free Radic. Res.* **2006**, *40*, 223–231. [CrossRef] [PubMed]
22. Lee, J.; Jung, E.; Koh, J.; Kim, Y.S.; Park, D. Effect of rosmarinic acid on atopic dermatitis. *J. Dermatol.* **2008**, *35*, 768–771. [CrossRef] [PubMed]

23. Takahashi, R.; Ono, K.; Takamura, Y.; Mizuguchi, M.; Ikeda, T.; Nishijo, H.; Yamada, M. Phenolic compounds prevent the oligomerization of alpha-synuclein and reduce synaptic toxicity. *J. Neurochem.* **2015**, *134*, 943–955. [CrossRef] [PubMed]
24. Ono, K.; Li, L.; Takamura, Y.; Yoshiike, Y.; Zhu, L.; Han, F.; Mao, X.; Ikeda, T.; Takasaki, J.; Nishijo, H.; et al. Phenolic compounds prevent amyloid β-protein oligomerization and synaptic dysfunction by site-specific binding. *J. Biol. Chem.* **2012**, *287*, 14631–14643. [CrossRef] [PubMed]
25. Yagi, H.; Kusaka, E.; Hongo, K.; Mizobata, T.; Kawata, Y. Amyloid fibril formation of alpha-synuclein is accelerated by preformed amyloid seeds of other proteins: Implications for the mechanism of transmissible conformational diseases. *J. Biol. Chem.* **2005**, *280*, 38609–38616. [CrossRef] [PubMed]
26. Narhi, L.; Wood, S.J.; Steavenson, S.; Jiang, Y.; Wu, G.M.; Anafi, D.; Kaufman, S.A.; Martin, F.; Sitney, K.; Denis, P.; et al. Both familial Parkinson's disease mutations accelerate alpha-synuclein aggregation. *J. Biol. Chem.* **1999**, *274*, 9843–9846. [CrossRef] [PubMed]
27. Yamakawa, M.Y.; Uchino, K.; Watanabe, Y.; Adachi, T.; Nakanishi, M.; Ichino, H.; Hongo, K.; Mizobata, T.; Kobayashi, S.; Nakashima, K.; et al. Anthocyanin suppresses the toxicity of Aβ deposits through diversion of molecular forms in in vitro and in vivo models of Alzheimer's disease. *Nutr. Neurosci.* **2016**, *19*, 32–42. [CrossRef]
28. Yamamoto, H.; Fukui, N.; Adachi, M.; Saiki, E.; Yamasaki, A.; Matsumura, R.; Kuroyanagi, D.; Hongo, K.; Mizobata, T.; Kawata, Y. Human Molecular Chaperone Hsp60 and Its Apical Domain Suppress Amyloid Fibril Formation of α-Synuclein. *Int. J. Mol. Sci.* **2019**, *21*, 47. [CrossRef]
29. Erkan, N.; Ayranci, G.; Ayranci, E. Antioxidant activities of rosemary (Rosmarinus Officinalis L.) extract, blackseed (Nigella sativa L.) essential oil, carnosic acid, rosmarinic acid and sesamol. *Food Chem.* **2008**, *110*, 76–82. [CrossRef]
30. Ono, K.; Yamada, M. Antioxidant compounds have potent anti-fibrillogenic and fibril-destabilizing effects for alpha-synuclein fibrils in vitro. *J. Neurochem.* **2006**, *97*, 105–115. [CrossRef]
31. Bieschke, J.; Russ, J.; Friedrich, R.P.; Ehrnhoefer, D.E.; Wobst, H.; Neugebauer, K.; Wanker, E.E. EGCG remodels mature alpha-synuclein and amyloid-beta fibrils and reduces cellular toxicity. *Proc. Natl. Acad. Sci. USA* **2010**, *107*, 7710–7715. [CrossRef] [PubMed]
32. Hamaguchi, T.; Ono, K.; Murase, A.; Yamada, M. Phenolic compounds prevent Alzheimer's pathology through different effects on the amyloid-beta aggregation pathway. *Am. J. Pathol.* **2009**, *175*, 2557–2565. [CrossRef] [PubMed]
33. Ono, K.; Hirohata, M.; Yamada, M. Ferulic acid destabilizes preformed β-amyloid fibrils in vitro. *Biochem. Biophys. Res. Commun.* **2005**, *336*, 444–449. [CrossRef] [PubMed]
34. Wang, S.; Wang, Y.; Su, Y.; Zhou, W.; Yang, S.; Zhang, R.; Zhao, M.; Li, Y.; Zhang, Z.; Zhan, D.; et al. Rutin inhibits β-amyloid aggregation and cytotoxicity, attenuates oxidative stress, and decreases the production of nitric oxide and proinflammatory cytokines. *NeuroToxicology* **2012**, *33*, 482–490. [CrossRef] [PubMed]
35. Durairajan, S.S.K.; Yuan, Q.; Xie, L.; Chan, W.; Kum, W.; Koo, I.; Liu, C.; Song, Y.; Huang, J.; Klein, W.L.; et al. Salvianolic acid B inhibits Aβ fibril formation and disaggregates preformed fibrils and protects against Aβ-induced cytotoxicty. *Neurochem. Int.* **2008**, *52*, 741–750. [CrossRef]
36. Mroczko, B.; Groblewska, M.; Litman-Zawadzka, A. The Role of Protein Misfolding and Tau Oligomers (TauOs) in Alzheimer's Disease (AD). *Int. J. Mol. Sci.* **2019**, *20*, 4661. [CrossRef]
37. Siposova, K.; Kozar, T.; Huntosova, V.; Tomkova, S.; Musatov, A. Inhibition of amyloid fibril formation and disassembly of pre-formed fibrils by natural polyphenol rottlerin. *Biochimica et biophysica acta. Proteins Proteom.* **2019**, *1867*, 259–274. [CrossRef]
38. Ono, K.; Yoshiike, Y.; Takashima, A.; Hasegawa, K.; Naiki, H.; Yamada, M. Potent anti-amyloidogenic and fibril-destabilizing effects of polyphenols in vitro: Implications for the prevention and therapeutics of Alzheimer's disease. *J. Neurochem.* **2003**, *87*, 172–181. [CrossRef]
39. Ono, K.; Hasegawa, K.; Naiki, H.; Yamada, M. Anti-amyloidogenic activity of tannic acid and its activity to destabilize Alzheimer's beta-amyloid fibrils in vitro. *Biochim. Biophys. Acta* **2004**, *1690*, 193–202. [CrossRef]
40. Cheng, B.; Gong, H.; Xiao, H.; Petersen, R.B.; Zheng, L.; Huang, K. Inhibiting toxic aggregation of amyloidogenic proteins: A therapeutic strategy for protein misfolding diseases. *Biochim. Biophys. Acta* **2013**, *1830*, 4860–4871. [CrossRef]

41. Sato, M.; Murakami, K.; Uno, M.; Nakagawa, Y.; Katayama, S.; Akagi, K.; Masuda, Y.; Takegoshi, K.; Irie, K. Site-specific inhibitory mechanism for amyloid β42 aggregation by catechol-type flavonoids targeting the Lys residues. *J. Biol. Chem.* **2013**, *288*, 23212–23224. [CrossRef] [PubMed]
42. Lorenzen, N.; Nielsen, S.B.; Yoshimura, Y.; Vad, B.S.; Andersen, C.B.; Betzer, C.; Kaspersen, J.D.; Christiansen, G.; Pedersen, J.S.; Jensen, P.H.; et al. How epigallocatechin gallate can inhibit α-synuclein oligomer toxicity in vitro. *J. Biol. Chem.* **2014**, *289*, 21299–21310. [CrossRef] [PubMed]
43. Taniguchi, S.; Suzuki, N.; Masuda, M.; Hisanaga, S.; Iwatsubo, T.; Goedert, M.; Hasegawa, M. Inhibition of heparin-induced tau filament formation by phenothiazines, polyphenols, and porphyrins. *J. Biol. Chem.* **2005**, *280*, 7614–7623. [CrossRef] [PubMed]
44. Hase, T.; Shishido, S.; Yamamoto, S.; Yamashita, R.; Nukima, H.; Taira, S.; Toyoda, T.; Abe, K.; Hamaguchi, T.; Ono, K.; et al. Rosmarinic acid suppresses Alzheimer's disease development by reducing amyloid β aggregation by increasing monoamine secretion. *Sci. Rep.* **2019**, *9*, 8711. [CrossRef]

Publisher's Note: MDPI stays neutral with regard to jurisdictional claims in published maps and institutional affiliations.

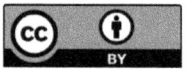 © 2020 by the authors. Licensee MDPI, Basel, Switzerland. This article is an open access article distributed under the terms and conditions of the Creative Commons Attribution (CC BY) license (http://creativecommons.org/licenses/by/4.0/).

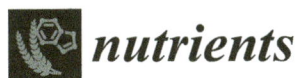

Article

Maternal Protein Restriction in Rats Alters the Expression of Genes Involved in Mitochondrial Metabolism and Epitranscriptomics in Fetal Hypothalamus

Morgane Frapin [1], Simon Guignard [1], Dimitri Meistermann [2], Isabelle Grit [1], Valentine S. Moullé [1], Vincent Paillé [1], Patricia Parnet [1] and Valérie Amarger [1,*]

[1] Nantes Université, INRAE, IMAD, CRNH-O, UMR 1280, PhAN, F-44000 Nantes, France; morgane.frapin@univ-nantes.fr (M.F.); simon.guignard@inserm.fr (S.G.); isabelle.grit@univ-nantes.fr (I.G.); valentine.moulle@inrae.fr (V.S.M.); vincent.paille@univ-nantes.fr (V.P.); patricia.parnet@univ-nantes.fr (P.P.)
[2] Nantes Université, INSERM, UMR 1064-CRTI, ITUN, F-44000 Nantes, France; dimitri.meistermann@univ-nantes.fr
* Correspondence: valerie.amarger@univ-nantes.fr

Received: 17 April 2020; Accepted: 13 May 2020; Published: 19 May 2020

Abstract: Fetal brain development is closely dependent on maternal nutrition and metabolic status. Maternal protein restriction (PR) is known to be associated with alterations in the structure and function of the hypothalamus, leading to impaired control of energy homeostasis and food intake. The objective of this study was to identify the cellular and molecular systems underlying these effects during fetal development. We combined a global transcriptomic analysis on the fetal hypothalamus from a rat model of maternal PR with in vitro neurosphere culture and cellular analyses. Several genes encoding proteins from the mitochondrial respiratory chain complexes were overexpressed in the PR group and mitochondrial metabolic activity in the fetal hypothalamus was altered. The level of the N6-methyladenosine epitranscriptomic mark was reduced in the PR fetuses, and the expression of several genes involved in the writing/erasing/reading of this mark was indeed altered, as well as genes encoding several RNA-binding proteins. Additionally, we observed a higher number of neuronal-committed progenitors at embryonic day 17 (E17) in the PR fetuses. Together, these data strongly suggest a metabolic adaptation to the amino acid shortage, combined with the post-transcriptional control of protein expression, which might reflect alterations in the control of the timing of neuronal progenitor differentiation.

Keywords: maternal nutrition; protein restriction; fetal brain; hypothalamus; differentiation; neurogenesis; transcriptomics; epitranscriptomics; mitochondria

1. Introduction

The impact of altered nutrient availability on brain development during the perinatal period is widely acknowledged and is corroborated by both observations on humans and animal studies. Fetal malnutrition may be the consequence of an imbalanced maternal nutrition or placenta deficiency [1,2], with both possibly resulting in Intra Uterine Growth Restriction (IUGR) and a risk of preterm birth. In addition, very preterm infants often experience poor early postnatal growth, characterized by a deficit of lean mass [3]. This is often associated with neurological impairments during infancy [3,4]. Poor fetal growth is also known to confer a risk of developing metabolic diseases in adulthood according to the thrifty phenotype hypothesis [5], with the consequence being the impaired control of energy homeostasis. The hypothalamus, because of its central role in the regulation of energy homeostasis and food intake, has been intensely studied using animal models. Malnutrition in the perinatal period is associated with impaired hypothalamus development as well as altered leptin and insulin signaling, leading to defects in the control of food intake [6–9]. However, although the impact of perinatal nutrition on postnatal development of the hypothalamus and its functional consequences have been widely described [7,10], little is known about alterations that may take place during the morphogenesis of the fetal hypothalamus, probably because of the enormous complexity of the anatomy and functionality characterizing this brain region [11].

The development of the hypothalamus starts during early embryonic development with anterior–posterior patterning of the developing neural tube. The numerous nuclei of the hypothalamus are generated between E11 and E17 embryonic days in rodents [11,12]. This morphogenesis step is followed after birth, during the first two weeks of life in rodents, by the organization of nuclei that connect to each other and towards other regions of the brain [13].

The different cell types found in the hypothalamic nuclei originate from undifferentiated dividing neural progenitor cells (NPCs) residing in the ventricular zone of the brain, a transient embryonic layer of tissue. These NPCs, also named radial glial (RG) cells, are derived from neuroepithelial cells and give rise to committed neuronal and glial progenitors that migrate and differentiate according to a strictly defined program. In rodents, hypothalamic neurogenesis occurs prenatally between E12 and E17 and precedes astrogenesis that takes place during the postnatal period [13,14]. Because cell number and neurogenesis are determined during the prenatal period, the fetal environment, including maternal nutrition and metabolic status, may impact these processes, as already demonstrated by several studies on hippocampal and cortical tissues (reviewed in [15]). For instance, fetal malnutrition was associated with an alteration in the level of neuronal proliferation, maintenance and apoptosis of hippocampal cells [16,17]. Maternal protein restriction has been shown to reduce the proliferation of neural stem cells and to influence progenitor cell fate during embryonic cortex development in mice, resulting in increased cortex thickness [18].

Neural stem cells show a spectacular plasticity in their capacity to differentiate into a variety of cell types. This confers to the developing brain a great adaptability but also a high sensitivity to external cues. Hypothalamic progenitor cells were shown to respond in vitro to environmental stimuli such as the neurotrophic hormones insulin and leptin [19] or the endocrine disruptor Bisphenol A [20].

However, even if the impact of the perinatal environment on hypothalamus development is now clearly established, the underlying mechanisms remain largely unexplored. The proliferation and differentiation of neural stem cells and progenitors is strongly based on the precise control of the expression of specific genes, including pluripotency genes and lineage-specific genes. The maintenance in an undifferentiated state or the commitment into neuronal or glial differentiation requires a complex interplay between external cues, transcription factors, DNA-binding proteins, epigenetic control of gene expression and possibly other, as yet uncharacterized, mechanisms [21]. Overall, evidence is growing that gene expression is finely regulated both at the transcriptional and translational level. Given all this complexity, it makes sense that environmental factors can act on many levels.

The objective of this study was to identify early determinants of the impact of maternal protein restriction on hypothalamic development and to characterize, at the molecular level, early indicators of an impaired development. We use a well-characterized rat model of maternal protein restriction during gestation, which was designed to mimic placental defects, often resulting in the altered transfer of amino acids between mother and child [22]. We have previously shown that protein deficiency during gestation and lactation results in alterations in the development of the hypothalamus, leading to defects in the control of food intake [8,9] and metabolic alterations during adulthood [23].

Our strategy was to analyze fetal hypothalami at E17, which approximately represents the end of neurogenesis in rats [11,12]. Using 3′ digital gene expression sequencing (DGE-seq) for differential gene expression analysis, pathway enrichment analysis and N6-methyladenosine (m6A) RNA methylation assay, we have sought to identify possible molecular targets of fetal undernutrition that underlie alterations of in neurogenesis process in the hypothalamus.

2. Materials and Methods

2.1. Animals

All experiments were carried out in accordance with current guidelines of the local animal welfare committee and were approved by the Animal Ethics Committee of Pays de La Loire under reference 2016112412253439/APAFIS 7768. Nulliparous female Sprague–Dawley rats were purchased from Janvier Labs (Le Genest Saint Isle, France) and delivered to our facilities at the age of 7/8 weeks. On arrival, rats were housed (two per cage) under controlled conditions (22 °C, 12 h/12 h dark/light cycle) with free access to a standard diet (A04, SAFE-diets, Augy, France). After one week of acclimation, the estrous cycle was determined by vaginal smears and female rats in early estrous were mated overnight with a male. The presence of spermatozoa was verified the next day through vaginal smears and, when positive, this day was considered embryonic day 0 (E0). Pregnant rats were housed individually and randomly assigned to two experimental groups receiving either a control (C) diet containing 20% protein or a protein-restricted (PR) diet containing 8% protein (UPAE, Jouy-en-Josas, France). A detailed composition of the diets was described in [24]. At embryonic day 17 (E17), dams were anesthetized with 4% isoflurane and fetuses were sampled by caesarian section. Fetuses and placentas were weighed and brains were rapidly removed and dissected under a binocular magnifier to collect the hypothalamus. Some hypothalami were snap frozen in liquid nitrogen and stored at −80 °C for transcriptomic and proteomic analysis, while others were collected in cold PBS containing 2% glucose for cell biology experiments.

2.2. In Vitro Culture of Neurospheres from E17 Hypothalamus

For each litter, we collected six hypothalami to prepare neurospheres. After one wash in 2 mL of sterile PBS containing 2% glucose, hypothalami were mechanically triturated in 1 mL of NeuroCult Basal Medium (STEMCELL Technologies Inc., Vancouver, BC, Canada) using a 1 mL micropipette until a single-cell suspension was obtained. The cell suspension was then filtered on a 40 μm cell strainer (Greiner Bio-one International GmBH, Kremsmünster, Austria) and centrifuged at 500× g for 5 min. Cell pellets were resuspended in NeuroCult Basal Medium and viable cells were counted on a hemocytometer after eosin staining. All cells from one hypothalamus were seeded in a T-12.5 cm^2 tissue culture flask containing 5 mL of Complete NeuroCult^{TM} Proliferation Medium and incubated at 37 °C and 5% CO_2. The obtained neurospheres were passed after 3 days in vitro. Briefly, cell passages were done by centrifuging neurospheres at 90× g for 5 min and incubating pellets with 200 μL of Accutase (STEMCELL Technologies Inc.) followed by gentle trituration to obtain single-cell suspensions. Cells were washed in NeuroCult Basal Medium, centrifuged at 500× g for 5 min and resuspended in NeuroCult Basal Medium, Complete NeuroCult^{TM} Proliferation Medium or Complete NeuroCult^{TM} Differentiation Medium, depending on the following experiment.

2.3. Proliferation Test Using BrdU

Cell proliferation was measured with a BrdU Cell Proliferation colorimetric ELISA Kit (ab126556, Abcam, Cambridge, UK) following the manufacturer's manual. This experiment was performed on passaged cells following neurosphere culture. Briefly, 20,000 cells resuspended in 100 μL of Complete NeuroCult^{TM} Proliferation Medium were seeded in coated 96-well plates, incubated with 20 μL of 1× BrdU Reagent at 37 °C and 5% CO_2 for 24 h and fixed with the provided solution. Fixed cells were incubated with anti-BrdU primary antibody, horseradish peroxidase-conjugated secondary antibody and tetramethybenzidine (TMB) substrate and absorbance at 450 nm was measured using a Varioskan LUX (ThermoFisher Scientific, Waltham, MA, USA).

2.4. Immunocytochemistry

Immature and mature neurons, undifferentiated cells and proliferative cell proportions were determined by immunochemistry using anti-TUJ1 (1:1000; MMS-435P-100 Eurogentec, Liège, Belgium), anti-MAP2 (1:100; #4542 Cell Signaling Technology, Leiden, The Netherlands), anti-NES (1:250; ab92391, Abcam) and anti-Ki67 (1:250; ab66155, Abcam) antibodies, respectively. Immunocytochemistry was performed on cells obtained after hypothalamus dissociation and on neurosphere cells resuspended in NeuroCult Basal Medium. Cells were fixed on Lab-Tek™ II Chamber Slide™ System (154534, ThermoFisher Scientific) with PBS and 4% paraformaldehyde (PFA). Blocking was done with an incubation step with PBS, 3% Bovine Serum Albumin (BSA) and 0.2% Triton for 1 h at room temperature and primary antibodies were added overnight at 4 °C. After three washings with PBS, secondary antibodies: Alexa 647-conjugated donkey anti-mouse (1:1000; 715-605-150, Jackson, Cambridge, UK), Alexa 647- conjugated donkey anti-rabbit (1:1000; 711-606-152, Jackson, Cambridge, UK) and biotin-conjugated goat anti-rabbit (1:1000; A24541, ThermoFisher Scientific were added and incubated for 1 h. After three washes, streptavidin Alexa 568 (1:1000; s11226, Molecular Probes, Eugene, OR, USA) was added to the wells containing biotinylated secondary antibodies. Cells were then incubated for 5 min at room temperature with DAPI (1/10,000; D3571 Molecular probes) and washed. The chambers were removed and the slides were mounted in VECTASHIELD® Vibrance™ Antifade Mounting Medium (Vector Laboratories, Burlingame, CA, USA). Pictures of each well were obtained using ×20 magnification on Zeiss Axio Imager.M2m microscope and positive cells for each marker were automatically counted with an ImageJ [25] script based on object detection using signal intensity.

2.5. Mitochondrial Membrane Potential Determination

For each litter, two hypothalami were collected in cold PBS and 2% glucose was used to determine mitochondrial membrane potential using MitoTracker Red CMXRos (ThermoFisher Scientific) staining. Cell dissociation and counting were performed as previously described for cell culture. About 20,000 viable cells were incubated 30 min with Mitotracker Red CMXRos (500 nM). Cells were then centrifuged at 700× g for 3 min and resuspended in PBS before the fluorescence was read in Varioskan LUX (ThermoFisher Scientific) (Ex 579 nm, Em 599 nm). The values of the fluorescence were normalized to the number of viable cells seeded.

2.6. Western Blotting

Proteins were extracted from E17 fetal hypothalami stored at −80 °C with lysis buffer containing Radio Immunoprecipitation Assay (RIPA) lysis buffer (EMD Millipore Corp, Burlington, MA, USA), protease inhibitor and phosphatase I and II inhibitor (Sigma-Aldrich, Saint-Louis, MO, USA). Lysis buffer was added to each sample then hypothalami were shredded (Precellys® Ozyme, 2 × 15 s at 5000 rpm) and centrifuged at 5590× g for 5 min at 4 °C. Protein concentrations were measured with Pierce™ BCA Protein Assay Kit (ThermoFisher Scientific) and 25 µg of proteins per sample were used for Western Blot. For subsequent labelling with the CSDE1 antibody, proteins were denatured with a heating step at 95 °C for 5 min with Laemmli Sample Buffer (Bio-Rad, Hercules, CA, USA) whereas, for the OXPHOS antibody, proteins were not denatured as recommended by the manufacturer. Proteins from the extracts were separated on a 4%–15% precast polyacrylamide gel (Bio-Rad) then transferred onto nitrocellulose membrane with the Trans-Blot Turbo Transfer System (Bio-Rad). For the membranes that were subsequently labelled with the OXPHOS antibody, total proteins were stained using the Revert™ 700 Total Protein Stain (LI-COR Biosciences, Lincoln, NE, USA) following the manufacturer recommendations. The total amount of proteins per sample was quantified on the Odyssey (LI-COR Biosciences) using Image Studio Ver 5.2 (LI-COR Biosciences) and the EMPIRIA Studio software Ver 1.2 (LI-COR Biosciences) and used for normalization. The Revert stain was removed from the membrane using the Revert Reversal Solution before the incubation with the antibody. Membranes were then blocked in TBST containing 5% dried fat-free milk and incubated overnight with primary antibodies anti-CSDE1 (1:1000; ab 201688,), anti-β-ACTIN (1:7,500; A5441, Sigma-Aldrich) or anti-OXPHOS cocktail (1:250; ab 110413, Abcam) then one hour with secondary antibodies goat anti-rabbit IgG DyLight 800 (1:10,000, SA5-10036, ThermoFisher Scientific), goat anti-mouse IgG DyLight 680 (1:10,000, 35519, ThermoFisher Scientific) and goat anti-mouse IgG Dylight

800 (1:10,000, SA5610176, ThermoFisher Scientific). Immunolabelling was then revealed on the Odyssey (LI-COR Biosciences) using Image Studio Lite Ver 5.2 (LI-COR Biosciences). For the experiment with the anti-CSDE1 antibody, normalization of the signal was performed using the anti-β-ACTIN antibody.

2.7. m6A RNA Methylation Assay

The total amount of m6A in total RNA was measured using the m6A RNA Methylation Assay Kit (Fluorometric) (ab 233491, Abcam), following the manufacturer manual. For each sample, 200 ng of total RNA from E17 hypothalamus preparation were used.

2.8. 3'DGE Library Preparation, Differential Gene Expression Analysis and Enrichment Analysis

Total RNA and DNA were extracted simultaneously from hypothalami stored at −80 °C using NucleoSpin® RNA columns and RNA/DNA buffer set (Macherey–Nagel, Hoerdt, France) following the manufacturer's manual. Transcriptomic analysis was performed using 3'DGE (Digital Gene Expression)-sequencing in accordance with [26]. Briefly, mRNA libraries were prepared from 10 ng of total RNA from 96 individuals (eight males and eight females from each experimental group collected at three different ages (E17, D0 and D130)). Poly(A) mRNA tails were tagged using universal primers, sample-specific barcodes and a unique molecular identifier (UMI) and cDNA synthesis was performed using template-switching reverse transcriptase. Samples were then pooled, amplified and fragmented using a transposon fragmentation method that enriches for 3' ends of cDNA. Fragments ranging from 350–800 bp were selected and sequenced on an Illumina Hiseq 2500. Paired-end sequencing was performed using a Hiseq Rapid SBS kit v2 50 cycles (FC-402-4022) and a Hiseq Rapid PE Cluster kit v2 (PE-402-4022). The first read of 16 bp corresponds to the sample-specific barcode and the second read of 57 bp to the mRNA in the 5' 3' direction. Alignments were done on RefSeq rat mRNA sequences (Rn6) by using BWA (version 0.7.15-0). The number of unique UMI associated with each RefSeq gene was counted. Only genes with three or more reads per sample in at least four samples were kept in the count table. Normalization and differential gene expression analyses were processed using DESeq2 (version 1.24.0) [27] with a correction for sex effect. Data from the 96 samples were used for normalization and differential expression analysis was performed separately for each age. Functional enrichment was done using FGSEA [28,29] from Gene Ontology (GO) [30], Kyoto Encyclopedia of Genes and Genomes (KEGG) [31] and Reactome [32] databases. The datasets generated for this study can be found at the European Nucleotide Archive (ENA) under the accession PRJEB35794.

2.9. Mitochondrial DNA Quantification Using qPCR

Mitochondrial DNA was quantified by quantitative PCR using primers designed against the mitochondrial *CytB* gene (Forward 5'-TTCCGCCCAATCACCCAAATC-3', Reverse 5'-GCTGAT GGAGGCTAGTTGGCC-3') and normalized against the geometric mean of the amplification signal from two nuclear genes: *Gapdh* (Forward 5'-TTCAACGGCACAGTCAAGG-3', Reverse (5'-CTCAGCACCAGCATCACC-3') and *Zfx-Zfy* (5'-AAGCATATGAAGACCCACAG-3', Reverse 5'-CTTCGGAATCCTTTCTTGCAG-3'). Ten ng of total DNA were amplified in a total volume of 15 µL using the iTaq™ Universal SYBR® Green Supermix (Biorad) and 0.25 µM of each primer following the manufacturer's instructions, in a CFX Connect™ Real Time PCR Detection System (Biorad). A relative amount of mitochondrial DNA was quantified using the $2^{-\Delta\Delta Ct}$ method.

2.10. Statistics

Either a Mann–Whitney or t-test was used to evaluate differences between groups and a two-way analysis of variance (ANOVA) was used to additionally assess sex effects. For each experiment, the tests are indicated in Figure and Table legends. The statistical analyses were performed using R software (version 3.6).

3. Results

3.1. Fetal and Placenta Weight at E17 Did Not Differ between Control and PR Fetuses

The number of pups per litter and weight gain during gestation did not vary between the control and PR dams (Table 1). Fetal and placenta weight were recorded immediately after caesarian section. Females weighed about 5% less than males in both control and PR groups, but there was no difference between the two groups in both sexes (Table 1). Placenta weight and Placenta–Fetus Ratio (PFR) were not impacted by maternal nutrition and fetus sex.

Table 1. Litter and fetus characteristics at embryonic day 17 (E17).

	Controls		Protein Restricted		p-Value
Litter Size	13.00 ± 3.39 ($n = 13$)		14.13 ± 2.61 ($n = 15$)		0.50 *
Maternal Weight Gain (g)	112.39 ± 17.77 ($n = 13$)		99.47 ± 21.12 ($n = 13$)		0.16 *
Fetal Weight (g)	♀($n = 32$) 0.76 ± 0.05	♂($n = 38$) 0.79 ± 0.05	♀($n = 54$) 0.77 ± 0.07	♂($n = 36$) 0.81 ± 0.06	Group: 0.41 [#] Sex: <0.0001 [#]
Placenta Weight (g)	0.39 ± 0.06 ($n = 70$)		0.40 ± 0.07 ($n = 81$)		0.85 *
PFR (Placenta–Fetus Ratio)	0.51 ± 0.09 ($n = 70$)		0.52 ± 0.10 ($n = 81$)		0.83 *

* Mann–Whitney test; [#] two-way ANOVA test.

3.2. Hypothalami from PR Fetuses Contained a Lower Number of Cells

The hypothalami from 129 fetuses (69 PR and 60 C) from 13 different litters were immediately dissociated into single cells. Cell number and viability were determined using a hematocytometer before subsequent analyses or cell culture. The percentage of viable cells was not different between both groups (control: 65.76 ± 10.39, PR: 68.39 ± 12.81, t-test $p = 0.21$). The total number of cells per hypothalamus was significantly lower in the PR group ($6.7 \pm 3.2 \times 10^5$) compared to the control group ($7.8 \pm 2.9 \times 10^5$) (two-way ANOVA group effect $p = 0.04$) (Figure 1). There was no difference between males and females.

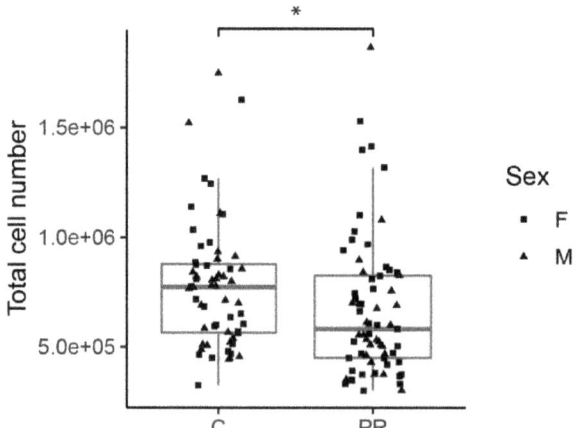

Figure 1. Total number of cells obtained from each E17 fetal hypothalamus after mechanical dissociation. The cells were counted on a hemocytometer (PR: $n = 27$ males and 42 females C: $n = 32$ males and 28 females). (two-way ANOVA: group effect * $p = 0.04$, sex effect $p = 0.35$) (boxplot: median, first and third quartiles).

3.3. The Proportion of the Several Cell Populations Present in E17 Hypothalami Did Not Differ between Control and PR Fetuses

In order to assess the impact of maternal diet on the proportion of the different cell types present in the hypothalamus at E17, dissociated cells were fixed on glass plates, stained with antibodies directed against Nestin, beta-III-tubulin, MAP2 and the proliferation marker KI67 and automatically counted after photomicrograph acquisition. Each cell type marker was counted on about 6000 cells per sample. The proportion of proliferating Ki67-positive cells was on average 82% in both groups. Nestin+ cells, representing undifferentiated NSCs and progenitors, accounted for about 60% of the cells (Figure 2). Beta-III-tubulin +cells, i.e., neural progenitors and young neurons accounted for 20% to 50% of the cells in both groups (Figure 2). Nestin and beta-III-tubulin markers were expressed at different levels in early or late progenitors but, based on this marker, we were not able to distinguish these two populations and therefore we could not accurately determine the level of these two types of progenitors. In contrast, more mature neurons, expressing MAP2, accounted for about 30% of the cells (Figure 2). Interestingly, although we observed a high inter-individual variability in the number of beta-III-tubulin+ and MAP2+ cells, the relative proportion of these two populations remained equal. We did not observe any significant difference between control and PR fetuses regarding the proportion of the different cell types, but a rather high inter-individual variability was observed that may alter the statistical power. This was especially true for Ki67+ cells, probably because Ki67 expression depends on the cellular cycle phase. Labelling experiments using a glial progenitor and astrocyte marker, GFAP, did not detect any positive cells at this early stage (data not shown).

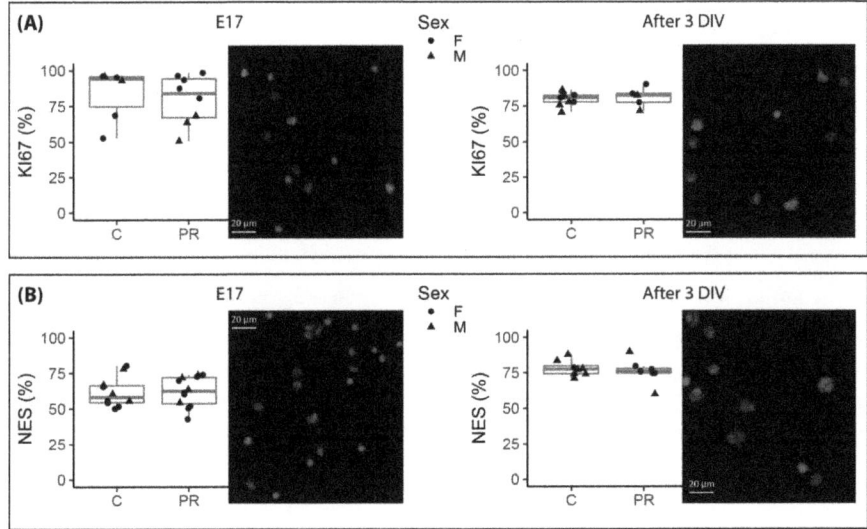

Figure 2. *Cont.*

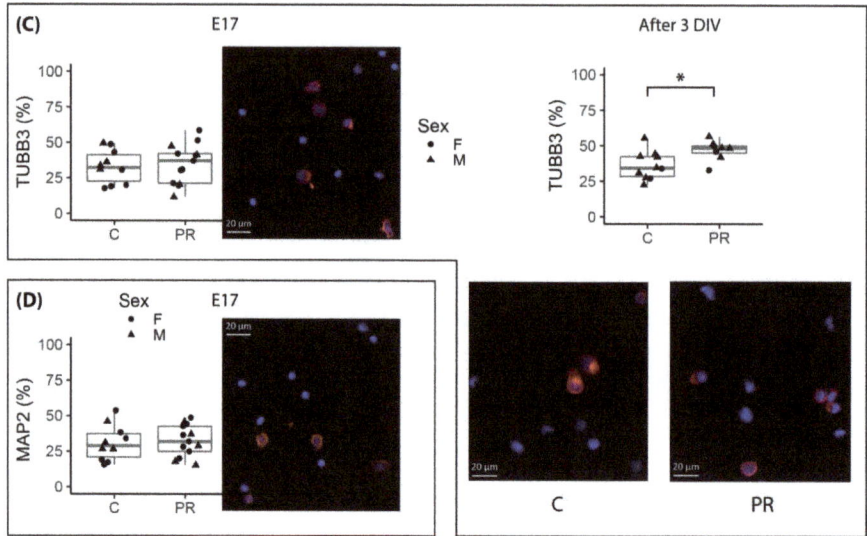

Figure 2. Neural cell type proportions in total hypothalamic cells sampled at E17 and after three days in vitro (3 DIV) labelled by immunocytochemistry and automatically counted on microscopy images. Each marker is illustrated by images obtained by optical microscopy (scale bars, 20 μm). Red and orange labelling is for markers of interest, Ki67 (**A**), Nestin (**B**), TUJ1 = TUBB3 (**C**) and MAP2 (**D**) and nucleus are labelled with DAPI in blue (n = 6–13 per group). Group and sex effects were tested using two-way ANOVA, * group effect p = 0.02. Non-significant p values are not mentioned. (boxplot: median, first and third quartiles).

3.4. Neurosphere Cultures from PR E17 Hypothalami Contained a Higher Number of Committed Neuronal Progenitors after Three Days of Proliferation In Vitro

For a subset of E17 hypothalami, dissociated cells were allowed to grow in vitro and form neurospheres. The purpose of neurosphere culture was to select and increase the number of cells that have the ability to proliferate, i.e., stem cells and progenitors. We deliberately limited the culture time to 3 days in order to minimize the biases introduced by a longer culture and preserve the initial intrinsic properties of the cells. After three days of culture, the proportion of proliferating Ki67+ cells was about 80% and rather homogeneous between samples (Figure 2). The number of Nestin+ cells was significantly higher in the neurospheres compared to the E17 hypothalami (76% versus 60% on average, $p = 1.4 \times 10^{-5}$), which was expected since neurosphere culture allows the selection of stem and progenitor cells. There was no difference between the control and PR fetuses regarding the proportion of Ki67+ and Nestin+ cells (Figure 2). A higher proportion of committed neuronal progenitors (beta-III-tubulin+) was present in the neurospheres coming from PR (47% on average) than control fetuses (36%) (two-way ANOVA group effect p = 0.02).

3.5. Neurospheres Cultures Did Not Show Any Proliferation Potential Difference between Control and PR Fetuses

Neurospheres were passaged after three days in culture and BrdU was added to the culture media for 24 h in order to test the cell proliferation capacities. There was no difference between groups in the amount of BrdU-incorporated (data not shown).

3.6. The Expression of More than 400 Genes Was Altered in PR E17 Fetal Hypothalamus

Because cell differentiation relies on the precise control of gene expression, we performed a global transcriptomic analysis using the digital gene expression sequencing (DGE-seq) approach. This technique is based on the sequencing of the 3′ end of mRNAs and is known to be highly sensitive for gene expression quantification but does not give any transcript-splicing information [26]. The experiment was performed on hypothalami of 16 individuals (eight males and eight females) from each experimental group collected at three different ages (E17, D0 and D130). However, because the objective of the present study was to evaluate the impact of maternal PR on fetal hypothalamus development, only the data from E17 fetuses will be presented here. An average of 3.4 million reads per sample was obtained and about 1.1 million reads with a single UMI were assigned to a known gene after alignment on the RefSeq transcript database. A total of 11,244 expressed transcripts were detected from the 18,946 transcripts from the RefSeq database (including the genes from the mitochondrial genome) (Supplementary Table S1). Among these, 6723 genes for which the normalized number of reads per E17 fetus was at least 10 were identified. The number of reads per gene varied from 10 to 21,000.

A total of 440 genes (247 Up and 193 Down) were differentially expressed between the control and PR fetuses (adjusted p-value (padj) < 0.05) (Supplementary Table S1). Males and females were analyzed together and the data were corrected for sex effects. A volcano plot comparison showed that the magnitude of expression changes between both groups was relatively small, with log2 Fold Change (log2FC) ranging from −0.82 to 0.67, which means a fold change ranging from 0.56 to 1.6 (Figure 3). On the MA plot displaying the log2FC in relation to the level of expression, it appeared that the genes that were upregulated in the PR group had, on average, a higher expression level than genes that were downregulated (Figure 3). Among the 100 most-expressed genes (base mean > 1300 reads), 15 were upregulated in the PR group whereas none were downregulated. *Atp6*, *CytB* and *Cox2* were among the four genes with the highest expression rate, they are all encoded by the mitochondrial genome, involved in mitochondrial respiratory chain and were upregulated in the PR group (*Atp6*: log2FC = 0.2-padj = 0.04, *Cox2*: log2FC = 0.16-padj = 0.03 and *CytB*: log2FC = 0.18-padj = 0.09) (Figure 3) (Supplementary Table S1).

The top 20 up- and downregulated genes in the PR group compared to the control group are presented in Tables A1 and A2 together with information regarding their function. Several genes potentially involved in the regulation of cell cycle, proliferation and cell migration were present in both lists (*Ube2n*, *Chrac1* and *Marcks* were upregulated, *Fgfr1op*, *Eps15*, *Robo1* and *Myo18a* were downregulated). Four genes encode RNA-binding proteins that are involved in RNA degradation, stability and translation (*Csde1*, *Cirbp*, *Rbm7* and *Qk*). In particular, *Csde1* and *Cirbp* genes, which play an essential role in the control of neuron differentiation, were highly expressed and upregulated in the PR group. Interestingly, several genes involved in the control of redox homeostasis and mitochondrial metabolism were also upregulated (*Coa5*, *Coq7*, *Mterf1*, *LOC100174910*).

A Fast Gene Set Enrichment Analysis (FGSEA) was performed in order to identify gene families and/or metabolic pathways significantly impacted by the maternal diet. Briefly, the principle of this method is to rank the genes according to the significance of their differential expression and fold change and to test which pathways are significantly enriched in genes that are globally up- and/or downregulated [33]. We used several databases (KEGG, Reactome, GO) that are partly redundant but more or less complete in order to conduct an exhaustive search of metabolic pathways and cellular processes that may be impacted by the maternal diet. A total of 585 pathways were significantly enriched (enrichment adjusted p.value < 0.05) (Supplementary Table S2). The FGSEA analysis generates a Normalized Enrichment Score (NES) which reflects the degree to which a gene set is overrepresented at the extremes of the ranked list of genes [33]. A selection of the top pathways is presented on Figure 4. Pathways with an NES > 0 or NES < 0 contain genes that are predominantly over- or under-expressed, respectively, in the PR group compared to the control group.

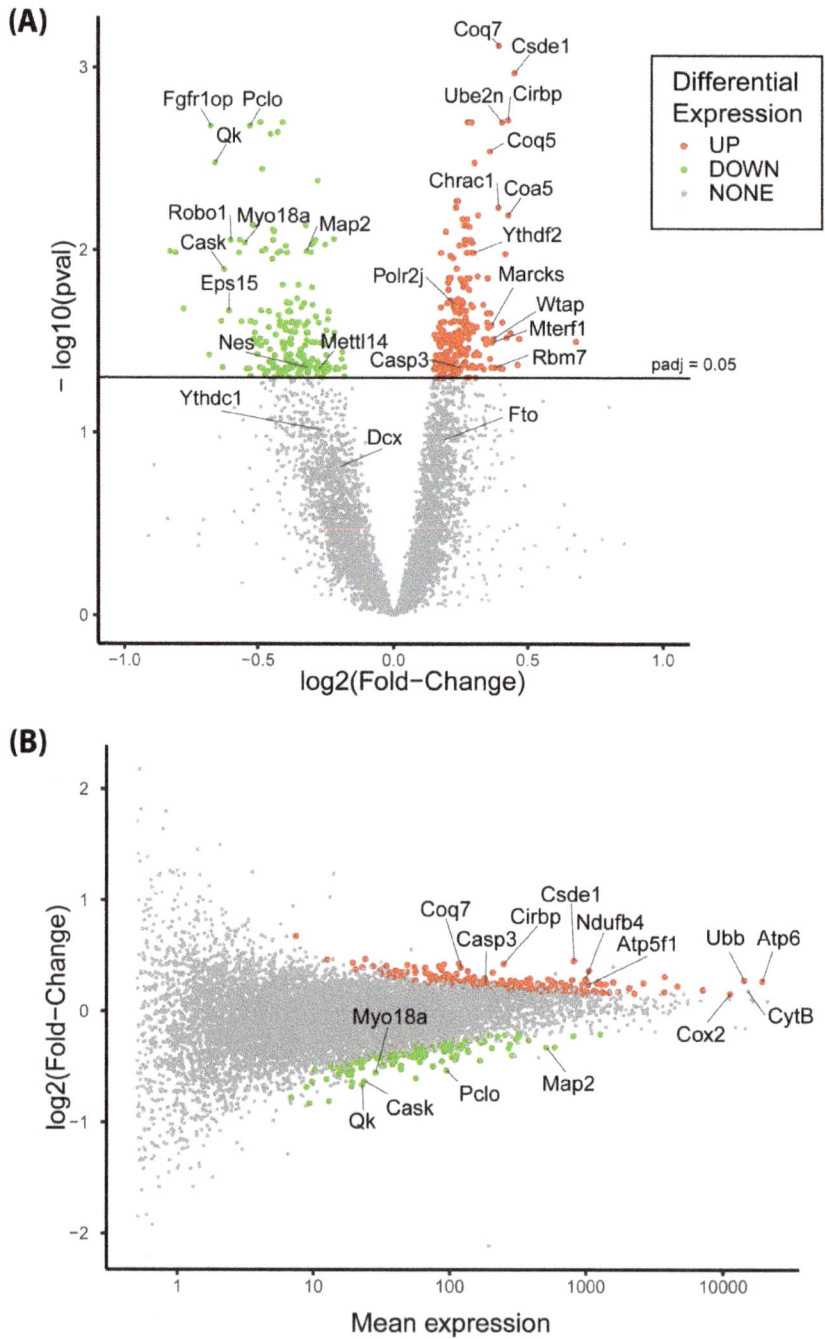

Figure 3. Volcano plot (**A**) and MA plot (**B**) of differentially expressed genes at E17 in the protein restriction (PR) group compared to Control group (PR: n = eight males + eight females, C: n = eight males + eight females). (padj = adjusted *p*-value from Deseq2 analysis). Mean expression corresponds to the average normalized read number.

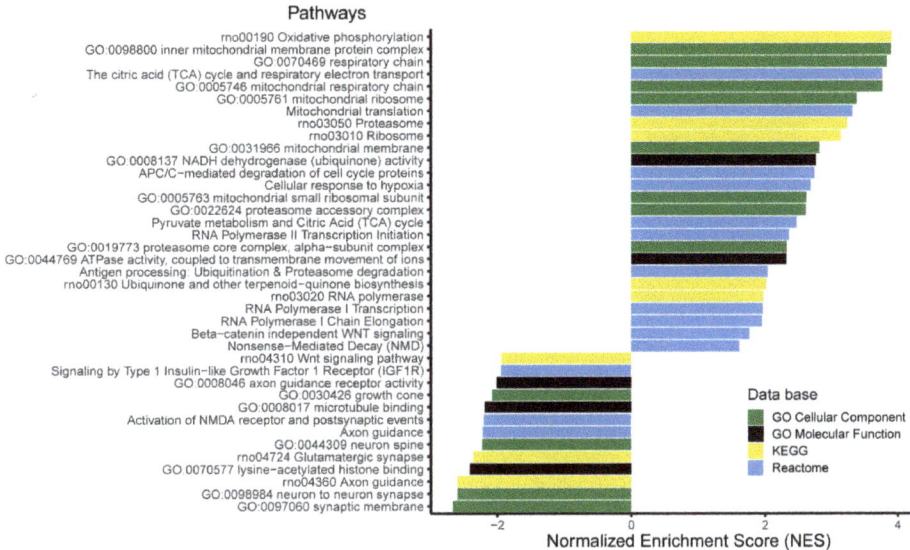

Figure 4. Selection of the gene families and metabolic pathways significantly enriched in differentially expressed genes (Fast Gene Set Enrichment Analysis (FGSEA), padj < 0.05). The pathways with a Normalized Enrichment Score (NES) > 0 are enriched in genes upregulated in the PR group and pathways with an NES < 0 are enriched in genes downregulated in the PR group.

A large number of pathways related to mitochondrial energy metabolism were significantly enriched with an NES > 0 (Figure 4, Supplementary Table S2). These pathways contain the genes encoding proteins of the mitochondrial respiratory chain complexes, including NADH dehydrogenase (*Ndufa1*, *Ndufa12*, *Ndufa13*, *Ndufa2*, *Ndufa4*, *Ndufa5*, *Ndufa7*, *Ndufab1*, *Ndufb4*, *Ndufb8*, *Ndufv2*), ATP synthase (*Atp5f1*, *Atp5f1c*, *Atp5mf*, *Atp5pf*, *Atp6*) and ubiquinone synthase (*Coq5*, *Coq7*). Genes encoding enzymes from the Tricarboxylic Acid (TCA) cycle and pyruvate metabolism were also significantly over expressed in the PR fetuses, as well as genes encoding mitochondrial ribosomal proteins (*Mrpl17*, *Mrpl27*, *Mrpl30*, *Mrpl35*, *Mrpl50*, *Mrpl51*, *Mrpl53*, *Mrps11*, *Mrps18c*) that are involved in mitochondrial translation.

Several pathways related to the proteasome complex were significantly enriched in upregulated genes (Figure 4). The *Ubb* gene, encoding the ubiquitin protein, which forms a polymerized chain that binds to target proteins and shuttles them to the proteasome, was also upregulated in the PR group. In addition, several genes encoding the subunits of the RNA polymerase II (*Polr2e*, *Polr2i*, *Polr2j*) and proteins associated with RNA transcription (*Ccnh*, *Taf6*, *Taf9*, *H3f3b*, *Tbp*) were over-expressed in the PR group, as illustrated by the enrichment of RNA polymerase-related pathways.

The enriched pathways with an NES < 0, i.e., containing genes that were downregulated in the PR group were predominantly related to neurogenesis, axonal growth and synaptogenesis (Figure 4), including the Wnt signaling pathway, a key element in neurodevelopment [34].

3.7. Mitochondrial Membrane Potential Was Enhanced in the Hypothalamus of E17 PR Fetuses

In order to validate, at the cellular level, the relevance of the observed upregulation of several genes related to the mitochondrial oxidative phosphorylation metabolism, we quantified the mitochondrial membrane potential by using a MitoTracker staining method on total cells dissociated immediately after sampling the E17 fetal hypothalami. The MitoTracker molecules diffuse through the inner membrane of active mitochondria, in proportion to their membrane potential, making it possible to quantify the mitochondrial membrane potential. We observed a significantly higher mitochondrial membrane potential in the hypothalamus cells from the PR E17 fetuses (Figure 5).

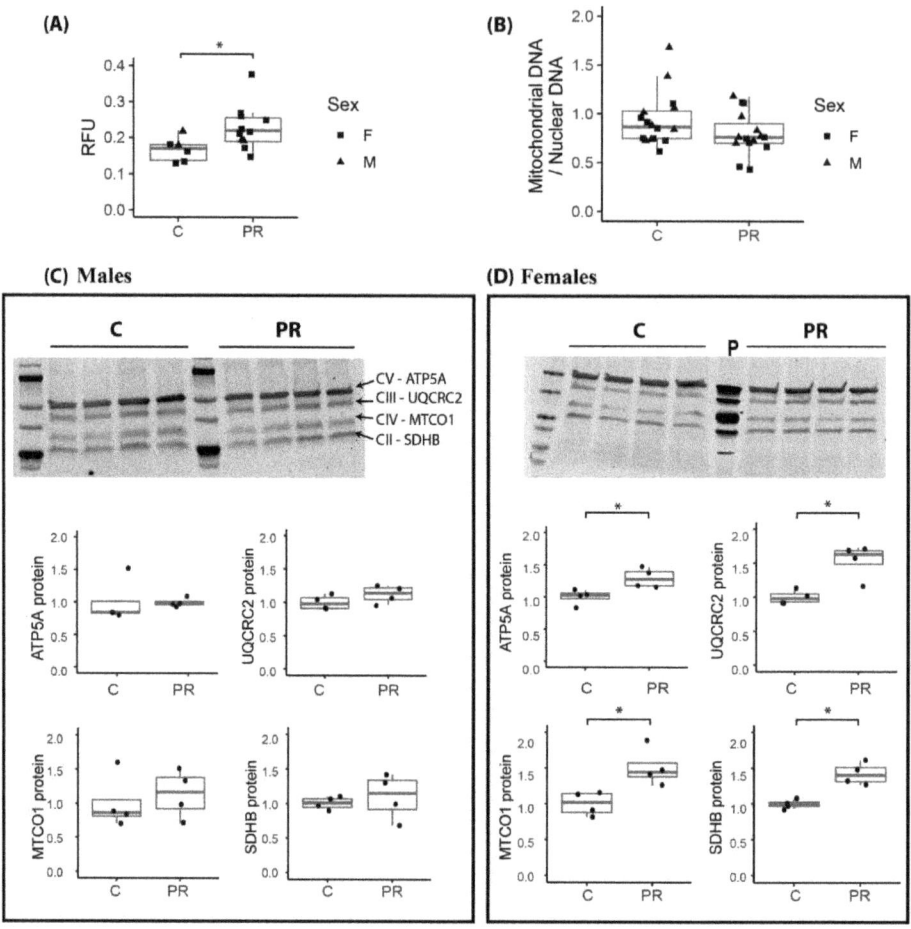

Figure 5. Mitochondrial membrane potential, DNA and protein quantification from total E17 fetal hypothalamus. (**A**) Mitochondrial membrane potential was quantified in dissociated total fetal hypothalamus cells by MitoTracker Red CMXRos and expressed in Relative Fluorescence Units (RFU)/lived cells x 1000 (C: n = two males + four females, PR: n = two males + nine females) (two-way ANOVA: group effect * $p = 0.04$, sex effect $p = 0.91$). (**B**) Mitochondrial DNA was quantified using qPCR amplification on total DNA from E17 whole hypothalamus of the mitochondrial *CytB* gene and normalized with two nuclear genes *Gapdh* and *Zfx-Zfy*. (**C,D**) Four proteins from the mitochondrial respiratory chain complexes (SDHB, MTCO1, UQCRC2 and ATP5A from Complexes II, III, IV and V, respectively) were quantified using Western blot on total proteins from E17 total hypothalamus in four males (**C**) and four females (**D**) from each group. Total protein stain was used for normalization. (Mann Whitney * $p < 0.05$) (p: Positive control = mitochondrial protein extract from rat heart tissue lysate (Abcam ab110341)) (boxplot: median, first and third quartiles).

Then, we quantified mitochondrial DNA in E17 fetal hypothalamus, in order to check if the increase in gene expression could be due to a higher number of mitochondrial genome copy numbers and therefore a higher number of mitochondria per cell (Figure 5B). There was no difference in the amount of mitochondrial DNA between the control and PR fetuses, which suggests that the difference in gene expression level were linked to mitochondrial activity rather than number.

We also quantified, at the protein level, four proteins, SDHB, UQCRC2, MTCO1 and ATP5A, from the complexes II, III, IV and V, of the mitochondrial respiratory chain, respectively (Figure 5C,D). The four proteins were significantly overexpressed in females from the PR group (Figure 5D) whereas there was no difference between control and PR males (Figure 5C).

3.8. The Csde1 Gene, a Major Regulator of Neuronal Differentiation, Was Upregulated in the PR Group

Among the top 20 upregulated genes (Table A1), the *Csde1* gene encodes an RNA-binding protein implicated in the post-transcriptional regulation of a subset of cellular mRNA and was recently shown to prevent neural differentiation [35]. *Csde1* was highly expressed in the fetal hypothalamus (mean normalized read count = 817) and its expression level was about 35% higher in the PR group (log2FC = 0.45, padj = 0.001). Since CSDE1 protein is known to regulate the translation of its own mRNA, the amount of transcript does not necessarily reflect the amount of protein [35]. Therefore, we quantified the amount of CSDE1 protein in fetal hypothalamus using Western Blot and observed a significantly higher level of the protein in the PR group in accordance with the level of mRNA expression, but there was no effect due to the sex (Figure 6).

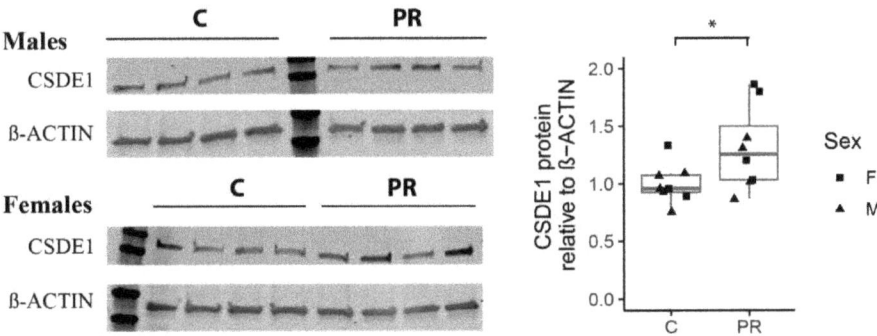

Figure 6. Quantification of the CSDE1 protein in E17 fetal Hypothalamus using Western blot. (PR: n = four males + four females, C: n = four males + four females) (ANOVA, group effect * p = 0.04, sex-effet p = 0.18) (boxplot: median, first and third quartiles).

3.9. The m6A Epitranscriptomic Mark Was Altered in the PR Fetuses

The expression of a family of genes involved in the writing/erasing/reading of the m6A epitranscriptomic mark was impacted by maternal PR. The m6A mark is the most abundant modification of mRNA and its involvement in many developmental processes; in particular, neural stem cell fate and neurodevelopment are attracting increasing interest. The *Wtap*, *Mettl14* and *Mettl3* genes encode proteins that constitute the methylation complex in charge of the writing of the m6A mark, whereas the *Fto* and *Alkbh5* encode the erasers that suppress it. The *Mettl14* gene was significantly under-expressed in the PR group (log2FC = −0.27, padj = 0.04), whereas the *Wtap* gene was over-expressed (log2FC = 0.37, padj = 0.03) and the *Mettl3* gene was unchanged (Figure 7A). In addition, the *Fto* gene showed a tendency to be slightly overexpressed in the PR group (log2FC = 0.18, padj = 0.10), and the *Ythdf2* gene, encoding an m6A reader that reduces mRNA stability, was also significantly overexpressed in the PR group (log2FC = 0.29, padj = 0.01) whereas the *Ythdc1* gene, encoding a reader protein involved in mRNA splicing, was slightly under-expressed (log2FC = −0.27, padj = 0.10) in the PR group (Figure 7A).

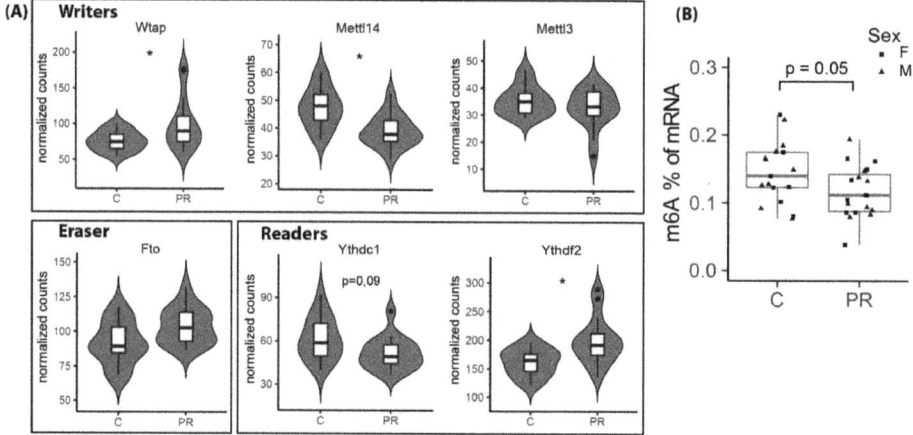

Figure 7. (**A**) Normalized expression level of the genes from the m6A epitranscriptomic machinery obtained using DESeq2 on E17 Hypothalamic RNA sequenced in DGE-seq (PR: n = eight males + eight females, C: n = eight males + eight females) (adjusted p-value from Deseq2 analysis: * padj < 0.05). (**B**) Quantification of the percentage of m6A in total RNA from E17 fetal hypothalamus using m6A immunodetection assay (PR: n = 10 males + nine females, C: n = 10 males + seven females) (two-way ANOVA group effect p = 0.05, sex effect p = 0.73) (boxplot: median, first and third quartiles).

In relation to the variation in the expression of this family of genes, we next quantified the global level of m6A in the mRNAs from E17 fetal hypothalamus. For that purpose, we used an ELISA-based kit involving an antibody specifically designed against the m6A mark. The percentage of m6A in total mRNA varied from 0.08 to 0.20 and was lower in the PR group (p = 0.05), but was not influenced by sex (Figure 7B).

4. Discussion

In this study, we used a well-characterized model of maternal protein restriction during gestation to identify gene families and physiological pathways that were altered in the fetal hypothalamus in response to the maternal PR diet.

The impact of an imbalanced maternal diet on the proliferation and differentiation capacities of neural stem cells during embryo and fetal development is now clearly established [18,36–38]. Our observations on the cells sampled on E17 fetuses and grown in vitro as neurospheres confirmed these alterations. The total number of cells after dissociation of the fetal hypothalami was lower in the PR group, which may reflect reduced proliferation in an earlier period in the PR group. In addition, we observed, after three days of proliferation in vitro, a higher proportion of TUBB3+ cells in the PR group, which may reflect that E17 PR fetuses had initially a higher number of committed neuronal progenitors that proliferated in culture. Similarly, Gould et al. [18] showed that low protein diet throughout gestation was associated with an increase in the number of late neural progenitors in mice brain but tempered by increased apoptosis. Further investigation would be required in order to establish whether this was also the case in our model.

Interestingly, the proportion of cells expressing NES and MAP2 were not different between groups whereas the genes encoding these proteins were under-expressed in the PR group. This may be related to the fact that the level of expression of these genes varies throughout the differentiation process, from early to late progenitors until differentiated neurons. Therefore, the difference in expression level might reflect an alteration in the timing of differentiation which cannot be seen in the immunochemistry experiments that do not distinguish between cells that have variable levels of gene expression. Additionally, we cannot exclude post-transcriptional control of expression.

E17 corresponds approximately to the time when neurogenesis is complete and residual NPCs start to differentiate into astrocytes [13,14]. Indeed, no cell was GFAP-positive at E17 and the *Gfap* gene was not expressed. The switch between neurogenesis and astrocytogenesis is based upon a complex interaction between external signals and a cell-intrinsic program via a strict control of gene expression. This interaction first requires nutrient sensing and detection of metabolic and hormonal signals coming from the mother and the placenta and then the activation of regulatory pathways that control cell differentiation. By using a large scale transcriptomic approach on whole fetal hypothalamus, we highlighted several metabolic pathways and molecular regulation systems that were impacted by maternal PR and led us to propose some mechanistic hypotheses in order to explain alterations of various neurodevelopment processes.

Our data suggested an alteration of the mitochondrial respiratory chain activity in the PR group, as evidenced both by the over-expression of genes encoding the complexes of the respiratory chain and several enzymes from the pyruvate and citric acid metabolism as well as the increased mitochondrial membrane potential of the E17 hypothalamic cells. Mitochondrial DNA copy number was not different between control and PR fetal hypothalamus, suggesting that the difference in the respiratory activity was not a consequence of a major shift in the number of mitochondria, but possibly a difference in their metabolic activity. One interesting observation that would require to be extended to other proteins from the respiratory chain complexes was the fact that the protein level of four of these proteins was increased mostly in females. Although brain mitochondrial metabolism is known to differ between adult males and females both in human and rodents [39,40], there is, to our knowledge, no data in the literature regarding sex effect on mitochondria dynamics and metabolism in the developing fetal brain. Only the testosterone surge occurring around birth in male mice was shown to impact the synthesis of the mitochondrial-specific phospholipid cardiolipin [41].

Mitochondria dynamics is closely associated with cell fate and differentiation process during brain development. Mitochondria structure and metabolism change throughout the differentiation process [42]. At the metabolic level, while energy production relies mostly on glycolysis in undifferentiated cells, it progressively switches to oxidative phosphorylation throughout neural differentiation in order to meet the higher energy requirements of the differentiated neurons [42]. It has also been illustrated that mitochondria dynamics and metabolic shift precede and functionally regulate neuronal differentiation [43].

Several evidences have already established a link between PR during early life and alterations in the mitochondrial metabolism at a later stage of life. Maternal PR was shown to be associated with (1) impaired mitochondrial metabolism in the brain of adult rat offspring [44] and (2) alteration in the expression level of several proteins from the mitochondrial respiratory chain complexes in the hypothalamus of pre-weaned rat [45]. In addition, in human, mitochondrial metabolism is altered in the placenta of neonates suffering from Intra Uterine Growth Restriction that is often the result of a reduced provision of nutrients to the fetus [46]. Oxidative stress that may results from impaired mitochondrial function is indeed evoked as a major programming mechanism in the increased risk of chronic degenerative diseases induced by neonatal protein restriction [47]. However, although the consequences of neonatal PR on mitochondrial metabolism and oxidative stress on several tissues after birth are widely acknowledged, the link between PR, mitochondrial metabolism in fetal brain and an impaired neurodevelopment is, to our knowledge, not documented. Are mitochondria of neural stem/progenitor cells able to function as nutritional sensors and integrate very early on signals from their environment? In a mice model of maternal protein restriction, Eckert et al. [48] demonstrated that, as early as E3.5, the blastocyst was able to sense maternal metabolic alterations, including deficiency in essential amino acids, within uterine fluid and they showed evidence of the implication of the mammalian Target of Rapamycin Complex 1 (mTORC1) signaling pathway in this process. Mitochondrial activity reflects the energetic status of the cells and mitochondria architecture was recently suggested to play an important role in bioenergetics adaptation to metabolic demands [49]. Therefore, mitochondria dynamics constitute a way for the cell to adapt to nutrient shortage or excess.

For instance, nutrient shortage was shown to result in the fusion of mitochondria associated with increased oxidative phosphorylation, which is for the cell the most efficient way to produce ATP [50].

Our data are not sufficient to conclude that mitochondrial respiratory chain activity was definitely increased in the fetal hypothalamus of the PR group and additional experiments are certainly required to confirm this hypothesis. For instance, it could be interesting to measure mitochondrial mass and ROS production. However, the combination of our results regarding this point, together with what is already known about the link between mitochondrial activity and neuronal differentiation strongly supports the impact of maternal PR on these processes.

How the mitochondrial adaptive mechanism, linked to nutrient shortage, interacts with the program of differentiation of neural cells remains to be clarified.

The ubiquitin gene and several genes encoding the subunits of the proteasome complex were also upregulated in the PR fetal hypothalamus. The UPS (Ubiquitin Proteasome System) is closely associated with the mitochondrial metabolism. Mitochondria need the UPS for the removal of proteins that are damaged by ROS (Reactive Oxygen Species) and the proteasome function requires ATP [51]. These two functions are especially important in neuronal function and differentiation [52–54] as well as adult neurogenesis [55]. Although the precise mechanisms of the role of the amino acid sensing pathway mTORC1 in the activation of the proteasome activity in situation of nutrient shortage are still under debate [56], these two major pathways are obviously interconnected [57], suggesting that they may interact in the response of neural cells to amino acid shortage. Cellular response to nutrient shortage may also involve autophagy, another major stress-response system that is closely linked to the mTORC1 detection system and which was shown to be important for neuronal development and axon growth [58]. We did not find evidence of alterations in the expression of genes involved in the autophagy in our model but we did notice enrichment in upregulated genes from the lysosome pathway (Table S2).

Epigenetic control of chromatin conformation [59,60], DNA-binding proteins [61] and transcription factors [62–64] are among the best known molecular actors of the highly complex process of neuronal differentiation. Their action is itself modulated by factors related to the metabolic status of the cell via the remodeling of chromatin [65]. Recently, post-transcriptional control was highlighted as a new layer of regulation in the determinism of cell fate and differentiation, particularly in the brain [66]. Post transcriptional regulation include (1) chemical modifications of mRNA such as epitranscriptomic marks and (2) RNA-binding proteins that are involved in mRNA stability, turn-over, trafficking, degradation and translation.

We have shown, in our large-scale transcriptomic study, and confirmed (by the quantification of m6A) that the expression of several genes from the m6A epitranscriptomic machinery was significantly disturbed in the PR fetuses and that this was linked to a decrease in the global level of m6A. The m6A epitranscriptomic mark is the major mRNA modification identified so far and is associated with the control of various aspects of mRNA functions including stability, degradation, trafficking, splicing and translation [67]. The brain is the tissue where this mark is the highest and it is especially present in mRNAs implicated in transcriptional regulation, cell adhesion, axon guidance and synaptogenesis [68]. In addition, Yoon et al. [69] recently demonstrated that depleting the writing of the m6A mark by inactivation of the *Mettl14* gene in the embryonic brain of mice prolongs neurogenesis postnatally. This was associated with a decrease in the turnover of mRNAs encoding proteins involved in cell cycle, neurogenesis, and neuronal differentiation. The action of the m6A mark is mediated through interaction with different RNA-binding proteins that specifically recognize methylated or unmethylated mRNAs and will subsequently promote transcript fate [67]. Interestingly, the m6A mark was demonstrated to be involved in the action of the Fragile X Mental Retardation Protein (FMRP) which is an RNA-binding protein with a major role in synapse function [68] and that was shown to be over-expressed in the cortex of mice that suffered from fetal protein restriction [18]. Although the expression of the *Fmr1* gene was not altered in our model, the *Fxr1* gene was downregulated in the PR group. Since this gene also encodes an RNA-binding protein that was recently shown to control the translation of the mitochondrial

Cox2 gene [70] and since *Cox 2* was one of the most expressed and significantly upregulated genes in the PR group, a possible link could exist between the m6A mark, RNA-binding proteins and mitochondrial function. On the other hand, FTO protein, which acts as a m6A demethylase, was shown to have a role in the cellular sensing of amino acids via the mTORC1 pathway and this activity was associated with its demethylase function [71]. In addition, the mTORC1 pathway was demonstrated to mediate the link between nutrient shortage and the control of protein synthesis at the post transcriptional level [66]. Interestingly, the mRNAs that are regulated by this system are enriched for the consensus motif of the m6A epitranscriptomic mark [66]. All these elements converge to propose the m6A mark as a major actor in the impact of amino acid deficiency on hypothalamus development.

The role of post-transcriptional regulation in the consequences of PR on the timing of neurogenesis was also suggested by the over-expression at both the transcription and translation levels of CSDE1 in the PR group. The CSDE1 protein was recently shown to be a master regulator of neuronal differentiation, by regulating, at the translational level, the expression of a large number of genes [35]. The expression of CSDE1 decreases throughout differentiation and modulates the transcriptional landscape by controlling the expression of key regulators of cell fate and neuronal differentiation. Therefore, the overexpression of both the gene and the protein that we observed in the PR group may reflect a delay in the neuronal differentiation process that may be consistent with a higher number of neuronal progenitors.

The DGE-seq approach was rather helpful for the detection of the pathways impacted by maternal diet. Of course, transcriptomic data do not always reflect the amount of proteins, but the DGE-seq approach is rather straightforward and more sensitive that a proteomics approach for the detection of mild effects. The proof is that we have indeed been able to identify key players in post-transcriptional regulation who are certainly involved in the impact of fetal nutrition in the precise control of neuronal differentiation. We made the choice to focus here on metabolic pathways and gene families that were, in our opinion, relevant regarding the physiological and cellular alterations observed in our model, but the transcriptomic approach also identified many other genes that certainly may require further investigation. The magnitude of gene expression change between PR and control fetuses was rather modest. However, major cellular pathways related to energy metabolism and neuronal differentiation have been impacted, so we believe that even mild disturbances can have repercussions on a process as precise and finely regulated as neuronal differentiation.

5. Conclusions

In conclusion, our study identified a number of cellular and molecular pathways that could link an environmental event such as PR to alterations in cellular metabolism, leading to early alterations of neuronal development and subsequent impaired hypothalamus function. These hypotheses certainly require further investigation, but we believe that a global approach like ours could be useful in obtaining an overview of all biological systems, including nutrient detection, energy metabolism and the control of transcription/translation, which could link nutritional status to the regulation of cell differentiation, especially in models where the effects are mild and multiple.

Supplementary Materials: The following are available online at http://www.mdpi.com/2072-6643/12/5/1464/s1. Table S1: DESeq2 output [27] obtained from the differential gene expression analysis. BaseMean column indicates mean of normalized counts for each gene at all ages used for DGE-seq (E17, D0 and D130). BaseMeanE17 column indicates mean of normalized counts for each gene only at E17. Padj: adjusted *p*-value. DE: Differential Expression (UP: PR > C padj < 0.05; DOWN: PR < C padj < 0.05; NONE: padj > 0.05). Table S2: FGSEA (Fast Gene Set Enrichment Analysis) output [29] obtained from functional enrichment analysis using Reactome, KEGG and GO databases.

Author Contributions: Conceptualization, M.F., V.P., P.P. and V.A.; Data curation, M.F. and D.M.; Formal analysis, M.F., D.M. and V.A.; Funding acquisition, P.P. and V.A.; Investigation, M.F., S.G., I.G., V.S.M. and V.A.; Methodology, M.F., I.G. and V.A.; Project administration, V.A.; Resources, P.P. and V.A.; Software, D.M.; Supervision, P.P. and V.A.; Validation, M.F. and V.A.; Writing—Original draft, M.F. and V.A.; Writing—Review & Editing, M.F., V.S.M., V.P., P.P. and V.A. All authors have read and agreed to the published version of the manuscript.

Funding: This work was funded by INRAE. M.F. is supported by a PhD fellowship from INRAE and Région Pays de la Loire and VSM by a postdoc fellowship from the Fondation pour la Recherche Médicale (ARF20170938730).

Acknowledgments: We thank MicroPICell facility (SFR François Bonamy, Nantes Université, INSERM, CNRS) for their help in microscopy and especially Magalie Feyeux for image analysis, and GenoBIRD facility (SFR François Bonamy, Nantes Université, INSERM, CNRS) for the sequencing and primary analysis of the DGE-seq experiments. We are grateful to Blandine Castellano, Diane Beuzelin, and Laurent David for technical help and advice.

Conflicts of Interest: The authors declare no conflict of interest. The funders had no role in the design of the study; in the collection, analyses, or interpretation of data; in the writing of the manuscript, or in the decision to publish the results.

Appendix A

Table A1. Top 20 upregulated genes in the protein-restricted group.

Gene Symbol	Log2FC	Padj	Base Mean	Full Name	Function(s) *
Slc35c2	0.469	0.031	24.122	Solute carrier family 35 member C2	May play a role in cellular response to tissue hypoxia
Ppcs	0.463	0.042	12.650	Phosphopantothenoylcysteine synthetase	Involved in the biosynthesis of coenzyme A, a precursor of Acetyl CoA
Csde1	0.452	0.001	817.685	Cold shock domain containing E1	RNA-binding protein—prevents neuronal differentiation in neural stem cells
Nipa2	0.437	0.028	19.597	Nipa magnesium transporter 2	Non-imprinted gene in Prader–Willi/Angelman syndrome region
Coa5	0.429	0.006	117.035	Cytochrome C oxydase assembly factor 5	Involved in the mitochondrial complex IV assembly
Cirbp	0.428	0.002	250.612	Cold inducible RNA-binding protein	Essential for embryonic gastrulation and neural development
Hs6st1	0.423	0.030	91.038	Heparan-sulfate 6-O-sulfotransferase 1	Critical for normal neuronal development, may play a role in neuron branching
LOC100174910	0.418	0.010	48.852	Glutaredoxin-like protein	Involved in oxidation-reduction process. May be involved in cell redox homeostasis
Wdr83	0.407	0.044	34.218	WD repeat domain-containing protein 83	Involved in response to hypoxia
Tmem53	0.406	0.025	27.565	Transmembrane protein 53	
Ube2n	0.405	0.002	83.937	Ubiquitin conjugating enzyme E2N	Involved in protein ubiquitination. Plays a role in the control of cell cycle and differentiation
Tmcc2	0.397	0.044	55.090	Transmembrane and coiled-coil domains protein 2	Expressed in endoplasmic reticulum
Sec23b	0.395	0.044	23.013	COPII coat complex component	Involved in protein transport from endoplasmic reticulum
Coq7	0.393	0.001	120.626	coenzyme Q7 hydroxylase	Involved in ubiquinone synthesis, in mitochondrial respiratory metabolism
Chrac1	0.391	0.006	66.458	Chromatin accessibility complex protein 1	Histone-fold protein that binds DNA. May be involved in cell growth and survival
Rbm7	0.377	0.044	20.552	RNA-binding protein 7	Member of the exosome targeting complex, involved in RNA degradation
Wtap	0.373	0.031	87.528	WT1 associated protein	Member of the complex that mediate m6A methylation of RNAs
Mterf1	0.367	0.032	30.933	Mitochondrial transcription termination factor 1	DNA-binding protein, involved in termination of mitochondrial transcription
Marcks	0.365	0.026	1055.600	Myristoylated alanine rich protein kinase C substrate	Binds protein of cytoskeleton, may be involved in cell migration
Pqlc1	0.365	0.044	39.620	Solute carrier family 66 member 2	Involved in phospholipid translocation

*: from the UNIPROT database (www.uniprot.org) [72] and the NCBI/Gene database (www.ncbi.nlm.nih.gov/gene) [73].

Table A2. Top 20 downregulated genes in the protein-restricted group.

Gene Symbol	log2FC	Padj	Base Mean	Full Name	Function(s) *
Brsk1	−0.807	0.010	13.066	Serine Threonine protein kinase	Role in polarization of neurons and centrosome duplication
Fgfr1op	−0.676	0.002	19.199	FGFR1 oncogen partner	Required for anchoring microtubules to the centrosomes. Involved in cell proliferation
Qk	−0.658	0.003	22.941	Quaking	RNA-binding protein that regulates pre-mRNA splicing, export, stability and translation. Involved in oligodendrogenesis
Tcf20	−0.636	0.024	19.373	Transcription factor 20	Transcriptional activator. May be involved in neurodevelopment
Cask	−0.625	0.013	23.749	Calcium/calmodulin dependent serine protein kinase	Involved in synaptic membrane protein anchoring. Contributes to neurodevelopment
Eps15	−0.607	0.021	12.515	Epidermal growth factor receptor pathway substrate 15	Involved in cell growth regulation. May be involved in the control of cell proliferation
Robo1	−0.600	0.009	56.779	Roundabout guidance receptor 1	Involved in axon guidance and neuronal precursor cell migration
Fam168a	−0.569	0.010	19.145	Also known as Tcrp1	Involved in cancer chemotherapy resistance
Iqgap1	−0.566	0.009	18.290	IQ motif containing GTPase activating protein 1	Regulates the assembly and dynamic if the cytoskeleton. May promote neurite outgrowth.
Phactr3	−0.560	0.025	15.498	Phosphatase and actin regulator 3	Associated with the nuclear scaffold in proliferating cells
Myo18a	−0.548	0.009	28.595	Myosin 18A	Associated with the Golgi. May be required for cell migration
Sesn3	−0.541	0.045	17.734	Sestrin 3	Required for regulation of glucose and insulin regulation. May be involved in the protection against oxidative stress
Kcnma1	−0.530	0.044	16.245	Potassium calcium-activated channel subfamily M alpha 1	Involved in the control of neuron excitability
Pclo	−0.529	0.002	95.164	Piccolo presynaptic cytomatrix protein	Involved in synaptogenesis
Mgat3	−0.526	0.024	19.383	beta−1,4-mannosyl-glycoprotein 4 beta-N-Acetylglucosaminyltransferase	May be involved in response to oxidative stress in brain and in cell migration regulation
Timp3	−0.526	0.049	10.279	TIMP metallopeptidase inhibitor 3	
Taok1	−0.518	0.007	43.989	Serine Threonine protein kinase TAO1	Acts as a regulator of cytoskeleton stability. May be involved in the induction of apoptosis
Nlgn1	−0.515	0.031	15.813	Neuroligin 1	Neuronal cell surface protein. May be involved in the formation and remodeling of synapses
Kpnb1	−0.511	0.025	18.776	Karyopherin subunit beta 1	Involved in nuclear protein import, including ribosomal proteins and histone H1
Slmap	−0.510	0.028	14.084	Sarcolemma associated protein	Membrane associated protein

*: from the UNIPROT database (www.uniprot.org) [72] and the NCBI/Gene database (www.ncbi.nlm.nih.gov/gene) [73].

References

1. Katz, J.; Lee, A.C.; Kozuki, N.; Lawn, J.E.; Cousens, S.; Blencowe, H.; Ezzati, M.; Bhutta, Z.A.; Marchant, T.; Willey, B.A.; et al. Mortality risk in preterm and small-for-gestational-age infants in low-income and middle-income countries: A pooled country analysis. *Lancet* **2013**, *382*, 417–425. [CrossRef]
2. Sibley, C.P.; Brownbill, P.; Dilworth, M.; Glazier, J.D. Review: Adaptation in placental nutrient supply to meet fetal growth demand: Implications for programming. *Placenta* **2010**, *31*, S70–S74. [CrossRef]
3. Frondas-Chauty, A.; Simon, L.; Flamant, C.; Hanf, M.; Darmaun, D.; Roze, J.C. Deficit of Fat Free Mass in Very Preterm Infants at Discharge is Associated with Neurological Impairment at Age 2 Years. *J. Pediatr.* **2018**, *196*, 301–304. [CrossRef]

4. Ehrenkranz, R.A.; Dusick, A.M.; Vohr, B.R.; Wright, L.L.; Wrage, L.A.; Poole, W.K. Growth in the neonatal intensive care unit influences neurodevelopmental and growth outcomes of extremely low birth weight infants. *Pediatrics* **2006**, *117*, 1253–1261. [CrossRef]
5. Barker, D.J. Adult consequences of fetal growth restriction. *Clin. Obstet. Gynecol.* **2006**, *49*, 270–283. [CrossRef]
6. Delahaye, F.; Breton, C.; Risold, P.Y.; Enache, M.; Dutriez-Casteloot, I.; Laborie, C.; Lesage, J.; Vieau, D. Maternal perinatal undernutrition drastically reduces postnatal leptin surge and affects the development of arcuate nucleus proopiomelanocortin neurons in neonatal male rat pups. *Endocrinology* **2008**, *149*, 470–475. [CrossRef]
7. Bouret, S.G. Role of early hormonal and nutritional experiences in shaping feeding behavior and hypothalamic development. *J. Nutr.* **2010**, *140*, 653–657. [CrossRef]
8. Coupe, B.; Amarger, V.; Grit, I.; Benani, A.; Parnet, P. Nutritional programming affects hypothalamic organization and early response to leptin. *Endocrinology* **2010**, *151*, 702–713. [CrossRef]
9. Coupe, B.; Grit, I.; Hulin, P.; Randuineau, G.; Parnet, P. Postnatal growth after intrauterine growth restriction alters central leptin signal and energy homeostasis. *PLoS ONE* **2012**, *7*, e30616. [CrossRef]
10. Dearden, L.; Bouret, S.G.; Ozanne, S.E. Sex and gender differences in developmental programming of metabolism. *Mol. Metab.* **2018**, *15*, 8–19. [CrossRef]
11. Bedont, J.L.; Newman, E.A.; Blackshaw, S. Patterning, specification, and differentiation in the developing hypothalamus. *Wiley Interdiscip. Rev. Dev. Biol.* **2015**, *4*, 445–468. [CrossRef]
12. Markakis, E.A. Development of the neuroendocrine hypothalamus. *Front. Neuroendocr.* **2002**, *23*, 257–291. [CrossRef]
13. Bouret, S.G. Nutritional programming of hypothalamic development: Critical periods and windows of opportunity. *Int. J. Obes. Suppl.* **2012**, *2*, S19–S24. [CrossRef]
14. Gotz, M.; Huttner, W.B. The cell biology of neurogenesis. *Nat. Rev. Mol. Cell Biol.* **2005**, *6*, 777–788. [CrossRef]
15. Moody, L.; Chen, H.; Pan, Y.X. Early-Life Nutritional Programming of Cognition-The Fundamental Role of Epigenetic Mechanisms in Mediating the Relation between Early-Life Environment and Learning and Memory Process. *Adv. Nutr.* **2017**, *8*, 337–350. [CrossRef]
16. Val-Laillet, D.; Besson, M.; Guerin, S.; Coquery, N.; Randuineau, G.; Kanzari, A.; Quesnel, H.; Bonhomme, N.; Bolhuis, J.E.; Kemp, B.; et al. A maternal Western diet during gestation and lactation modifies offspring's microbiota activity, blood lipid levels, cognitive responses, and hippocampal neurogenesis in Yucatan pigs. *FASEB J.* **2017**, *31*, 2037–2049. [CrossRef]
17. Staples, M.C.; Fannon, M.J.; Mysore, K.K.; Dutta, R.R.; Ongjoco, A.T.; Quach, L.W.; Kharidia, K.M.; Somkuwar, S.S.; Mandyam, C.D. Dietary restriction reduces hippocampal neurogenesis and granule cell neuron density without affecting the density of mossy fibers. *Brain Res.* **2017**, *1663*, 59–65. [CrossRef]
18. Gould, J.M.; Smith, P.J.; Airey, C.J.; Mort, E.J.; Airey, L.E.; Warricker, F.D.M.; Pearson-Farr, J.E.; Weston, E.C.; Gould, P.J.W.; Semmence, O.G.; et al. Mouse maternal protein restriction during preimplantation alone permanently alters brain neuron proportion and adult short-term memory. *Proc. Natl. Acad. Sci. USA* **2018**, *115*, 7398–7407. [CrossRef]
19. Desai, M.; Li, T.; Ross, M.G. Fetal hypothalamic neuroprogenitor cell culture: Preferential differentiation paths induced by leptin and insulin. *Endocrinology* **2011**, *152*, 3192–3201. [CrossRef]
20. Desai, M.; Ferrini, M.G.; Han, G.; Jellyman, J.K.; Ross, M.G. In vivo maternal and in vitro BPA exposure effects on hypothalamic neurogenesis and appetite regulators. *Environ. Res.* **2018**, *164*, 45–52. [CrossRef]
21. Cariaga-Martinez, A.E.; Gutierrez, K.J.; Alelu-Paz, R. The Vast Complexity of the Epigenetic Landscape during Neurodevelopment: An Open Frame to Understanding Brain Function. *Int. J. Mol. Sci.* **2018**, *19*, 1333. [CrossRef]
22. Tran, N.T.; Amarger, V.; Bourdon, A.; Misbert, E.; Grit, I.; Winer, N.; Darmaun, D. Maternal citrulline supplementation enhances placental function and fetal growth in a rat model of IUGR: Involvement of insulin-like growth factor 2 and angiogenic factors. *J. Matern.-Fetal Neonatal Med.* **2017**, *30*, 1906–1911. [CrossRef]
23. Martin Agnoux, A.; Antignac, J.P.; Simard, G.; Poupeau, G.; Darmaun, D.; Parnet, P.; Alexandre-Gouabau, M.C. Time-window dependent effect of perinatal maternal protein restriction on insulin sensitivity and energy substrate oxidation in adult male offspring. *Am. J. Physiol. Regul. Integr. Comp. Physiol.* **2014**, *307*, R184–R197. [CrossRef]

24. Sevrin, T.; Alexandre-Gouabau, M.C.; Castellano, B.; Aguesse, A.; Ouguerram, K.; Ngyuen, P.; Darmaun, D.; Boquien, C.Y. Impact of Fenugreek on Milk Production in Rodent Models of Lactation Challenge. *Nutrients* **2019**, *11*, 2571. [CrossRef]
25. Schindelin, J.; Arganda-Carreras, I.; Frise, E.; Kaynig, V.; Longair, M.; Pietzsch, T.; Preibisch, S.; Rueden, C.; Saalfeld, S.; Schmid, B.; et al. Fiji: An open-source platform for biological-image analysis. *Nat. Methods* **2012**, *9*, 676–682. [CrossRef]
26. Soumillon, M.; Cacchiarelli, D.; Semrau, S. Characterization of directed differentiation by high-throughput single-cell RNA-Seq. *BioRxiv* **2014**, BioRxiv:003236. Available online: https://www.biorxiv.org/content/early/2014/03/05/003236 (accessed on 26 November 2014).
27. Love, M.I.; Huber, W.; Anders, S. Moderated estimation of fold change and dispersion for RNA-seq data with DESeq2. *Genome Biol.* **2014**, *15*, 550. [CrossRef]
28. Kilens, S.; Meistermann, D.; Moreno, D.; Chariau, C.; Gaignerie, A.; Reignier, A.; Lelievre, Y.; Casanova, M.; Vallot, C.; Nedellec, S.; et al. Parallel derivation of isogenic human primed and naive induced pluripotent stem cells. *Nat. Commun.* **2018**, *9*, 360. [CrossRef]
29. Korotkevich, G.; Sukhov, V.; Sergushichev, A. Fast gene set enrichment analysis. *BioRxiv* **2019**, BioRxiv:060012. Available online: https://www.biorxiv.org/content/10.1101/060012v2 (accessed on 22 October 2019).
30. The Gene Ontology, C. The Gene Ontology Resource: 20 years and still GOing strong. *Nucleic Acids Res.* **2019**, *47*, D330–D338. [CrossRef]
31. Kanehisa, M.; Goto, S. KEGG: Kyoto encyclopedia of genes and genomes. *Nucleic Acids Res.* **2000**, *28*, 27–30. [CrossRef]
32. Jassal, B.; Matthews, L.; Viteri, G.; Gong, C.; Lorente, P.; Fabregat, A.; Sidiropoulos, K.; Cook, J.; Gillespie, M.; Haw, R.; et al. The reactome pathway knowledgebase. *Nucleic Acids Res.* **2020**, *48*, D498–D503. [CrossRef] [PubMed]
33. Subramanian, A.; Tamayo, P.; Mootha, V.K.; Mukherjee, S.; Ebert, B.L.; Gillette, M.A.; Paulovich, A.; Pomeroy, S.L.; Golub, T.R.; Lander, E.S.; et al. Gene set enrichment analysis: A knowledge-based approach for interpreting genome-wide expression profiles. *Proc. Natl. Acad. Sci. USA* **2005**, *102*, 15545–15550. [CrossRef] [PubMed]
34. Mulligan, K.A.; Cheyette, B.N. Wnt signaling in vertebrate neural development and function. *J. Neuroimmune Pharmacol.* **2012**, *7*, 774–787. [CrossRef] [PubMed]
35. Ju Lee, H.; Bartsch, D.; Xiao, C.; Guerrero, S.; Ahuja, G.; Schindler, C.; Moresco, J.J.; Yates, J.R.; Gebauer, F.; Bazzi, H.; et al. A post-transcriptional program coordinated by CSDE1 prevents intrinsic neural differentiation of human embryonic stem cells. *Nat. Commun.* **2017**, *8*, 1456. [CrossRef] [PubMed]
36. Coupe, B.; Dutriez-Casteloot, I.; Breton, C.; Lefevre, F.; Mairesse, J.; Dickes-Coopman, A.; Silhol, M.; Tapia-Arancibia, L.; Lesage, J.; Vieau, D. Perinatal undernutrition modifies cell proliferation and brain-derived neurotrophic factor levels during critical time-windows for hypothalamic and hippocampal development in the male rat. *J. Neuroendocr.* **2009**, *21*, 40–48. [CrossRef]
37. Amarger, V.; Lecouillard, A.; Ancellet, L.; Grit, I.; Castellano, B.; Hulin, P.; Parnet, P. Protein content and methyl donors in maternal diet interact to influence the proliferation rate and cell fate of neural stem cells in rat hippocampus. *Nutrients* **2014**, *6*, 4200–4217. [CrossRef]
38. Desai, M.; Li, T.; Ross, M.G. Hypothalamic neurosphere progenitor cells in low birth-weight rat newborns: Neurotrophic effects of leptin and insulin. *Brain Res.* **2011**, *1378*, 29–42. [CrossRef]
39. Guevara, R.; Santandreu, F.M.; Valle, A.; Gianotti, M.; Oliver, J.; Roca, P. Sex-dependent differences in aged rat brain mitochondrial function and oxidative stress. *Free. Radic. Biol. Med.* **2009**, *46*, 169–175. [CrossRef]
40. Gaignard, P.; Frechou, M.; Liere, P.; Therond, P.; Schumacher, M.; Slama, A.; Guennoun, R. Sex differences in brain mitochondrial metabolism: Influence of endogenous steroids and stroke. *J. Neuroendocr.* **2018**, *30*, e12497. [CrossRef]
41. Acaz-Fonseca, E.; Ortiz-Rodriguez, A.; Lopez-Rodriguez, A.B.; Garcia-Segura, L.M.; Astiz, M. Developmental Sex Differences in the Metabolism of Cardiolipin in Mouse Cerebral Cortex Mitochondria. *Sci. Rep.* **2017**, *7*, 43878. [CrossRef]
42. Khacho, M.; Harris, R.; Slack, R.S. Mitochondria as central regulators of neural stem cell fate and cognitive function. *Nat. Rev. Neurosci.* **2019**, *20*, 34–48. [CrossRef] [PubMed]

43. Khacho, M.; Clark, A.; Svoboda, D.S.; Azzi, J.; MacLaurin, J.G.; Meghaizel, C.; Sesaki, H.; Lagace, D.C.; Germain, M.; Harper, M.E.; et al. Mitochondrial Dynamics Impacts Stem Cell Identity and Fate Decisions by Regulating a Nuclear Transcriptional Program. *Cell Stem Cell* **2016**, *19*, 232–247. [CrossRef] [PubMed]
44. Ferreira, D.J.S.; Pedroza, A.A.; Braz, G.R.F.; Fernandes, M.P.; Lagranha, C.J. Mitochondrial dysfunction: Maternal protein restriction as a trigger of reactive species overproduction and brainstem energy failure in male offspring brainstem. *Nutr. Neurosci.* **2018**, *22*, 778–788. [CrossRef]
45. Alexandre-Gouabau, M.C.; Bailly, E.; Moyon, T.L.; Grit, I.C.; Coupe, B.; Le Drean, G.; Rogniaux, H.J.; Parnet, P. Postnatal growth velocity modulates alterations of proteins involved in metabolism and neuronal plasticity in neonatal hypothalamus in rats born with intrauterine growth restriction. *J. Nutr. Biochem.* **2011**, *23*, 140–152. [CrossRef]
46. Guitart-Mampel, M.; Juarez-Flores, D.L.; Youssef, L.; Moren, C.; Garcia-Otero, L.; Roca-Agujetas, V.; Catalan-Garcia, M.; Gonzalez-Casacuberta, I.; Tobias, E.; Milisenda, J.C.; et al. Mitochondrial implications in human pregnancies with intrauterine growth restriction and associated cardiac remodelling. *J. Cell. Mol. Med.* **2019**, *23*, 3962–3973. [CrossRef]
47. Martin-Gronert, M.S.; Ozanne, S.E. Mechanisms underlying the developmental origins of disease. *Rev. Endocr. Metab. Disord.* **2012**, *13*, 85–92. [CrossRef]
48. Eckert, J.J.; Porter, R.; Watkins, A.J.; Burt, E.; Brooks, S.; Leese, H.J.; Humpherson, P.G.; Cameron, I.T.; Fleming, T.P. Metabolic induction and early responses of mouse blastocyst developmental programming following maternal low protein diet affecting life-long health. *PLoS ONE* **2012**, *7*, e52791. [CrossRef]
49. Liesa, M.; Shirihai, O.S. Mitochondrial dynamics in the regulation of nutrient utilization and energy expenditure. *Cell Metab.* **2013**, *17*, 491–506. [CrossRef]
50. Gomes, L.C.; Di Benedetto, G.; Scorrano, L. During autophagy mitochondria elongate, are spared from degradation and sustain cell viability. *Nat. Cell Biol.* **2011**, *13*, 589–598. [CrossRef]
51. Ross, J.M.; Olson, L.; Coppotelli, G. Mitochondrial and Ubiquitin Proteasome System Dysfunction in Ageing and Disease: Two Sides of the Same Coin? *Int. J. Mol. Sci.* **2015**, *16*, 19458–19476. [CrossRef]
52. Ekstrand, M.I.; Terzioglu, M.; Galter, D.; Zhu, S.; Hofstetter, C.; Lindqvist, E.; Thams, S.; Bergstrand, A.; Hansson, F.S.; Trifunovic, A.; et al. Progressive parkinsonism in mice with respiratory-chain-deficient dopamine neurons. *Proc. Natl. Acad. Sci. USA* **2007**, *104*, 1325–1330. [CrossRef] [PubMed]
53. Cook, C.; Petrucelli, L. A critical evaluation of the ubiquitin-proteasome system in Parkinson's disease. *Biochim. Biophys. Acta-Mol. Basis Dis.* **2009**, *1792*, 664–675. [CrossRef] [PubMed]
54. Sahu, I.; Nanaware, P.; Mane, M.; Mulla, S.W.; Roy, S.; Venkatraman, P. Role of a 19S Proteasome Subunit-PSMD10(Gankyrin) in Neurogenesis of Human Neuronal Progenitor Cells. *Int. J. Stem Cells* **2019**, *12*, 463. [CrossRef]
55. Niu, X.; Zhao, Y.; Yang, N.; Zhao, X.; Zhang, W.; Bai, X.; Li, A.; Yang, W.; Lu, L. Proteasome activation by insulin-like growth factor-1/nuclear factor erythroid 2-related factor 2 signaling promotes exercise-induced neurogenesis. *Stem Cells* **2019**, *38*, 246–260. [CrossRef]
56. Adegoke, O.A.J.; Beatty, B.E.; Kimball, S.R.; Wing, S.S. Interactions of the super complexes: When mTORC1 meets the proteasome. *Int. J. Biochem. Cell Biol.* **2019**, *117*, 105638. [CrossRef]
57. Chantranupong, L.; Sabatini, D.M. Cell biology: The TORC1 pathway to protein destruction. *Nature* **2016**, *536*, 155–156. [CrossRef]
58. Lee, K.M.; Hwang, S.K.; Lee, J.A. Neuronal autophagy and neurodevelopmental disorders. *Exp. Neurobiol.* **2013**, *22*, 133–142. [CrossRef]
59. Sanosaka, T.; Namihira, M.; Nakashima, K. Epigenetic mechanisms in sequential differentiation of neural stem cells. *Epigenetics* **2009**, *4*, 89–92. [CrossRef]
60. Juliandi, B.; Abematsu, M.; Nakashima, K. Epigenetic regulation in neural stem cell differentiation. *Dev. Growth Differ.* **2010**, *52*, 493–504. [CrossRef]
61. Tsujimura, K.; Abematsu, M.; Kohyama, J.; Namihira, M.; Nakashima, K. Neuronal differentiation of neural precursor cells is promoted by the methyl-CpG-binding protein MeCP2. *Exp. Neurol.* **2009**, *219*, 104–111. [CrossRef]
62. Saito, A.; Kanemoto, S.; Kawasaki, N.; Asada, R.; Iwamoto, H.; Oki, M.; Miyagi, H.; Izumi, S.; Sanosaka, T.; Nakashima, K.; et al. Unfolded protein response, activated by OASIS family transcription factors, promotes astrocyte differentiation. *Nat. Commun.* **2012**, *3*, 967. [CrossRef] [PubMed]

63. Imayoshi, I.; Kageyama, R. bHLH factors in self-renewal, multipotency, and fate choice of neural progenitor cells. *Neuron* **2014**, *82*, 9–23. [CrossRef] [PubMed]
64. Imayoshi, I.; Isomura, A.; Harima, Y.; Kawaguchi, K.; Kori, H.; Miyachi, H.; Fujiwara, T.; Ishidate, F.; Kageyama, R. Oscillatory control of factors determining multipotency and fate in mouse neural progenitors. *Science* **2013**, *342*, 1203–1208. [CrossRef] [PubMed]
65. Berger, S.L.; Sassone-Corsi, P. Metabolic Signaling to Chromatin. *Cold Spring Harb. Perspect. Biol.* **2016**, *8*, a019463. [CrossRef]
66. Baser, A.; Skabkin, M.; Kleber, S.; Dang, Y.; Gulculer Balta, G.S.; Kalamakis, G.; Gopferich, M.; Ibanez, D.C.; Schefzik, R.; Lopez, A.S.; et al. Onset of differentiation is post-transcriptionally controlled in adult neural stem cells. *Nature* **2019**, *566*, 100–104. [CrossRef]
67. Widagdo, J.; Anggono, V. The m6A-epitranscriptomic signature in neurobiology: From neurodevelopment to brain plasticity. *J. Neurochem.* **2018**, *147*, 137–152. [CrossRef]
68. Chang, M.; Lv, H.; Zhang, W.; Ma, C.; He, X.; Zhao, S.; Zhang, Z.W.; Zeng, Y.X.; Song, S.; Niu, Y.; et al. Region-specific RNA m(6)A methylation represents a new layer of control in the gene regulatory network in the mouse brain. *Open Biol.* **2017**, *7*, 170166. [CrossRef]
69. Yoon, K.J.; Ringeling, F.R.; Vissers, C.; Jacob, F.; Pokrass, M.; Jimenez-Cyrus, D.; Su, Y.; Kim, N.S.; Zhu, Y.; Zheng, L.; et al. Temporal Control of Mammalian Cortical Neurogenesis by m(6)A Methylation. *Cell* **2017**, *171*, 877–889.e17. [CrossRef]
70. Li, X.C.; Song, M.F.; Sun, F.; Tian, F.J.; Wang, Y.M.; Wang, B.Y.; Chen, J.H. Fragile X-related protein 1 (FXR1) regulates cyclooxygenase-2 (COX-2) expression at the maternal-fetal interface. *Reprod. Fertil. Dev.* **2018**, *30*, 1566–1574. [CrossRef]
71. Gulati, P.; Cheung, M.K.; Antrobus, R.; Church, C.D.; Harding, H.P.; Tung, Y.C.; Rimmington, D.; Ma, M.; Ron, D.; Lehner, P.J.; et al. Role for the obesity-related FTO gene in the cellular sensing of amino acids. *Proc. Natl. Acad. Sci. USA* **2013**, *110*, 2557–2562. [CrossRef]
72. UniProt, C. UniProt: A worldwide hub of protein knowledge. *Nucleic Acids Res.* **2019**, *47*, D506–D515. [CrossRef]
73. Coordinators, N.R. Database resources of the National Center for Biotechnology Information. *Nucleic Acids Res.* **2018**, *46*, D8–D13. [CrossRef] [PubMed]

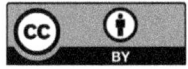

© 2020 by the authors. Licensee MDPI, Basel, Switzerland. This article is an open access article distributed under the terms and conditions of the Creative Commons Attribution (CC BY) license (http://creativecommons.org/licenses/by/4.0/).

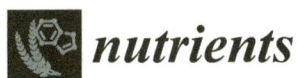

Article

Maternal Diet Influences the Reinstatement of Cocaine-Seeking Behavior and the Expression of Melanocortin-4 Receptors in Female Offspring of Rats

Dawid Gawliński, Kinga Gawlińska, Małgorzata Frankowska and Małgorzata Filip *

Maj Institute of Pharmacology Polish Academy of Sciences, Department of Drug Addiction Pharmacology, Smętna Street 12, 31-343 Kraków, Poland; gawlin@if-pan.krakow.pl (D.G.); kingaw@if-pan.krakow.pl (K.G.); frankow@if-pan.krakow.pl (M.F.)
* Correspondence: mal.fil@if-pan.krakow.pl

Received: 12 April 2020; Accepted: 14 May 2020; Published: 19 May 2020

Abstract: Recent studies have emphasized the role of the maternal diet in the development of mental disorders in offspring. Substance use disorder is a major global health and economic burden. Therefore, the search for predisposing factors for the development of this disease can contribute to reducing the health and social damage associated with addiction. In this study, we focused on the impact of the maternal diet on changes in melanocortin-4 (MC-4) receptors as well as on behavioral changes related to cocaine addiction. Rat dams consumed a high-fat diet (HFD), high-sugar diet (HSD, rich in sucrose), or mixed diet (MD) during pregnancy and lactation. Using an intravenous cocaine self-administration model, the susceptibility of female offspring to cocaine reward and cocaine-seeking propensities was evaluated. In addition, the level of MC-4 receptors in the rat brain structures related to cocaine reward and relapse was assessed. Modified maternal diets did not affect cocaine self-administration in offspring. However, the maternal HSD enhanced cocaine-seeking behavior in female offspring. In addition, we observed that the maternal HSD and MD led to increased expression of MC-4 receptors in the nucleus accumbens, while increased MC-4 receptor levels in the dorsal striatum were observed after exposure to the maternal HSD and HFD. Taken together, it can be concluded that a maternal HSD is an important factor that triggers cocaine-seeking behavior in female offspring and the expression of MC-4 receptors.

Keywords: cocaine self-administration; high-fat diet; high-sugar diet; maternal diet; pregnancy and lactation; melanocortin-4 receptor; offspring brain; rat offspring

1. Introduction

In the global population, every fourth person suffers from mental illnesses throughout their life, the most common of which are depression, anxiety, substance (alcohol, drugs) use disorder, and schizophrenia [1–3]. Substance use disorder is a chronic brain disorder associated with the uncontrolled exploration and use of drugs, leading to devastating health consequences and a destructive impact on the familial, social, and professional aspects of a patient's life. In addition, even after long periods of abstinence, this disease is characterized by high susceptibility to relapse in response to stress and to cues or contexts associated with drugs [4].

Recent studies have focused on the contribution of a properly balanced maternal diet during intrauterine growth and early childhood in the development of the central nervous system of offspring. In fact, exposure to excessive or insufficient amounts of macronutrients (fats, sugars, proteins) can lead to morphological, molecular, and functional changes in the brains of offspring, predisposing them to the occurrence of behavioral disorders and mental diseases, such as increased impulsiveness, depression, or anxiety, which further predispose them to the risk of developing substance use disorders later in life [5–9]. A maternal diet rich in fat provokes increased consumption and preference for palatable but unhealthy food in offspring [10–12], increased nicotine and ethanol self-administration [13,14], and disturbed behavioral reactions in animals regarding the administration of psychostimulant substances (reduced locomotor activity and amphetamine-induced behavioral sensitization) [15]. In turn, a maternal diet rich in fructose or sucrose induces an increase in the amount of alcohol consumed by the offspring [16]. Together, these studies confirm the positive relationship between the maternal diet and the offspring's susceptibility to drugs; however, there is still a lack of data on the relationship between the composition of the maternal diet and the development of cocaine use disorder (one of the most used drugs in the world among psychostimulants) [17]. Increasing knowledge about the predisposing factors for the development of mental disorders, including psychostimulant addiction, may contribute to reducing the health, social, and economic damage associated with these diseases in the future. Most literature provide data on the role of maternal obesity induced by high-calorie food on the development of the central nervous system in offspring. By limiting the modified types of diets only to pregnancy and lactation, our research will allow to indicate the period of intrauterine development and early childhood more specifically as a key factor in the development of the brain and behavioral disorders in adult offspring. Because the melanocortin system in the brain acts through melanocortin-4 (MC-4) receptors, which are located in brain regions that represent part of the reward system [18,19] and control (among other things) nutritional behavior, memory, positive enhancement, and emotions [20–22], these receptors were selected as a potential molecular biomarker of mechanisms underlying the cocaine susceptible phenotype in rat offspring induced by maternal nutrition. The relationship between maternal diet, MC-4 receptors and cocaine self-administration was demonstrated in recent studies by our group [23]. We showed, among other results, that a maternal high sugar-diet (HSD) significantly affects the expression of MC-4 receptors in the brains of male offspring following chronic cocaine self-administration or an abstinence period. Moreover, administration of an MC-4 receptor antagonist reduced cocaine- and cue-induced reinstatement of cocaine-seeking behavior; concurrently, male offspring that had received maternal nutrition from an HSD were more sensitive to the anti-relapsing effects of an MC-4 receptor antagonist than control male offspring [23].

In light of the above data and the small number of studies on the pathogenesis of developing addiction in females compared to studies in males, the purpose of this study was to determine the role of a maternal high-fat diet (HFD), HSD, and mixed diet (MD; rich in carbohydrate and fat) during pregnancy and lactation (critical periods in early life) on the behavioral and neurochemical changes in female offspring in the aspect of cocaine addiction. For this purpose, using the animal model of intravenous self-administration, we have comprehensively characterized the impact of a modified maternal diet on changes in the phenotype of offspring assessed at various stages of addiction: the acquisition and maintenance of cocaine addiction; abstinence; and the strength of cocaine-seeking behavior to cue- and cocaine-induced priming. In addition, at the molecular level, we evaluated the role of diet modifications during pregnancy and lactation on changes in MC-4 receptor protein expression in the synaptosomal fraction of brain structures related to cocaine addiction (the prefrontal cortex, dorsal striatum, nucleus accumbens, ventral tegmental area, and hypothalamus) in young adult female offspring.

2. Materials and Methods

2.1. Animals and Diets

All experiments were performed in accordance with the guidelines of the European Directive 2010/63/EU and were approved by the 2nd Local Institutional Animal Care and Use Committee (Maj Institute of Pharmacology Polish Academy of Sciences, Kraków, Poland; approval number 1270/2015; 42/2017). Every effort was made to minimize suffering and the number of animals used.

Wistar rats from Charles River (Germany) were housed in standard plastic rodent cages in a room maintained at 22 ± 2 °C and 55 ± 10% humidity under a 12 h light–dark cycle (lights on at 6:00 a.m.). Unless otherwise specified, animals had free access to water and food. Nulliparous female rats (200–240 g), after the acclimatization period and during the proestrus phase (smears from females were collected daily to determine the estrous cycle phase), were mated with males overnight, and pregnancy was confirmed by examining vaginal smears for the presence of sperm. Pregnant females ($n = 10$/group) were then individually housed and randomly assigned to four groups: control diet (CD; cat# VRF1; Special Diets Services, UK) or special diets purchased from Altromin (Germany): HFD (cat# C1057 mod.), HSD (cat# C1010), or MD (cat# C1011). The composition of the diets used in the study is presented in Table 1.

Table 1. Macronutrient profiles (expressed as a percentage of energy) and energy values of the control and modified diets used in this study.

	Control Diet (CD)	High-Fat Diet (HFD)	High-Sugar Diet (HSD)	Mixed Diet (MD)
Carbohydrate	65%	25%	70%	56%
Sucrose	4.6%		44%	18%
Fat	13%	60%	12%	28%
Protein	22%	15%	18%	16%
Total energy	3.4 kcal/g	5.3 kcal/g	3.8 kcal/g	3.9 kcal/g

Dams consumed these diets ad libitum during the gestation (21 days) and lactation periods (21 days). Dam body weight and food intake were monitored every third day. Litter sizes were normalized to 9–12 pups. After weaning, offspring were separated according to sex, housed six per cage, and fed a CD. Female offspring were used in the present study. The experimental design and timeline of the study are illustrated in Figure 1.

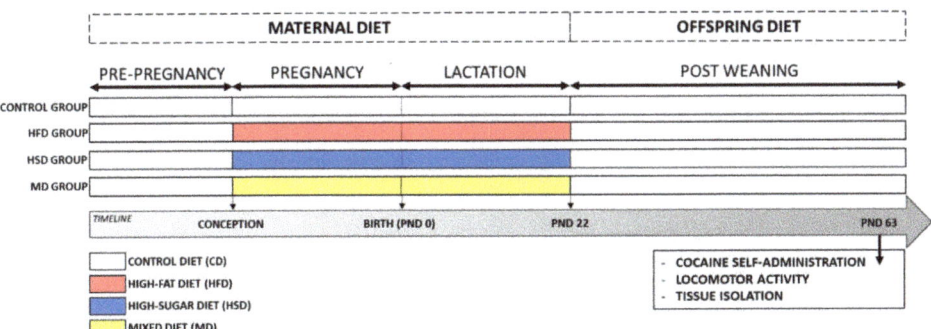

Figure 1. Experimental design and timeline. Dams were fed a control diet (CD) or one of the three modified diets: high-fat (HFD), high-sugar (HSD), or mixed (MD; rich in carbohydrate and fat) during pregnancy and lactation. Female offspring were divided into three cohorts and at postnatal day (PND) 63, they were assessed by tissue isolation and biochemical analyses, via the cocaine self-administration study and for locomotor activity.

2.2. Behavioral Procedures

2.2.1. Drugs

Cocaine hydrochloride (Toronto Research Chemicals, North York, ON, Canada) was dissolved in sterile 0.9% NaCl. The cocaine solution was administered intravenously or intraperitoneally. In a volume of 0.1 mL/infusion or 1 mL/kg, respectively.

2.2.2. Cocaine Self-Administration Procedure

Catheter Implantation and Initial Lever-Press Training

At PND 53, female rats (n = 12 for each group) were anaesthetized with ketamine HCl (75 mg/kg; Bioketan; Biowet, Puławy, Poland) and xylazine (5 mg/kg; Sedazin; Biowet, Puławy, Poland) and chronically implanted with a silastic catheter in the external jugular vein, as described previously [24]. After surgery, meloxicam subcutaneously (0.5 mg/kg; Metacam; Boehringer Ingelheim Vetmedica GmbH, Ingelheim am Rhein, Germany) was administered, and animals were kept individually in standard home cages water and food ad libitum. Each day, catheters were flushed with 0.1 mL of saline solution containing heparin (70 U/mL; Polfa, Warszawa, Poland) or 0.1 mL of cephazolin solution (10 mg/mL; Biochemie GmbH, Kundl, Austria). After seven days of recovery, animals were food-deprived for 18–20 h (with free access to water) and were then trained to press a lever during 2-h daily sessions under the fixed ratio (FR) 1 schedule of sweetened milk reinforcement for two days. Throughout the two training days, food was limited to 70% of the rats' free-feeding amount.

Cocaine Self-Administration

Female offspring at PND 63 began lever pressing for cocaine reinforcement during the 2-h daily sessions performed six days/week (maintenance) for a total of three weeks, and from that time, they were given free access to food throughout the remainder of the experiment. Rats were trained to self-administer cocaine in described previously [25] standard operant chambers (Med-Associates, Fairfax, VT, USA) in contact with an infusion pump (Model 3.33 RPM, Med-Associates, Fairfax, VT, USA) according to two experimental protocols: (a) a stable dose of cocaine (0.5 mg/kg/infusion) and an increased schedule of reinforcement (FR1–5) or (b) increased cocaine doses (0.25–1 mg/kg/infusion) and a stable FR1 schedule of reinforcement. Each schedule was completed by pressing the "active" lever resulting in a 5 s infusion of cocaine and a 5 s presentation of the stimulus complex, which consisted of an activation of the white stimulus light directly above the "active" lever and a tone from the generator (2000 Hz; 15 dB above the ambient noise level). Following each infusion, there was a 20 s time-out period during which the response was recorded but had no programmed consequences. An "inactive" lever response never activated the infusion pump.

Progressive Ratio Test

After the final experimental cocaine session described above, rats were tested for the self-administration of cocaine under the progressive ratio (PR) schedule of reinforcement, and this session lasted 4 h. During the PR session, the delivery of intravenous cocaine was contingent on an increasing number of responses incremented through the following progression: 1–603 [26]. Breakpoints were defined as the number of completed ratios in the series over 4 h.

Extinction

After cocaine self-administration (see above), the rats previously used for the two different cocaine self-administration protocols were used in the extinction training/reinstatement tests. During the extinction sessions, the animals had 1-h daily sessions with neither a cocaine delivery (exchanged to saline) nor tone and light stimuli (conditioned stimuli).

Reinstatement of Cocaine-Seeking

After 10 days of extinction training, animals were evaluated for the response reinstatement induced by either a conditioned cue (the tone and light associated with cocaine self-administration) or a noncontingent presentation of a self-administered reinforcement (2.5 or 10 mg/kg cocaine, intraperitoneal). The order of the cocaine priming injections was counterbalanced according to a Latin square design, and the test sessions were separated by at least 2–3 baseline sessions of extinction training. During the 2-h reinstatement tests, presses of the active lever resulted in the intravenous infusion of saline.

2.2.3. Locomotor Activity

Spontaneous motor activity was recorded individually for each drug-naïve rat from the subset at PND 63 in Opto-Varimex cages (43 cm × 44 cm, Columbus Instruments, Columbus, OH, USA) and analyzed using Auto-Track software (Columbus Instruments, Columbus, OH, USA) as described previously [24]. The locomotor activity of rats was defined as horizontal activity and was presented as the distance traveled in cm during 5-, 30-, and 120-min trials.

2.3. Biochemical Analysis

2.3.1. Brain Tissue Collection

For biochemical analysis, at PND 63, a subset of drug-naïve female offspring rats was sacrificed by rapid decapitation, and the brains were promptly removed. Relevant brain structures were dissected according to the rat brain atlas [27] and isolated on ice-cold glass plates, immediately frozen on dry ice and stored at −80 °C for enzyme-linked immunosorbent assay (ELISA) analyses. To avoid the potential effect of stress on molecular changes in the brain, animals were not fasting before decapitation. All samples were collected between 9:00–12:00 (a.m.).

2.3.2. Melancortin-4 Receptor Expression

MC-4 receptor expression was determined in the synaptosomal fraction The brain tissue samples were homogenized using a sonicator (EpiShear™ Probe Sonicator; Active Motif, Carlsbad, CA, USA) in 10% (w/v) of 0.32 M sucrose HEPES buffer (containing 145 mM NaCl, 5 mM KCl, 2 mM $CaCl_2$, 1 mM $MgCl_2$, 5 mM glucose, and 5 mM HEPES) with a protease inhibitor cocktail (Complete, Roche, Mannheim, Germany). Later, suspended tissue was homogenized with a Dounce tissue grinder. The homogenate was centrifuged at 4 °C for 10 min at 600× g. The supernatant was then diluted 1:1 with 1.3 M sucrose HEPES buffer to obtain a suspension at a final concentration of 0.8 M sucrose. This suspension was further centrifuged twice in a series of washes with HEPES buffer at 4 °C for 15 min at 12,000× g. The supernatant was discarded each time. The pellet was suspended in RIPA buffer (containing a protease inhibitor, PMSF and 0.2% Triton X-100) and centrifuged at 4 °C for 30 min at 20,000× g [28]. The supernatant containing the synaptosomal fraction was frozen overnight at −20 °C and was used for further analyses the following day.

The levels of MC-4 receptors in the synaptosomal fraction of the prefrontal cortex (including the infralimbic, prelimbic, and cingulate cortices; Bregma: 5.2–2.7 mm), dorsal striatum, nucleus accumbens, ventral tegmental area, and hypothalamus were measured using ELISA kits (cat# E11964R; Wuhan EIAab Science Co., Wuhan, China) according to the manufacturer's protocols. Duplicate aliquots of 100 µL of each sample along with MC-4 receptor standards (0, 0.312, 0.625, 1.25, 2.5, 5, 10, and 20 ng/mL) were transferred to precoated 96-well ELISA plates. The absorbance was measured at a wavelength of $\lambda = 450$ nm using a Multiskan Spectrum spectrophotometer (Thermo LabSystems, Philadelphia, PA, USA). The concentration of MC-4 receptors was calculated from a standard curve and expressed as ng/mg of protein. Bicinchoninic acid assay (BCA) protein assay kits (Thermo Scientific, Rockford, IL, USA) were used (the Pierce™ BCA Protein Assay Kit for the prefrontal cortex, dorsal striatum and nucleus accumbens or the Micro BCA™ Protein Assay kit for the ventral tegmental area and hypothalamus) to determine the protein concentrations.

2.4. Statistical Analysis

Animals that had problems with the catheters during the recovery or experimental periods were excluded from the data analysis. All data are expressed as the mean ± standard error of mean (SEM). Statistical analyses were performed with either one-, two-, or multi-way analysis of variance (ANOVA), with the terms of the repeated measure analysis dependent on the experiment, using Statistica version 12 software (StatSoft, Tulsa, OK, USA). Post hoc Dunnett's or Newman–Keuls tests were used to analyze differences between group means. $p < 0.05$ was considered statistically significant.

3. Results

3.1. Maternal Body Weight, Caloric Intake and Litter Size

The effects of the modified diets on changes in dam body weight and caloric intake during pregnancy and lactation are shown in Supplemental Figure S1. A two-way ANOVA for repeated measures showed significant effects of maternal diet × day interactions ($F(51, 1324) = 2.515$, $p < 0.01$). We observed that dams consumed MD had lower body weight gain in the last days of lactation compared to that of the control group. In addition, it was shown that modified diet consumption resulted in a change in caloric intake during pregnancy ($F(3, 36) = 4.754$, $p < 0.01$) and lactation ($F(3, 36) = 20.660$, $p < 0.001$). Females fed an HSD consumed more calories during pregnancy ($p < 0.05$), while during lactation, significantly more calories were consumed by dams from the HFD group ($p < 0.01$), in contrast to females fed MD, in which a decrease in the average daily caloric intake was observed ($p < 0.01$; Figure S1b). At the same time, modified maternal diets did not affect the litter size ($F(3, 36) = 0.873$, $p = 0.464$; Figure S1c) or birth weight of female offspring ($F(3, 124) = 1.585$, $p = 0.196$; Figure S1d).

3.2. Expression of MC-4 Receptors

The influence of maternal diet on the level of MC-4 receptors in the synaptosomal fraction of brain structures related to cocaine addiction (the prefrontal cortex, dorsal striatum, nucleus accumbens, ventral tegmental area, and hypothalamus) at PND 63 in the naïve female offspring was assessed (Figure 2).

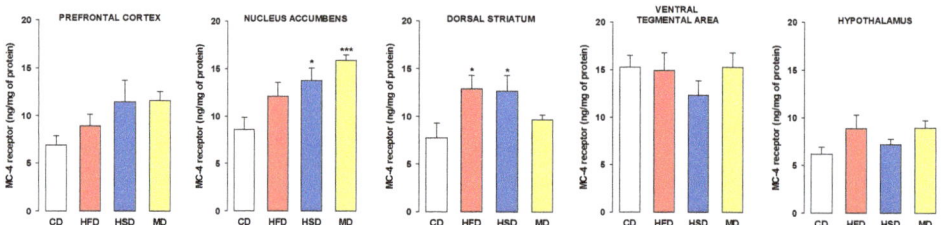

Figure 2. Effects of maternal diet during pregnancy and lactation on melanocortin-4 (MC-4) receptor expression in the synaptosomal fraction of the prefrontal cortex, nucleus accumbens, dorsal striatum, ventral tegmental area, and hypothalamus in female offspring rats at PND 63. The results are expressed as the mean (±SEM). $n = 8$ rats/group. Data were analyzed by one-way analysis of variance (ANOVA) followed by Dunnett's post hoc test. * $p < 0.05$, *** $p < 0.001$ versus the control diet (CD) group. HSD, high-sugar diet; HFD, high-fat diet; MD, mixed diet.

We observed that modified maternal diets during pregnancy and lactation evoked changes in MC-4 receptors in the synaptosomal fraction in the nucleus accumbens ($F(3, 28) = 6.604$, $p < 0.01$) and dorsal striatum ($F(3, 28) = 3.359$, $p < 0.05$), but not in the prefrontal cortex ($F(3, 28) = 2.493$, $p = 0.081$), ventral tegmental area (F(3, 28) = 0.148, p = 0.930) or hypothalamus (F(3, 28) = 2.128, p = 0.119) in female offspring. Post hoc analysis showed that a maternal HSD or MD during pregnancy and lactation increased the expression of MC-4 receptors in the female nucleus accumbens ($p < 0.05$ and $p < 0.001$, respectively), and a maternal HFD or HSD increased its expression within the dorsal striatum ($p < 0.05$).

3.3. Locomotor Activity

Spontaneous locomotor activity, recorded for 5, 30, and 120 min, did not differ between female offspring whose mothers consumed different diets, CD, HFD, HSD, or MD, during pregnancy and lactation (Table 2).

Table 2. Locomotor activity of female offspring at postnatal day 63.

		CD	HFD	HSD	MD	
Distance traveled (cm)	5 min	1064.93 ± 63.75	1031.16 ± 56.43	1112.13 ± 71.78	1018.53 ± 60.86	F(3, 44) = 0.435, p = 0.729
	30 min	3130.32 ± 214.53	3332.69 ± 223.62	3210.91 ± 145.59	3070.44 ± 217.69	F(3, 44) = 0.313, p = 0.816
	120 min	5262.90 ± 380.66	4979.64 ± 284.89	5615.37 ± 603.51	5392.65 ± 562.38	F(3, 44) = 0.311, p = 0.817

Distance traveled (cm) was measured after 5, 30, and 120 min in female offspring whose mothers were fed a high-fat (HFD), high-sugar (HSD), or mixed diet (MD) during pregnancy and lactation. The results are expressed as the mean (±SEM). n = 12 rats/group. Data were analyzed by one-way analysis of variance (ANOVA) versus the control diet (CD) group.

3.4. Cocaine Self-Administration

The impact of maternal diets during pregnancy and lactation on cocaine self-administration in female offspring rats in two experimental protocols (stable dose of drug reinforcement and an increased reinforcement schedule, or an increased dose of the drug with a stable reinforcement schedule) was studied.

3.4.1. Stable Cocaine Dose and Increased Reinforcement Schedule

Figure 3a shows the number of active and inactive lever presses (upper panels) and the number of infusions (lower panels) during three sequential weeks with increasing FR schedules of reinforcement (FR1–5) and a stable dose of cocaine (0.5 mg/kg/infusion) for the female offspring from the CD, HFD, HSD, and MD groups. Multi-way ANOVA for repeated measures did not show significant effects of maternal diet × session × lever interactions during the eighteen days of cocaine self-administration (F(51, 1324) = 0.515, p = 0.998). In addition, we did not find differences between the effect of maternal diet on the number of cocaine infusions during the three weeks of self-administration, as demonstrated by a two-way ANOVA for repeated measures (F(51, 663) = 1.112, p = 0.280). Despite the lack of statistically significant differences, a reduced amount of infusions can be seen in the first and second weeks of self-administration in female offspring exposed to a maternal HSD.

3.4.2. Increased Cocaine Dose and Stable Reinforcement Schedule

The number of active and inactive lever presses (upper panels) and the number of cocaine infusions (lower panels) for the increasing doses of cocaine (0.25, 0.5 and 1 mg/kg/infusion) with a stable FR1 reinforcement schedule during the entire experiment are shown in Figure 4a. We observed that the active and inactive lever presses of female offspring whose mothers were fed modified diets during pregnancy and lactation did not differ significantly from the lever presses conducted by the control diet group in this protocol. Multi-way ANOVA for repeated measures did not reveal significant maternal diet × session × lever interactions during the eighteen sessions of cocaine self-administration (F(51, 1428) = 0.896, p = 0.682). A two-way ANOVA for repeated measures also showed no significant changes in the number of cocaine infusion (F(51, 714) = 0.989, p = 0.497) in offspring.

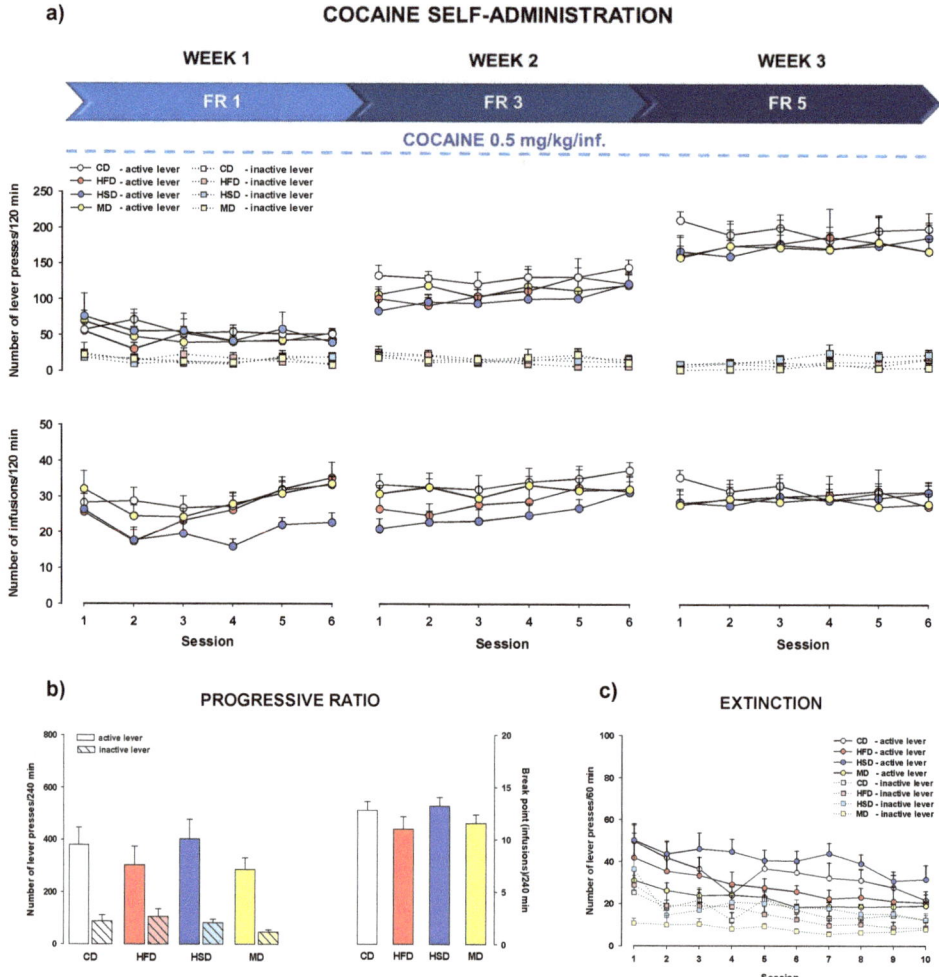

Figure 3. (**a**) Effects of a maternal high-fat (HFD), high-sugar (HSD), or mixed (MD) diet during pregnancy and lactation on the acquisition/maintenance of cocaine (0.5 mg/kg/infusion) self-administration with increasing fixed ratio (FR) schedules of reinforcement (FR1–5) in female offspring rats. (**b**) Effects of the modified maternal diets on cocaine self-administration with a progressive ratio schedule in female offspring day after the last session of cocaine self-administration under an increasing schedule of reinforcement (FR1–5) and a stable dose of cocaine (0.5 mg/kg/infusion). (**c**) Effects of the modified maternal diets upon self-administration extinction with a fixed dose of cocaine (0.5 mg/kg/infusion) and an increased schedule of reinforcement (FR1–5) in female offspring rats. Numbers of active and inactive lever presses and cocaine infusions are expressed as the mean (±SEM). The number of animals in each group was as follows: CD ($n = 11$), HFD ($n = 10$), HSD ($n = 10$), MD ($n = 12$). CD, control diet.

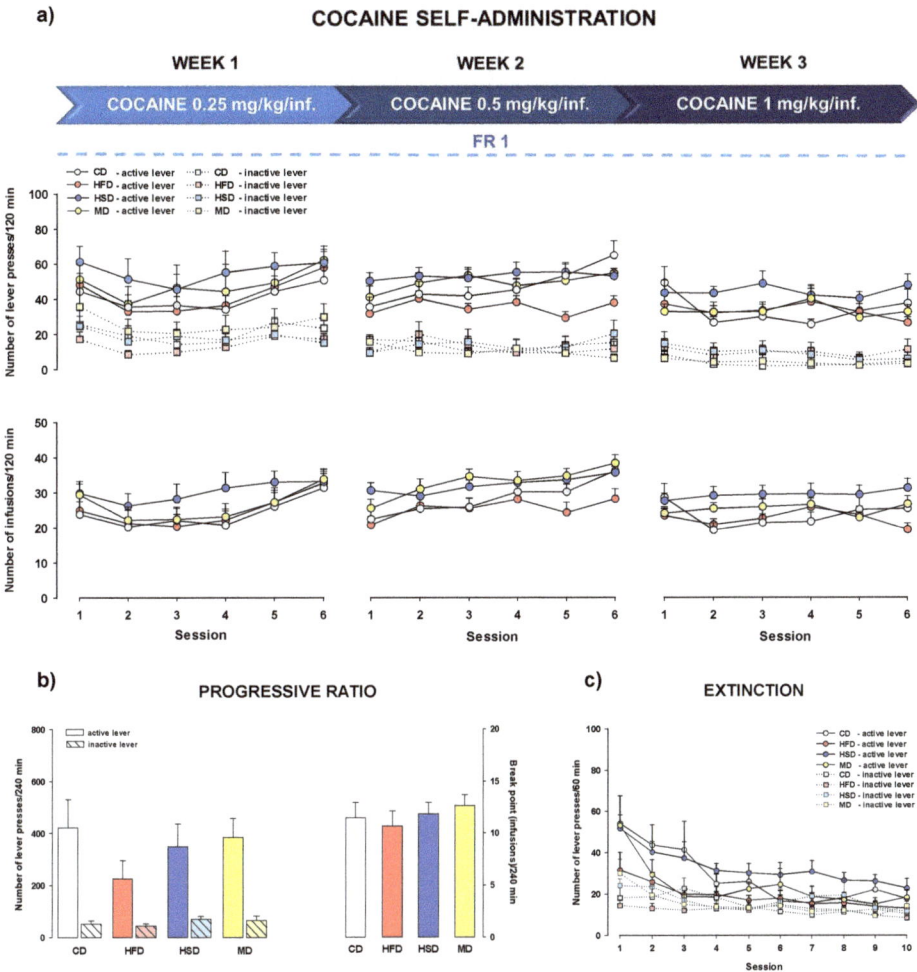

Figure 4. (**a**) Effects of a maternal high-fat (HFD), high-sugar (HSD), or mixed (MD) diet during pregnancy and lactation on the acquisition/maintenance of cocaine (0.25–1 mg/kg/infusion) self-administration with a stable FR1 schedule of reinforcement in female offspring rats. (**b**) Effects of the modified maternal diets on cocaine self-administration with a progressive ratio schedule in female offspring day after the last session of cocaine self-administration with a stable FR1 schedule of reinforcement and an increasing dose of cocaine (0.25–1 mg/kg/infusion). (**c**) Effects of the modified maternal diets on self-administration extinction with increased doses of cocaine (0.25–1 mg/kg/infusion) and a stable FR1 schedule of reinforcement in female offspring rats. Numbers of active and inactive lever presses and cocaine infusions are expressed as the mean (±SEM). The number of animals in each group was as follows: cocaine self-administration CD ($n = 12$), HFD ($n = 11$), HSD ($n = 11$), MD ($n = 12$); extinction training CD ($n = 11$), HFD ($n = 10$), HSD ($n = 10$), MD ($n = 12$). CD, control diet.

3.5. PR Schedule of Cocaine Reinforcement

The female offspring from the HFD, HSD, and MD groups did not differ from the control group in the break point during cocaine self-administration under the PR reinforcement schedule following an increasing schedule of reinforcement and a stable dose of cocaine ($F(3, 39) = 1.222$, $p = 0.315$).

Animals did not differ in active and inactive lever presses during cocaine (0.5 mg/kg/infusion) self-administration in the PR protocol (F(3, 78) = 0.637, p = 0.594; Figure 3b).

Maternal exposure to HFD, HSD, or MD did not change behavioral readouts in female offspring in cocaine (1 mg/kg/infusion) self-administration in the PR scheme following a stable FR1 reinforcement schedule and an increasing dose of cocaine (number of cocaine infusions (F(3, 42) = 0.406, p = 0.749); number of active and inactive lever presses (F(3, 84) = 0.804, p = 0.495; Figure 4b).

3.6. Extinction Training

Extinction training was introduced to all rats after cocaine self-administration. After substituting saline for cocaine, a progressive drop in lever responses was observed over the extinction sessions for the CD, HFD, HSD, and MD groups. In the female offspring trained to self-administer cocaine (0.5 mg/kg/infusion) with the increased FR1–5 schedule of reinforcement, a multi-way ANOVA for repeated measures did not show significant effects of maternal diets on extinguished active lever pressing (F(27, 702) = 0.545, p = 0.972; Figure 3c). Rats from mothers fed different diets did not differ in their extinction of active lever responses (F(27, 702) = 0.442, p = 0.994) following cocaine (from 0.25 to 1 mg/kg/infusion) with the FR1 reinforcement schedule (Figure 4c).

3.7. Reinstatement of Cocaine-Seeking Behavior

Following 10 days of extinction training, all groups of female rats were tested for response reinstatement induced by the cocaine-associated cue or cocaine (2.5 or 10 mg/kg, intraperitoneal).

3.7.1. Relapse after Stable Cocaine Dose and Increased Reinforcement Schedule

Figure 5a shows the number of active and inactive lever presses in offspring that were previously subjected to self-administered cocaine (0.5 mg/kg/infusion) with the increased FR schedule of reinforcement. Statistical analysis demonstrated that in female offspring, modified maternal diets changed cue-induced reinstatement (F(3, 78) = 3.453, p < 0.05) as well as cocaine-induced reinstatement for a cocaine dose of 2.5 mg/kg (F(3, 78) = 4.670, p < 0.01). Furthermore, there was no significant difference in the strength of the recurrence of cocaine-seeking behavior between the CD group and the tested diets for cocaine doses of 10 mg/kg (F(3, 78) = 1.661, p = 0.182). Post hoc tests indicated an increase in active lever responses only in female offspring from the HSD group upon re-exposure on cue or intraperitoneal cocaine administration at a dose of 2.5 mg/kg (p < 0.01 and p < 0.001, respectively).

3.7.2. Relapse after Increased Cocaine Dose and Stable Reinforcement Schedule

The number of active and inactive lever responses in animals that were previously trained to self-administer increasing cocaine doses (0.25–1 mg/kg/infusion) with a stable FR1 schedule of reinforcement is shown in Figure 5b. We found that a maternal HFD, HSD, and MD did not significantly change the female offspring relapse strength after re-exposure to cocaine-associated cues (F(3, 78) = 1.895, p = 0.448) and cocaine (2.5 mg/kg) compared to that of the control animals (F(3, 78) = 1.990, p = 0.122). However, differences in active lever presses were observed after cocaine was administered at a dose of 10 mg/kg (F(3, 78) = 3.043, p < 0.05). The HSD female offspring pressed the active lever more times during the test (p < 0.05) compared to the number of presses performed by the CD group.

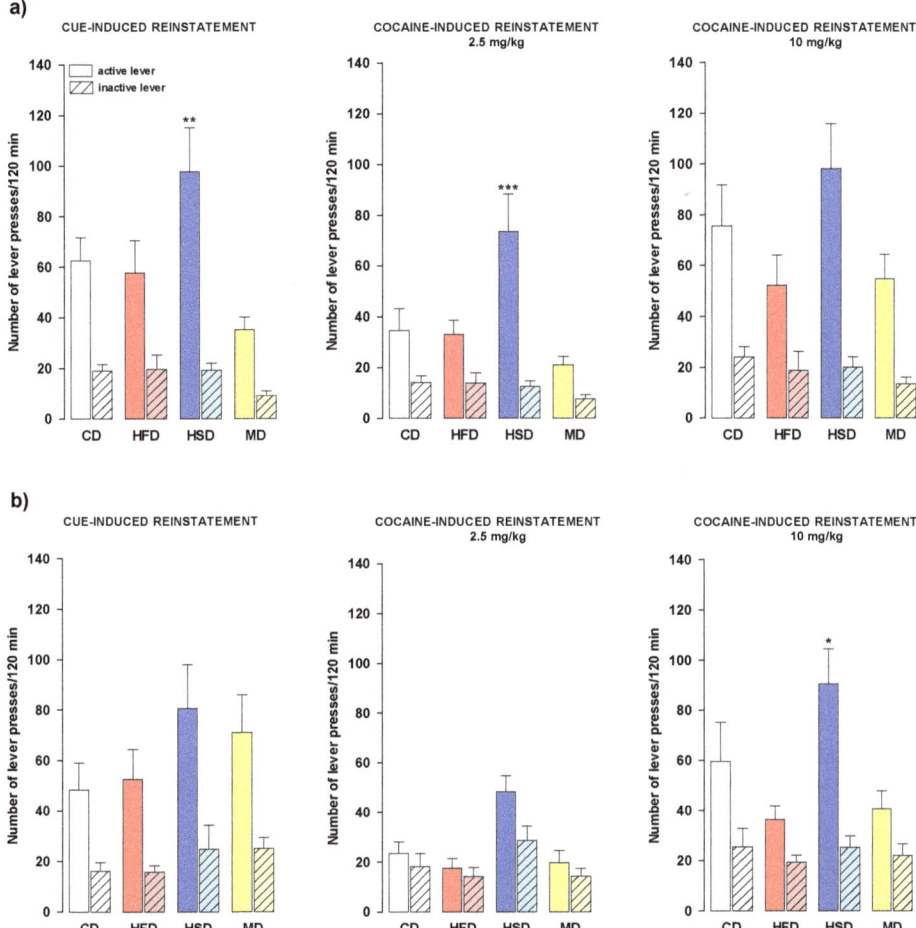

Figure 5. Effects of a maternal high-fat (HFD), high-sugar (HSD), or mixed (MD) diet during pregnancy and lactation on reinstatement of the cocaine-seeking behavior induced by the cue (CUE; tone + light) and the drug in female rat offspring. Drug-induced reinstatement was triggered by the administration of cocaine (2.5 or 10 mg/kg, i.p.). (**a**) Tests were performed after cocaine (0.5 mg/kg/infusion) self-administration with an increasing schedule of reinforcement (FR1–5) and 10 days of extinction training. (**b**) Tests were performed after cocaine (0.25–1 mg/kg/infusion) self-administration with a stable FR1 schedule of reinforcement and 10 days of extinction training. The numbers of active and inactive lever presses are expressed as the mean (±SEM). The number of animals each group was as follows: CD ($n = 11$), HFD ($n = 10$), HSD ($n = 10$), MD ($n = 12$). Data were analyzed by two-way ANOVA and the post hoc Newman–Keuls test. * $p < 0.05$, ** $p < 0.01$, *** $p < 0.001$ versus the control diet (CD) group.

4. Discussion

In this study, we showed that a modified maternal diet during pregnancy and the lactation period is an important factor inducing impairments at the behavioral and neurochemical levels and a cocaine-seeking prone phenotype in female offspring. We focused on females due to the observed differences in addiction to psychoactive substances in relation to sex (e.g., women are more likely to relapse than men) [29] as well as the smaller number of studies assessing the effect of maternal nutrition on behavioral changes in female offspring compared to the number of studies regarding male offspring. The results of this work are the first to indicate that a modification in the composition of maternal diet, particularly an increased amount of carbohydrates (mainly sucrose) consumed during fetal development and early childhood, results in an increased relapse of cocaine-seeking behavior and in increased levels of MC-4 receptors in selected brain structures in female offspring.

Human research indicates that both obesity and the consumption of an HFD increases total food consumption and the risk of alcohol [30,31] and nicotine addictions [32]. Recently, an increasing number of preclinical studies focused mainly on maternal HFDs have proven that nutrition may predispose offspring to an increased intake of palatable food [10,11,33], drinking alcohol [16,34,35], nicotine [14], or simultaneous ethanol and nicotine [13] self-administration. In this paper, a series of behavioral tests using an animal model of intravenous cocaine self-administration to determine the female offspring phenotype after exposure to modified maternal diets were performed. We showed that the predisposition to cocaine self-administration in female rats from a CD, HFD, HSD, or MD groups was similar and did not depend on the schedule of reinforcement or the dose range of cocaine. In fact, the animals did not differ significantly in the number of presses on the active and inactive levers or the number of drug infusions during the acquisition/maintenance phase in either the cocaine motivational scoring protocol (FR1–5) while testing the rewarding effects of the drug (cocaine 0.25–1 mg/kg/infusion) or during the following test using the PR schedule to assess animals' motivation. Moreover, following three weeks of exposure to cocaine self-administration, no changes in female behavior were noted during the drug abstinence period. In other words, modified maternal diets during pregnancy and lactation did not influence either the rewarding or motivational aspects of cocaine intake in female offspring.

Substance use disorder is a debilitating chronic brain disease characterized by high susceptibility to relapse in response to stress or stimuli associated with previous drug use, even after a long period of abstinence [4]. Approximately 40–60% of human addicts entering therapy return to using addictive substances within the first year of treatment [36]. Due to the serious problem of relapse concerning effective addiction therapy, our main finding was that in comparison to the control groups, the females consuming an HSD, depending on the protocol of cocaine self-administration, evoked a higher reinstatement following re-exposure to the cue associated with the previous cocaine infusions or the presentation of the cocaine-priming dose (10 mg/kg). Interestingly, cocaine at a dose of 2.5 mg/kg, which normally does not cause relapse (subthreshold dose), also significantly enhanced the active lever presses in the female offspring of mothers that had consumed an HSD. It seems, therefore, that the increased potency of cocaine relapse in offspring exposed to a maternal HSD may depend not only on the conditions of individual development, but also on the pattern of drug use before abstinence. Moreover, in both schedule protocols, there was no change in the rats' responses to the inactive lever, which suggests the specificity of the observed behavioral responses. Additionally, naïve female offspring from diet-exposed groups showed similar spontaneous locomotor activity, which means that the rats' motor activity was not affected by the maternal diets and that the observed changes in cocaine-seeking behavior are specific. Our findings showed that the effect of a maternal HSD during pregnancy and lactation on the severity of a cocaine relapse is not dependent on sex, as a similar increase in the reinstatement of drug-seeking behavior was found in male offspring [23].

Behavioral studies emphasize that prenatal exposure to cocaine causes increased self-administration of cocaine [37–39] or alcohol [40] in offspring. Data from human observations indicate that exposure to cocaine in utero leads to the earlier and more frequent use of drugs (cocaine, marijuana, alcohol, and nicotine) by offspring in adolescence and early adulthood [41–44]. On the other hand, the literature provides evidence that the consumption of a natural reward, such as sugar, manifests similar neurochemical effects in the brain as the use of most addictive psychoactive substances. Within the central reward system, an increased dopamine level was observed [45–48], as was the altered expression of dopamine receptors [49–51] or the adaptive reduction of dopamine levels as a result of chronic exposure to a sweet, natural reward [52]. In addition, behavioral changes characteristic of drug addiction were observed similar to the neurochemical responses to natural rewards and psychoactive substances. These included, among others, increased sugar consumption [53] or increased animal responses to a conditional stimulus associated with prior sucrose self-harvesting [54] after a period of abstinence. Hence, the abuse of tasty foods or drugs is not the only way to induce similar neurochemical and behavioral changes. Preclinical studies emphasize that exposure to a modified maternal diet during intrauterine development, as well as addictive substances, also significantly affects the offspring reward system being formed and its behavior later in life. Exposure to a diet rich in energy (e.g., an HFD or western-type diet) during pregnancy and lactation induced increased cocaine-induced place preference in the conditioned place preference (CPP) test, alcohol consumption, sensitivity to amphetamine administration, and preference for fat, and at the molecular level changes in dopaminergic brain signaling in juvenile and adult offspring [10,12,35,55]. There is also evidence of the interaction of natural rewards (e.g., sucrose) and addictive substances such as cocaine [56–58], methamphetamine [59], or alcohol [60]. For example, sensitization of behavioral responses occurs following cocaine administration and prolonged activity involving addictive substances in rats having intermittent access to granulated sucrose compared to the behavioral responses in animals consuming only standard laboratory feed [56]. This may suggest that maternal exposure to an increased amount of sucrose relative to a CD during pregnancy and early childhood, which is crucial for normal brain development, may lead to hypersensitivity between the natural reward (sugars) and the psychostimulants in offspring. Hence, female offspring of mothers that consumed an HSD may be more sensitive to conditional and unconditional stimuli associated with previous positive enhancements experienced during cocaine self-administration.

One of the neurochemical mechanisms that can potentially explain the offspring's behavior to cocaine may be associated with changes in the melanocortin system induced by a modified maternal diet. In fact, female offspring of mothers that consumed an HSD demonstrated increased cocaine-seeking behavior irrespective of the protocol, and the drug-naïve young adults female originating from mothers that consumed an HSD showed an upregulation of MC-4 receptors in the synaptosomal fraction of the nucleus accumbens and dorsal striatum, the brain regions linked to drug-seeking behavior [61,62]. Similarly, increased levels of accumbal MC-4 receptors were observed in female offspring exposed to an MD or in the dorsal striatum in the HFD group, but such changes did not provoke behavioral changes. This indicates the complexity of the factors involved in cocaine-seeking behavior or that behavioral changes manifest only when disturbance within MC-4 receptors occurs in several structures of the reward system. The simultaneous change in the expression of MC-4 receptors within the nucleus accumbens and dorsal striatum may lead to different activities of these structures than that observed in members of the CD group after exposure to conditional and unconditional stimuli, which may contribute to the observed intensification of the reinstatement of cocaine-seeking behavior in these animals. Previous studies assessing the effect of HFD intake by mothers before conception and during pregnancy and lactation showed reduced MC-4 mRNA expression in the female hypothalamus of offspring immediately after lactation (PND 20) [63]. Our findings demonstrate that switching to a CD after weaning, on one hand, can restore the basal level of MC-4 receptors in the hypothalamus, but the maternal diet leading to distant neurochemical consequences occurring in the nucleus accumbens and dorsal striatum does not disappear during the lifetime of the offspring.

The changes within the MC-4 receptors observed in the rat brain regions associated with the dopamine mesocorticolimbic system seem to be particularly important, as the brain structure is strongly associated with psychostimulant reward effects [64] and is involved in cue-, cocaine-, or stress-inducing reinstatement [65,66], supplementing existing knowledge about the interaction of psychoactive substances and MC-4 receptors. Recent studies have shown a decrease in the activity of agouti-related protein (AgRP) and proopiomelanocortin (POMC) neurons in the hypothalamus after the administration of cocaine, amphetamine, and nicotine, which suggests that not only reward pathways but also neuronal pathways associated with maintaining homeostasis affect the enhancement of these substances [67]. Typically, passively administered cocaine resulted in an increase in MC-4 receptor mRNA levels in the striatum, hippocampus, and hypothalamus [68,69]. Moreover, administration of the MC-4 receptor antagonist SHU-9119 to the nucleus accumbens reduced low-dose cocaine self-administration (0.125–0.25 mg/kg/infusion), cocaine-induced CPP, and the reinstatement of cocaine-seeking behavior [69]. On the other hand, the blockade of central MC-3/4 receptors with AgRP resulted in the blockade of acute and sensitized locomotor responses to cocaine [70]. Our recent data showed differences in the levels of MC-4 receptors within the prefrontal cortex, nucleus accumbens, dorsal striatum, and amygdala between CD and HSD male offspring after three weeks of cocaine self-administration and 10 days of extinction [23]. The data suggest that a maternal HSD during pregnancy and lactation interferes with the adaptive mechanisms in the brains of male offspring, during which abstinence can restore melanocortin signaling homeostasis after cocaine exposure. Current evidence suggests that MC-4 receptor activity may affect behavioral aspects of the cocaine response through interaction and modulation of the dopaminergic system [71–75].

In summary, the described results emphasize the important role of a maternal diet rich in sugars during fetal development and early childhood in the predisposition of female offspring to cocaine-seeking behavior in adult life. Moreover, an altered amount of macronutrients in the maternal diet disrupts the proper expression of MC-4 receptors in brain structures involved in cocaine relapse in female offspring, thus leading to a stronger response to exposure to conditioned and unconditioned stimuli combined with earlier cocaine self-administration.

Supplementary Materials: The following are available online at http://www.mdpi.com/2072-6643/12/5/1462/s1, Figure S1: Effects of a high-fat (HFD), high-sugar (HSD), or mixed (MD) diet on (a) maternal body weight changes (as a percentage of weight gain compared to start weight) and (b) average daily energy intake during pregnancy and lactation. Effects of the modified maternal diets on (c) litter size and (d) birth body weight of female offspring.

Author Contributions: D.G. designed and performed the study, analyzed the data and writing the manuscript. K.G. and M.F. (Małgorzata Frankowska) performed the study, analyzed the data and contributed to writing the manuscript. M.F. (Małgorzata Filip) conceived, designed and coordinated the study and contributed to writing the manuscript. All authors have read and agreed to the published version of the manuscript.

Funding: This study was funded by National Science Centre (Kraków, Poland), research grant UMO-2016/21/B/NZ4/00203.

Conflicts of Interest: The authors declare no conflict of interest.

References

1. Degenhardt, L.; Charlson, F.; Ferrari, A.; Santomauro, D.; Erskine, H.; Mantilla-Herrara, A.; Whiteford, H.; Leung, J.; Naghavi, M.; Griswold, M.; et al. The global burden of disease attributable to alcohol and drug use in 195 countries and territories, 1990–2016: A systematic analysis for the Global Burden of Disease Study 2016. *Lancet Psychiatry* **2018**, *5*, 987–1012. [CrossRef]
2. O'Rourke, M.; Wrigley, C.; Hammond, S. Violence within mental health services: How to enhance risk management. *Risk Manag. Healthc. Policy* **2018**, *11*, 159–167. [CrossRef] [PubMed]
3. Uher, R.; Zwicker, A. Etiology in psychiatry: Embracing the reality of poly-gene-environmental causation of mental illness. *World Psychiatry* **2017**, *16*, 121–129. [CrossRef] [PubMed]
4. Mukhara, D.; Banks, M.L.; Neigh, G.N. Stress as a risk factor for substance use disorders: A mini-review of molecular mediators. *Front. Behav. Neurosci.* **2018**, *12*, 309. [CrossRef]
5. Edlow, A.G. Maternal obesity and neurodevelopmental and psychiatric disorders in offspring. *Prenat. Diagn.* **2017**, *37*, 95–110. [CrossRef]
6. Gawlińska, K.; Gawliński, D.; Przegaliński, E.; Filip, M. Maternal high-fat diet during pregnancy and lactation provokes depressive-like behavior and influences the irisin/brain-derived neurotrophic factor axis and inflammatory factors in male and female offspring in rats. *J. Physiol. Pharmacol.* **2019**, *70*, 407–411. [CrossRef]
7. Rivera, H.M.; Christiansen, K.J.; Sullivan, E.L. The role of maternal obesity in the risk of neuropsychiatric disorders. *Front. Neurosci.* **2015**, *9*, 194. [CrossRef]
8. Sullivan, E.L.; Nousen, E.K.; Chamlou, K.A. Maternal high fat diet consumption during the perinatal period programs offspring behavior. *Physiol. Behav.* **2014**, *123*, 236–242. [CrossRef]
9. Sullivan, E.L.; Riper, K.M.; Lockard, R.; Valleau, J.C. Maternal high-fat diet programming of the neuroendocrine system and behavior. *Horm. Behav.* **2015**, *76*, 153–161. [CrossRef]

10. Naef, L.; Moquin, L.; Dal Bo, G.; Giros, B.; Gratton, A.; Walker, C.D. Maternal high-fat intake alters presynaptic regulation of dopamine in the nucleus accumbens and increases motivation for fat rewards in the offspring. *Neuroscience* **2011**, *176*, 225–236. [CrossRef]
11. Ong, Z.Y.; Muhlhausler, B.S. Maternal "junk-food" feeding of rat dams alters food choices and development of the mesolimbic reward pathway in the offspring. *FASEB J.* **2011**, *25*, 2167–2179. [CrossRef] [PubMed]
12. Paradis, J.; Boureau, P.; Moyon, T.; Nicklaus, S.; Parnet, P.; Paillé, V. Perinatal western diet consumption leads to profound plasticity and GABAergic phenotype changes within hypothalamus and reward pathway from birth to sexual maturity in rat. *Front. Endocrinol.* **2017**, *8*, 216. [CrossRef] [PubMed]
13. Karatayev, O.; Lukatskaya, O.; Moon, S.H.; Guo, W.R.; Chen, D.; Algava, D.; Abedi, S.; Leibowitz, S.F. Nicotine and ethanol co-use in Long-Evans rats: Stimulatory effects of perinatal exposure to a fat-rich diet. *Alcohol* **2015**, *49*, 479–489. [CrossRef]
14. Morganstern, I.; Lukatskaya, O.; Moon, S.-H.; Guo, W.-R.; Shaji, J.; Karatayev, O.; Leibowitz, S.F. Stimulation of nicotine reward and central cholinergic activity in Sprague–Dawley rats exposed perinatally to a fat-rich diet. *Psychopharmacology* **2013**, *230*, 509–524. [CrossRef] [PubMed]
15. Naef, L.; Srivastava, L.; Gratton, A.; Hendrickson, H.; Owens, S.M.; Walker, C.D. Maternal high fat diet during the perinatal period alters mesocorticolimbic dopamine in the adult rat offspring: Reduction in the behavioral responses to repeated amphetamine administration. *Psychopharmacology (Berl.)* **2008**, *197*, 83–94. [CrossRef] [PubMed]
16. Bocarsly, M.E.; Barson, J.R.; Hauca, J.M.; Hoebel, B.G.; Leibowitz, S.F.; Avena, N.M. Effects of perinatal exposure to palatable diets on body weight and sensitivity to drugs of abuse in rats. *Physiol. Behav.* **2012**, *107*, 568–575. [CrossRef]
17. Favrod-Coune, T.; Broers, B. The Health Effect of Psychostimulants: A Literature Review. *Pharmaceuticals* **2010**, *3*, 2333–2361. [CrossRef]
18. Alvaro, J.D.; Tatro, J.B.; Quillan, J.M.; Fogliano, M.; Eisenhard, M.; Lerner, M.R.; Nestler, E.J.; Duman, R.S. Morphine down-regulates melanocortin-4 receptor expression in brain regions that mediate opiate addiction. *Mol. Pharmacol.* **1996**, *50*, 583–591.
19. Lindblom, J.; Schiöth, H.B.; Larsson, A.; Wikberg, J.E.S.; Bergström, L. Autoradiographic discrimination of melanocortin receptors indicates that the MC3 subtype dominates in the medial rat brain. *Brain Res.* **1998**, *810*, 161–171. [CrossRef]
20. Adan, R.A.H.; Tiesjema, B.; Hillebrand, J.J.G.; La Fleur, S.E.; Kas, M.J.H.; De Krom, M. The MC4 receptor and control of appetite. *Br. J. Pharmacol.* **2006**, *149*, 815–827. [CrossRef]
21. Chaki, S.; Okuyama, S. Involvement of melanocortin-4 receptor in anxiety and depression. *Peptides* **2005**, *26*, 1952–1964. [CrossRef]
22. Cone, R.D. Anatomy and regulation of the central melanocortin system. *Nat. Neurosci.* **2005**, *8*, 571–578. [CrossRef]
23. Gawliński, D.; Gawlińska, K.; Frankowska, M.; Filip, M. Maternal high-sugar diet changes offspring vulnerability to reinstatement of cocaine-seeking behavior: Role of melanocortin-4 receptors. *FASEB J.* (in press). [CrossRef]
24. Jastrzębska, J.; Frankowska, M.; Szumiec, Ł.; Sadakierska-Chudy, A.; Haduch, A.; Smaga, I.; Bystrowska, B.; Daniel, W.A.; Filip, M. Cocaine self-administration in Wistar-Kyoto rats: A behavioral and biochemical analysis. *Behav. Brain Res.* **2015**, *293*, 62–73. [CrossRef] [PubMed]
25. Frankowska, M.; Miszkiel, J.; Pomierny-Chamioło, L.; Pomierny, B.; Giannotti, G.; Suder, A.; Filip, M. Alternation in dopamine D_2-like and metabotropic glutamate type 5 receptor density caused by differing housing conditions during abstinence from cocaine self-administration in rats. *J. Psychopharmacol.* **2019**, *33*, 372–382. [CrossRef] [PubMed]
26. Richardson, N.R.; Roberts, D.C.S. Progressive ratio schedules in drug self-administration studies in rats: A method to evaluate reinforcing efficacy. *J. Neurosci. Methods* **1996**, *66*, 1–11. [CrossRef]
27. Paxinos, G.; Watson, C. *The Rat Brain in Stereotaxic Coordinates*, 4th ed.; Academic Press: San Diego, CA, USA, 1998.
28. Kamat, P.K.; Kalani, A.; Tyagi, N. Method and validation of synaptosomal preparation for isolation of synaptic membrane proteins from rat brain. *MethodsX* **2014**, *1*, 102–107. [CrossRef]
29. Becker, J.B.; McClellan, M.L.; Reed, B.G. Sex differences, gender and addiction. *J. Neurosci. Res.* **2017**, *95*, 136–147. [CrossRef]

30. Kesse, E.; Clavel-Chapelon, F.; Slimani, N.; van Liere, M.; E3N Group. Do eating habits differ according to alcohol consumption? Results of a study of the French cohort of the European Prospective Investigation into Cancer and Nutrition (E3N-EPIC). *Am. J. Clin. Nutr.* **2001**, *74*, 322–327. [CrossRef]
31. Sansone, R.A.; Sansone, L.A. Obesity and substance misuse: Is there a relationship? *Innov. Clin. Neurosci.* **2013**, *10*, 30–35.
32. Hussaini, A.E.; Nicholson, L.M.; Shera, D.; Stettler, N.; Kinsman, S. Adolescent Obesity as a Risk Factor for High-Level Nicotine Addiction in Young Women. *J. Adolesc. Health* **2011**, *49*, 511–517. [CrossRef] [PubMed]
33. Chang, G.-Q.; Gaysinskaya, V.; Karatayev, O.; Leibowitz, S.F. Maternal high-fat diet and fetal programming: Increased proliferation of hypothalamic peptide-producing neurons that increase risk for overeating and obesity. *J. Neurosci.* **2008**, *28*, 12107–12119. [CrossRef] [PubMed]
34. Cabanes, A.; de Assis, S.; Gustafsson, J.-A.; Hilakivi-Clarke, L. Maternal High n-6 Polyunsaturated Fatty Acid Intake during Pregnancy Increases Voluntary Alcohol Intake and Hypothalamic Estrogen Receptor Alpha and Beta Levels among Female Offspring. *Dev. Neurosci.* **2000**, *22*, 488–493. [CrossRef] [PubMed]
35. Peleg-Raibstein, D.; Sarker, G.; Litwan, K.; Krämer, S.D.; Ametamey, S.M.; Schibli, R.; Wolfrum, C. Enhanced sensitivity to drugs of abuse and palatable foods following maternal overnutrition. *Transl. Psychiatry* **2016**, *6*, e911. [CrossRef]
36. McLellan, A.T.; Lewis, D.C.; O'Brien, C.P.; Kleber, H.D. Drug dependence, a chronic medical illness implications for treatment, insurance, and outcomes evaluation. *J. Am. Med. Assoc.* **2000**, *284*, 1689–1695. [CrossRef]
37. Hecht, G.S.; Spear, N.E.; Spear, L.P. Alterations in the reinforcing efficacy of cocaine in adult rats following prenatal exposure to cocaine. *Behav. Neurosci.* **1998**, *112*, 410–418. [CrossRef]
38. Keller, R.W.; LeFevre, R.; Raucci, J.; Carlson, J.N.; Glick, S.D. Enhanced cocaine self-administration in adult rats prenatally exposed to cocaine. *Neurosci. Lett.* **1996**, *205*, 153–156. [CrossRef]
39. Rocha, B.A.; Mead, A.N.; Kosofsky, B.E. Increased vulnerability to self-administer cocaine in mice prenatally exposed to cocaine. *Psychopharmacology* **2002**, *163*, 221–229. [CrossRef]
40. Kelley, B.M.; Middaugh, L.D. Ethanol self-administration and motor deficits in adult C57BL/6J mice exposed prenatally to cocaine. *Pharmacol. Biochem. Behav.* **1996**, *55*, 575–584. [CrossRef]
41. Delaney-Black, V.; Chiodo, L.M.; Hannigan, J.H.; Greenwald, M.K.; Janisse, J.; Patterson, G.; Huestis, M.A.; Partridge, R.T.; Ager, J.; Sokol, R.J. Prenatal and postnatal cocaine exposure predict teen cocaine use. *Neurotoxicol. Teratol.* **2011**, *33*, 110–119. [CrossRef]
42. Frank, D.A.; Rose-Jacobs, R.; Crooks, D.; Cabral, H.J.; Gerteis, J.; Hacker, K.A.; Martin, B.; Weinstein, Z.B.; Heeren, T. Adolescent initiation of licit and illicit substance use: Impact of intrauterine exposures and post-natal exposure to violence. *Neurotoxicol. Teratol.* **2011**, *33*, 100–109. [CrossRef] [PubMed]
43. Minnes, S.; Singer, L.; Min, M.O.; Wu, M.; Lang, A.; Yoon, S. Effects of prenatal cocaine/polydrug exposure on substance use by age 15. *Drug Alcohol. Depend.* **2014**, *134*, 201–210. [CrossRef] [PubMed]
44. Richardson, G.A.; De Genna, N.M.; Goldschmidt, L.; Larkby, C.; Donovan, J.E. Prenatal cocaine exposure: Direct and indirect associations with 21-year-old offspring substance use and behavior problems. *Drug Alcohol Depend.* **2019**, *195*, 121–131. [CrossRef] [PubMed]
45. Bassareo, V.; Cucca, F.; Frau, R.; Di Chiara, G. Differential activation of accumbens shell and core dopamine by sucrose reinforcement with nose poking and with lever pressing. *Behav. Brain Res.* **2015**, *294*, 215–223. [CrossRef]
46. Bassareo, V.; Cucca, F.; Frau, R.; Di Chiara, G. Monitoring dopamine transmission in the rat nucleus accumbens shell and core during acquisition of nose-poking for sucrose. *Behav. Brain Res.* **2015**, *287*, 200–206. [CrossRef]
47. Hajnal, A.; Smith, G.P.; Norgren, R. Oral sucrose stimulation increases accumbens dopamine in the rat. *Am. J. Physiol. Regul. Integr. Comp. Physiol.* **2004**, *286*, 31–37. [CrossRef]
48. Rada, P.; Avena, N.M.; Hoebel, B.G. Daily bingeing on sugar repeatedly releases dopamine in the accumbens shell. *Neuroscience* **2005**, *134*, 737–744. [CrossRef]
49. Bello, N.T.; Lucas, L.R.; Hajnal, A. Repeated sucrose access influences dopamine D2 receptor density in the striatum. *Neuroreport* **2002**, *13*, 1575–1578. [CrossRef]
50. Colantuoni, C.; Schwenker, J.; McCarthy, J.; Rada, P.; Ladenheim, B.; Cadet, J.-L.; Schwartz, G.J.; Moran, T.H.; Hoebel, B.G. Excessive sugar intake alters binding to dopamine and mu-opioid receptors in the brain. *Neuroreport* **2001**, *12*, 3549–3552. [CrossRef]

51. Spangler, R.; Wittkowski, K.M.; Goddard, N.L.; Avena, N.M.; Hoebel, B.G.; Leibowitz, S.F. Opiate-like effects of sugar on gene expression in reward areas of the rat brain. *Mol. Brain Res.* **2004**, *124*, 134–142. [CrossRef]
52. Ahmed, S.; Kashem, M.A.; Sarker, R.; Ahmed, E.U.; Hargreaves, G.A.; McGregor, I.S. Neuroadaptations in the striatal proteome of the rat following prolonged excessive sucrose intake. *Neurochem. Res.* **2014**, *39*, 815–824. [CrossRef] [PubMed]
53. Avena, N.M.; Long, K.A.; Hoebel, B.G. Sugar-dependent rats show enhanced responding for sugar after abstinence: Evidence of a sugar deprivation effect. *Physiol. Behav.* **2005**, *84*, 359–362. [CrossRef] [PubMed]
54. Grimm, J.W.; Fyall, A.M.; Osincup, D.P. Incubation of sucrose craving: Effects of reduced training and sucrose pre-loading. *Physiol. Behav.* **2005**, *84*, 73–79. [CrossRef] [PubMed]
55. Bayol, S.A.; Farrington, S.J.; Stickland, N.C. A maternal "junk food" diet in pregnancy and lactation promotes an exacerbated taste for "junk food" and a greater propensity for obesity in rat offspring. *Br. J. Nutr.* **2007**, *98*, 843–851. [CrossRef]
56. Gosnell, B.A. Sucrose intake enhances behavioral sensitization produced by cocaine. *Brain Res.* **2005**, *1031*, 194–201. [CrossRef]
57. Lenoir, M.; Serre, F.; Cantin, L.; Ahmed, S.H. Intense sweetness surpasses cocaine reward. *PLoS ONE* **2007**, *2*, e698. [CrossRef]
58. Li, Y.Q.; LE, Q.M.; Yu, X.C.; Ma, L.; Wang, F.F. Sucrose reward promotes rats' motivation for cocaine. *Sheng Li Xue Bao* **2016**, *68*, 233–240. [CrossRef]
59. Caprioli, D.; Zeric, T.; Thorndike, E.B.; Venniro, M. Persistent palatable food preference in rats with a history of limited and extended access to methamphetamine self-administration. *Addict. Biol.* **2015**, *20*, 913–926. [CrossRef]
60. Culleré, M.E.; Spear, N.E.; Molina, J.C. Prenatal ethanol increases sucrose reinforcement, an effect strengthened by postnatal association of ethanol and sucrose. *Alcohol* **2014**, *48*, 25–33. [CrossRef]
61. Pacchioni, A.M.; Gabriele, A.; See, R.E. Dorsal striatum mediation of cocaine-seeking after withdrawal from short or long daily access cocaine self-administration in rats. *Behav. Brain Res.* **2011**, *218*, 296–300. [CrossRef]
62. Scofield, M.D.; Heinsbroek, J.A.; Gipson, C.D.; Kupchik, Y.M.; Spencer, S.; Smith, A.C.W.; Roberts-Wolfe, D.; Kalivas, P.W. The Nucleus Accumbens: Mechanisms of Addiction across Drug Classes Reflect the Importance of Glutamate Homeostasis. *Pharmacol. Rev.* **2016**, *68*, 816–871. [CrossRef] [PubMed]
63. Nguyen, L.T.; Saad, S.; Tan, Y.; Pollock, C.; Chen, H. Maternal high-fat diet induces metabolic stress response disorders in offspring hypothalamus. *J. Mol. Endocrinol.* **2017**, *59*, 81–92. [CrossRef] [PubMed]
64. Everitt, B.J.; Wolf, M.E. Psychomotor stimulant addiction: A neural systems perspective. *J. Neurosci.* **2002**, *22*, 3312–3320. [CrossRef] [PubMed]
65. Farrell, M.R.; Schoch, H.; Mahler, S.V. Modeling cocaine relapse in rodents: Behavioral considerations and circuit mechanisms. *Prog. Neuro-Psychopharmacol. Biol. Psychiatry* **2018**, *87*, 33–47. [CrossRef]
66. Stewart, J. Psychological and neural mechanisms of relapse. *Philos. Trans. R. Soc. Lond. B Biol. Sci.* **2008**, *363*, 3147–3158. [CrossRef]
67. Alhadeff, A.L.; Goldstein, N.; Park, O.; Klima, M.L.; Vargas, A.; Betley, J.N. Natural and Drug Rewards Engage Distinct Pathways that Converge on Coordinated Hypothalamic and Reward Circuits. *Neuron* **2019**, *103*, 891–908. [CrossRef]
68. Alvaro, J.D.; Taylor, J.R.; Duman, R.S.; Iadarola, M.; Nestler, E. Molecular and behavioral interactions between central melanocortins and cocaine. *J. Pharmacol. Exp. Ther.* **2003**, *304*, 391–399. [CrossRef]
69. Hsu, R.; Taylor, J.R.; Newton, S.S.; Alvaro, J.D.; Haile, C.; Han, G.; Hruby, V.J.; Nestler, E.J.; Duman, R.S. Blockade of melanocortin transmission inhibits cocaine reward. *Eur. J. Neurosci.* **2005**, *21*, 2233–2242. [CrossRef]
70. Alserda, E.; Adan, R.A.H.; Ramakers, G.M.J. Repeated agouti related peptide (83–132) injections inhibit cocaine-induced locomotor sensitisation, but not via the nucleus accumbens. *Eur. J. Pharmacol.* **2013**, *719*, 187–191. [CrossRef]
71. Cui, H.; Lutter, M. The expression of MC4Rs in D1R neurons regulates food intake and locomotor sensitization to cocaine. *Genes Brain Behav.* **2013**, *12*, 658–665. [CrossRef]
72. Dietrich, M.O.; Bober, J.; Ferreira, J.G.; Tellez, L.A.; Mineur, Y.S.; Souza, D.O.; Gao, X.-B.; Picciotto, M.R.; Araújo, I.; Liu, Z.-W.; et al. AgRP neurons regulate development of dopamine neuronal plasticity and nonfood-associated behaviors. *Nat. Neurosci.* **2012**, *15*, 1108–1110. [CrossRef] [PubMed]

73. Lim, B.K.; Huang, K.W.; Grueter, B.A.; Rothwell, P.E.; Malenka, R.C. Anhedonia requires MC4R-mediated synaptic adaptations in nucleus accumbens. *Nature* **2012**, *487*, 183–189. [CrossRef] [PubMed]
74. Lindblom, J.; Opmane, B.; Mutulis, F.; Mutule, I.; Petrovska, R.; Klusa, V.; Bergström, L.; Wikberg, J.E. The MC4 receptor mediates alpha-MSH induced release of nucleus accumbens dopamine. *Neuroreport* **2001**, *12*, 2155–2158. [CrossRef] [PubMed]
75. Sánchez, M.S.; Barontini, M.; Armando, I.; Celis, M.E. Correlation of increased grooming behavior and motor activity with alterations in nigrostriatal and mesolimbic catecholamines after alpha-melanotropin and neuropeptide glutamine-isoleucine injection in the rat ventral tegmental area. *Cell. Mol. Neurobiol.* **2001**, *21*, 523–533. [CrossRef]

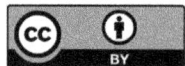

© 2020 by the authors. Licensee MDPI, Basel, Switzerland. This article is an open access article distributed under the terms and conditions of the Creative Commons Attribution (CC BY) license (http://creativecommons.org/licenses/by/4.0/).

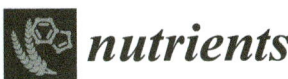 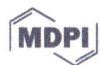

Review

Beneficial Effects of Exogenous Ketogenic Supplements on Aging Processes and Age-Related Neurodegenerative Diseases

Zsolt Kovács [1], Brigitta Brunner [1,2], and Csilla Ari [3,4,*]

1. Department of Biology, Savaria University Centre, ELTE Eötvös Loránd University, Károlyi Gáspár tér 4., 9700 Szombathely, Hungary; zskovacsneuro@gmail.com (Z.K.); brunnerb28@gmail.com (B.B.)
2. Faculty of Sciences, Institute of Biology, University of Pécs, Ifjúság Str. 6, 7624 Pécs, Hungary
3. Behavioral Neuroscience Research Laboratory, Department of Psychology, University of South Florida, 4202 E. Fowler Ave, PCD 3127, Tampa, FL 33620, USA
4. Ketone Technologies LLC, 2780 E. Fowler Ave. #226, Tampa, FL 33612, USA
* Correspondence: csari2000@yahoo.com; Tel.: +1-(813)-2409725

Citation: Kovács, Z.; Brunner, B.; Ari, C. Beneficial Effects of Exogenous Ketogenic Supplements on Aging Processes and Age-Related Neurodegenerative Diseases. *Nutrients* 2021, *13*, 2197. https://doi.org/10.3390/nu13072197

Academic Editor: M. Hasan Mohajeri

Received: 26 May 2021
Accepted: 24 June 2021
Published: 26 June 2021

Publisher's Note: MDPI stays neutral with regard to jurisdictional claims in published maps and institutional affiliations.

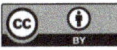

Copyright: © 2021 by the authors. Licensee MDPI, Basel, Switzerland. This article is an open access article distributed under the terms and conditions of the Creative Commons Attribution (CC BY) license (https://creativecommons.org/licenses/by/4.0/).

Abstract: Life expectancy of humans has increased continuously up to the present days, but their health status (healthspan) was not enhanced by similar extent. To decrease enormous medical, economical and psychological burden that arise from this discrepancy, improvement of healthspan is needed that leads to delaying both aging processes and development of age-related diseases, thereby extending lifespan. Thus, development of new therapeutic tools to alleviate aging processes and related diseases and to increase life expectancy is a topic of increasing interest. It is widely accepted that ketosis (increased blood ketone body levels, e.g., β-hydroxybutyrate) can generate neuroprotective effects. Ketosis-evoked neuroprotective effects may lead to improvement in health status and delay both aging and the development of related diseases through improving mitochondrial function, antioxidant and anti-inflammatory effects, histone and non-histone acetylation, β-hydroxybutyrylation of histones, modulation of neurotransmitter systems and RNA functions. Administration of exogenous ketogenic supplements was proven to be an effective method to induce and maintain a healthy state of nutritional ketosis. Consequently, exogenous ketogenic supplements, such as ketone salts and ketone esters, may mitigate aging processes, delay the onset of age-associated diseases and extend lifespan through ketosis. The aim of this review is to summarize the main hallmarks of aging processes and certain signaling pathways in association with (putative) beneficial influences of exogenous ketogenic supplements-evoked ketosis on lifespan, aging processes, the most common age-related neurodegenerative diseases (Alzheimer's disease, Parkinson's disease and amyotrophic lateral sclerosis), as well as impaired learning and memory functions.

Keywords: ketogenic supplement; ketosis; aging; lifespan; neurodegenerative disease; learning; memory

1. Introduction

Aging processes result in irreversible decline of normal physiological functions (time-dependent functional decline) and age-related diseases. It has been demonstrated that several genes and environmental factors can modulate cellular functions leading to the appearance of ageing hallmarks, such as cellular senescence, mitochondrial dysfunction, loss of proteostasis, telomere attrition, deregulated nutrient sensing, stem cell exhaustion and epigenetic alterations [1,2]. These changes may generate, for example, chronic inflammation and aging that leads to increased risk for age-related chronic diseases, such as neurodegenerative diseases (e.g., Alzheimer's disease), osteoporosis, cardiovascular diseases, cancer, diabetes, sarcopenia and osteoarthritis [1,2].

A worldwide increase in elderly population has been predicted, as about 9% of people were over the age of 65 in 2019, which number was predicted to increase to approximately 17% by 2050 [3,4]. Human lifespan is increasing, as a result of more and more effective therapeutic tools and improvement in living conditions, but the health status of patients is not improving by the same intensity. Thus, the prevalence of age-related diseases, such as neurodegenerative diseases are continuously increasing each year [5,6] and the consequences of aging processes and related diseases generate enormous medical, psychological and economical burden for humanity [7]. To decrease the negative consequences of aging processes and related diseases, thereby to mitigate their negative effects on health and the economy, several drugs were developed that are undergoing clinical trials. For example, rapamycin and its analogues [8–10], metformin [11,12], sirtuin (SIRT) activators [13,14] and senolytics (for elimination of senescent cells) [15] can modulate aging mechanisms, and, as a consequence, increase lifespan and decrease risk for age-related diseases. However, to prevent, alleviate and delay age-related processes and diseases, to extend health span and to improve the quality of life of elderly population, development of safer and more effective drugs and therapeutic tools are needed.

Exogenous ketogenic supplements (EKSs), such as ketone esters (KEs, e.g., R,S-1,3-butanediol—acetoacetate diester), ketone salts (KSs, e.g., Na^+/K^+—β-hydroxybutyrate/βHB mineral salt), and medium chain triglycerides (MCTs/MCT oils containing, e.g., about 60% caprylic triglyceride and 40% capric triglyceride) have been proven effective when used together with normal diet to induce and maintain an increased blood ketone body level (ketosis) [16–20]. It has been demonstrated that the level of EKSs-induced ketosis may change by age and gender [21]. Ketone bodies (e.g., βHB and acetoacetate) can enter to the central nervous system (CNS) via monocarboxylate transporters and can be used for ATP (adenosine triphosphate) synthesis via the Krebs-cycle in brain cells [22–25]. It has been demonstrated that EKSs can generate rapid (0.5–6 h after administration) and mild to moderate [19,26–29] therapeutic ketosis (about 1–7 mM) [30,31]. In order to sustain therapeutic ketosis leading to positive outcome, administration of different amounts of EKSs must be repeated for several days or up to several months depending on the disease, the dose and type of EKSs. For example, administration of 30 g MCT drink/day for 6 months and 75 g KE/day for 4 weeks were able to evoke beneficial effects in patients with mild cognitive impairment and type 2 diabetes, respectively [32,33]. However, it has been suggested that not only these, but other EKSs may be effective and safe ketone body precursors for the treatment of diseases in humans through increased βHB level (ketosis) [29,32,34,35]. It has been demonstrated that EKSs are well-tolerated and safe (with mild adverse effects, if any) [19,26,28,29,33,36]. Moreover, administration of EKSs can circumvent both dietary restrictions and adverse effects of ketogenic diets (e.g., nephrolithiasis, constipation and hyperlipidemia) [37]. Thus, administration of EKSs may be a safe and effective alternative metabolic therapy to the ketogenic diet.

It has also been demonstrated that administration of EKSs-generated therapeutic ketosis may evoke beneficial effects on CNS diseases [34,38,39]. For example, KEs, KSs and MCT oils can evoke anti-seizure and anti-epileptic effects [36,40–42], anxiolytic influence [26,43,44], regeneration of nervous system injuries [45] and alleviating effects on neurodegenerative diseases (such as Alzheimer's disease) [41,46–48]. These beneficial effects were induced likely through ketosis-evoked neuroprotective effects, for example, by improved mitochondrial functions, enhanced ATP levels, decreased inflammatory processes and decreased oxidative stress [23,24,34,49,50]. Moreover, ketone bodies may modulate aging processes thereby extend lifespan and delay the development of age-related diseases, such as neurodegenerative diseases. In fact, it has been demonstrated that not only ketogenic diets, but also administration of EKSs can increase and maintain blood ketone body level [19,26–29], which ketone bodies, such as βHB, may promote anti-aging effects [35,51,52]. Moreover, it was demonstrated that βHB, as an endogenous ligand molecule, can activate the hydroxycarboxylic acid receptor 2 (HCAR2 or GPR109A receptor) [53,54]. HCAR2 receptors are expressed not only in macrophages, but also in the brain cells, mainly in microglia, as well as astrocytes and neurons [54–56]. Thus, βHB molecule via, for example, HCAR2 receptors can modulate not only physiological, but also pathophysiological processes in the brain that are connected to aging and neurodegenerative diseases [55,57,58]. Based on the literature, increase of βHB level may be the main factor contributing to the beneficial effects on aging, lifespan and age-related diseases after administration of EKSs. Indeed, it has been demonstrated that βHB decreased the senescence associated secretory phenotype (SASP) of mammals [59] and extended the lifespan of *C. elegans* [60]. Consequently, in this review paper we focused on βHB-generated alleviating effects. Although limited evidence supports the alleviating influence of EKSs on lifespan, aging processes and related CNS diseases, we can hypothesize that EKSs-evoked increase in blood βHB level can modulate (alleviate) aging processes and improve symptoms of age-related diseases through their neuroprotective effects, therefore may delay both aging and the development of related diseases and extend lifespan.

This review discusses the hallmarks of aging and putative anti-aging molecular mechanisms (pathways) by which EKSs may be able to exert their beneficial effects on lifespan, healthspan, aging, the most common age-related neurodegenerative diseases (Alzheimer's disease, Parkinson's disease and amyotrophic lateral sclerosis), as well as learning and memory.

2. Main Features of Aging Processes

It has been demonstrated that aging is the most common risk factor for emergence of neurodegenerative diseases [2]. Indeed, as life expectancy of humans increase, more and more people suffer from different types of neurodegenerative diseases, such as Alzheimer's disease [61]. Moreover, it has been demonstrated that development and incidence of the most common neurodegenerative diseases, Alzheimer's disease (e.g., characterized by extracellular senile, amyloid-β/Aβ plaque and neurofibrillary tangle/hyperphosphorylated and misfolded Tau accumulation in the brain; impairment of learning and memory), Parkinson's diseases (e.g., characterized by the accumulation of α-synuclein and the loss of dopaminergic neurons; tremors and muscle rigidity) and amyotrophic lateral sclerosis (e.g., accumulation of TAR DNA-binding protein 43; progressive degeneration of motor neurons a motor defects; muscle weakness) are promoted by aging [6,62–64]. It has also been also demonstrated that aging hallmarks, such as reduced telomere length and/or genomic instability, epigenetic alterations, mitochondrial dysfunction, cellular senescence, loss of proteostasis, changes in activity of nutrient sensing pathways and intercellular communication, as well as stem cell exhaustion can be detected in Alzheimer's disease, Parkinson's disease and amyotrophic lateral sclerosis. However, in amyotrophic lateral sclerosis, the reduced telomere length, genomic instability, cellular senescence and changes in intercellular communication may be the main contributing factors [63,64]. Thus, in this chapter, we shortly characterize the main aging hallmarks and their connection with the development of the above-mentioned age-related neurodegenerative diseases. Moreover, based on the literature (e.g., administration and effects of senomorphic drugs and caloric restriction) we present the main signaling pathways contributing to the modulation of aging processes, suggesting that inhibition or activation of these pathways may be used for delaying not only aging, but also related neurodegenerative diseases, improve impaired learning and memory functions, as well as to promote lifespan.

2.1. Nutrient Sensing Pathways

Changes in activity of nutrient sensing pathways may have a role in aging and development of age-related diseases. It has been demonstrated that caloric restriction and fasting can attenuate aging, expand lifespan, generate neuroprotective effects and prevent age-related diseases through energy (nutrient) sensing insulin/insulin-like growth factor (IGF) 1 (IIS) pathway, AMP (adenosine monophosphate) activated serine-threonine protein kinase (AMPK), Sirtuin 1 (SIRT1) and transcriptional factor FOXOs (Forkhead box Os) [65–68]. Previous studies show that caloric restriction can decrease IGF, insulin, glucose and amino acid levels, whereas increase NAD^+ (nicotinamide adenine dinucleotide) and AMP levels (Figure 1). These alterations are sensed by the (i) IIS pathway, activated by increased IGF and glucose levels; (ii) AMPK, which senses low energy states via increased

AMP levels; (iii) SIRT1, which also senses low energy states via increased NAD$^+$ levels (NAD$^+$-dependent protein deacetylase); and (iv) mechanistic target of rapamycin (mTOR), which senses high amino acid levels leading to stress resistance, oxidative metabolism, enhanced DNA repair, epigenetic stability and increase in longevity [69–71].

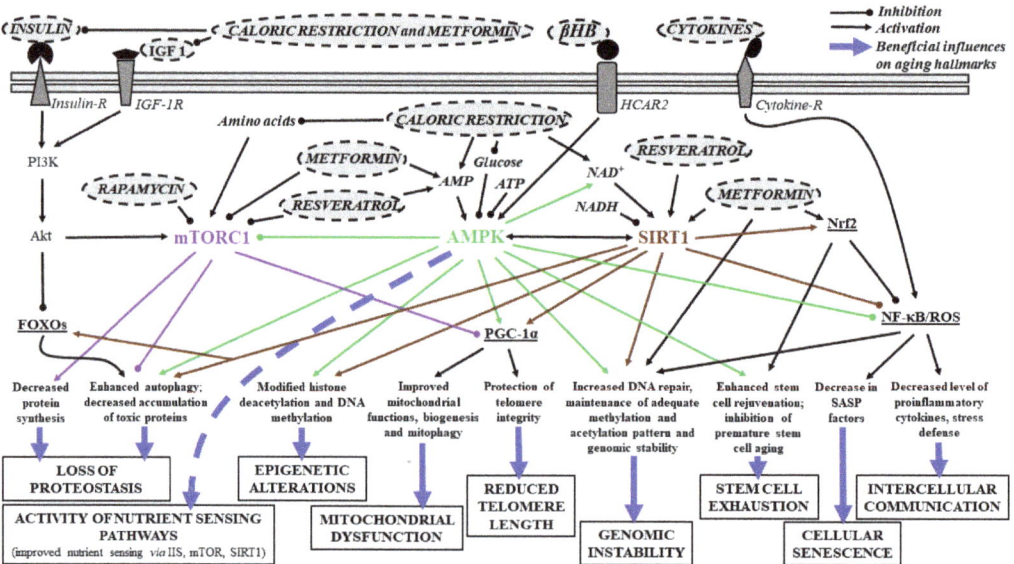

Figure 1. Main downstream signaling pathways and some effects, by which different senomorphic drugs (e.g., metformin), interventions (e.g., caloric restriction) and, theoretically, exogenous ketogenic supplements-evoked ketosis (βHB) can improve age-dependent impaired processes (aging hallmarks). Abbreviations: Akt, Akt kinase/protein kinase B; AMPK, AMP activated serine-threonine protein kinase; ATP, adenosine triphosphate; βHB, beta-hydroxybutyrate; FOXOs, Forkhead box Os; HCAR2, hydroxycarboxylic acid receptor 2; IGF 1, insulin-like growth factor 1; mTORC1, mechanistic target of rapamycin C1; NAD$^+$, nicotinamide adenine dinucleotide; NADH, nicotinamide adenine dinucleotide (NAD) + hydrogen (H); NF-κB, nuclear factor kappa-light-chain-enhancer of activated B cells; Nrf2, nuclear factor erythroid 2-related factor 2; PGC-1α, peroxisome proliferator-activated receptor gamma (PPARγ) coactivator-1α; PI3K, phosphatidyl inositol-3-kinase; ROS, reactive oxygen species; SASP, senescence associated secretory phenotype; SIRT1, Sirtuin 1.

Reduced activity of the IIS pathways can extend lifespan [72], similarly to the mTOR inhibitor rapamycin-evoked increase in lifespan [9]. It was also demonstrated that decreased IIS signaling reduced the aggregation-mediated toxicity of the Aβ1–42 (amyloid β-peptide 1–42), suggesting that decreased insulin signaling may be protective against abnormal aggregation of proteins in neurodegenerative diseases, such as Alzheimer's disease [73]. Moreover, mTOR (a serine/threonine protein kinase) is the main regulator of cellular growth and mass accumulation, which contains mTORC1 and mTORC2 complexes [6]. mTORC1 is able to integrate signals from nutrients, growth factors, energy, and oxygen level in order to promote cell proliferation and growth (e.g., enhancement of energy metabolism/glycolysis and nucleotide, protein, as well as lipid synthesis and inhibition of catabolism/autophagy) [74,75] (Figure 1). Indeed, for example, mTORC1 supports protein synthesis by phosphorylation of S6K1 (ribosomal protein S6 kinase 1) and 4EBP1 (eukaryotic translation initiation factor 4E binding protein 1) molecules, which processes may be activated by Akt kinase (protein kinase B) [6,75,76] (Figure 1). Moreover, mTORC1 can suppress autophagy via inhibition of ULK1 (Uncoordinated/Unc-51-like kinase 1) by which impedes the cellular homeostasis maintaining processes (e.g., providing nutrients under starvation and removing damaged organelles and misfolded proteins) [75,77]. Thus, inhibition of mTORC1 effects on autophagy may be an important tool to decrease age-dependent processes (aging hallmarks, such as loss of proteostasis) and promoting longevity [6] (Figure 1). It was also demonstrated that mTORC2 has a role in the cytoskeleton reorganization (connected to cell growth) and cell survival modulation [75,78].

SIRTs and AMPK also have a role in the modulation of lifespan. Activation of AMPK mediated pathways by low energy levels has a role in inhibition of glucose production, increase in activity of beta-oxidation (fat burning) and promotion of mitochondrial functions and mitochondrial biogenesis [79,80] (Figure 1). AMPK exerts its effect on energy metabolism by phosphorylation of, for example, (i) ACCs (acetyl-CoA carboxylases), such as ACC1, which ACC1 inhibition lead to enhancement of fatty acid oxidation/mitochondrial-oxidation and suppression of lipogenesis; and (ii) the transcription factor SREBP1 (sterol regulatory element-binding protein 1). The inhibitory effect of AMPK results in reduced fatty acid synthesis [80]. It was suggested that AMPK activation may be a promising anti-aging therapeutic target, for example, by improvement of mitochondrial dysfunction. AMPK activation not only decreased the activity of anabolic pathways and increased activity of catabolic pathways leading to increase of activity of energy (ATP)-generating pathways and decrease in energy (ATP)-consuming processes, but also increased lifespan in diabetic patients [79,80]. Moreover, increase in AMPK activity decreases the expression of proinflammatory cytokines, therefore modulate intercellular communication (Figure 1) by inhibition of advanced-glycation end products (AGEs)-evoked increase in the level of transcription factor NF-κB (nuclear factor kappa-light-chain-enhancer of activated B cells) mRNA and protein [81]. However, AMPK activation may suppress inflammation through the inflammatory response inducer NF-κB by other pathways, for example, through triggering of inhibitory activity of SIRT1, PGC-1α (peroxisome proliferator-activated receptor γ/PPARγ coactivator 1α), FOXOs and p53 (transcription factor tumor suppressor protein 53) on NF-κB-signaling or via inhibition of NF-κB activator ER (endoplasmic reticulum) stress and oxidative stress [82]. Moreover, AMPK is able to increase PGC-1α activity not only directly (by phosphorylation, before subsequent deacetylation of PGC1-α by SIRT1) [83], but also via arrest of PGC-1α inhibitory effect of mTORC1 [66] (Figure 1).

It has also been demonstrated that caloric restriction may exert its effect on lifespan through SIRTs [84], thus SIRTs are considered as putative anti-aging factors. SIRTs, such as SIRT1 and SIRT3 are able to sense low energy levels via detection of high NAD^+ levels. SIRTs are Class III HDACs histone deacetylases, which enzymes use coenzyme NAD^+ to remove acyl groups of proteins, such as acetyl-lysine residues of histones and non-histones, such as PGC-1α, FOXOs, p53 and NF-κB [69,85]. Under nutrient deprivation (caloric restriction), the level of a nutrient-sensing deacetylase SIRT1 is elevated (which, e.g., increases hepatic glucose production through PGC-1α), but its level reduced by overfeeding [86,87]. It has been demonstrated that activation (overexpression) of SIRT1 may increase lifespan and have an alleviating role in all age-related processes (hallmarks) (Figure 1) and several diseases, such as neurodegenerative diseases [88–90]. Indeed, SIRT1 expression was found to decrease with age, for example in the brain [91]. Moreover, it was also demonstrated that decreased level of SIRT1 in microglia can lead to cognitive decline (Tau-mediated memory deficits) in aging and neurodegeneration by upregulation of IL-1β (interleukin-1β) [91]. It was also demonstrated that caloric restriction can attenuate Alzheimer's disease progression, for example, by decreasing the accumulation of Aβ plaque [92] and promote longevity and healthy aging [93] likely via SIRT1 activation [93–95], whereas higher caloric intake may increase the risk of the development of Alzheimer's disease [96]. Reduction of SIRT1 levels was also demonstrated in parietal cortex in patients with Alzheimer's disease, which was associated with the accumulation of Aβ and Tau [97], whereas activation of SIRT1 can suppress α-synuclein aggregation [98]. It has been demonstrated that SIRT1-evoked neuroprotection may evoke not only decrease in excitotoxicity and neurodegeneration [99,100], but also improved healthspan and extended lifespan likely through activation of PGC-1α (regulation of mitochondrial biogenesis) (Figure 1) and FOXOs (enhancing stress response via autophagy, resistance to oxidative stress and DNA damage and FOXO3's ability to induce cell cycle arrest), as well as inhibition of p53 (regulation of apoptosis and cell cycle) and SREBP1 (regulation of lipid metabolism) activation [6,88,101,102]. These pathways can lead to alleviating effects in neurodegenerative diseases, such as Alzheimer's disease and amyotrophic lateral sclerosis via, for example, SIRT1-generated deacetylation (and activation) of PGC-1α [94]. It has been demonstrated that SIRT1 is able to inhibit cell aging via p53 (deacetylation thereby inhibition of both p53 and its proapoptotic activity) [103] and can modulate development (fate) of neural progenitor cells [104]. It was also demonstrated that cellular NAD^+ level decreased with age (evoked by, e.g., accumulated DNA damages during aging) leading to decreased SIRT activity, mitochondrial dysfunction [88,105] and development of age-related diseases, such as neurodegenerative diseases [106]. Consequently, therapeutic tools, such as administration of different drugs and metabolic therapies, which increase NAD^+ level can evoke alleviating effects on aging-related processes and diseases, as well as promote longevity [6,106] (Figure 1).

It was also demonstrated that mutation, lacking, genetic variants or inactivation of insulin/IGF-1 receptor, as well as caloric restriction (inhibiting insulin/IGF-1 signaling) (Figure 1) extends the lifespan, not only in different animals, such as mice, but also in humans [6,107,108] via PI3K (phosphatidyl inositol-3-kinase)/Akt/FOXOs pathway promoting stress defense. Under these conditions (e.g., caloric restriction-evoked decrease in insulin level) unphosphorylated FOXOs can be transported to the nucleus to promote the transcription of several genes (namely, their phosphorylation impedes their translocation to the nucleus) leading to increased stress resistance, cell cycle arrest, damage repair and increased longevity (lifespan) [72,109].

2.2. Telomere Shortening and Genome Instability

Reduced length of repetitive ribonucleoprotein sequences at the distal ends of eukaryotic chromosomes (telomere) during cell division was demonstrated during physiological ("natural") aging of mammals [110]. However, if the length of telomeres is too short it can cause damage of the DNA molecules, cellular senescence, mitochondrial dysfunctions (decreased mitochondrial biogenesis and functions, as well as increased ROS/reactive oxygen species level via p53-evoked repression of PGC-1α/β), and inflammation thereby aging [110–112]. It was also suggested that activation of telomerase activity not only enhances the survival time and increase lifespan of mammals [3,113], but also may be favorable for cancer cell development (by decreased senescence and immortalization) [2,114]. Thus, shorter telomeres- and low (if any) telomerase activity-evoked senescence can prevent tumorigenesis at least in animals with long lifespan [2]. It was also suggested that telomere attrition may have a role in development of age-related neurodegenerative diseases, such as Alzheimer's disease [111]. AMPK and SIRT1 can attenuate age-related telomere shortening through PGC-1α (Figure 1) suggesting beneficial role of AMPK/SIRT1 activation on neurodegenerative diseases [115].

Not only telomere shortening, but also chromosomal aneuploidy, somatic mutations and copy mutations may have a role in DNA damage [116]. Moreover, defects of DNA repair mechanisms (such as base excision repair), mitochondrial DNA mutation and perturbations of the nuclear lamina may also generate genome instability (accumulation of genetic damage), cell dysfunction and aging via senescence [63,117–119], which processes may evoke (or have a role in) age-related diseases [78]. Indeed, DNA damage can trigger the onset of neurodegenerative diseases, such as Parkinson's disease and amyotrophic lateral sclerosis [120]. Changes in integrity and stability of DNA can be evoked through both exogenous effects (e.g., by chemical, physical and biological agents) and endogenous influences (e.g., by increase in ROS level and DNA replication errors) [118]. SIRT1 have a positive influence on DNA repair thereby genomic instability (Figure 1), suggesting alleviating effect of SIRT1 activation on neurodegenerative diseases [115].

2.3. Epigenetic Alterations

The epigenome contains molecular switches by which genes may be activated or inhibited during the entire lifetime [121]. It was demonstrated that epigenetic alterations, such as changes in DNA methylation patterns (which methylation is inversely proportional to gene activation), chromatin remodeling, expression of non-coding RNAs and posttranslational histone modifications may also promote aging processes [78,122]. For example, it has been demonstrated that (hyper)methylation of promoter sequences of the genes (and in general on the DNA) can lead to silencing of genes related to, for example, apoptosis [123], whereas DNA hypomethylation promotes gene activation [124,125]. It was also demonstrated that changes in the pattern of DNA methylation (hypermethylation or hypomethylation) by age may be important in the mechanism of aging [126] and used as an aging clock (e.g., a link between methylcytosine/DNA methylation and age was demonstrated) [125,127]. Both global decrease of DNA methylation (which hypomethylation may induce age-associated genomic instability and loss of telomere integrity) and site-specific hypermethylation of promoter sequences were observed by age [122–124,128]. A previous study showed that age-induced hypomethylation was corrected by caloric restriction [129].

It has been suggested that caloric restriction can upregulate SIRT1 transcription leading to increase in histone deacetylation and methylation of DNA, which effects may compensate the decrease in both SIRT1 activity and DNA methylation, as well as increase in histone acetylation by age and increase lifespan (e.g., by maintenance of adequate DNA methylation pattern and genomic stability) [90,130] (Figure 1). Histone acetyl transferases (HATs) can attach acetyl groups to histones leading to increased positive charge, and attenuation of interaction with DNA, and thereby enhancing DNA transcription. Conversely, HDACs can remove acetyl groups from histones, which effect enhances interaction between histones and DNA resulting decreased transcription. Consequently, antagonists of HDACs may facilitate DNA transcription [131,132]. Based on these results above, expression of genes can be blocked (silenced) through not only methylation of DNA (e.g., methylation of promoter sequences of genes), but also deacetylation of histones, which continuous silencing of genes may be an important factor in progressive aging [123]. Moreover, histone methylation and demethylation (by histone methyl transferases and demethylases) and histone acetylation and deacetylation (by HATs and HDACs) can modulate lifespan, aging and age-related diseases [124,133,134]. For example, SIRT1-evoked deacetylation of Nk2 homeobox 1 can extend lifespan and delay aging processes in mice [133]. It has been demonstrated that inhibitors of HDACs (Classes I, II and IV HDACs), such as Trichostatin A, may be effective in the treatment of neurodegenerative diseases and the extension of lifespan [135,136]. Moreover, HDAC inhibitors decreased death of motor neurons, enhanced motor performance, increased the survival time and resulted in life extension in a mice model of amyotrophic lateral sclerosis [137], restored fear learning, decreased Aβ accumulation and improved cognitive performance in mouse models of Alzheimer's disease [138,139] and generated neuroprotection in a model of Parkinson's disease [140]. It was also suggested that miRNAs (microRNAs; a class of small non-coding silencing RNAs, which have a role in regulation of mRNA translation) may promote longevity and have a role in both neurodegeneration and age-related neurodegenerative diseases [141,142]. For example, hippocampal upregulation of miR-181 and related decrease of SIRT1 expression and, as a result, reduction of synaptic plasticity was demonstrated in a mouse model of Alzheimer's disease [143]. As a response to severe, persistent DNA damage (e.g., by oxidative stress), activated poly(ADP-ribose)-polymerase-1 (PARP-1) adds ADP-ribose units to histones leading to the promotion of chromatin relaxation [144], enhances PARylation (generating PAR polymers as epigenetic effect) at sites of DNA damage (alteration) [63] and induce neuronal cell death via modulation of gene expression and mitochondrial dysfunction [145]. Moreover, excess PARP1 activation was demonstrated in aging and neurodegenerative diseases resulting mitochondrial dysfunction, neuroinflammation and dysregulation of autophagy (and mitophagy; e.g., via mTOR activation) [144,146]. For example, PARP1 enhances inflammation via NF-κB, decreased NAD$^+$ level and SIRT1 activity and has a role in telomere shortening and, as a consequence, enhances senescence, leading to neurodegeneration and reduced lifespan [144,146,147]. As SIRT1 activity decreased by age [91], under this condition, both acetylation (activation) of PARP1, and PAPR1-evoked neuroinflammation may be increased. However, to retain its own functions via preservation of NAD$^+$ levels, SIRT1 is able to deactivate (deacetylate) Parp1 [148]. Moreover, increased expression and excessive activation of PARP1 was demonstrated in Parkinson's disease, Alzheimer's disease and amyotrophic lateral sclerosis [145,149,150]. As it was demonstrated, Aβ and α-synuclein accumulation may generate activation of PAPR1 via, for example, increased level of ROS; thus, enhanced PARP1 activity aggravates Alzheimer's disease and Parkinson's disease symptoms by promotion of Aβ and α-synuclein aggregation, respectively [145,149]. Consequently, PARP1 inhibition can alleviate neuroinflammation, dysregulation of autophagy and mitochondrial dysfunction thereby inhibit development of inflammation(age)-related neurodegenerative diseases (or alleviate their symptoms), for example via SIRT1 activation [146,151]. It was also demonstrated that increase in βHB level can evoke epigenetic (posttranslational) gene regulation by β-hydroxybutyrylation of histones resulting regulation of gene expression thereby adaptation of cells to altered cellular energy source [152].

2.4. Mitochondrial Dysfunction

Mitochondrial dysfunction is associated with the decline of mitochondrial activity, such as defect of respiratory chain, decrease in ATP synthesis and level, as well as increase in ROS production. This hallmark of aging may be evoked by, for example, decreased mitochondrial biogenesis, defective mitophagy and mtDNA mutations leading to processes (e.g., enhancement of inflammatory processes), which can reduce lifespan, enhance aging and the risk of age-related diseases [69,153]. Indeed, it has been demonstrated that decrease in mitochondrial functions or damage of mitochondria may also be in the background of the development of neurodegenerative diseases [154] through excessive ROS formation leading to inflammation and genomic instability. These processes can enhance cellular senescence, aging processes and development of age-related diseases [154]. It was also demonstrated, that increased level of ROS may generate protective, homeostatic (alleviating) processes (e.g., on lifespan limiting cellular processes via ROS-dependent, protective, stress-response pathways), but, by aging progress, above a certain level ROS can evoke (aggravate) age-related damages [155]. It was demonstrated that autophagy (and mitophagy) declined with age [156], which can generate accumulation of damaged mitochondria thereby increased inflammation (e.g., via increased ROS level-evoked activation of NLRP3/NOD-like receptor pyrin domain 3 and NF-κB), cell death (e.g., through activation of caspases and mitochondrial permeability transition/mPT pore by excess ROS) and DNA damage (by ROS leading to increase in apoptotic signaling, such as p53) [153]. Moreover, it has been demonstrated that defects in mitochondria and autophagy (thereby aggregation of not only α-synuclein and Aβ peptide, but also impaired mitochondria) may have a role in development of neurodegenerative diseases, such as Parkinson's disease and Alzheimer's disease [153,156–158]. Thus, drugs or interventions, such as caloric restriction, which are able to promote autophagy and mitophagy, therefore inhibit mitochondrial dysfunction, ROS production, aggregation of toxic proteins, inflammation, cell death and cell senescence, can delay age-related degeneration, extend healthy lifespan and alleviate neurodegenerative diseases [159–161]. Indeed, for example, it was demonstrated that SIRT1 has a role in elimination of damaged mitochondria via autophagy (by enhanced activity of autophagy proteins) [162–164] and in mitochondrial biogenesis (increase in mitochondrial biogenesis) via increased transcriptional cofactor PGC-1α activity [87] (Figure 1), whereas a mitochondrial deacetylase SIRT3 controls (decreases) ROS level by enhancement of antioxidant activity of superoxide dismutase 2 (SOD2) during caloric restriction, leading to increased oxidative stress resistance [165]. Moreover, it was also demonstrated that increased SIRT3 activity can suppress mPT pore formation by which it can prevent mitochondrial dysfunctions [166]. It was also demonstrated that PGC-1α activation can enhance mitochondrial biogenesis and improve mitochondrial energy metabolism, therefore increasing lifespan and protecting against neurodegenerative diseases [167]. PGC-1α can bind and co-activate the transcription factor PPARγ (belongs to the superfamily of nuclear receptors) and promotes not only mitochondrial biogenesis, but also SOD and catalase activity, glucose metabolism and oxidative phosphorylation [162,168–170], whereas reduces the level of NF-κB and pro-inflammatory cytokines [171,172], as well as Aβ generation [173,174]. Indeed, reduced level of PGC1-α can result in decreased mitochondrial respiration and enhanced inflammatory processes [175]. Moreover, mitochondrial uncoupling via the overexpression of uncoupling protein 1 (UCP1) may also increase the lifespan [176].

2.5. Altered Intercellular Communication: Increased Inflammatory Processes

Aging processes are also connected to dysregulation of cell-cell connectivity and intercellular communication leading to, among others, sterile (activation of immune response without appearance of pathogens), chronic, low-grade inflammation (named "inflammaging") with activation of NF-κB, as well as increased synthesis and release of proinflammatory cytokines (e.g., IL-1β and TNF-α/tumor necrosis factor-α) [69,125,177,178]. Increase in inflammatory processes and proinflammatory cytokine levels can also enhance (trigger) aging processes, for example, through increased activation of intracellular multiprotein sensor NLRP3 inflammasome, senescent cells-evoked release of proinflammatory cytokines and NF-κB level and signaling [177,179,180]. Autophagy failure in old organisms (e.g., decrease in activity of autophagy), and in patients with Alzheimer's disease and Parkinson's disease [181,182] were also demonstrated. It was suggested that aging (e.g., decreased autophagy by age) can stimulate NF-κB signaling, which transcription factor NF-κB (similar to increase in ROS by mitochondria and aggregation of Aβ) stimulate inflammatory processes, for example, via increased NLRP3 expression and IL-1β release [161,179,183–185], whereas autophagic uptake of damaged mitochondria (resulting decrease in ROS level) suppresses NLRP3 stimulation [161]. Thus, it was suggested that autophagy may generate an anti-inflammatory effect by inhibition of NLRP3 inflammasome thereby mitigating the NLRP3-evoked cleavage of pro-IL-1β to its active form/IL-1β by caspase-1 [186,187] leading to delay in aging processes [180].

Moreover, responsiveness of AMPK signaling decreased by age [180,188], which mitigates its inhibitory activity on NF-κB signaling [82] (Figure 1) and impairs autophagic activity leading to increased oxidative stress and activation of inflammasomes [180] and can attenuate lifespan [82]. As mTORC1 is able to inhibit autophagy (e.g., mitophagy or macroautophagy of altered proteins) all of drugs or interventions, which are able to inhibit mTORC1 (e.g., caloric restriction leading to mTOR inhibition) may be potent delayer of aging processes and enhancer of lifespan via inhibition of inflammation [180] (Figure 1), by which can alleviate not only neuroinflammation, but also neurodegeneration and related diseases, such as Alzheimer's disease, Parkinson's disease and amyotrophic lateral sclerosis [183,189]. Indeed, inhibition of NF-κB signaling was able to prevent age-associated features in mouse models extending their longevity [190].

2.6. Cellular Senescence

Cellular senescence can be evoked by intracellular and extracellular, genomic and epigenomic harmful stimuli and damages resulting hallmarks of aging (e.g., age-related stress: oxidative stress and telomere shortening; metabolic, as well as ER stress; mitochondrial dysfunction, loss of proteostasis) [191–193]. One of the main features of aging is the enhancement of cellular senescence (irreversible cell-cycle arrest regulated by, e.g., telomere attrition/DNA damage-evoked p53-dependent DNA-damage response, in which p53 is activated). Excessive accumulation of senescent cells, which cells decrease tissue regeneration and resistant to apoptosis (e.g., by upregulation of antiapoptotic Bcl-2/B cell lymphoma-2 family proteins resulting resistance to apoptosis-inducing signals), can evoke harmful processes on surrounding cells by secretion of proinflammatory agents (SASP factors, e.g., IL-1β,) and other components (e.g., IGF-1) [2,191,194,195]. For example, previous studies show that acute administration of IGF-1 can promote cell proliferation and survival whereas prolonged administration of IGF-1 promotes cell growth arrest and senescence (and the latter, enhances aging processes and inhibits tumorigenesis) via through SIRT1 inhibition and increased p53 activity (by increased acetylation) [196] and suppression of autophagy (e.g., via mTOR) [197] (Figure 1). Indeed, SIRT1 can inhibit not only DNA-damage, but also cellular senescence via deacetylation (inhibition) of p53 resulting anti-aging effects [198]. In contrast with cellular senescence, cellular quiescence occurs when nutrition or growth factor levels are very low (or lack) leading to a reversible cell-cycle arrest. In this state the cells may impede initiation of cell senescence [199] and has a role in maintenance of stemness [200]. However, in relation to maintaining cellular balance, senescence of cells is a double-edged sword [2]. For example, cellular senescence can reduce liver fibrosis [201], promote tissue repair and has a role in not only physiological, but also pathophysiological processes (e.g., embryogenesis and wound healing) [195] and prevent cancer development [202], but exaggerated attenuation of processes of cell senescence and accumulation of senescent cells can generate (or enhance) aging, and, as a consequence, development of age related diseases, such as Alzheimer's disease and cancer [192,195,203–205]. Thus, medication of cellular senescence needs careful attention. Under glucose deprived condition, AMPK-induced p53 activation potentiates cellular survival (p53-dependent metabolic arrest), but excessive (lasting) AMPK activation leads to enhanced p53-dependent cellular senescence [206,207]. However, not only SIRT1, but also AMPK activation can improve cellular senescence via, for example, inhibition of proinflammatory mediators [5,81,82] (Figure 1).

2.7. Loss of Proteostasis and Stem Cell Exhaustion

Impaired protein homeostasis (loss of proteostasis) by age may also be in the background of aging and related diseases (e.g., neurodegenerative diseases) leading to dysregulation of protein synthesis, degradation and protein aggregation, disaggregation, assembly, folding and trafficking [208]. For example, activity of ubiquitin-proteasome system and autophagy decreased with age [209], whereas increased activity of proteostasis network (e.g., enhanced autophagy) extended the healthspan and lifespan [210]. Inhibition of mTOR pathways (e.g., by caloric restriction through decreased protein synthesis and activation of autophagy) may improve protein homeostasis and extend lifespan [211,212] (Figure 1). It has been demonstrated that maintained mitochondrial proteostasis prolonged lifespan and reduced Aβ protein aggregation in Alzheimer's disease models [213]. Moreover, decreased activity of autophagy-lysosomal pathway may have a role in the development of both Alzheimer's disease and Parkinson's disease and other neurodegenerative diseases [77]. Indeed, activation of mitophagy (by which autophagy-lysosomal pathway remove damaged/dysfunctional mitochondria) was able to increase lifespan in worms and reverse cognitive deficits in models of Alzheimer's disease [214,215]. AMPK activation may participate in maintenance of proteostasis via inhibition of mTOR and phosphorylation of eIF2α (eukaryotic initiation factor 2α; resulting attenuation of protein synthesis) and via activation of autophagy [79,80] (Figure 1). Moreover, it was also demonstrated that autophagy may be enhanced via inhibition of mTOR by SIRT1 [216] (Figure 1). Thus, activation of AMPK/SIRT1 and inhibition of mTOR (mTORC1, but not mTORC2 because the latter is required for autophagy) activity may be a promising target in anti-aging therapy [77]. Indeed, aging and age-associated diseases can upregulate mTORC1 [69].

Stem cell exhaustion may have a role in aging and appearance of age-related diseases through loss of regenerative ability of cells, tissues and organs. For example, activity and number of hematopoietic cells and intestinal stem cells are decreased by age leading to decrease in lymphoid cell number and adaptive immune response, increase in risk of anemia development and myeloid cell number, as well as malfunctions in intestinal functions [217,218]. Moreover, age-dependent decrease in function of other stem cells, such as neuronal stem cells was also demonstrated [71]. It was suggested that stem cell aging may be evoked by several factors, such as DNA damage and mutation, cellular senescence, defects in proteostasis, mitochondrial dysfunction and telomere attrition [63,71].

Thus, we can conclude that activation of AMPK/SIRTs-modulated signaling pathways, inhibition of mTOR effects (e.g., by inhibition of IIS pathway) and modulation of gene expression (e.g., by HDAC inhibitors) can alleviate aging processes (hallmarks) through direct and indirect manner (e.g., improvement of one of aging hallmarks, such as telomere attrition can improve other aging hallmarks, such as senescence and mitochondrial dysfunction), leading to extended lifespan and delay the appearance of neurodegenerative diseases.

2.8. Effects of Senotherapeutic Drugs on Aging Hallmarks and Neurodegenerative Diseases: Main Signaling Pathways

It has been demonstrated that elimination of senescent cells by senolytics (such as senolytic cocktails containing quercetin and dasatinib) can evoke alleviating effects on age-related diseases, such as Alzheimer's disease and Parkinson's disease and improve healthspan in aged humans [192,203,219]. Another senotherapeutic strategy is the administration of senomorphics (e.g., metformin and rapamycin) to alleviate (abolish) features of senescence (e.g., decrease in production and release of SASP factors) (Figure 1) without elimination of senescent cells, which may delay both aging and development of age-related diseases [194]. It was suggested that mTOR has a role in, among others, lifespan control [220]. Indeed, rapamycin (sirolimus; as an mTOR inhibitor) (Figure 1) is able to decrease the risk of development of age-related diseases, such as neurodegenerative diseases, to improve age-related decrease in memory and learning functions and to extend longevity [74,220]. Rapamycin decreased accumulation of Aβ and Tau leading to decreased loss of neurons, attenuated neuroinflammation and alleviated cognitive dysfunction in mouse models of Alzheimer's disease [221]. Resveratrol also promotes clearance of Aβ peptides [95], likely via inhibition of mTOR and activation of AMPK [5] and prevents cognitive impairment [222] in different cell lines and models of Alzheimer's disease. Thus, these results suggest that resveratrol and rapamycin exert its neuroprotective, alleviating effect on health span, lifespan and age-associated diseases likely by modulation of autophagy and proteostasis (via mTOR inhibition), as well as inflammation, among others [211,212,220] (Figure 1). Rapamycin and metformin (an antidiabetic drug, which reduces IGF levels, insulin resistance and insulin level) reduced accumulation of α-synuclein and improved behavioral impairments in models of Parkinson's disease [74,220,223]. Moreover, metformin inhibits the mitochondrial electron transport chain (ETC complex I: NADH/ubiquinone oxidoreductase; thereby oxidative phosphorylation), consequently, cytoplasmic AMP/ATP and ADP/ATP ratios were increased resulting direct activation (phosphorylation) of AMPK [224,225] and decrease in ROS level [226]. Activation of AMPK (e.g., by metformin) (Figure 1) enhances mitochondrial biogenesis (via SIRT1/PGC-1α) and lipid beta-oxidation (via ACCs), inhibits hepatic glucose production and alleviates proteostasis (via mTOR inhibition), enhances autophagy (via mTOR inhibition and activation of ULK1), evokes hypoglycemia (decreasing plasma glucose levels, e.g., via improved hepatic insulin sensitivity leading to decrease in hepatic glucose production), improves nutrient sensing (via IIS/mTOR/SIRT1 pathways), inhibits NF-κB, improves DNA repair and decreases the level of proinflammatory cytokines (e.g., via activation of SIRT1) [6,12,225–228] leading to alleviating effects on aging-processes and related neurodegenerative diseases. As AMPK-independent influences, metformin is able to inhibit ROS production (via, e.g., inhibition of mitochondrial ETC and activation of antioxidant transcription factor nuclear factor erythroid 2-related factor 2/Nrf2) (Figure 1), enhance autophagy (through direct inhibition of mTOR), enhance SIRT1 activity (especially when NAD^+ level highly reduced), activate DNA-damage-like response (and facilitates DNA repair likely via p53), attenuate NF-κB signaling and synthesis (release) of proinflammatory cytokines, inhibit SASP factors via Nrf2 and decrease level of insulin and IGF-1 levels thereby insulin/IGF-1 signaling (by which decreases mTOR activity) [66,86,225,229–232]. All of these processes can increase lifespan and evoke alleviating effects on both ageing and age-related diseases, such as Alzheimer's disease and Parkinson's disease [224,225,233]. Moreover, metformin is able to inhibit premature stem cell aging (via Nrf2), enhance stem cell rejuvenation (through AMPK) [234], affect histone modifications (e.g., via activation of SIRT1, inhibition of Class II HDACs and HAT phosphorylation) through AMPK-dependent and independent pathways [235], increase the levels of several miRNAs, which are implicated in the regulation of aging and cellular senescence, likely via AMPK [236] and reduce telomere shortening (e.g., via AMKP/PGC-1α/telomeric repeat-containing RNA/TERRA pathway; TERRA is transcribed from telomeres and has an important role in protection of telomere integrity) [225,237,238] (Figure 1). Indeed, it was demonstrated that, activation of AMPK can both enhance gene expression (e.g., by phosphorylation/inactivation of HDACs and activation of HAT1-evoked acetylation of histones) and inhibit gene transcription (e.g., via enhanced cellular NAD^+ levels, and, as a consequence, increased SIRT1 deacetylation activity) [235]. Moreover, resveratrol can also extend lifespan and prevent neurodegenerative diseases [239]. For example, resveratrol can generate anti-inflammatory and anti-oxidative effects (e.g., decreases level of ROS, p53, NF-κB and proinflammatory cytokines, such as TNF-α and IL-1β) [5] and increase mean life expectancy and maximal life span in models of Alzheimer's disease [240]. Moreover, resveratrol improved motor neuron function and extended the lifespan in a mouse model of amyotrophic lateral sclerosis [241]. It was suggested that resveratrol may exert its effects via activation of AMPK/SIRT1-modulated pathways [242] (Figure 1) by which this drug can deacetylate several substrates, such as p53, PGC-1α, FOXOs (e.g., FOXO3) and SREBP1 leading to induction of cell cycle arrest, mitochondrial biogenesis, DNA repair, oxidative stress response, autophagy and regulation of lipid metabolism [6,101,243]. For example, SIRT1 can decrease ROS and NF-κB-evoked effects (e.g., neuroinflammation) via Nrf2 [5] (Figure 1). However, it was also suggested that not only SIRT1, but also PGC1-α can increase the expression of Nrf2 [244,245] and AMPK enhances the nuclear translocation of the Nrf2 [246]. Based on these results, more effective sirtuin-activating compounds were developed, such as SRT2104, which drug may be a promising anti-aging drug (e.g., it increased lifespan and decreased inflammatory processes) [247]. Other natural products, such as curcumin, berberine and quercetin [6] can also generate positive effects on lifespan (by slowing aging), age and age-related diseases, for example, through AMPK activation and mTOR inhibition (e.g., to induce autophagy), activation of SIRT1 (to promote mitochondrial biogenesis) and anti-inflammatory effects [74,248–250].

Thus, administration of senotherapeutic drugs suggests that therapeutic tools and drugs, which are able to modify aging processes through activation or inhibition of certain signaling pathways can also delay development (or improve symptoms) of neurodegenerative diseases (such as Alzheimer's disease, Parkinson's disease and amyotrophic lateral sclerosis), improve memory and learning functions, as well as extend longevity.

3. Alleviating Effects of Ketosis on Lifespan, Aging and Age-Related Neurodegenerative Diseases

3.1. Ketosis-Evoked Neuroprotective Effects and Downstream Signaling Pathways

It has been demonstrated that ketosis and administration of βHB (as an alternative energy fuel to glucose) can increase mitochondrial ATP production and ATP release leading to increased extracellular level of purine nucleoside adenosine (via metabolism of ATP) [251–253]. Adenosine can activate its receptors leading to reduced oxidative stress (ROS level) [254] and reduce inflammatory processes [255]. Indeed, as enhanced level of ROS may activate (open) mPT pore thereby uncouple electron transport system from ATP production, βHB-evoked decrease in ROS production [94] can improve mitochondrial respiration and ATP production [49]. It was also suggested that therapeutic ketosis can increase the inhibitory GABAergic effects [22,256], decrease glutamate release and glutamate-induced neuronal excitability [256,257] and modulate (increase) the level of dopamine, adrenaline, noradrenaline and serotonin [258,259].

As an epigenetic gene regulator, βHB can inhibit the activity of the classical HDAC family (Class I and Class IIa HDACs) leading to enhanced acetylation of histone residues, thereby DNA can be accessed for transcription factors, such as FOXO3A [53,132,260]. FOXO3A generates enhanced expression of various antioxidants genes, enhances mitochondrial homeostasis (e.g., by regulation of mitochondrial biogenesis and ATP synthesis) and decreases oxidative stress [260,261]. Moreover, decrease in oxidative stress can also be generated by βHB-evoked inhibition of HDACs via attenuation of ER stress [262]. It has also been demonstrated, that the expression of brain-derived neurotrophic factor (BDNF) may be increased through βHB-evoked inhibition of HDACs [263] by which βHB evokes anti-inflammatory effects (via inhibition of both NLRP3, NF-κB and proinflammatory cytokine levels) [264,265], increases mitochondrial respiration and ATP levels [266], enhances the activity of anti-oxidant enzymes (such as SOD), and protects tissues against glutamate-induced excitotoxicity [267,268]. It has been also demonstrated that βHB can modulate gene expression through promotion of histone and non-histone acetylation by HATs [266,269]. Moreover, βHB is able to directly bind to an RNA-binding protein hnRNP A1 (heterogeneous nuclear ribonucleoprotein A1), which protein regulates, for example, RNA processing and function, as well as stabilization of mRNA [59,270,271].

Previous studies showed that βHB, through HCAR2, activates AMPK leading to NAD$^+$-generation, which increases activity of SIRTs (e.g., SIRT1 and SIRT3; βHB/HCAR2/NAD$^+$/SIRTs pathways) [272] (Figure 1) and thereby evoke neuroprotective effects [53,83,273,274]. Through both βHB/HCAR2/AMPK/SIRT1/NF-κB pathway and βHB/HCAR2/AMPK/mTOR pathway, βHB may generate anti-inflammatory effects by, for example, inhibition of proinflammatory transcription factor NF-κB and enhancement of autophagy, respectively [55,272,275], leading to decreased level of proinflammatory agents (e.g., TNF-α, IL-1β) [50,55,57,276]. βHB/HCAR2/AMPK/SIRT1/FOXO3A pathway can evoke antioxidant influences, thereby decrease in oxidative stress by increased expression of genes of the antioxidants (e.g., manganese superoxide dismutase/MnSOD: βHB/HCAR2/AMPK/SIRT1/FOXO3A/MnSOD pathway) [164,277]. Ketone bodies increase the expression of not only HCAR2 [278,279], but also SIRTs (e.g., SIRT1 and SIRT3) and PGC1-α [164,278,280]. These results suggest that both βHB/HCAR2/AMPK/SIRT1/PGC1-α and βHB/HCAR2/AMPK/SIRT3/PGC1-α pathways can function in the CNS. Indeed, neuroprotective influences of PGC1-α (e.g., anti-inflammatory effects and promotion of mitochondrial functions) can be modulated through not only SIRT1, but also SIRT3 [278,281–283]. It was also suggested that βHB-evoked effects on mitochondrial functions (e.g., mitochondrial biogenesis) may be generated through βHB/HDAC/BDNF/PGC1-α pathway [284]. Moreover, ketosis can enhance the expression of PPARs and the activity of the Nrf2 in the brain likely through βHB/HCAR2/AMPK/Nrf2 or βHB/HCAR2/AMPK/SIRTs/PGC1-α/Nrf2 pathway [285–287]. It has been suggested that ketosis may enhance expression of UCPs, therefore decrease the production of ROS [23,288,289] and defend mitochondria and mitochondrial functions (e.g., by reduction of oxidative stress) through activation of βHB/HCAR2/AMPK/SIRT3/PGC1-α/UCP1 pathway [283] and/or βHB/HCAR2/AMPK/SIRT3/PGC1-α/UCP2 pathway [278]. Moreover, not only ketosis (βHB), but also decrease in glucose level can mitigate inflammatory processes through decreased NLRP3 inflammasome activity. Namely, βHB is an endogenous inhibitor of NLRP3 inflammasome, likely via βHB/NLRP3/IL-1R (IL-1 receptor)/NF-κB pathway, whereas increased glucose level may enhance activity of NLRP3 and inflammatory processes. In addition, enhanced glucose level generally increases insulin level leading to decrease in ketone body synthesis [290–292]. EKSs were proven to decrease glucose levels [21,26,28,36,293], thereby they may increase activity of AMPK/SIRTs signaling pathways and inhibit mTOR-evoked effects (Figure 1).

Thus, based on previous studies, βHB/HCAR2/AMPK/SIRT1/NF-κB, βHB/HCAR2/AMPK/mTOR and βHB/NLRP3/IL-1R/NF-κB pathways (anti-inflammatory effects), βHB/HCAR2/AMPK/SIRT1/FOXO3A pathway (improving mitochondrial functions, anti-oxidant influences), βHB/HCAR2/AMPK/SIRT1/PGC1-α/Nrf2, HCAR2/AMPK/SIRT3/PGC1-α/Nrf2 and HCAR2/AMPK/Nrf2 pathways (improving mitochondrial functions, anti-oxidant and anti-inflammatory effects), βHB/HDAC/BDNF/PGC1-α pathway (improving mitochondrial functions; anti-oxidant and anti-inflammatory influences), βHB/HCAR2/AMPK/SIRT3/PGC1-α/UCP1 and/or βHB/HCAR2/AMPK/SIRT3/PGC1-α/UCP2 pathways (anti-oxidant and anti-inflammatory effects, improving mitochondrial functions) and modulatory effects of βHB on neurotransmission (e.g., purinergic, GABAergic, dopaminergic, noradrenergic and glutamatergic systems), gene expression (e.g., enhanced acetylation of histone residues via βHB/HDACs, promotion of histone and non-histone acetylation through βHB/HATs and hydroxybutyrylation of histones) and RNA functions (e.g., via RNA-biding proteins) may be activated during ketosis (Figure 2). Consequently, EKSs-evoked ketosis (increase in blood βHB levels) may influence all of above mentioned (e.g., mTOR-, AMPK- and SIRTs-evoked) downstream signaling pathways and modulatory effects, which can lead to generation of alleviating effects (e.g., anti-inflammatory effects) on age-related processes (aging hallmarks) (Figures 1 and 2). Moreover, theoretically, EKSs-generated modulation of these signaling pathways and effects may be able to improve symptoms and/or delay development of not only aging-related hallmarks (such as changes in activity of nutrient sensing pathways, shortening of telomere, genomic instability, epigenetic alterations, mitochondrial dysfunction, altered intercellular communication, cellular senescence, loss of proteostasis and stem cell exhaustion), but also age-associated neurodegenerative diseases, and to extend lifespan (through both increased βHB level- and decreased glucose level-evoked changes in activity of several signaling pathways) (Figures 1 and 2).

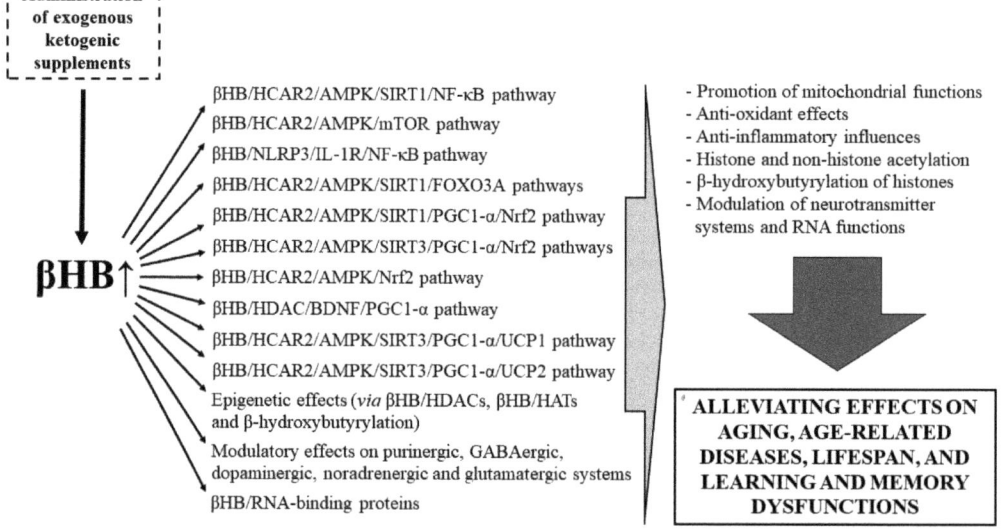

Figure 2. Signaling pathways and effects by which exogenous ketogenic supplements-generated ketosis (βHB) may extend lifespan, delay both aging and development of neurodegenerative diseases, and improve learning and memory dysfunctions. Abbreviations: AMPK, AMP activated serine-threonine protein kinase; βHB, beta-hydroxybutyrate; BDNF, brain-derived neurotrophic factor; FOXO, Forkhead box O; HATs, histone acetyltransferases; HCAR2, hydroxycarboxylic acid receptor 2; HDAC, histone deacetylase; IL-1R, IL-1 receptor; mTOR, mechanistic target of rapamycin; NF-κB, nuclear factor kappa-light-chain-enhancer of activated B cells; NLRP3, NOD-like receptor pyrin domain 3; Nrf2, nuclear factor erythroid 2-related factor 2; PGC1-α, peroxisome proliferator-activated receptor gamma (PPARγ) coactivator-1α; ROS, reactive oxygen species; SIRT, sirtuin; UCP, uncoupling protein.

3.2. Beneficial Effects of EKSs-Evoked Ketosis (βHB) on Lifespan, Aging, Age-Related Diseases, as Well as Learning and Memory Dysfunctions

Administration of βHB generated anti-aging and life-extending effects in *C. elegans* [22,60]. This result suggests that lifespan extension by βHB may also be mediated in mammals through signaling pathways similar to *C. elegans* [60,294], likely by activation of AMPK/SIRT1/mTOR/FOXOs/Nrf2 pathways, HDAC inhibition (and related increase in FOXOs activity) or reduction of insulin signaling pathway activity (Figures 1 and 2). Indeed, for example, it was demonstrated that inhibition of IIS pathways, thereby activation of FOXOs are important processes for lifespan extension [295] and FOXO3A gene is strongly associated with human longevity [296]. Increase in autophagy by caloric (or dietary) restriction can enhance lifespan not only in *C. elegans*, but also in mammals through similar pathways, which may also be activated by administration of EKSs, such as KEs and KSs. For example, in mammals, this effect may be mediated through βHB-evoked inhibition of mTOR activity, activation of FOXOs (via both activation of SIRT1 and direct inhibition of Akt), and ketone body metabolism-evoked decrease in blood glucose and insulin levels, which also decrease the activity of IIS pathways [52,77,180,297,298]. Moreover, long-lived animals showed decrease in mitochondrial ROS production [299] suggesting both inverse correlation between longevity and mitochondrial ROS production (and mitochondrial DNA damage) [52,299] and βHB-evoked enhancement of longevity (lifespan) (Figures 1 and 2). It was also suggested that ketogenic diet (likely through ketogenic diet-generated ketosis/elevated blood βHB, at least partly) can reduce midlife mortality [300], extends longevity and healthspan in adult mice [51], increased lifespan in *Kcna1*-null mice [301] and decreased senescence may be partly through β-hydroxybutyrylation-evoked decrease in p53 activity (in addition, β-hydroxybutyrylation also can attenuate acetylation of p53, because β-hydroxybutyrylation interferes with acetylation) [302]. These results suggest that βHB-generated activation of different signaling pathways may have a role in modulation of aging processes, thereby both lifespan and healthspan. Indeed, it was demonstrated that βHB can alleviate cellular senescence through increased autophagy and decreased plasma insulin level and inflammatory processes in male rats [303], likely through AMPK/SIRT1 pathways (Figure 1). It has also been demonstrated that increased level of blood βHB can delay the age-related processes, for example, by inhibition of SASP, thereby senescence, likely through βHB/hnRNP A1-binding-evoked increase in binding of hnRNP A1 and Oct4 (embryonic stem cell regulator octamer-binding transcriptional factor 4) leading to stabilization of Oct4 mRNA (complex formation with Oct4 mRNA and upregulation of Oct4 expression) and SIRT1 mRNAs [59,304]. βHB-evoked activation of Oct4 not only triggers (maintains) quiescent state of cells (e.g., AMPK activation and mTOR inhibition), but also decreases induction of senescent state of cells (e.g., reduction of the blood level of a pro-senescence marker IL-1α and SASP expression) leading to protection of cells against senescence, and likely, induction of autophagy [59]. These results above suggest that, indeed, EKSs(βHB)-evoked ketosis can alleviate aging-processes (aging hallmarks), at least theoretically, through βHB-evoked activation of AMPK/SIRT1 or SIRT3 downstream signaling pathways (e.g., βHB/HCAR2/AMPK/SIRT1/NF-κB pathway), inhibition of mTOR- (e.g., βHB/HCAR2/AMPK/mTOR pathway) and NLRP3/IL-1R-generated effects, HDAC inhibition, β-hydroxybutyrylation and hnRNP A1-binding (Figures 1 and 2) leading to improved healthspan, delayed aging, thereby extended lifespan.

A great deal of evidence suggests that progression of aging processes by age can lead to not only emergence of aging hallmarks, but also enhanced risk for development of neurodegenerative diseases and impaired learning and memory functions through, for example, mitochondrial dysfunction, epigenetic alterations and enhanced inflammation, which processes may be alleviated by EKSs-generated ketosis (βHB) (Figures 1 and 2). For example, impaired mitochondrial functions, increased oxidative stress and neuronal injury were demonstrated in different CNS diseases, such as Alzheimer's disease, Parkinson's disease and amyotrophic lateral sclerosis [305–308]. Moreover, mitochondrial dysfunction-evoked increase in ROS level may enhance inflammatory processes [309,310], leading to impaired cognitive functions, for example in patients with neurodegenerative diseases (e.g., Alzheimer's disease) [311–313]. It has been suggested that ketogenic diet- and EKSs-evoked ketosis can improve or prevent impaired cognitive functions, learning and memory, for example, via enhanced mitochondrial respiration and antioxidant mechanisms [49,314–317]. Indeed, not only ketogenic diet (and related ketosis) and βHB, but also KE, KS and MCT supplementation improved cognitive functions, learning and memory, as well as their age-related decline in animal models of Alzheimer's disease and patients with Alzheimer's disease or mild cognitive impairment [32,43,47,50,317–320] (Table 1), in a mouse model of Angelman syndrome [41] and in old animals and elderly humans [321,322]. EKSs may exert these beneficial effects via increased ketone body level, which can improve mitochondrial functions. For example, increased level of βHB can compensate glucose hypometabolism-generated decrease in energy source in human and restore ATP synthesis [16,289,318,319,323]. In fact, glucose hypometabolism may contribute to the development of, for example, Alzheimer's disease [324,325]. It has also been demonstrated that MCT supplementation-evoked improvement in cognitive functions was observed in patients with mild to moderate Alzheimer's disease or mild cognitive impairment without apolipoprotein E (*APOE*) ε4 allele [326,327], but the mechanism of action of *APOE*-ε4 status on MCT/ketosis-generated alleviating effects was not identified. Moreover, improved learning and memory was also demonstrated in relation to ketone bodies-evoked decrease in both oxidative stress and intracellular A$β_{42}$ accumulation, and increased mitochondrial complex I activity in models of Alzheimer's disease [50,328,329] (Table 1). It was demonstrated that βHB can protect neurons and alleviate symptoms in models of not only Alzheimer's disease, but also Parkinson's disease [328,330], likely via improvement of mitochondrial function (e.g., by increased ATP synthesis) and activation of other neuroprotective mechanisms, leading to improvement (or protection) in neurodegeneration, motor functions (e.g., tremor) and impaired cognition [258,259,328,331]. Moreover, indeed, βHB administration can decrease aggregation of α-synuclein and delay the toxicity of Aβ [60]. Ketogenic diet- and EKSs-generated ketosis, βHB or the Deanna protocol, containing (among others) MCTs, can also generate alleviating effects on (i) motor neurons and motor performance in preclinical rodent models, such as animal models of amyotrophic lateral sclerosis [48,332–336] and (ii) dopaminergic neurons and motor performance in animal models of Parkinson's disease [55,258] likely through improved mitochondrial function and ATP synthesis (Table 1). Dysregulation of different neurotransmitter systems may have a role in the pathophysiology of neurodegenerative diseases, for example, in animal models and patients with impaired motor function (e.g., dopaminergic dysfunction; GABA and glutamate imbalance) [337–340], Parkinson's disease (e.g., decrease in serotonin level and increase in glutamatergic transmission), Alzheimer's disease (decreased cholinergic neurotransmission) and both Alzheimer's disease and Parkinson's disease (deficits in dopaminergic signaling) [337,339,341–343]. Moreover, dysfunctions in neurotransmitter systems (e.g., GABAergic, glutamatergic and cholinergic) can lead to impaired learning and memory [340,342,344]. It has also been demonstrated that dysregulation of acetylation and deacetylation can lead to neurodegenerative diseases (such as Alzheimer's disease, Parkinson's diseases, amyotrophic lateral sclerosis) and learning and memory deficits [345–348]. Moreover, HDAC inhibitors can improve symptoms or impede development of Parkinson's disease, Alzheimer's disease, amyotrophic lateral sclerosis and restore learning and memory functions [347,349–352]. Low BDNF levels were demonstrated in patients with Alzheimer's disease, which decrease in BDNF level correlates with loss of cognitive functions [353,354], suggesting that ketosis (elevated blood βHB levels) can exert its beneficial effects on Alzheimer's disease and cognitive functions, among others, through HDAC/BDNF system leading to enhancement of alleviating BDNF effects (e.g., by stimulation of hippocampal neurogenesis) [355]. Thus, EKSs (via ketosis/βHB) can exert alleviating effects on neurodegenerative diseases, learning and memory functions through modulation of not only mitochondrial functions and inflammatory processes, but also neurotransmitter systems and via epigenetic modification (Figure 2). Indeed, for example, it was suggested that EKSs may be able to prevent or improve neurodegenerative diseases and learning and memory, among others, through HDAC inhibition [30].

Table 1. Beneficial effects of beta-hydroxybutyrate (βHB), ketone esters (KEs) and medium chain triglycerides (MCTs) on neurodegenerative diseases as well as impaired motor, memory and learning functions in in vivo studies.

Name (Components)	Dose and Route of Administration	Treatment Duration	Model Organism (Species)	Significant Increase in Blood βHB Level	Main Findings	Ref.
Beta-hydroxybutyrate (βHB)						
βHB (DL-β-Hydroxybutyric acid sodium salt)	1.5 mmol/kg/day (subcutaneous administration, 0.25 µL/h)	4 weeks	A mouse model of Alzheimer's disease (5XFAD)	No data	Improved learning and memory; attenuated Aβ accumulation	[50]
βHB + acetoacetate	600 mg βHB/kg/day + 150 mg acetoacetate/kg/day (subcutaneous injection)	2 months	A mouse model of Alzheimer's disease (APPSwInd)	Yes	Improved cognitive performance; reduced Aβ accumulation	[329]
βHB	0.4, 0.8, or 1.6 mmol/kg/day (subcutaneous administration, 1 µL/h)	28 days	LPS-induced Parkinson's disease rat model	No data	Beneficial effects on motor dysfunction; protection of dopaminergic neurons	[55]
βHB (D-βHB)	0.4, 0.8, or 1.6 mmol/kg/day (subcutaneous administration, 1 µL/h)	1 week	MPTP-induced Parkinson's disease mouse model	Yes	Improved motor performance; decrease in MPTP-induced dopaminergic neurodegeneration	[258]
Ketone esters (KEs)						
KE (R,S-1,3-butanediol acetoacetate diester: BD-AcAc₂; standard rodent chow mixed at 10% BD-AcAc₂ by volume and 1% saccharin)	Ad libitum (oral intake)	8 weeks	A mouse model of Angelman syndrome (UBE3A^{tm1Alb} null mutation mice)	Yes	Improved motor coordination, learning and memory	[41]
KE (comprised of D-β-hydroxybutyrate and (R)-1,3-butanediol; 125 g KE/1000 g diet)	Animals were fed a 4 to 5 g pellet/animal at approximately 06:00 hours each day (oral intake)	8 months	A mouse model of Alzheimer's disease (3xTgAD)	Yes	Improvements in performance on learning and memory tests; decreased Aβ and hyperphosphorylated tau deposition	[43]
KE [ketone monoester, (R)-3-hydroxybutyl (R)-3-hydroxybutyrate] + MCT and coconut oil (CO) mixture (4:3)	Normal diet + 28.7 g of the KE thrice daily + 165 mL/day of the MCT/CO mixture (oral intake)	20 months	A patient with Alzheimer's disease dementia	Yes	Improving behavior as well as cognitive and daily-activity performance	[47]

Table 1. Cont.

Name (Components)	Dose and Route of Administration	Treatment Duration	Model Organism (Species)	Significant Increase in Blood βHB Level	Main Findings	Ref.
Medium chain triglycerides (MCTs)						
MCT (97% caprylic acid + 3% capric acid; a normal diet supplemented with 5.5% MCT)	Dogs were fed once/day for about one hour; about 200 g supplemented diet/day/animal (oral intake)	8 months	Aged dogs	Yes	Improvements in learning ability and attention	[322]
MCT (the diet was mixed with Deanna protocol/DP at 22% by weight; DP contained 10% MCT high in caprylic acid)	Ad libitum (oral intake)	6–10 weeks	A mouse model of Amyotrophic lateral sclerosis (SOD1-G93A)	No	Better motor performance, improved (lower) neurological scores and extended survival time	[332]
MCT (a diet in which 35% of the calories was derived from triheptanoin)	Ad libitum (oral intake)	24 weeks	A mouse model of Amyotrophic lateral sclerosis (SOD1-G93A)	Yes	Protection against motor neuron loss; improved motor function	[48]
MCT [a diet containing 10% (w/w) caprylic acid]	Ad libitum; about 3 g diet/day was consumed/animal (oral intake)	About 12 weeks	A mouse model of Amyotrophic lateral sclerosis (SOD1-G93A)	Yes	Protection against motor neuron loss; improved motor function	[336]
MCT (NeoBee 895, >95% of the fatty acids are caprylic acid; the remainder consists of caproic and capric acids)	40 mL MCT (oral intake)	Single administration	Adult subjects with Alzheimer's disease or mild cognitive impairment	Yes	Improvement in cognitive functions (in patients without APOE ε4 allele)	[327]
MCT (AC-1202, an MCT composed of glycerin and, almost entirely, caprylic acid, NeoBee 895)	Normal diet + 20 g MCT/day/patient (oral intake)	3 months	Humans with mild to moderate Alzheimer's disease	Yes	Improvement in cognitive performance (in patients without APOE ε4 allele)	[326]
MCT (50 g Ketogenic meal, Ketonformula containing 20 g of MCTs: 15 g caprylic acid + 5 g capric acid)	50 g ketogenic meal (oral intake)	Single administration	Humans; elderly, non-demented	Yes	Positive effects on working memory, visual attention, and task switching	[321]
MCT (MCT drink: a 12% emulsion of Captex 355, containing 60% caprylic acid and 40% capric acid)	Normal diet + 15 g MCT twice/day/patient in a ketogenic drink (oral intake)	6 months	Humans; aged participants with mild cognitive impairment	Yes	Improved executive function, memory, and language	[32]
MCT (MCT oil, Nestle™)	Normal diet + 56 g MCT/day/patient (oral intake)	24 weeks	Humans; adults with mild cognitive impairment	Yes	Improved memory	[320]

Abbreviations: 5XFAD, β-amyloid precursor protein and presenilin-1 double-transgenic mouse; Aβ, amyloid β; APOE, apolipoprotein E; APPSwInd, a transgenic mouse, express a mutant form of the human amyloid protein precursor (APP) with the APP KM670/671NL (Swedish) and APP V717F (Indiana) mutations; LPS, lipopolysaccharide; MPTP, 1-methyl-4-phenyl-1,2,3,6-tetrahydropyridine; UBE3A^tm1Alb, a mouse with Ube3A (ubiquitin protein ligase E3A) knock-out mutation; 3xTgAD, a mouse with APP KM670/671NL (Swedish), MAPT P301L and PSEN1 M146V mutations; SOD1-G93A, a transgenic mouse with a G93A mutant form of human superoxide dismutase (SOD1).

HCAR2 ligands can generate alleviating effects on Parkinson's disease, Alzheimer's disease, impaired learning, memory and motor functions, as well as amyotrophic lateral sclerosis via anti-inflammatory effects [43,50,57,258], suggesting that EKSs-evoked ketosis (βHB) exerts its alleviating effects on learning, memory, as well as age and age-related diseases through βHB/HCAR2-evoked downstream signaling (Figure 2). Indeed, previous studies show that ketosis (βHB) may evoke therapeutic effects in the treatment of Alzheimer's disease, Parkinson's disease and amyotrophic lateral sclerosis and enhance learning and memory through anti-inflammatory effects induced by HCAR2 [50,55,57,58,275,279]. It was also demonstrated that enhanced expression of proinflammatory cytokines and oxidative stress have a role in the development of Alzheimer's disease [276,356,357], Parkinson's disease [55,276,356,357], amyotrophic lateral sclerosis [356–358], impaired motor functions [337,359] and impairment of learning and memory [309,310,360]. Thus, ketosis may also improve symptoms of neurodegenerative diseases, motor, learning and memory dysfunctions through anti-inflammatory and anti-oxidative effects via HCAR2 [50,275,361] (Figure 2). It has been demonstrated that SIRT1 levels were decreased in neurodegenerative diseases, such as Alzheimer's disease and Parkinson's disease [97,362] suggesting alleviating effects of SIRT1 activation-modulated pathway(s) in the treatment of neurodegenerative diseases [363]. It was also suggested that activation of SIRT1-dependent pathways can modulate learning and memory by which ketone bodies may be able to improve both learning and memory functions [327]. Indeed, overexpression of SIRT1 was protective against learning and memory impairment in animal models of Alzheimer's disease [364,365] and increased SIRT1 activity could promote memory processes, whereas SIRT1 knockout animals showed impaired cognitive abilities [366,367]. Moreover, activation of SIRT1 generated protective influences in mouse models of amyotrophic lateral sclerosis (e.g., enhanced biogenesis of mitochondria and suppressed deterioration of motor neurons) [94,368,369], preserved dopaminergic neurons in a mouse model of Parkinson's disease [370] and evoked protection against Aβ plaque formation in mouse models of Alzheimer's disease [94,371] likely via, for example, SIRT1/PGC1-α/MnSOD pathway [173,372]. In fact, it has been demonstrated that PGC1-α-deficiency may be in connection with neurodegenerative lesions [373], and decreased PGC1-α expression may be one of the most important factors in the development of both Parkinson's disease [374,375] and Alzheimer's disease [174,376]. Moreover, PPARγ agonist pioglitazone (an antidiabetic agent) and overexpression of PGC1-α were able to improve symptoms of amyotrophic lateral sclerosis in mouse models [377,378] and other PPARγ agonists can improve not only symptoms of neurodegenerative diseases (e.g., Parkinson's disease, Alzheimer's disease and amyotrophic lateral sclerosis), but also impaired cognitive functions, learning and memory [379,380]. As oxidative stress has a role in the pathophysiology of neurodegenerative diseases, such as Parkinson's disease, Nrf2 thereby, for example, AMPK/SIRT1/Nrf2 pathway may be an important therapeutic target in the treatment of these diseases [381,382]. Moreover, it was also suggested that activation of SIRT3/PGC1-α/MnSOD pathways could also generate alleviating effect on Parkinson's disease, Alzheimer's disease, and amyotrophic lateral sclerosis [383–385]. Consequently, indeed, EKSs-generated ketosis (βHB) can alleviate or delay development of neurodegenerative diseases, and improve learning and memory dysfunctions likely through different βHB/HCAR2/AMPK-modulated downstream signaling pathways (Figure 2).

4. Conclusions

A great deal of evidence suggests that EKSs-generated ketosis may improve healthspan, therefore can delay ageing and the onset of age-related neurodegenerative diseases, as well as learning and memory dysfunctions through neuroprotective effects. In spite of the overwhelming amount of promising mechanistic findings, only a limited number of studies focused on and demonstrated the beneficial effects of EKSs-evoked ketosis on lifespan, aging-processes, age-related diseases and impaired learning and memory functions. However, their beneficial effects on healthspan and lifespan—likely through improving mitochondrial functions, anti-oxidant effects, anti-inflammatory influences, and modulation of histone and non-histone acetylation, as well as neurotransmitter systems-, can be hypothesized. Indeed, it has been suggested that EKSs-evoked ketosis may alter the activity of different downstream signaling pathways (e.g., AMPK-, SIRTs- and mTOR-modulated pathways) and modulatory effects, through which not only senotherapeutic drugs, but also ketosis (βHB) can improve symptoms and delay development of age-related hallmarks, age-associated neurodegenerative diseases and learning and memory dysfunctions, and extend lifespan. Consequently, administration of EKSs may be a potential therapeutic tool as an adjuvant therapeutics in combination with different therapeutic drugs (such as metformin and rapamycin) for regenerative medicine to enhance effectivity of drugs to rejuvenate aging hallmarks, decrease the risk for age-related neurodegenerative diseases and increase the healthspan of the aging human population. However, modulating ageing processes and related diseases by administration of EKSs needs careful attention, because insufficient clinical data is available currently on its positive effects, efficacy and safety, regarding this specific application. Thus, long-term studies are needed to investigate the exact mechanisms of action by which EKSs-evoked ketosis modulate aging processes, age-related diseases, learning and memory functions, healthspan and lifespan. Moreover, in order to develop effective treatments for patients with different age-related diseases more studies are needed to identify the most effective doses, administration routes, treatment duration and different formulations of EKSs.

Author Contributions: Writing—original draft, Z.K., and B.B.; Writing—review and editing, C.A. All authors have read and agreed to the published version of the manuscript.

Funding: This work was supported by ELTE BDPK Excellence Program 12/2020 (to Zsolt Kovács) and Ketone Technologies LLC. The funding body had no influence on writing the manuscript.

Institutional Review Board Statement: Not applicable.

Informed Consent Statement: Not applicable.

Data Availability Statement: Not applicable.

Conflicts of Interest: Patent: #10980764, University of South Florida, C.A., D.P.D. "Exogenous ketone supplements for reducing anxiety-related behavior"; Non-provisional patents: Ari, C., Arnold P., D'Agostino, D.P. Technology Title: "Elevated Blood Ketone Levels by Ketogenic Diet or Exogenous Ketone Supplements Induced Increased Latency of Anesthetic Induction" USF Ref. No. 16A018PR ; Ari, C., Arnold P., D'Agostino, D.P. Technology Title: "Exogenous Ketone Supplementation Improved Motor Function in Sprague-Dawley Rats." USF Ref. No: 16A019; Ari, C., Arnold P., D'Agostino, D.P. Technology Title: "Lowering of Blood Glucose in Exercising and Non-Exercising Rats Following Administration of Exogenous Ketones and Ketone Formulas." USF Ref. No: 16A049; Ari, C., Arnold P., D'Agostino, D.P. Technology Title: "Neuroregeneration improved by ketone." USF Ref. No: 16B128 (provisional patent); Ari, C., D'Agostino, D.P. Dean, J.B. Technology Title: "Delaying latency to seizure by combinations of ketone supplements." USF Ref. No: 16B138PR. C. Ari is co-owner of Ketone Technologies LLC, and owner of Fortis World LLC. These interests have been reviewed and managed by the University in accordance with its Institutional and Individual Conflict of Interest policies. All authors declare that there are no additional conflict of interest.

Abbreviations

Aβ: amyloid-β; ACCs, acetyl-CoA carboxylases; Akt, Akt kinase/protein kinase B; AMPK, AMP activated serine-threonine protein kinase; BDNF, brain-derived neurotrophic factor; βHB, beta-hydroxybutyrate; CNS, central nervous system; EKSs, exogenous ketogenic supplements; ER, endoplasmic reticulum; ETC, electron transport chain; FOXOs, Forkhead box Os; HATs, histone acetyltransferases; HCAR2, hydroxycarboxylic acid receptor 2; HDACs, histone deacetylases; hnRNP A1, heterogeneous nuclear ribonucleoprotein A1; IGF 1, insulin-like growth factor 1; IIS pathway, insulin/insulin-like growth factor (IGF) 1 pathway; IL-1β, interleukin-1β; IL-1R, IL-1 receptor; KE, ketone ester; KS, ketone salt; MCT, medium chain triglyceride; miRNAs, microRNAs; MnSOD, manganese superoxide dismutase; mPT pore, mitochondrial permeability transition pore; mTOR, mechanistic target of rapamycin; NAD⁺, nicotinamide adenine dinucleotide; NF-κB, nuclear factor kappa-light-chain-enhancer of activated B cells; NLRP3, NOD-like receptor pyrin domain 3; Nrf2, nuclear factor erythroid 2-related factor 2; Oct4, embryonic stem cell regulator octamer-binding transcriptional factor 4; p53, transcription factor tumor suppressor protein 53; PARP-1, poly(ADP-ribose)-polymerase-1; PGC-1α, peroxisome proliferator-activated receptor gamma (PPARγ) coactivator-1α; ROS, reactive oxygen species; SASP, senescence associated secretory phenotype; SIRT, Sirtuin; SOD, superoxide dismutase; SREBP1, sterol regulatory element-binding protein 1; TNF-α, tumor necrosis factor-α; UCP, uncoupling protein; ULK1, Uncoordinated/Unc-51-like kinase 1.

References

1. Campisi, J.; Kapahi, P.; Lithgow, G.J.; Melov, S.; Newman, J.C.; Verdin, E. From discoveries in ageing research to therapeutics for healthy ageing. *Nature* **2019**, *571*, 183–192. [CrossRef] [PubMed]
2. Li, Z.; Zhang, Z.; Ren, Y.; Wang, Y.; Fang, J.; Yue, H.; Ma, S.; Guan, F. Aging and age-related diseases: From mechanisms to therapeutic strategies. *Biogerontology* **2021**, *22*, 165–187. [CrossRef] [PubMed]
3. Sen, A.; Capelli, V.; Husain, M. Cognition and dementia in older patients with epilepsy. *Brain* **2018**, *141*, 1592–1608. [CrossRef]
4. United Nations, Department of Economic and Social Affairs, Population Division. *World Population Ageing 2019: Highlights*; United Nations: New York, NY, USA, 2019; ISBN 978-92-1-148325-3.
5. Drygalski, K.; Fereniec, E.; Koryciński, K.; Chomentowski, A.; Kiełczewska, A.; Odrzygóźdź, C.; Modzelewska, B. Resveratrol and Alzheimer's disease. From molecular pathophysiology to clinical trials. *Exp. Gerontol.* **2018**, *113*, 36–47. [CrossRef]
6. Yang, C.; Zhang, W.; Dong, X.; Fu, C.; Yuan, J.; Xu, M.; Liang, Z.; Qiu, C.; Xu, C. A natural product solution to aging and aging-associated diseases. *Pharmacol. Ther.* **2020**, *216*, 107673. [CrossRef] [PubMed]
7. De Magalhães, J.P.; Stevens, M.; Thornton, D. The Business of Anti-Aging Science. *Trends Biotechnol.* **2017**, *35*, 1062–1073. [CrossRef] [PubMed]
8. Anisimov, V.N.; Zabezhinski, M.A.; Popovich, I.G.; Piskunova, T.S.; Semenchenko, A.V.; Tyndyk, M.L.; Yurova, M.N.; Rosenfeld, S.V.; Blagosklonny, M.V. Rapamycin increases lifespan and inhibits spontaneous tumorigenesis in inbred female mice. *Cell Cycle* **2011**, *10*, 4230–4236. [CrossRef] [PubMed]
9. Bitto, A.; Ito, T.K.; Pineda, V.V.; LeTexier, N.J.; Huang, H.Z.; Sutlief, E.; Tung, H.; Vizzini, N.; Chen, B.; Smith, K.; et al. Transient rapamycin treatment can increase lifespan and healthspan in middle-aged mice. *Elife* **2016**, *5*, e16351. [CrossRef]
10. Mannick, J.B.; Morris, M.; Hockey, H.P.; Roma, G.; Beibel, M.; Kulmatycki, K.; Watkins, M.; Shavlakadze, T.; Zhou, W.; Quinn, D.; et al. TORC1 inhibition enhances immune function and reduces infections in the elderly. *Sci. Transl. Med.* **2018**, *10*, eaaq1564. [CrossRef] [PubMed]
11. Bannister, C.A.; Holden, S.E.; Jenkins-Jones, S.; Morgan, C.L.; Halcox, J.P.; Schernthaner, G.; Mukherjee, J.; Currie, C.J. Can people with type 2 diabetes live longer than those without? A comparison of mortality in people initiated with metformin or sulphonylurea monotherapy and matched, non-diabetic controls. *Diabetes Obes. Metab.* **2014**, *16*, 1165–1173. [CrossRef]
12. Barzilai, N.; Crandall, J.P.; Kritchevsky, S.B.; Espeland, M.A. Metformin as a Tool to Target Aging. *Cell Metab.* **2016**, *23*, 1060–1065. [CrossRef] [PubMed]
13. Bonkowski, M.S.; Sinclair, D.A. Slowing ageing by design: The rise of NAD⁺ and sirtuin-activating compounds. *Nat. Rev. Mol. Cell Biol.* **2016**, *17*, 679–690. [CrossRef]
14. Kane, A.E.; Sinclair, D.A. Sirtuins and NAD⁺ in the Development and Treatment of Metabolic and Cardiovascular Diseases. *Circ. Res.* **2018**, *123*, 868–885. [CrossRef] [PubMed]
15. Kirkland, J.L.; Tchkonia, T.; Zhu, Y.; Niedernhofer, L.J.; Robbins, P.D. The Clinical Potential of Senolytic Drugs. *J. Am. Geriatr. Soc.* **2017**, *65*, 2297–2301. [CrossRef] [PubMed]
16. Brownlow, M.L.; Jung, S.H.; Moore, R.J.; Bechmann, N.; Jankord, R. Nutritional Ketosis Affects Metabolism and Behavior in Sprague-Dawley Rats in Both Control and Chronic Stress Environments. *Front. Mol. Neurosci.* **2017**, *10*, 129. [CrossRef]
17. Brunengraber, H. Potential of ketone body esters for parenteral and oral nutrition. *Nutrition* **1997**, *13*, 233–235. [CrossRef]
18. Clarke, K.; Tchabanenko, K.; Pawlosky, R.; Carter, E.; Knight, N.S.; Murray, A.J.; Cochlin, L.E.; King, M.T.; Wong, A.W.; Roberts, A.; et al. Oral 28-day and developmental toxicity studies of (R)-3-hydroxybutyl (R)-3-hydroxybutyrate. *Regul. Toxicol. Pharmacol.* **2012**, *63*, 196–208. [CrossRef]
19. Clarke, K.; Tchabanenko, K.; Pawlosky, R.; Carter, E.; Todd King, M.; Musa-Veloso, K.; Ho, M.; Roberts, A.; Robertson, J.; Vanitallie, T.B.; et al. Kinetics, safety and tolerability of (R)-3-hydroxybutyl (R)-3-hydroxybutyrate in healthy adult subjects. *Regul. Toxicol. Pharmacol.* **2012**, *63*, 401–408. [CrossRef]
20. Schönfeld, P.; Wojtczak, L. Short- and medium-chain fatty acids in energy metabolism: The cellular perspective. *J. Lipid Res.* **2016**, *57*, 943–954. [CrossRef]
21. Kovács, Z.; Brunner, B.; D'Agostino, D.P.; Ari, C. Age- and Sex-Dependent Modulation of Exogenous Ketone Supplement-Evoked Effects on Blood Glucose and Ketone Body Levels in Wistar Albino Glaxo Rijswijk Rats. *Front. Neurosci.* **2021**, *14*, 618422. [CrossRef]

22. Achanta, L.B.; Rae, C.D. β-Hydroxybutyrate in the Brain: One Molecule, Multiple Mechanisms. *Neurochem. Res.* **2017**, *42*, 35–49. [CrossRef]
23. Koppel, S.J.; Swerdlow, R.H. Neuroketotherapeutics: A modern review of a century-old therapy. *Neurochem. Int.* **2018**, *117*, 114–125. [CrossRef] [PubMed]
24. Newman, J.C.; Verdin, E. Ketone bodies as signaling metabolites. *Trends Endocrinol. Metab.* **2014**, *25*, 42–52. [CrossRef] [PubMed]
25. Soto-Mota, A.; Norwitz, N.G.; Clarke, K. Why a d-β-hydroxybutyrate monoester? *Biochem. Soc. Trans.* **2020**, *48*, 51–59. [CrossRef]
26. Ari, C.; Kovács, Z.; Juhasz, G.; Murdun, C.; Goldhagen, C.R.; Koutnik, A.P.; Poff, A.M.; Kesl, S.L.; D'Agostino, D.P. Exogenous Ketone Supplements Reduce Anxiety-Related Behavior in Sprague-Dawley and Wistar Albino Glaxo/Rijswijk Rats. *Front. Mol. Neurosci.* **2016**, *9*, 137. [CrossRef]
27. Kesl, S.L.; Poff, A.M.; Ward, N.P.; Fiorelli, T.N.; Ari, C.; Van Putten, A.J.; Sherwood, J.W.; Arnold, P.; D'Agostino, D.P. Effects of exogenous ketone supplementation on blood ketone, glucose, triglyceride, and lipoprotein levels in Sprague-Dawley rats. *Nutr. Metab.* **2016**, *13*, 9. [CrossRef]
28. Myette-Côté, É.; Neudorf, H.; Rafiei, H.; Clarke, K.; Little, J.P. Prior ingestion of exogenous ketone monoester attenuates the glycaemic response to an oral glucose tolerance test in healthy young individuals. *J. Physiol.* **2018**, *596*, 1385–1395. [CrossRef] [PubMed]
29. Stubbs, B.J.; Cox, P.J.; Evans, R.D.; Santer, P.; Miller, J.J.; Faull, O.K.; Magor-Elliott, S.; Hiyama, S.; Stirling, M.; Clarke, K. On the Metabolism of Exogenous Ketones in Humans. *Front. Physiol.* **2017**, *8*, 848. [CrossRef]
30. Hashim, S.A.; VanItallie, T.B. Ketone body therapy: From the ketogenic diet to the oral administration of ketone ester. *J. Lipid Res.* **2014**, *55*, 1818–1826. [CrossRef]
31. McDonald, T.J.; Cervenka, M.C. Lessons learned from recent clinical trials of ketogenic diet therapies in adults. *Curr. Opin. Clin. Nutr. Metab. Care* **2019**, *22*, 418–424. [CrossRef]
32. Fortier, M.; Castellano, C.A.; St-Pierre, V.; Myette-Côté, É.; Langlois, F.; Roy, M.; Morin, M.C.; Bocti, C.; Fulop, T.; Godin, J.P.; et al. A ketogenic drink improves cognition in mild cognitive impairment: Results of a 6-month RCT. *Alzheimers Dement.* **2021**, *17*, 543–552. [CrossRef]
33. Soto-Mota, A.; Norwitz, N.G.; Evans, R.; Clarke, K.; Barber, T.M. Exogenous ketosis in patients with type 2 diabetes: Safety, tolerability and effect on glycaemic control. *Endocrinol. Diabetes Metab.* **2021**, e00264. [CrossRef]
34. Camberos-Luna, L.; Massieu, L. Therapeutic strategies for ketosis induction and their potential efficacy for the treatment of acute brain injury and neurodegenerative diseases. *Neurochem. Int.* **2020**, *133*, 104614. [CrossRef]
35. Han, Y.M.; Ramprasath, T.; Zou, M.H. β-hydroxybutyrate and its metabolic effects on age-associated pathology. *Exp. Mol. Med.* **2020**, *52*, 548–555. [CrossRef] [PubMed]
36. Kovács, Z.; D'Agostino, D.P.; Dobolyi, A.; Ari, C. Adenosine A1 Receptor Antagonism Abolished the Anti-seizure Effects of Exogenous Ketone Supplementation in Wistar Albino Glaxo Rijswijk Rats. *Front. Mol. Neurosci.* **2017**, *10*, 235. [CrossRef]
37. Branco, A.F.; Ferreira, A.; Simões, R.F.; Magalhães-Novais, S.; Zehowski, C.; Cope, E.; Silva, A.M.; Pereira, D.; Sardão, V.A.; Cunha-Oliveira, T. Ketogenic diets: From cancer to mitochondrial diseases and beyond. *Eur. J. Clin. Investig.* **2016**, *46*, 285–298. [CrossRef]
38. Kim, D.Y.; Simeone, K.A.; Simeone, T.A.; Pandya, J.D.; Wilke, J.C.; Ahn, Y.; Geddes, J.W.; Sullivan, P.G.; Rho, J.M. Ketone bodies mediate antiseizure effects through mitochondrial permeability transition. *Ann. Neurol.* **2015**, *78*, 77–87. [CrossRef] [PubMed]
39. Kovács, Z.; D'Agostino, D.P.; Diamond, D.; Kindy, M.S.; Rogers, C.; Ari, C. Therapeutic Potential of Exogenous Ketone Supplement Induced Ketosis in the Treatment of Psychiatric Disorders: Review of Current Literature. *Front. Psychiatry* **2019**, *10*, 363. [CrossRef]
40. Berk, B.A.; Law, T.H.; Packer, R.M.A.; Wessmann, A.; Bathen-Nöthen, A.; Jokinen, T.S.; Knebel, A.; Tipold, A.; Pelligand, L.; Meads, Z.; et al. A multicenter randomized controlled trial of medium-chain triglyceride dietary supplementation on epilepsy in dogs. *J. Vet. Intern. Med.* **2020**, *34*, 1248–1259. [CrossRef]
41. Ciarlone, S.L.; Grieco, J.C.; D'Agostino, D.P.; Weeber, E.J. Ketone ester supplementation attenuates seizure activity, and improves behavior and hippocampal synaptic plasticity in an Angelman syndrome mouse model. *Neurobiol. Dis.* **2016**, *96*, 38–46. [CrossRef]
42. D'Agostino, D.P.; Pilla, R.; Held, H.E.; Landon, C.S.; Puchowicz, M.; Brunengraber, H.; Ari, C.; Arnold, P.; Dean, J.B. Therapeutic ketosis with ketone ester delays central nervous system oxygen toxicity seizures in rats. *Am. J. Physiol. Regul. Integr. Comp. Physiol.* **2013**, *304*, 829–836. [CrossRef]
43. Kashiwaya, Y.; Bergman, C.; Lee, J.H.; Wan, R.; King, M.T.; Mughal, M.R.; Okun, E.; Clarke, K.; Mattson, M.P.; Veech, R.L. A ketone ester diet exhibits anxiolytic and cognition-sparing properties, and lessens amyloid and tau pathologies in a mouse model of Alzheimer's disease. *Neurobiol. Aging* **2013**, *34*, 1530–1539. [CrossRef]
44. Kovács, Z.; D'Agostino, D.P.; Ari, C. Anxiolytic Effect of Exogenous Ketone Supplementation Is Abolished by Adenosine A1 Receptor Inhibition in Wistar Albino Glaxo/Rijswijk Rats. *Front. Behav. Neurosci.* **2018**, *12*, 29. [CrossRef]
45. Ari, C.; Zippert, M.; D'Agostino, D.P. Neuroregeneration improved by ketones. *FASEB J.* **2018**, *32*, 545–549. [CrossRef]
46. Ari, C.; Pilla, R.; D'Agostino, D. Nutritional/metabolic therapies in animal models of amyotrophic lateral sclerosis, Alzheimer's disease, and seizures. In *Bioactive Nutraceuticals and Dietary Supplements in Neurological and Brain Disease*; Ross Watson, R., Preedy, V.R., Eds.; Academic Press: New York, NY, USA, 2015; pp. 449–459. ISBN 978-0-12-411462-3.
47. Newport, M.T.; VanItallie, T.B.; Kashiwaya, Y.; King, M.T.; Veech, R.L. A new way to produce hyperketonemia: Use of ketone ester in a case of Alzheimer's disease. *Alzheimers Dement.* **2015**, *11*, 99–103. [CrossRef] [PubMed]

48. Tefera, T.W.; Wong, Y.; Barkl-Luke, M.E.; Ngo, S.T.; Thomas, N.K.; McDonald, T.S.; Borges, K. Triheptanoin Protects Motor Neurons and Delays the Onset of Motor Symptoms in a Mouse Model of Amyotrophic Lateral Sclerosis. *PLoS ONE* **2016**, *11*, e0161816. [CrossRef]
49. Maalouf, M.; Rho, J.M.; Mattson, M.P. The neuroprotective properties of calorie restriction, the ketogenic diet, and ketone bodies. *Brain Res. Rev.* **2009**, *59*, 293–315. [CrossRef]
50. Wu, Y.; Gong, Y.; Luan, Y.; Li, Y.; Liu, J.; Yue, Z.; Yuan, B.; Sun, J.; Xie, C.; Li, L.; et al. BHBA treatment improves cognitive function by targeting pleiotropic mechanisms in transgenic mouse model of Alzheimer's disease. *FASEB J.* **2020**, *34*, 1412–1429. [CrossRef]
51. Roberts, M.N.; Wallace, M.A.; Tomilov, A.A.; Zhou, Z.; Marcotte, G.R.; Tran, D.; Perez, G.; Gutierrez-Casado, E.; Koike, S.; Knotts, T.A.; et al. A Ketogenic Diet Extends Longevity and Healthspan in Adult Mice. *Cell Metab.* **2017**, *26*, 539–546. [CrossRef]
52. Veech, R.L.; Bradshaw, P.C.; Clarke, K.; Curtis, W.; Pawlosky, R.; King, M.T. Ketone bodies mimic the life span extending properties of caloric restriction. *IUBMB Life* **2017**, *69*, 305–314. [CrossRef]
53. Newman, J.C.; Verdin, E. β-hydroxybutyrate: Much more than a metabolite. *Diabetes Res. Clin. Pract.* **2014**, *106*, 173–181. [CrossRef]
54. Rahman, M.; Muhammad, S.; Khan, M.A.; Chen, H.; Ridder, D.A.; Müller-Fielitz, H.; Pokorná, B.; Vollbrandt, T.; Stölting, I.; Nadrowitz, R.; et al. The β-hydroxybutyrate receptor HCA2 activates a neuroprotective subset of macrophages. *Nat. Commun.* **2014**, *5*, 3944. [CrossRef]
55. Fu, S.P.; Wang, J.F.; Xue, W.J.; Liu, H.M.; Liu, B.R.; Zeng, Y.L.; Li, S.N.; Huang, B.X.; Lv, Q.K.; Wang, W.; et al. Anti-inflammatory effects of BHBA in both in vivo and in vitro Parkinson's disease models are mediated by GPR109A-dependent mechanisms. *J. Neuroinflamm.* **2015**, *12*, 9. [CrossRef]
56. Rezq, S.; Abdel-Rahman, A.A. Central GPR109A Activation Mediates Glutamate-Dependent Pressor Response in Conscious Rats. *J. Pharmacol. Exp. Ther.* **2016**, *356*, 456–465. [CrossRef]
57. Graff, E.C.; Fang, H.; Wanders, D.; Judd, R.L. Anti-inflammatory effects of the hydroxycarboxylic acid receptor 2. *Metabolism* **2016**, *65*, 102–113. [CrossRef]
58. Wakade, C.; Chong, R.; Bradley, E.; Thomas, B.; Morgan, J. Upregulation of GPR109A in Parkinson's disease. *PLoS ONE* **2014**, *9*, e109818. [CrossRef] [PubMed]
59. Han, Y.M.; Bedarida, T.; Ding, Y.; Somba, B.K.; Lu, Q.; Wang, Q.; Song, P.; Zou, M.H. β-Hydroxybutyrate Prevents Vascular Senescence through hnRNP A1-Mediated Upregulation of Oct4. *Mol. Cell* **2018**, *71*, 1064–1078. [CrossRef] [PubMed]
60. Edwards, C.; Canfield, J.; Copes, N.; Rehan, M.; Lipps, D.; Bradshaw, P.C. D-beta-hydroxybutyrate extends lifespan in C. elegans. *Aging* **2014**, *6*, 621–644. [CrossRef]
61. Trevisan, K.; Cristina-Pereira, R.; Silva-Amaral, D.; Aversi-Ferreira, T.A. Theories of Aging and the Prevalence of Alzheimer's Disease. *Biomed. Res. Int.* **2019**, *2019*, 9171424. [CrossRef] [PubMed]
62. Ascherio, A.; Schwarzschild, M.A. The epidemiology of Parkinson's disease: Risk factors and prevention. *Lancet Neurol.* **2016**, *15*, 1257–1272. [CrossRef]
63. Hou, Y.; Dan, X.; Babbar, M.; Wei, Y.; Hasselbalch, S.G.; Croteau, D.L.; Bohr, V.A. Ageing as a risk factor for neurodegenerative disease. *Nat. Rev. Neurol.* **2019**, *15*, 565–581. [CrossRef] [PubMed]
64. Pandya, V.A.; Patani, R. Decoding the relationship between ageing and amyotrophic lateral sclerosis: A cellular perspective. *Brain* **2020**, *143*, 1057–1072. [CrossRef]
65. Broughton, S.; Partridge, L. Insulin/IGF-like signalling, the central nervous system and aging. *Biochem. J.* **2009**, *418*, 1–12. [CrossRef]
66. Klement, R.J.; Fink, M.K. Dietary and pharmacological modification of the insulin/IGF-1 system: Exploiting the full repertoire against cancer. *Oncogenesis* **2016**, *5*, e193. [CrossRef]
67. Martin, B.; Mattson, M.P.; Maudsley, S. Caloric restriction and intermittent fasting: Two potential diets for successful brain aging. *Ageing Res. Rev.* **2006**, *5*, 332–353. [CrossRef]
68. Santos, J.; Leitão-Correia, F.; Sousa, M.J.; Leão, C. Dietary Restriction and Nutrient Balance in Aging. *Oxid. Med. Cell Longev.* **2016**, *2016*, 4010357. [CrossRef] [PubMed]
69. López-Otín, C.; Blasco, M.A.; Partridge, L.; Serrano, M.; Kroemer, G. The hallmarks of aging. *Cell* **2013**, *153*, 1194–1217. [CrossRef] [PubMed]
70. Nugent, S.; Tremblay, S.; Chen, K.W.; Ayutyanont, N.; Roontiva, A.; Castellano, C.A.; Fortier, M.; Roy, M.; Courchesne-Loyer, A.; Bocti, C.; et al. Brain glucose and acetoacetate metabolism: A comparison of young and older adults. *Neurobiol. Aging* **2014**, *35*, 1386–1395. [CrossRef] [PubMed]
71. Schultz, M.B.; Sinclair, D.A. When stem cells grow old: Phenotypes and mechanisms of stem cell aging. *Development* **2016**, *143*, 3–14. [CrossRef]
72. Mathew, R.; Pal Bhadra, M.; Bhadra, U. Insulin/insulin-like growth factor-1 signalling (IIS) based regulation of lifespan across species. *Biogerontology* **2017**, *18*, 35–53. [CrossRef]
73. Cohen, E.; Bieschke, J.; Perciavalle, R.M.; Kelly, J.W.; Dillin, A. Opposing activities protect against age-onset proteotoxicity. *Science* **2006**, *313*, 1604–1610. [CrossRef] [PubMed]
74. Li, J.; Kim, S.G.; Blenis, J. Rapamycin: One drug, many effects. *Cell Metab.* **2014**, *19*, 373–379. [CrossRef] [PubMed]
75. Saxton, R.A.; Sabatini, D.M. mTOR Signaling in Growth, Metabolism, and Disease. *Cell* **2017**, *168*, 960–976. [CrossRef] [PubMed]

76. Johnson, S.C.; Rabinovitch, P.S.; Kaeberlein, M. mTOR is a key modulator of ageing and age-related disease. *Nature* **2013**, *493*, 338–345. [CrossRef] [PubMed]
77. Menzies, F.M.; Fleming, A.; Caricasole, A.; Bento, C.F.; Andrews, S.P.; Ashkenazi, A.; Füllgrabe, J.; Jackson, A.; Jimenez Sanchez, M.; Karabiyik, C.; et al. Autophagy and Neurodegeneration: Pathogenic Mechanisms and Therapeutic Opportunities. *Neuron* **2017**, *93*, 1015–1034. [CrossRef] [PubMed]
78. Sen, P.; Shah, P.P.; Nativio, R.; Berger, S.L. Epigenetic Mechanisms of Longevity and Aging. *Cell* **2016**, *166*, 822–839. [CrossRef]
79. Carling, D. The AMP-activated protein kinase cascade—A unifying system for energy control. *Trends Biochem. Sci.* **2004**, *29*, 18–24. [CrossRef]
80. Steinberg, G.R.; Kemp, B.E. AMPK in Health and Disease. *Physiol. Rev.* **2009**, *89*, 1025–1078. [CrossRef]
81. Chung, M.M.; Nicol, C.J.; Cheng, Y.C.; Lin, K.H.; Chen, Y.L.; Pei, D.; Lin, C.H.; Shih, Y.N.; Yen, C.H.; Chen, S.J.; et al. Metformin activation of AMPK suppresses AGE-induced inflammatory response in hNSCs. *Exp. Cell Res.* **2017**, *352*, 75–83. [CrossRef]
82. Salminen, A.; Hyttinen, J.M.; Kaarniranta, K. AMP-activated protein kinase inhibits NF-κB signaling and inflammation: Impact on healthspan and lifespan. *J. Mol. Med.* **2011**, *89*, 667–676. [CrossRef]
83. Cantó, C.; Gerhart-Hines, Z.; Feige, J.N.; Lagouge, M.; Noriega, L.; Milne, J.C.; Elliott, P.J.; Puigserver, P.; Auwerx, J. AMPK regulates energy expenditure by modulating NAD+ metabolism and SIRT1 activity. *Nature* **2009**, *458*, 1056–1060. [CrossRef]
84. Kapahi, P.; Kaeberlein, M.; Hansen, M. Dietary restriction and lifespan: Lessons from invertebrate models. *Ageing Res. Rev.* **2017**, *39*, 3–14. [CrossRef]
85. He, W.; Newman, J.C.; Wang, M.Z.; Ho, L.; Verdin, E. Mitochondrial sirtuins: Regulators of protein acylation and metabolism. *Trends Endocrinol. Metab.* **2012**, *23*, 467–476. [CrossRef]
86. Gillum, M.P.; Kotas, M.E.; Erion, D.M.; Kursawe, R.; Chatterjee, P.; Nead, K.T.; Muise, E.S.; Hsiao, J.J.; Frederick, D.W.; Yonemitsu, S.; et al. SirT1 regulates adipose tissue inflammation. *Diabetes* **2011**, *60*, 3235–3245. [CrossRef]
87. Rodgers, J.T.; Lerin, C.; Haas, W.; Gygi, S.P.; Spiegelman, B.M.; Puigserver, P. Nutrient control of glucose homeostasis through a complex of PGC-1alpha and SIRT1. *Nature* **2005**, *434*, 113–118. [CrossRef]
88. Imai, S.; Guarente, L. NAD+ and sirtuins in aging and disease. *Trends Cell Biol.* **2014**, *24*, 464–471. [CrossRef] [PubMed]
89. Morigi, M.; Perico, L.; Benigni, A. Sirtuins in Renal Health and Disease. *J. Am. Soc. Nephrol.* **2018**, *29*, 1799–1809. [CrossRef]
90. Wątroba, M.; Dudek, I.; Skoda, M.; Stangret, A.; Rzodkiewicz, P.; Szukiewicz, D. Sirtuins, epigenetics and longevity. *Ageing Res. Rev.* **2017**, *40*, 11–19. [CrossRef]
91. Cho, S.H.; Chen, J.A.; Sayed, F.; Ward, M.E.; Gao, F.; Nguyen, T.A.; Krabbe, G.; Sohn, P.D.; Lo, I.; Minami, S.; et al. SIRT1 deficiency in microglia contributes to cognitive decline in aging and neurodegeneration via epigenetic regulation of IL-1β. *J. Neurosci.* **2015**, *35*, 807–818. [CrossRef] [PubMed]
92. Patel, N.V.; Gordon, M.N.; Connor, K.E.; Good, R.A.; Engelman, R.W.; Mason, J.; Morgan, D.G.; Morgan, T.E.; Finch, C.E. Caloric restriction attenuates Abeta-deposition in Alzheimer transgenic models. *Neurobiol. Aging* **2005**, *26*, 995–1000. [CrossRef] [PubMed]
93. Wang, J.; Fivecoat, H.; Ho, L.; Pan, Y.; Ling, E.; Pasinetti, G.M. The role of Sirt1: At the crossroad between promotion of longevity and protection against Alzheimer's disease neuropathology. *Biochim. Biophys. Acta* **2010**, *1804*, 1690–1694. [CrossRef]
94. Kim, D.; Nguyen, M.D.; Dobbin, M.M.; Fischer, A.; Sananbenesi, F.; Rodgers, J.T.; Delalle, I.; Baur, J.A.; Sui, G.; Armour, S.M.; et al. SIRT1 deacetylase protects against neurodegeneration in models for Alzheimer's disease and amyotrophic lateral sclerosis. *EMBO J.* **2007**, *26*, 3169–3179. [CrossRef] [PubMed]
95. Marambaud, P.; Zhao, H.; Davies, P. Resveratrol promotes clearance of Alzheimer's disease amyloid-beta peptides. *J. Biol. Chem.* **2005**, *280*, 37377–37382. [CrossRef]
96. Luchsinger, J.A.; Tang, M.X.; Shea, S.; Mayeux, R. Caloric intake and the risk of Alzheimer disease. *Arch. Neurol.* **2002**, *59*, 1258–1263. [CrossRef] [PubMed]
97. Julien, C.; Tremblay, C.; Emond, V.; Lebbadi, M.; Salem, N., Jr.; Bennett, D.A.; Calon, F. Sirtuin 1 reduction parallels the accumulation of tau in Alzheimer disease. *J. Neuropathol. Exp. Neurol.* **2009**, *68*, 48–58. [CrossRef] [PubMed]
98. Oosterhof, N.; Dekens, D.W.; Lawerman, T.F.; van Dijk, M. Yet another role for SIRT1: Reduction of α-synuclein aggregation in stressed neurons. *J. Neurosci.* **2012**, *32*, 6413–6414. [CrossRef] [PubMed]
99. Araki, T.; Sasaki, Y.; Milbrandt, J. Increased nuclear NAD biosynthesis and SIRT1 activation prevent axonal degeneration. *Science* **2004**, *305*, 1010–1013. [CrossRef]
100. Virgili, M.; Contestabile, A. Partial neuroprotection of in vivo excitotoxic brain damage by chronic administration of the red wine antioxidant agent, trans-resveratrol in rats. *Neurosci. Lett.* **2000**, *281*, 123–126. [CrossRef]
101. Brunet, A.; Sweeney, L.B.; Sturgill, J.F.; Chua, K.F.; Greer, P.L.; Lin, Y.; Tran, H.; Ross, S.E.; Mostoslavsky, R.; Cohen, H.Y.; et al. Stress-dependent regulation of FOXO transcription factors by the SIRT1 deacetylase. *Science* **2004**, *303*, 2011–2015. [CrossRef]
102. Zhao, L.; Cao, J.; Hu, K.; He, X.; Yun, D.; Tong, T.; Han, L. Sirtuins and their Biological Relevance in Aging and Age-Related Diseases. *Aging Dis.* **2020**, *11*, 927–945. [CrossRef]
103. Vaziri, H.; Dessain, S.K.; Ng Eaton, E.; Imai, S.I.; Frye, R.A.; Pandita, T.K.; Guarente, L.; Weinberg, R.A. hSIR2(SIRT1) functions as an NAD-dependent p53 deacetylase. *Cell* **2001**, *107*, 149–159. [CrossRef]
104. Prozorovski, T.; Schulze-Topphoff, U.; Glumm, R.; Baumgart, J.; Schröter, F.; Ninnemann, O.; Siegert, E.; Bendix, I.; Brüstle, O.; Nitsch, R.; et al. Sirt1 contributes critically to the redox-dependent fate of neural progenitors. *Nat. Cell Biol.* **2008**, *10*, 385–394. [CrossRef] [PubMed]

105. Chang, H.C.; Guarente, L. SIRT1 mediates central circadian control in the SCN by a mechanism that decays with aging. *Cell* **2013**, *153*, 1448–1460. [CrossRef] [PubMed]
106. Yaku, K.; Okabe, K.; Nakagawa, T. NAD metabolism: Implications in aging and longevity. *Ageing Res. Rev.* **2018**, *47*, 1–17. [CrossRef] [PubMed]
107. Blüher, M.; Kahn, B.B.; Kahn, C.R. Extended longevity in mice lacking the insulin receptor in adipose tissue. *Science* **2003**, *299*, 572–574. [CrossRef]
108. Kenyon, C.J. The genetics of ageing. *Nature* **2010**, *464*, 504–512. [CrossRef] [PubMed]
109. Greer, E.L.; Brunet, A. Different dietary restriction regimens extend lifespan by both independent and overlapping genetic pathways in *C. elegans*. *Aging Cell* **2009**, *8*, 113–127. [CrossRef]
110. Zhu, Y.; Liu, X.; Ding, X.; Wang, F.; Geng, X. Telomere and its role in the aging pathways: Telomere shortening, cell senescence and mitochondria dysfunction. *Biogerontology* **2019**, *20*, 1–16. [CrossRef]
111. Herrmann, M.; Pusceddu, I.; März, W.; Herrmann, W. Telomere biology and age-related diseases. *Clin. Chem. Lab. Med.* **2018**, *56*, 1210–1222. [CrossRef]
112. Sahin, E.; DePinho, R.A. Axis of ageing: Telomeres, p53 and mitochondria. *Nat. Rev. Mol. Cell Biol.* **2012**, *13*, 397–404. [CrossRef]
113. Bernardes de Jesus, B.; Vera, E.; Schneeberger, K.; Tejera, A.M.; Ayuso, E.; Bosch, F.; Blasco, M.A. Telomerase gene therapy in adult and old mice delays aging and increases longevity without increasing cancer. *EMBO Mol. Med.* **2012**, *4*, 691–704. [CrossRef] [PubMed]
114. Shay, J.W. Role of Telomeres and Telomerase in Aging and Cancer. *Cancer Discov.* **2016**, *6*, 584–593. [CrossRef]
115. Palacios, J.A.; Herranz, D.; De Bonis, M.L.; Velasco, S.; Serrano, M.; Blasco, M.A. SIRT1 contributes to telomere maintenance and augments global homologous recombination. *J. Cell Biol.* **2010**, *191*, 1299–1313. [CrossRef] [PubMed]
116. Tiwari, V.; Wilson, D.M., 3rd. DNA Damage and Associated DNA Repair Defects in Disease and Premature Aging. *Am. J. Hum. Genet.* **2019**, *105*, 237–257. [CrossRef]
117. Foo, M.X.R.; Ong, P.F.; Dreesen, O. Premature aging syndromes: From patients to mechanism. *J. Dermatol. Sci.* **2019**, *96*, 58–65. [CrossRef] [PubMed]
118. Hoeijmakers, J.H. DNA damage, aging, and cancer. *N. Engl. J. Med.* **2009**, *361*, 1475–1485. [CrossRef] [PubMed]
119. Kauppila, T.E.S.; Bratic, A.; Jensen, M.B.; Baggio, F.; Partridge, L.; Jasper, H.; Grönke, S.; Larsson, N.G. Mutations of mitochondrial DNA are not major contributors to aging of fruit flies. *Proc. Natl. Acad. Sci. USA* **2018**, *115*, 9620–9629. [CrossRef]
120. Thanan, R.; Oikawa, S.; Hiraku, Y.; Ohnishi, S.; Ma, N.; Pinlaor, S.; Yongvanit, P.; Kawanishi, S.; Murata, M. Oxidative stress and its significant roles in neurodegenerative diseases and cancer. *Int. J. Mol. Sci.* **2014**, *16*, 193–217. [CrossRef]
121. Feinberg, A.P.; Tycko, B. The history of cancer epigenetics. *Nat. Rev. Cancer* **2004**, *4*, 143–153. [CrossRef]
122. Kane, A.E.; Sinclair, D.A. Epigenetic changes during aging and their reprogramming potential. *Crit. Rev. Biochem. Mol. Biol.* **2019**, *54*, 61–83. [CrossRef]
123. Burzynski, S.R. Aging: Gene silencing or gene activation? *Med. Hypotheses* **2005**, *64*, 201–208. [CrossRef]
124. Ben-Avraham, D.; Muzumdar, R.H.; Atzmon, G. Epigenetic genome-wide association methylation in aging and longevity. *Epigenomics* **2012**, *4*, 503–509. [CrossRef]
125. Benayoun, B.A.; Pollina, E.A.; Brunet, A. Epigenetic regulation of ageing: Linking environmental inputs to genomic stability. *Nat. Rev. Mol. Cell Biol.* **2015**, *16*, 593–610. [CrossRef]
126. Hernandez, D.G.; Nalls, M.A.; Gibbs, J.R.; Arepalli, S.; van der Brug, M.; Chong, S.; Moore, M.; Longo, D.L.; Cookson, M.R.; Traynor, B.J.; et al. Distinct DNA methylation changes highly correlated with chronological age in the human brain. *Hum. Mol. Genet.* **2011**, *20*, 1164–1172. [CrossRef]
127. Waki, T.; Tamura, G.; Sato, M.; Motoyama, T. Age-related methylation of tumor suppressor and tumor-related genes: An analysis of autopsy samples. *Oncogene* **2003**, *22*, 4128–4133. [CrossRef]
128. Casillas, M.A., Jr.; Lopatina, N.; Andrews, L.G.; Tollefsbol, T.O. Transcriptional control of the DNA methyltransferases is altered in aging and neoplastically-transformed human fibroblasts. *Mol. Cell. Biochem.* **2003**, *252*, 33–43. [CrossRef] [PubMed]
129. Li, Y.; Liu, L.; Tollefsbol, T.O. Glucose restriction can extend normal cell lifespan and impair precancerous cell growth through epigenetic control of hTERT and p16 expression. *FASEB J.* **2010**, *24*, 1442–1453. [CrossRef] [PubMed]
130. Wakeling, L.A.; Ions, L.J.; Ford, D. Could Sirt1-mediated epigenetic effects contribute to the longevity response to dietary restriction and be mimicked by other dietary interventions? *Age* **2009**, *31*, 327–341. [CrossRef]
131. Alageel, A.; Tomasi, J.; Tersigni, C.; Brietzke, E.; Zuckerman, H.; Subramaniapillai, M.; Lee, Y.; Iacobucci, M.; Rosenblat, J.D.; Mansur, R.B.; et al. Evidence supporting a mechanistic role of sirtuins in mood and metabolic disorders. *Prog. Neuropsychopharmacol. Biol. Psychiatry* **2018**, *86*, 95–101. [CrossRef]
132. De Ruijter, A.J.; van Gennip, A.H.; Caron, H.N.; Kemp, S.; van Kuilenburg, A.B. Histone deacetylases (HDACs): Characterization of the classical HDAC family. *Biochem. J.* **2003**, *370*, 737–749. [CrossRef] [PubMed]
133. Satoh, A.; Brace, C.S.; Rensing, N.; Cliften, P.; Wozniak, D.F.; Herzog, E.D.; Yamada, K.A.; Imai, S. Sirt1 extends life span and delays aging in mice through the regulation of Nk2 homeobox 1 in the DMH and LH. *Cell Metab.* **2013**, *18*, 416–430. [CrossRef]
134. Siebold, A.P.; Banerjee, R.; Tie, F.; Kiss, D.L.; Moskowitz, J.; Harte, P.J. Polycomb Repressive Complex 2 and Trithorax modulate Drosophila longevity and stress resistance. *Proc. Natl. Acad. Sci. USA* **2010**, *107*, 169–174. [CrossRef]
135. Pasyukova, E.G.; Vaiserman, A.M. HDAC inhibitors: A new promising drug class in anti-aging research. *Mech. Ageing Dev.* **2017**, *166*, 6–15. [CrossRef] [PubMed]

136. Sharma, S.; Taliyan, R. Targeting histone deacetylases: A novel approach in Parkinson's disease. *Parkinsons Dis.* **2015**, *2015*, 303294. [CrossRef] [PubMed]
137. Yoo, Y.E.; Ko, C.P. Treatment with trichostatin A initiated after disease onset delays disease progression and increases survival in a mouse model of amyotrophic lateral sclerosis. *Exp. Neurol.* **2011**, *231*, 147–159. [CrossRef] [PubMed]
138. Ricobaraza, A.; Cuadrado-Tejedor, M.; Marco, S.; Pérez-Otaño, I.; García-Osta, A. Phenylbutyrate rescues dendritic spine loss associated with memory deficits in a mouse model of Alzheimer disease. *Hippocampus* **2012**, *22*, 1040–1050. [CrossRef]
139. Wiley, J.C.; Pettan-Brewer, C.; Ladiges, W.C. Phenylbutyric acid reduces amyloid plaques and rescues cognitive behavior in AD transgenic mice. *Aging Cell* **2011**, *10*, 418–428. [CrossRef]
140. Harrison, I.F.; Crum, W.R.; Vernon, A.C.; Dexter, D.T. Neurorestoration induced by the HDAC inhibitor sodium valproate in the lactacystin model of Parkinson's is associated with histone acetylation and up-regulation of neurotrophic factors. *Br. J. Pharmacol.* **2015**, *172*, 4200–4215. [CrossRef]
141. Grillari, J.; Grillari-Voglauer, R. Novel modulators of senescence, aging, and longevity: Small non-coding RNAs enter the stage. *Exp. Gerontol.* **2010**, *45*, 302–311. [CrossRef]
142. Nelson, P.T.; Wang, W.X.; Rajeev, B.W. MicroRNAs (miRNAs) in neurodegenerative diseases. *Brain Pathol.* **2008**, *18*, 130–138. [CrossRef]
143. Rodriguez-Ortiz, C.J.; Baglietto-Vargas, D.; Martinez-Coria, H.; LaFerla, F.M.; Kitazawa, M. Upregulation of miR-181 decreases c-Fos and SIRT-1 in the hippocampus of 3xTg-AD mice. *J. Alzheimers Dis.* **2014**, *42*, 1229–1238. [CrossRef]
144. Mao, K.; Zhang, G. The role of PARP1 in neurodegenerative diseases and aging. *FEBS J* **2021**. [CrossRef]
145. Martire, S.; Mosca, L.; d'Erme, M. PARP-1 involvement in neurodegeneration: A focus on Alzheimer's and Parkinson's diseases. *Mech. Ageing Dev.* **2015**, *146-148*, 53–64. [CrossRef] [PubMed]
146. Narne, P.; Pandey, V.; Simhadri, P.K.; Phanithi, P.B. Poly(ADP-ribose)polymerase-1 hyperactivation in neurodegenerative diseases: The death knell tolls for neurons. *Semin. Cell Dev. Biol.* **2017**, *63*, 154–166. [CrossRef] [PubMed]
147. Beneke, S.; Cohausz, O.; Malanga, M.; Boukamp, P.; Althaus, F.; Bürkle, A. Rapid regulation of telomere length is mediated by poly(ADP-ribose) polymerase-1. *Nucleic Acids Res.* **2008**, *36*, 6309–6317. [CrossRef] [PubMed]
148. Ye, T.J.; Lu, Y.L.; Yan, X.F.; Hu, X.D.; Wang, X.L. High mobility group box-1 release from H_2O_2-injured hepatocytes due to sirt1 functional inhibition. *World J. Gastroenterol.* **2019**, *25*, 5434–5450. [CrossRef]
149. Kam, T.I.; Mao, X.; Park, H.; Chou, S.C.; Karuppagounder, S.S.; Umanah, G.E.; Yun, S.P.; Brahmachari, S.; Panicker, N.; Chen, R.; et al. Poly(ADP-ribose) drives pathologic α-synuclein neurodegeneration in Parkinson's disease. *Science* **2018**, *362*, eaat8407. [CrossRef] [PubMed]
150. Rulten, S.L.; Rotheray, A.; Green, R.L.; Grundy, G.J.; Moore, D.A.; Gómez-Herreros, F.; Hafezparast, M.; Caldecott, K.W. PARP-1 dependent recruitment of the amyotrophic lateral sclerosis-associated protein FUS/TLS to sites of oxidative DNA damage. *Nucleic Acids Res.* **2014**, *42*, 307–314. [CrossRef] [PubMed]
151. Chini, C.C.S.; Tarragó, M.G.; Chini, E.N. NAD and the aging process: Role in life, death and everything in between. *Mol. Cell. Endocrinol.* **2017**, *455*, 62–74. [CrossRef]
152. Xie, Z.; Zhang, D.; Chung, D.; Tang, Z.; Huang, H.; Dai, L.; Qi, S.; Li, J.; Colak, G.; Chen, Y.; et al. Metabolic Regulation of Gene Expression by Histone Lysine β-Hydroxybutyrylation. *Mol. Cell* **2016**, *62*, 194–206. [CrossRef]
153. Green, D.R.; Galluzzi, L.; Kroemer, G. Mitochondria and the autophagy-inflammation-cell death axis in organismal aging. *Science* **2011**, *333*, 1109–1112. [CrossRef] [PubMed]
154. Moehle, E.A.; Shen, K.; Dillin, A. Mitochondrial proteostasis in the context of cellular and organismal health and aging. *J. Biol. Chem.* **2019**, *294*, 5396–5407. [CrossRef]
155. Hekimi, S.; Lapointe, J.; Wen, Y. Taking a "good" look at free radicals in the aging process. *Trends Cell Biol.* **2011**, *21*, 569–576. [CrossRef] [PubMed]
156. Lipinski, M.M.; Zheng, B.; Lu, T.; Yan, Z.; Py, B.F.; Ng, A.; Xavier, R.J.; Li, C.; Yankner, B.A.; Scherzer, C.R.; et al. Genome-wide analysis reveals mechanisms modulating autophagy in normal brain aging and in Alzheimer's disease. *Proc. Natl. Acad. Sci. USA* **2010**, *107*, 14164–14169. [CrossRef]
157. Winslow, A.R.; Chen, C.W.; Corrochano, S.; Acevedo-Arozena, A.; Gordon, D.E.; Peden, A.A.; Lichtenberg, M.; Menzies, F.M.; Ravikumar, B.; Imarisio, S.; et al. α-Synuclein impairs macroautophagy: Implications for Parkinson's disease. *J. Cell Biol.* **2010**, *190*, 1023–1037. [CrossRef] [PubMed]
158. Youle, R.J.; Narendra, D.P. Mechanisms of mitophagy. *Nat. Rev. Mol. Cell. Biol.* **2011**, *12*, 9–14. [CrossRef]
159. Gottlieb, R.A.; Mentzer, R.M. Autophagy during cardiac stress: Joys and frustrations of autophagy. *Annu. Rev. Physiol.* **2010**, *72*, 45–59. [CrossRef]
160. Madeo, F.; Tavernarakis, N.; Kroemer, G. Can autophagy promote longevity? *Nat. Cell Biol.* **2010**, *12*, 842–846. [CrossRef]
161. Zhou, R.; Yazdi, A.S.; Menu, P.; Tschopp, J. A role for mitochondria in NLRP3 inflammasome activation. *Nature* **2011**, *469*, 221–225. [CrossRef]
162. Herzig, S.; Shaw, R.J. AMPK: Guardian of metabolism and mitochondrial homeostasis. *Nat. Rev. Mol. Cell Biol.* **2018**, *19*, 121–135. [CrossRef]
163. Lee, I.H.; Cao, L.; Mostoslavsky, R.; Lombard, D.B.; Liu, J.; Bruns, N.E.; Tsokos, M.; Alt, F.W.; Finkel, T. A role for the NAD-dependent deacetylase Sirt1 in the regulation of autophagy. *Proc. Natl. Acad. Sci. USA* **2008**, *105*, 3374–3379. [CrossRef]

164. McCarty, M.F.; DiNicolantonio, J.J.; O'Keefe, J.H. Ketosis may promote brain macroautophagy by activating Sirt1 and hypoxia-inducible factor-1. *Med. Hypotheses* **2015**, *85*, 631–639. [CrossRef] [PubMed]
165. Qiu, X.; Brown, K.; Hirschey, M.D.; Verdin, E.; Chen, D. Calorie restriction reduces oxidative stress by SIRT3-mediated SOD2 activation. *Cell Metab.* **2010**, *12*, 662–667. [CrossRef]
166. Hafner, A.V.; Dai, J.; Gomes, A.P.; Xiao, C.Y.; Palmeira, C.M.; Rosenzweig, A.; Sinclair, D.A. Regulation of the mPTP by SIRT3-mediated deacetylation of CypD at lysine 166 suppresses age-related cardiac hypertrophy. *Aging* **2010**, *2*, 914–923. [CrossRef]
167. Halling, J.F.; Pilegaard, H. PGC-1α-mediated regulation of mitochondrial function and physiological implications. *Appl. Physiol. Nutr. Metab.* **2020**, *45*, 927–936. [CrossRef] [PubMed]
168. Austin, S.; St-Pierre, J. PGC1α and mitochondrial metabolism—emerging concepts and relevance in ageing and neurodegenerative disorders. *J. Cell Sci.* **2012**, *125*, 4963–4971. [CrossRef] [PubMed]
169. Cantó, C.; Auwerx, J. PGC-1alpha, SIRT1 and AMPK, an energy sensing network that controls energy expenditure. *Curr. Opin. Lipidol.* **2009**, *20*, 98–105. [CrossRef]
170. Puigserver, P.; Spiegelman, B.M. Peroxisome proliferator-activated receptor-gamma coactivator 1 alpha (PGC-1α): Transcriptional coactivator and metabolic regulator. *Endocr. Rev.* **2003**, *24*, 78–90. [CrossRef]
171. Scirpo, R.; Fiorotto, R.; Villani, A.; Amenduni, M.; Spirli, C.; Strazzabosco, M. Stimulation of nuclear receptor peroxisome proliferator-activated receptor-γ limits NF-κB-dependent inflammation in mouse cystic fibrosis biliary epithelium. *Hepatology* **2015**, *62*, 1551–1562. [CrossRef]
172. Tyagi, S.; Gupta, P.; Saini, A.S.; Kaushal, C.; Sharma, S. The peroxisome proliferator-activated receptor: A family of nuclear receptors role in various diseases. *J. Adv. Pharm. Technol. Res.* **2011**, *2*, 236–240. [CrossRef]
173. Qin, W.; Yang, T.; Ho, L.; Zhao, Z.; Wang, J.; Chen, L.; Zhao, W.; Thiyagarajan, M.; MacGrogan, D.; Rodgers, J.T.; et al. Neuronal SIRT1 activation as a novel mechanism underlying the prevention of Alzheimer disease amyloid neuropathology by calorie restriction. *J. Biol. Chem.* **2006**, *281*, 21745–21754. [CrossRef] [PubMed]
174. Qin, W.; Haroutunian, V.; Katsel, P.; Cardozo, C.P.; Ho, L.; Buxbaum, J.D.; Pasinetti, G.M. PGC-1alpha expression decreases in the Alzheimer disease brain as a function of dementia. *Arch. Neurol.* **2009**, *66*, 352–361. [CrossRef] [PubMed]
175. Eisele, P.S.; Salatino, S.; Sobek, J.; Hottiger, M.O.; Handschin, C. The peroxisome proliferator-activated receptor γ coactivator 1α/β (PGC-1) coactivators repress the transcriptional activity of NF-κB in skeletal muscle cells. *J. Biol. Chem.* **2013**, *288*, 2246–2260. [CrossRef]
176. Mookerjee, S.A.; Divakaruni, A.S.; Jastroch, M.; Brand, M.D. Mitochondrial uncoupling and lifespan. *Mech. Ageing Dev.* **2010**, *131*, 463–472. [CrossRef] [PubMed]
177. Franceschi, C.; Garagnani, P.; Parini, P.; Giuliani, C.; Santoro, A. Inflammaging: A new immune-metabolic viewpoint for age-related diseases. *Nat. Rev. Endocrinol.* **2018**, *14*, 576–590. [CrossRef]
178. Josephson, A.M.; Bradaschia-Correa, V.; Lee, S.; Leclerc, K.; Patel, K.S.; Muinos Lopez, E.; Litwa, H.P.; Neibart, S.S.; Kadiyala, M.; Wong, M.Z.; et al. Age-related inflammation triggers skeletal stem/progenitor cell dysfunction. *Proc. Natl. Acad. Sci. USA* **2019**, *116*, 6995–7004. [CrossRef]
179. Bauernfeind, F.; Ablasser, A.; Bartok, E.; Kim, S.; Schmid-Burgk, J.; Cavlar, T.; Hornung, V. Inflammasomes: Current understanding and open questions. *Cell. Mol. Life Sci.* **2011**, *68*, 765–783. [CrossRef]
180. Salminen, A.; Kaarniranta, K.; Kauppinen, A. Inflammaging: Disturbed interplay between autophagy and inflammasomes. *Aging* **2012**, *4*, 166–175. [CrossRef]
181. Martinez-Vicente, M.; Cuervo, A.M. Autophagy and neurodegeneration: When the cleaning crew goes on strike. *Lancet Neurol.* **2007**, *6*, 352–361. [CrossRef]
182. Nixon, R.A.; Yang, D.S. Autophagy failure in Alzheimer's disease–locating the primary defect. *Neurobiol. Dis.* **2011**, *43*, 38–45. [CrossRef] [PubMed]
183. Masters, S.L.; O'Neill, L.A. Disease-associated amyloid and misfolded protein aggregates activate the inflammasome. *Trends Mol. Med.* **2011**, *17*, 276–282. [CrossRef]
184. Salminen, A.; Huuskonen, J.; Ojala, J.; Kauppinen, A.; Kaarniranta, K.; Suuronen, T. Activation of innate immunity system during aging: NF-kB signaling is the molecular culprit of inflamm-aging. *Ageing Res. Rev.* **2008**, *7*, 83–105. [CrossRef]
185. Zhou, R.; Tardivel, A.; Thorens, B.; Choi, I.; Tschopp, J. Thioredoxin-interacting protein links oxidative stress to inflammasome activation. *Nat. Immunol.* **2010**, *11*, 136–140. [CrossRef] [PubMed]
186. Levy, M.; Thaiss, C.A.; Elinav, E. Taming the inflammasome. *Nat. Med.* **2015**, *21*, 213–215. [CrossRef]
187. Patel, M.N.; Carroll, R.G.; Galván-Peña, S.; Mills, E.L.; Olden, R.; Triantafilou, M.; Wolf, A.I.; Bryant, C.E.; Triantafilou, K.; Masters, S.L. Inflammasome Priming in Sterile Inflammatory Disease. *Trends Mol. Med.* **2017**, *23*, 165–180. [CrossRef] [PubMed]
188. Mihaylova, M.M.; Shaw, R.J. The AMPK signalling pathway coordinates cell growth, autophagy and metabolism. *Nat. Cell Biol.* **2011**, *13*, 1016–1023. [CrossRef] [PubMed]
189. Abdullah, A.; Mohd Murshid, N.; Makpol, S. Antioxidant Modulation of mTOR and Sirtuin Pathways in Age-Related Neurodegenerative Diseases. *Mol. Neurobiol.* **2020**, *57*, 5193–5207. [CrossRef]
190. Osorio, F.G.; Bárcena, C.; Soria-Valles, C.; Ramsay, A.J.; de Carlos, F.; Cobo, J.; Fueyo, A.; Freije, J.M.; López-Otín, C. Nuclear lamina defects cause ATM-dependent NF-κB activation and link accelerated aging to a systemic inflammatory response. *Genes Dev.* **2012**, *26*, 2311–2324. [CrossRef]

191. Amaya-Montoya, M.; Pérez-Londoño, A.; Guatibonza-García, V.; Vargas-Villanueva, A.; Mendivil, C.O. Cellular Senescence as a Therapeutic Target for Age-Related Diseases: A Review. *Adv. Ther.* **2020**, *37*, 1407–1424. [CrossRef]
192. Borghesan, M.; Hoogaars, W.M.H.; Varela-Eirin, M.; Talma, N.; Demaria, M. A Senescence-Centric View of Aging: Implications for Longevity and Disease. *Trends Cell Biol.* **2020**, *30*, 777–791. [CrossRef]
193. Campisi, J. Aging, cellular senescence, and cancer. *Annu. Rev. Physiol.* **2013**, *75*, 685–705. [CrossRef]
194. Di Micco, R.; Krizhanovsky, V.; Baker, D.; d'Adda di Fagagna, F. Cellular senescence in ageing: From mechanisms to therapeutic opportunities. *Nat. Rev. Mol. Cell Biol.* **2021**, *22*, 75–95. [CrossRef] [PubMed]
195. He, S.; Sharpless, N.E. Senescence in Health and Disease. *Cell* **2017**, *169*, 1000–1011. [CrossRef] [PubMed]
196. Tran, D.; Bergholz, J.; Zhang, H.; He, H.; Wang, Y.; Zhang, Y.; Li, Q.; Kirkland, J.L.; Xiao, Z.X. Insulin-like growth factor-1 regulates the SIRT1-p53 pathway in cellular senescence. *Aging Cell* **2014**, *13*, 669–678. [CrossRef]
197. Young, A.R.; Narita, M.; Ferreira, M.; Kirschner, K.; Sadaie, M.; Darot, J.F.; Tavaré, S.; Arakawa, S.; Shimizu, S.; Watt, F.M.; et al. Autophagy mediates the mitotic senescence transition. *Genes Dev.* **2009**, *23*, 798–803. [CrossRef]
198. Chen, C.; Zhou, M.; Ge, Y.; Wang, X. SIRT1 and aging related signaling pathways. *Mech. Ageing Dev.* **2020**, *187*, 111215. [CrossRef]
199. Salmenperä, P.; Karhemo, P.R.; Räsänen, K.; Laakkonen, P.; Vaheri, A. Fibroblast spheroids as a model to study sustained fibroblast quiescence and their crosstalk with tumor cells. *Exp. Cell Res.* **2016**, *345*, 17–24. [CrossRef]
200. Cai, J.; Weiss, M.L.; Rao, M.S. In search of "stemness". *Exp. Hematol.* **2004**, *32*, 585–598. [CrossRef]
201. Kim, K.H.; Chen, C.C.; Monzon, R.I.; Lau, L.F. Matricellular protein CCN1 promotes regression of liver fibrosis through induction of cellular senescence in hepatic myofibroblasts. *Mol. Cell Biol.* **2013**, *33*, 2078–2090. [CrossRef]
202. Collado, M.; Serrano, M. Senescence in tumours: Evidence from mice and humans. *Nat. Rev. Cancer* **2010**, *10*, 51–57. [CrossRef] [PubMed]
203. Chinta, S.J.; Woods, G.; Demaria, M.; Rane, A.; Zou, Y.; McQuade, A.; Rajagopalan, S.; Limbad, C.; Madden, D.T.; Campisi, J.; et al. Cellular Senescence Is Induced by the Environmental Neurotoxin Paraquat and Contributes to Neuropathology Linked to Parkinson's Disease. *Cell Rep.* **2018**, *22*, 930–940. [CrossRef]
204. Finkel, T.; Serrano, M.; Blasco, M.A. The common biology of cancer and ageing. *Nature* **2007**, *448*, 767–774. [CrossRef]
205. Wang, J.C.; Bennett, M. Aging and atherosclerosis: Mechanisms, functional consequences, and potential therapeutics for cellular senescence. *Circ. Res.* **2012**, *111*, 245–259. [CrossRef]
206. Cao, L.; Li, W.; Kim, S.; Brodie, S.G.; Deng, C.X. Senescence, aging, and malignant transformation mediated by p53 in mice lacking the Brca1 full-length isoform. *Genes Dev.* **2003**, *17*, 201–213. [CrossRef]
207. Jones, R.G.; Plas, D.R.; Kubek, S.; Buzzai, M.; Mu, J.; Xu, Y.; Birnbaum, M.J.; Thompson, C.B. AMP-activated protein kinase induces a p53-dependent metabolic checkpoint. *Mol. Cell* **2005**, *18*, 283–293. [CrossRef] [PubMed]
208. Balch, W.E.; Morimoto, R.I.; Dillin, A.; Kelly, J.W. Adapting proteostasis for disease intervention. *Science* **2008**, *319*, 916–919. [CrossRef]
209. Klaips, C.L.; Jayaraj, G.G.; Hartl, F.U. Pathways of cellular proteostasis in aging and disease. *J. Cell Biol.* **2018**, *217*, 51–63. [CrossRef] [PubMed]
210. Lapierre, L.R.; De Magalhaes Filho, C.D.; McQuary, P.R.; Chu, C.C.; Visvikis, O.; Chang, J.T.; Gelino, S.; Ong, B.; Davis, A.E.; Irazoqui, J.E.; et al. The TFEB orthologue HLH-30 regulates autophagy and modulates longevity in *Caenorhabditis elegans*. *Nat. Commun.* **2013**, *4*, 2267. [CrossRef]
211. Basisty, N.; Meyer, J.G.; Schilling, B. Protein Turnover in Aging and Longevity. *Proteomics* **2018**, *18*, e1700108. [CrossRef]
212. Wong, S.Q.; Kumar, A.V.; Mills, J.; Lapierre, L.R. Autophagy in aging and longevity. *Hum. Genet.* **2020**, *139*, 277–290. [CrossRef] [PubMed]
213. Sorrentino, V.; Romani, M.; Mouchiroud, L.; Beck, J.S.; Zhang, H.; D'Amico, D.; Moullan, N.; Potenza, F.; Schmid, A.W.; Rietsch, S.; et al. Enhancing mitochondrial proteostasis reduces amyloid-β proteotoxicity. *Nature* **2017**, *552*, 187–193. [CrossRef]
214. Fang, E.F.; Hou, Y.; Palikaras, K.; Adriaanse, B.A.; Kerr, J.S.; Yang, B.; Lautrup, S.; Hasan-Olive, M.M.; Caponio, D.; Dan, X.; et al. Mitophagy inhibits amyloid-β and tau pathology and reverses cognitive deficits in models of Alzheimer's disease. *Nat. Neurosci.* **2019**, *22*, 401–412. [CrossRef] [PubMed]
215. Ryu, D.; Mouchiroud, L.; Andreux, P.A.; Katsyuba, E.; Moullan, N.; Nicolet-Dit-Félix, A.A.; Williams, E.G.; Jha, P.; Lo Sasso, G.; Huzard, D.; et al. Urolithin A induces mitophagy and prolongs lifespan in *C. elegans* and increases muscle function in rodents. *Nat. Med.* **2016**, *22*, 879–888. [CrossRef]
216. Ou, X.; Lee, M.R.; Huang, X.; Messina-Graham, S.; Broxmeyer, H.E. SIRT1 positively regulates autophagy and mitochondria function in embryonic stem cells under oxidative stress. *Stem Cells* **2014**, *32*, 1183–1194. [CrossRef] [PubMed]
217. Goodell, M.A.; Rando, T.A. Stem cells and healthy aging. *Science* **2015**, *350*, 1199–1204. [CrossRef] [PubMed]
218. Keyes, B.E.; Fuchs, E. Stem cells: Aging and transcriptional fingerprints. *J. Cell. Biol.* **2018**, *217*, 79–92. [CrossRef]
219. Zhang, P.; Kishimoto, Y.; Grammatikakis, I.; Gottimukkala, K.; Cutler, R.G.; Zhang, S.; Abdelmohsen, K.; Bohr, V.A.; Misra Sen, J.; Gorospe, M.; et al. Senolytic therapy alleviates Aβ-associated oligodendrocyte progenitor cell senescence and cognitive deficits in an Alzheimer's disease model. *Nat. Neurosci.* **2019**, *22*, 719–728. [CrossRef]
220. Ehninger, D.; Neff, F.; Xie, K. Longevity, aging and rapamycin. *Cell. Mol. Life Sci.* **2014**, *71*, 4325–4346. [CrossRef]
221. Kaeberlein, M.; Galvan, V. Rapamycin and Alzheimer's disease: Time for a clinical trial? *Sci. Transl. Med.* **2019**, *11*, eaar4289. [CrossRef] [PubMed]

222. Sharma, M.; Gupta, Y.K. Chronic treatment with trans resveratrol prevents intracerebroventricular streptozotocin induced cognitive impairment and oxidative stress in rats. *Life Sci.* **2002**, *71*, 2489–2498. [CrossRef]
223. Lu, M.; Su, C.; Qiao, C.; Bian, Y.; Ding, J.; Hu, G. Metformin Prevents Dopaminergic Neuron Death in MPTP/P-Induced Mouse Model of Parkinson's Disease via Autophagy and Mitochondrial ROS Clearance. *Int. J. Neuropsychopharmacol.* **2016**, *19*, pyw047. [CrossRef] [PubMed]
224. Foretz, M.; Guigas, B.; Bertrand, L.; Pollak, M.; Viollet, B. Metformin: From mechanisms of action to therapies. *Cell Metab.* **2014**, *20*, 953–966. [CrossRef] [PubMed]
225. Kulkarni, A.S.; Gubbi, S.; Barzilai, N. Benefits of Metformin in Attenuating the Hallmarks of Aging. *Cell Metab.* **2020**, *32*, 15–30. [CrossRef]
226. Najafi, M.; Cheki, M.; Rezapoor, S.; Geraily, G.; Motevaseli, E.; Carnovale, C.; Clementi, E.; Shirazi, A. Metformin: Prevention of genomic instability and cancer: A review. *Mutat. Res. Genet. Toxicol. Environ. Mutagen.* **2018**, *827*, 1–8. [CrossRef]
227. Aatsinki, S.M.; Buler, M.; Salomäki, H.; Koulu, M.; Pavek, P.; Hakkola, J. Metformin induces PGC-1α expression and selectively affects hepatic PGC-1α functions. *Br. J. Pharmacol.* **2014**, *171*, 2351–2363. [CrossRef]
228. Prasad, S.; Sajja, R.K.; Kaisar, M.A.; Park, J.H.; Villalba, H.; Liles, T.; Abbruscato, T.; Cucullo, L. Role of Nrf2 and protective effects of Metformin against tobacco smoke-induced cerebrovascular toxicity. *Redox Biol.* **2017**, *12*, 58–69. [CrossRef]
229. Cuyàs, E.; Verdura, S.; Llorach-Parés, L.; Fernández-Arroyo, S.; Joven, J.; Martin-Castillo, B.; Bosch-Barrera, J.; Brunet, J.; Nonell-Canals, A.; Sanchez-Martinez, M.; et al. Metformin Is a Direct SIRT1-Activating Compound: Computational Modeling and Experimental Validation. *Front. Endocrinol.* **2018**, *9*, 657. [CrossRef]
230. Moiseeva, O.; Deschênes-Simard, X.; St-Germain, E.; Igelmann, S.; Huot, G.; Cadar, A.E.; Bourdeau, V.; Pollak, M.N.; Ferbeyre, G. Metformin inhibits the senescence-associated secretory phenotype by interfering with IKK/NF-κB activation. *Aging Cell* **2013**, *12*, 489–498. [CrossRef]
231. Tizazu, A.M.; Nyunt, M.S.Z.; Cexus, O.; Suku, K.; Mok, E.; Xian, C.H.; Chong, J.; Tan, C.; How, W.; Hubert, S.; et al. Metformin Monotherapy Downregulates Diabetes-Associated Inflammatory Status and Impacts on Mortality. *Front. Physiol.* **2019**, *10*, 572. [CrossRef]
232. Wang, C.; Liu, C.; Gao, K.; Zhao, H.; Zhou, Z.; Shen, Z.; Guo, Y.; Li, Z.; Yao, T.; Mei, X. Metformin preconditioning provide neuroprotection through enhancement of autophagy and suppression of inflammation and apoptosis after spinal cord injury. *Biochem. Biophys. Res. Commun.* **2016**, *477*, 534–540. [CrossRef] [PubMed]
233. Markowicz-Piasecka, M.; Sikora, J.; Szydłowska, A.; Skupień, A.; Mikiciuk-Olasik, E.; Huttunen, K.M. Metformin—A Future Therapy for Neurodegenerative Diseases: Theme: Drug Discovery, Development and Delivery in Alzheimer's Disease Guest Editor: Davide Brambilla. *Pharm. Res.* **2017**, *34*, 2614–2627. [CrossRef]
234. Fang, J.; Yang, J.; Wu, X.; Zhang, G.; Li, T.; Wang, X.; Zhang, H.; Wang, C.C.; Liu, G.H.; Wang, L. Metformin alleviates human cellular aging by upregulating the endoplasmic reticulum glutathione peroxidase 7. *Aging Cell* **2018**, *17*, e12765. [CrossRef]
235. Bridgeman, S.C.; Ellison, G.C.; Melton, P.E.; Newsholme, P.; Mamotte, C.D.S. Epigenetic effects of metformin: From molecular mechanisms to clinical implications. *Diabetes Obes. Metab.* **2018**, *20*, 1553–1562. [CrossRef]
236. Noren Hooten, N.; Martin-Montalvo, A.; Dluzen, D.F.; Zhang, Y.; Bernier, M.; Zonderman, A.B.; Becker, K.G.; Gorospe, M.; de Cabo, R.; Evans, M.K. Metformin-mediated increase in DICER1 regulates microRNA expression and cellular senescence. *Aging Cell* **2016**, *15*, 572–581. [CrossRef] [PubMed]
237. De Zegher, F.; Díaz, M.; Ibáñez, L. Association between Long Telomere Length and Insulin Sensitization in Adolescent Girls with Hyperinsulinemic Androgen Excess. *JAMA Pediatr.* **2015**, *169*, 787–788. [CrossRef]
238. Diman, A.; Boros, J.; Poulain, F.; Rodriguez, J.; Purnelle, M.; Episkopou, H.; Bertrand, L.; Francaux, M.; Deldicque, L.; Decottignies, A. Nuclear respiratory factor 1 and endurance exercise promote human telomere transcription. *Sci. Adv.* **2016**, *2*, e1600031. [CrossRef] [PubMed]
239. Bhullar, K.S.; Hubbard, B.P. Lifespan and healthspan extension by resveratrol. *Biochim. Biophys. Acta* **2015**, *1852*, 1209–1218. [CrossRef] [PubMed]
240. Porquet, D.; Casadesús, G.; Bayod, S.; Vicente, A.; Canudas, A.M.; Vilaplana, J.; Pelegrí, C.; Sanfeliu, C.; Camins, A.; Pallàs, M.; et al. Dietary resveratrol prevents Alzheimer's markers and increases life span in SAMP8. *Age* **2013**, *35*, 1851–1865. [CrossRef] [PubMed]
241. Mancuso, R.; del Valle, J.; Modol, L.; Martinez, A.; Granado-Serrano, A.B.; Ramirez-Núñez, O.; Pallás, M.; Portero-Otin, M.; Osta, R.; Navarro, X. Resveratrol improves motoneuron function and extends survival in SOD1(G93A) ALS mice. *Neurotherapeutics* **2014**, *11*, 419–432. [CrossRef]
242. Price, N.L.; Gomes, A.P.; Ling, A.J.; Duarte, F.V.; Martin-Montalvo, A.; North, B.J.; Agarwal, B.; Ye, L.; Ramadori, G.; Teodoro, J.S.; et al. SIRT1 is required for AMPK activation and the beneficial effects of resveratrol on mitochondrial function. *Cell Metab.* **2012**, *15*, 675–690. [CrossRef]
243. Morris, B.J. Seven sirtuins for seven deadly diseases of aging. *Free Radic. Biol. Med.* **2013**, *56*, 133–171. [CrossRef]
244. Choi, H.I.; Kim, H.J.; Park, J.S.; Kim, I.J.; Bae, E.H.; Ma, S.K.; Kim, S.W. PGC-1α attenuates hydrogen peroxide-induced apoptotic cell death by upregulating Nrf-2 via GSK3β inactivation mediated by activated p38 in HK-2 Cells. *Sci. Rep.* **2017**, *7*, 4319. [CrossRef]
245. Huang, K.; Gao, X.; Wei, W. The crosstalk between Sirt1 and Keap1/Nrf2/ARE anti-oxidative pathway forms a positive feedback loop to inhibit FN and TGF-β1 expressions in rat glomerular mesangial cells. *Exp. Cell Res.* **2017**, *361*, 63–72. [CrossRef] [PubMed]

246. Joo, M.S.; Kim, W.D.; Lee, K.Y.; Kim, J.H.; Koo, J.H.; Kim, S.G. AMPK Facilitates Nuclear Accumulation of Nrf2 by Phosphorylating at Serine 550. *Mol. Cell Biol.* **2016**, *36*, 1931–1942. [CrossRef]
247. Mercken, E.M.; Mitchell, S.J.; Martin-Montalvo, A.; Minor, R.K.; Almeida, M.; Gomes, A.P.; Scheibye-Knudsen, M.; Palacios, H.H.; Licata, J.J.; Zhang, Y.; et al. SRT2104 extends survival of male mice on a standard diet and preserves bone and muscle mass. *Aging Cell* **2014**, *13*, 787–796. [CrossRef] [PubMed]
248. Carullo, G.; Cappello, A.R.; Frattaruolo, L.; Badolato, M.; Armentano, B.; Aiello, F. Quercetin and derivatives: Useful tools in inflammation and pain management. *Future Med. Chem.* **2017**, *9*, 79–93. [CrossRef]
249. Feng, X.; Sureda, A.; Jafari, S.; Memariani, Z.; Tewari, D.; Annunziata, G.; Barrea, L.; Hassan, S.T.S.; Šmejkal, K.; Malaník, M.; et al. Berberine in Cardiovascular and Metabolic Diseases: From Mechanisms to Therapeutics. *Theranostics* **2019**, *9*, 1923–1951. [CrossRef] [PubMed]
250. Sarker, M.R.; Franks, S.F. Efficacy of curcumin for age-associated cognitive decline: A narrative review of preclinical and clinical studies. *Geroscience* **2018**, *40*, 73–95. [CrossRef]
251. Sato, K.; Kashiwaya, Y.; Keon, C.A.; Tsuchiya, N.; King, M.T.; Radda, G.K.; Chance, B.; Clarke, K.; Veech, R.L. Insulin, ketone bodies, and mitochondrial energy transduction. *FASEB J.* **1995**, *9*, 651–658. [CrossRef] [PubMed]
252. Sharma, A.K.; Rani, E.; Waheed, A.; Rajput, S.K. Pharmacoresistant Epilepsy: A Current Update on Non-Conventional Pharmacological and Non-Pharmacological Interventions. *J. Epilepsy Res.* **2015**, *5*, 1–8. [CrossRef]
253. VanItallie, T.B.; Nufert, T.H. Ketones: Metabolism's ugly duckling. *Nutr. Rev.* **2003**, *61*, 327–341. [CrossRef] [PubMed]
254. Almeida, C.G.; de Mendonça, A.; Cunha, R.A.; Ribeiro, J.A. Adenosine promotes neuronal recovery from reactive oxygen species induced lesion in rat hippocampal slices. *Neurosci. Lett.* **2003**, *339*, 127–130. [CrossRef]
255. Choudhury, H.; Chellappan, D.K.; Sengupta, P.; Pandey, M.; Gorain, B. Adenosine Receptors in Modulation of Central Nervous System Disorders. *Curr. Pharm. Des.* **2019**, *25*, 2808–2827. [CrossRef] [PubMed]
256. McNally, M.A.; Hartman, A.L. Ketone bodies in epilepsy. *J. Neurochem.* **2012**, *121*, 28–35. [CrossRef]
257. Juge, N.; Gray, J.A.; Omote, H.; Miyaji, T.; Inoue, T.; Hara, C.; Uneyama, H.; Edwards, R.H.; Nicoll, R.A.; Moriyama, Y. Metabolic control of vesicular glutamate transport and release. *Neuron* **2010**, *68*, 99–112. [CrossRef]
258. Tieu, K.; Perier, C.; Caspersen, C.; Teismann, P.; Wu, D.C.; Yan, S.D.; Naini, A.; Vila, M.; Jackson-Lewis, V.; Ramasamy, R.; et al. D-beta-hydroxybutyrate rescues mitochondrial respiration and mitigates features of Parkinson disease. *J. Clin. Investig.* **2003**, *112*, 892–901. [CrossRef]
259. Veech, R.L.; Todd King, M.; Pawlosky, R.; Kashiwaya, Y.; Bradshaw, P.C.; Curtis, W. The "great" controlling nucleotide coenzymes. *IUBMB Life* **2019**, *71*, 565–579. [CrossRef]
260. Shimazu, T.; Hirschey, M.D.; Newman, J.; He, W.; Shirakawa, K.; Le Moan, N.; Grueter, C.A.; Lim, H.; Saunders, L.R.; Stevens, R.D.; et al. Suppression of oxidative stress by β-hydroxybutyrate, an endogenous histone deacetylase inhibitor. *Science* **2013**, *339*, 211–214. [CrossRef]
261. Tseng, A.H.; Shieh, S.S.; Wang, D.L. SIRT3 deacetylates FOXO3 to protect mitochondria against oxidative damage. *Free Radic. Biol. Med.* **2013**, *63*, 222–234. [CrossRef]
262. Zhao, L.; Ackerman, S.L. Endoplasmic reticulum stress in health and disease. *Curr. Opin. Cell Biol.* **2006**, *18*, 444–452. [CrossRef] [PubMed]
263. Sleiman, S.F.; Henry, J.; Al-Haddad, R.; El Hayek, L.; Abou Haidar, E.; Stringer, T.; Ulja, D.; Karuppagounder, S.S.; Holson, E.B.; Ratan, R.R.; et al. Exercise promotes the expression of brain derived neurotrophic factor (BDNF) through the action of the ketone body β-hydroxybutyrate. *Elife* **2016**, *5*, e15092. [CrossRef]
264. Manning, B.D.; Cantley, L.C. AKT/PKB signaling: Navigating downstream. *Cell* **2007**, *129*, 1261–1274. [CrossRef]
265. Xu, D.; Lian, D.; Wu, J.; Liu, Y.; Zhu, M.; Sun, J.; He, D.; Li, L. Brain-derived neurotrophic factor reduces inflammation and hippocampal apoptosis in experimental Streptococcus pneumoniae meningitis. *J. Neuroinflamm.* **2017**, *14*, 156. [CrossRef]
266. Marosi, K.; Kim, S.W.; Moehl, K.; Scheibye-Knudsen, M.; Cheng, A.; Cutler, R.; Camandola, S.; Mattson, M.P. 3-Hydroxybutyrate regulates energy metabolism and induces BDNF expression in cerebral cortical neurons. *J. Neurochem.* **2016**, *139*, 769–781. [CrossRef] [PubMed]
267. Lau, D.; Bengtson, C.P.; Buchthal, B.; Bading, H. BDNF Reduces Toxic Extrasynaptic NMDA Receptor Signaling via Synaptic NMDA Receptors and Nuclear-Calcium-Induced Transcription of inhba/Activin A. *Cell Rep.* **2015**, *12*, 1353–1366. [CrossRef] [PubMed]
268. Mattson, M.P.; Lovell, M.A.; Furukawa, K.; Markesbery, W.R. Neurotrophic factors attenuate glutamate-induced accumulation of peroxides, elevation of intracellular Ca^{2+} concentration, and neurotoxicity and increase antioxidant enzyme activities in hippocampal neurons. *J. Neurochem.* **1995**, *65*, 1740–1751. [CrossRef]
269. Menzies, K.J.; Zhang, H.; Katsyuba, E.; Auwerx, J. Protein acetylation in metabolism—Metabolites and cofactors. *Nat. Rev. Endocrinol.* **2016**, *12*, 43–60. [CrossRef] [PubMed]
270. Guil, S.; Long, J.C.; Cáceres, J.F. hnRNP A1 relocalization to the stress granules reflects a role in the stress response. *Mol. Cell. Biol.* **2006**, *26*, 5744–5758. [CrossRef] [PubMed]
271. Jean-Philippe, J.; Paz, S.; Caputi, M. hnRNP A1: The Swiss army knife of gene expression. *Int. J. Mol. Sci.* **2013**, *14*, 18999–19024. [CrossRef]

272. Parodi, B.; Rossi, S.; Morando, S.; Cordano, C.; Bragoni, A.; Motta, C.; Usai, C.; Wipke, B.T.; Scannevin, R.H.; Mancardi, G.L.; et al. Fumarates modulate microglia activation through a novel HCAR2 signaling pathway and rescue synaptic dysregulation in inflamed CNS. *Acta Neuropathol.* **2015**, *130*, 279–295. [CrossRef]
273. Maalouf, M.; Sullivan, P.G.; Davis, L.; Kim, D.Y.; Rho, J.M. Ketones inhibit mitochondrial production of reactive oxygen species production following glutamate excitotoxicity by increasing NADH oxidation. *Neuroscience* **2007**, *145*, 256–264. [CrossRef] [PubMed]
274. Pawlosky, R.J.; Kemper, M.F.; Kashiwaya, Y.; King, M.T.; Mattson, M.P.; Veech, R.L. Effects of a dietary ketone ester on hippocampal glycolytic and tricarboxylic acid cycle intermediates and amino acids in a 3xTgAD mouse model of Alzheimer's disease. *J. Neurochem.* **2017**, *141*, 195–207. [CrossRef]
275. Offermanns, S.; Schwaninger, M. Nutritional or pharmacological activation of HCA(2) ameliorates neuroinflammation. *Trends Mol. Med.* **2015**, *21*, 245–255. [CrossRef]
276. Shabab, T.; Khanabdali, R.; Moghadamtousi, S.Z.; Kadir, H.A.; Mohan, G. Neuroinflammation pathways: A general review. *Int. J. Neurosci.* **2017**, *127*, 624–633. [CrossRef]
277. Norwitz, N.G.; Hu, M.T.; Clarke, K. The Mechanisms by Which the Ketone Body D-β-Hydroxybutyrate May Improve the Multiple Cellular Pathologies of Parkinson's disease. *Front. Nutr.* **2019**, *6*, 63. [CrossRef]
278. Hasan-Olive, M.M.; Lauritzen, K.H.; Ali, M.; Rasmussen, L.J.; Storm-Mathisen, J.; Bergersen, L.H. A Ketogenic Diet Improves Mitochondrial Biogenesis and Bioenergetics via the PGC1α-SIRT3-UCP2 Axis. *Neurochem. Res.* **2019**, *44*, 22–37. [CrossRef] [PubMed]
279. Zou, X.H.; Li, H.M.; Wang, S.; Leski, M.; Yao, Y.C.; Yang, X.D.; Huang, Q.J.; Chen, G.Q. The effect of 3-hydroxybutyrate methyl ester on learning and memory in mice. *Biomaterials* **2009**, *30*, 1532–1541. [CrossRef]
280. Scheibye-Knudsen, M.; Mitchell, S.J.; Fang, E.F.; Iyama, T.; Ward, T.; Wang, J.; Dunn, C.A.; Singh, N.; Veith, S.; Hasan-Olive, M.M.; et al. A high-fat diet and NAD+ activate Sirt1 to rescue premature aging in cockayne syndrome. *Cell Metab.* **2014**, *20*, 840–855. [CrossRef] [PubMed]
281. Houtkooper, R.H.; Auwerx, J. Exploring the therapeutic space around NAD+. *J. Cell Biol.* **2012**, *199*, 205–209. [CrossRef]
282. Kong, X.; Wang, R.; Xue, Y.; Liu, X.; Zhang, H.; Chen, Y.; Fang, F.; Chang, Y. Sirtuin 3, a new target of PGC-1alpha, plays an important role in the suppression of ROS and mitochondrial biogenesis. *PLoS ONE* **2010**, *5*, e11707. [CrossRef]
283. Shi, T.; Wang, F.; Stieren, E.; Tong, Q. SIRT3, a mitochondrial sirtuin deacetylase, regulates mitochondrial function and thermogenesis in brown adipocytes. *J. Biol. Chem.* **2005**, *280*, 13560–13567. [CrossRef] [PubMed]
284. Cheng, A.; Wan, R.; Yang, J.L.; Kamimura, N.; Son, T.G.; Ouyang, X.; Luo, Y.; Okun, E.; Mattson, M.P. Involvement of PGC-1α in the formation and maintenance of neuronal dendritic spines. *Nat. Commun.* **2012**, *3*, 1250. [CrossRef] [PubMed]
285. Jeong, E.A.; Jeon, B.T.; Shin, H.J.; Kim, N.; Lee, D.H.; Kim, H.J.; Kang, S.S.; Cho, Q.J.; Choi, W.S.; Roh, G.S. Ketogenic diet-induced peroxisome proliferator-activated receptor-γ activation decreases neuroinflammation in the mouse hippocampus after kainic acid-induced seizures. *Exp. Neurol.* **2011**, *232*, 195–202. [CrossRef] [PubMed]
286. Morris, G.; Puri, B.K.; Carvalho, A.; Maes, M.; Berk, M.; Ruusunen, A.; Olive, L. Induced Ketosis as a Treatment for Neuroprogressive Disorders: Food for Thought? *Int. J. Neuropsychopharmacol.* **2020**, *23*, 366–384. [CrossRef]
287. Simeone, T.A.; Matthews, S.A.; Samson, K.K.; Simeone, K.A. Regulation of brain PPARgamma2 contributes to ketogenic diet anti-seizure efficacy. *Exp. Neurol.* **2017**, *287*, 54–64. [CrossRef]
288. Kashiwaya, Y.; Pawlosky, R.; Markis, W.; King, M.T.; Bergman, C.; Srivastava, S.; Murray, A.; Clarke, K.; Veech, R.L. A ketone ester diet increases brain malonyl-CoA and Uncoupling proteins 4 and 5 while decreasing food intake in the normal Wistar Rat. *J. Biol. Chem.* **2010**, *285*, 25950–25956. [CrossRef]
289. Srivastava, S.; Kashiwaya, Y.; King, M.T.; Baxa, U.; Tam, J.; Niu, G.; Chen, X.; Clarke, K.; Veech, R.L. Mitochondrial biogenesis and increased uncoupling protein 1 in brown adipose tissue of mice fed a ketone ester diet. *FASEB J.* **2012**, *26*, 2351–2362. [CrossRef]
290. Bae, H.R.; Kim, D.H.; Park, M.H.; Lee, B.; Kim, M.J.; Lee, E.K.; Chung, K.W.; Kim, S.M.; Im, D.S.; Chung, H.Y. β-Hydroxybutyrate suppresses inflammasome formation by ameliorating endoplasmic reticulum stress via AMPK activation. *Oncotarget* **2016**, *7*, 66444–66454. [CrossRef]
291. Yamanashi, T.; Iwata, M.; Kamiya, N.; Tsunetomi, K.; Kajitani, N.; Wada, N.; Iitsuka, T.; Yamauchi, T.; Miura, A.; Pu, S.; et al. Beta-hydroxybutyrate, an endogenic NLRP3 inflammasome inhibitor, attenuates stress-induced behavioral and inflammatory responses. *Sci. Rep.* **2017**, *7*, 7677. [CrossRef]
292. Youm, Y.H.; Nguyen, K.Y.; Grant, R.W.; Goldberg, E.L.; Bodogai, M.; Kim, D.; D'Agostino, D.; Planavsky, N.; Lupfer, C.; Kanneganti, T.D.; et al. The ketone metabolite β-hydroxybutyrate blocks NLRP3 inflammasome-mediated inflammatory disease. *Nat. Med.* **2015**, *21*, 263–269. [CrossRef]
293. Ari, C.; Murdun, C.; Koutnik, A.P.; Goldhagen, C.R.; Rogers, C.; Park, C.; Bharwani, S.; Diamond, D.M.; Kindy, M.S.; D'Agostino, D.P.; et al. Exogenous Ketones Lower Blood Glucose Level in Rested and Exercised Rodent Models. *Nutrients* **2019**, *11*, 2330. [CrossRef]
294. Edwards, C.; Copes, N.; Bradshaw, P.C. D-β-hydroxybutyrate: An anti-aging ketone body. *Oncotarget* **2015**, *6*, 3477–3478. [CrossRef] [PubMed]
295. Kenyon, C. The first long-lived mutants: Discovery of the insulin/IGF-1 pathway for ageing. *Philos. Trans. R. Soc. Lond. B. Biol. Sci.* **2011**, *366*, 9–16. [CrossRef] [PubMed]

296. Willcox, B.J.; Donlon, T.A.; He, Q.; Chen, R.; Grove, J.S.; Yano, K.; Masaki, K.H.; Willcox, D.C.; Rodriguez, B.; Curb, J.D. FOXO3A genotype is strongly associated with human longevity. *Proc. Natl. Acad. Sci. USA* **2008**, *105*, 13987–13992. [CrossRef] [PubMed]
297. Hansen, M.; Chandra, A.; Mitic, L.L.; Onken, B.; Driscoll, M.; Kenyon, C. A role for autophagy in the extension of lifespan by dietary restriction in C. elegans. *PLoS Genet.* **2008**, *4*, e24. [CrossRef]
298. Yamada, T.; Zhang, S.J.; Westerblad, H.; Katz, A. β-Hydroxybutyrate inhibits insulin-mediated glucose transport in mouse oxidative muscle. *Am. J. Physiol. Endocrinol. Metab.* **2010**, *299*, 364–373. [CrossRef]
299. Barja, G. Free radicals and aging. *Trends Neurosci.* **2004**, *27*, 595–600. [CrossRef]
300. Newman, J.C.; Covarrubias, A.J.; Zhao, M.; Yu, X.; Gut, P.; Ng, C.P.; Huang, Y.; Haldar, S.; Verdin, E. Ketogenic Diet Reduces Midlife Mortality and Improves Memory in Aging Mice. *Cell Metab.* **2017**, *26*, 547–557.e8. [CrossRef]
301. Simeone, K.A.; Matthews, S.A.; Rho, J.M.; Simeone, T.A. Ketogenic diet treatment increases longevity in Kcna1-null mice, a model of sudden unexpected death in epilepsy. *Epilepsia* **2016**, *57*, 178–182. [CrossRef]
302. Liu, K.; Li, F.; Sun, Q.; Lin, N.; Han, H.; You, K.; Tian, F.; Mao, Z.; Li, T.; Tong, T.; et al. p53 β-hydroxybutyrylation attenuates p53 activity. *Cell Death Dis.* **2019**, *10*, 243. [CrossRef]
303. Habieb, M.E.; Mohamed, M.A.; El Gamal, D.M.; Hawas, A.M.; Mohamed, T.M. Anti-aging effect of DL-β-hydroxybutyrate against hepatic cellular senescence induced by D-galactose or γ-irradiation via autophagic flux stimulation in male rats. *Arch. Gerontol. Geriatr.* **2021**, *92*, 104288. [CrossRef] [PubMed]
304. Wang, H.; Han, L.; Zhao, G.; Shen, H.; Wang, P.; Sun, Z.; Xu, C.; Su, Y.; Li, G.; Tong, T.; et al. hnRNP A1 antagonizes cellular senescence and senescence-associated secretory phenotype via regulation of SIRT1 mRNA stability. *Aging Cell* **2016**, *15*, 1063–1073. [CrossRef] [PubMed]
305. Armada-Moreira, A.; Gomes, J.I.; Pina, C.C.; Savchak, O.K.; Gonçalves-Ribeiro, J.; Rei, N.; Pinto, S.; Morais, T.P.; Martins, R.S.; Ribeiro, F.F.; et al. Going the Extra (Synaptic) Mile: Excitotoxicity as the Road Toward Neurodegenerative Diseases. *Front. Cell. Neurosci.* **2020**, *14*, 90. [CrossRef]
306. Coyle, J.T.; Puttfarcken, P. Oxidative stress, glutamate, and neurodegenerative disorders. *Science* **1993**, *262*, 689–695. [CrossRef] [PubMed]
307. Holper, L.; Ben-Shachar, D.; Mann, J.J. Multivariate meta-analyses of mitochondrial complex I and IV in major depressive disorder, bipolar disorder, schizophrenia, Alzheimer disease, and Parkinson disease. *Neuropsychopharmacology* **2019**, *44*, 837–849. [CrossRef] [PubMed]
308. Mosconi, L.; de Leon, M.; Murray, J.; Lu, J.; Javier, E.; McHugh, P.; Swerdlow, R.H. Reduced mitochondria cytochrome oxidase activity in adult children of mothers with Alzheimer's disease. *J. Alzheimers Dis.* **2011**, *27*, 483–490. [CrossRef] [PubMed]
309. Lugrin, J.; Rosenblatt-Velin, N.; Parapanov, R.; Liaudet, L. The role of oxidative stress during inflammatory processes. *Biol. Chem.* **2014**, *395*, 203–230. [CrossRef] [PubMed]
310. Wu, Z.; Yu, J.; Zhu, A.; Nakanishi, H. Nutrients, Microglia Aging, and Brain Aging. *Oxid. Med. Cell Longev.* **2016**, *2016*, 7498528. [CrossRef]
311. Hatanpää, K.; Isaacs, K.R.; Shirao, T.; Brady, D.R.; Rapoport, S.I. Loss of proteins regulating synaptic plasticity in normal aging of the human brain and in Alzheimer disease. *J. Neuropathol. Exp. Neurol.* **1999**, *58*, 637–643. [CrossRef]
312. Rao, J.S.; Kellom, M.; Kim, H.W.; Rapoport, S.I.; Reese, E.A. Neuroinflammation and synaptic loss. *Neurochem. Res.* **2012**, *37*, 903–910. [CrossRef]
313. Scheff, S.W.; Price, D.A.; Schmitt, F.A.; Mufson, E.J. Hippocampal synaptic loss in early Alzheimer's disease and mild cognitive impairment. *Neurobiol. Aging* **2006**, *27*, 1372–1384. [CrossRef]
314. Appelberg, K.S.; Hovda, D.A.; Prins, M.L. The effects of a ketogenic diet on behavioral outcome after controlled cortical impact injury in the juvenile and adult rat. *J. Neurotrauma* **2009**, *26*, 497–506. [CrossRef]
315. Krikorian, R.; Shidler, M.D.; Dangelo, K.; Couch, S.C.; Benoit, S.C.; Clegg, D.J. Dietary ketosis enhances memory in mild cognitive impairment. *Neurobiol. Aging* **2012**, *33*, e19–e27. [CrossRef]
316. Maalouf, M.; Rho, J.M. Oxidative impairment of hippocampal long-term potentiation involves activation of protein phosphatase 2A and is prevented by ketone bodies. *J. Neurosci. Res.* **2008**, *86*, 3322–3330. [CrossRef]
317. Rusek, M.; Pluta, R.; Ułamek-Kozioł, M.; Czuczwar, S.J. Ketogenic Diet in Alzheimer's disease. *Int. J. Mol. Sci.* **2019**, *20*, 3892. [CrossRef] [PubMed]
318. Chatterjee, P.; Fernando, M.; Fernando, B.; Dias, C.B.; Shah, T.; Silva, R.; Williams, S.; Pedrini, S.; Hillebrandt, H.; Goozee, K.; et al. Potential of coconut oil and medium chain triglycerides in the prevention and treatment of Alzheimer's disease. *Mech. Ageing Dev.* **2020**, *186*, 111209. [CrossRef]
319. Fernando, W.M.; Martins, I.J.; Goozee, K.G.; Brennan, C.S.; Jayasena, V.; Martins, R.N. The role of dietary coconut for the prevention and treatment of Alzheimer's disease: Potential mechanisms of action. *Br. J. Nutr.* **2015**, *114*, 1–14. [CrossRef] [PubMed]
320. Rebello, C.J.; Keller, J.N.; Liu, A.G.; Johnson, W.D.; Greenway, F.L. Pilot feasibility and safety study examining the effect of medium chain triglyceride supplementation in subjects with mild cognitive impairment: A randomized controlled trial. *BBA Clin.* **2015**, *3*, 123–125. [CrossRef]
321. Ota, M.; Matsuo, J.; Ishida, I.; Hattori, K.; Teraishi, T.; Tonouchi, H.; Ashida, K.; Takahashi, T.; Kunugi, H. Effect of a ketogenic meal on cognitive function in elderly adults: Potential for cognitive enhancement. *Psychopharmacology* **2016**, *233*, 3797–3802. [CrossRef]

322. Pan, Y.; Larson, B.; Araujo, J.A.; Lau, W.; de Rivera, C.; Santana, R.; Gore, A.; Milgram, N.W. Dietary supplementation with medium-chain TAG has long-lasting cognition-enhancing effects in aged dogs. *Br. J. Nutr.* **2010**, *103*, 1746–1754. [CrossRef] [PubMed]
323. Pawlosky, R.J.; Kashiwaya, Y.; King, M.T.; Veech, R.L. A Dietary Ketone Ester Normalizes Abnormal Behavior in a Mouse Model of Alzheimer's Disease. *Int. J. Mol. Sci.* **2020**, *21*, 1044. [CrossRef] [PubMed]
324. Alexander, G.E.; Chen, K.; Pietrini, P.; Rapoport, S.I.; Reiman, E.M. Longitudinal PET Evaluation of Cerebral Metabolic Decline in Dementia: A Potential Outcome Measure in Alzheimer's Disease Treatment Studies. *Am. J. Psychiatry* **2002**, *159*, 738–745. [CrossRef]
325. Reiman, E.M.; Chen, K.; Alexander, G.E.; Caselli, R.J.; Bandy, D.; Osborne, D.; Saunders, A.M.; Hardy, J. Functional brain abnormalities in young adults at genetic risk for late-onset Alzheimer's dementia. *Proc. Natl. Acad. Sci. USA* **2004**, *101*, 284–289. [CrossRef] [PubMed]
326. Henderson, S.T.; Vogel, J.L.; Barr, L.J.; Garvin, F.; Jones, J.J.; Costantini, L.C. Study of the ketogenic agent AC-1202 in mild to moderate Alzheimer's disease: A randomized, double-blind, placebo-controlled, multicenter trial. *Nutr. Metab.* **2009**, *6*, 31. [CrossRef]
327. Reger, M.A.; Henderson, S.T.; Hale, C.; Cholerton, B.; Baker, L.D.; Watson, G.S.; Hyde, K.; Chapman, D.; Craft, S. Effects of beta-hydroxybutyrate on cognition in memory-impaired adults. *Neurobiol. Aging* **2004**, *25*, 311–314. [CrossRef]
328. Kashiwaya, Y.; Takeshima, T.; Mori, N.; Nakashima, K.; Clarke, K.; Veech, R.L. D-beta-hydroxybutyrate protects neurons in models of Alzheimer's and Parkinson's disease. *Proc. Natl. Acad. Sci. USA* **2000**, *97*, 5440–5444. [CrossRef]
329. Yin, J.X.; Maalouf, M.; Han, P.; Zhao, M.; Gao, M.; Dharshaun, T.; Ryan, C.; Whitelegge, J.; Wu, J.; Eisenberg, D.; et al. Ketones block amyloid entry and improve cognition in an Alzheimer's model. *Neurobiol. Aging* **2016**, *39*, 25–37. [CrossRef]
330. Singer, T.P.; Ramsay, R.R.; McKeown, K.; Trevor, A.; Castagnoli, N.E., Jr. Mechanism of the neurotoxicity of 1-methyl-4-phenylpyridinium (MPP+), the toxic bioactivation product of 1-methyl-4-phenyl-1,2,3,6-tetrahydropyridine (MPTP). *Toxicology* **1988**, *49*, 17–23. [CrossRef]
331. Vanitallie, T.B.; Nonas, C.; Di Rocco, A.; Boyar, K.; Hyams, K.; Heymsfield, S.B. Treatment of Parkinson disease with diet-induced hyperketonemia: A feasibility study. *Neurology* **2005**, *64*, 728–730. [CrossRef]
332. Ari, C.; Poff, A.M.; Held, H.E.; Landon, C.S.; Goldhagen, C.R.; Mavromates, N.; D'Agostino, D.P. Metabolic therapy with Deanna Protocol supplementation delays disease progression and extends survival in amyotrophic lateral sclerosis (ALS) mouse model. *PLoS ONE* **2014**, *9*, e103526. [CrossRef]
333. Ari, C.; Murdun, C.; Goldhagen, C.; Koutnik, A.P.; Bharwani, S.R.; Diamond, D.M.; Kindy, M.; D'Agostino, D.P.; Kovacs, Z. Exogenous Ketone Supplements Improved Motor Performance in Preclinical Rodent Models. *Nutrients* **2020**, *12*, 2459. [CrossRef]
334. Netzahualcoyotzi, C.; Tapia, R. Degeneration of spinal motor neurons by chronic AMPA-induced excitotoxicity in vivo and protection by energy substrates. *Acta Neuropathol. Commun.* **2015**, *3*, 27. [CrossRef]
335. Zhao, Z.; Lange, D.J.; Voustianiouk, A.; MacGrogan, D.; Ho, L.; Suh, J.; Humala, N.; Thiyagarajan, M.; Wang, J.; Pasinetti, G.M. A ketogenic diet as a potential novel therapeutic intervention in amyotrophic lateral sclerosis. *BMC Neurosci.* **2006**, *7*, 29. [CrossRef]
336. Zhao, W.; Varghese, M.; Vempati, P.; Dzhun, A.; Cheng, A.; Wang, J.; Lange, D.; Bilski, A.; Faravelli, I.; Pasinetti, G.M. Caprylic triglyceride as a novel therapeutic approach to effectively improve the performance and attenuate the symptoms due to the motor neuron loss in ALS disease. *PLoS ONE* **2012**, *7*, e49191. [CrossRef] [PubMed]
337. Abg Abd Wahab, D.Y.; Gau, C.H.; Zakaria, R.; Muthu Karuppan, M.K.; A-Rahbi, B.S.; Abdullah, Z.; Alrafiah, A.; Abdullah, J.M.; Muthuraju, S. Review on Cross Talk between Neurotransmitters and Neuroinflammation in Striatum and Cerebellum in the Mediation of Motor Behaviour. *Biomed. Res. Int.* **2019**, *14*, 1767203. [CrossRef] [PubMed]
338. Blasco, H.; Mavel, S.; Corcia, P.; Gordon, P.H. The glutamate hypothesis in ALS: Pathophysiology and drug development. *Curr. Med. Chem.* **2014**, *21*, 3551–3575. [CrossRef]
339. Brichta, L.; Greengard, P.; Flajolet, M. Advances in the pharmacological treatment of Parkinson's disease: Targeting neurotransmitter systems. *Trends Neurosci.* **2013**, *36*, 543–554. [CrossRef]
340. Tisch, S.; Silberstein, P.; Limousin-Dowsey, P.; Jahanshahi, M. The basal ganglia: Anatomy, physiology, and pharmacology. *Psychiatr. Clin.* **2004**, *27*, 757–799. [CrossRef]
341. D'Amelio, M.; Puglisi-Allegra, S.; Mercuri, N. The role of dopaminergic midbrain in Alzheimer's disease: Translating basic science into clinical practice. *Pharmacol. Res.* **2018**, *130*, 414–419. [CrossRef]
342. Huang, D.; Liu, D.; Yin, J.; Qian, T.; Shrestha, S.; Ni, H. Glutamate-glutamine and GABA in brain of normal aged and patients with cognitive impairment. *Eur. Radiol.* **2017**, *27*, 2698–2705. [CrossRef]
343. Stanciu, G.D.; Luca, A.; Rusu, R.N.; Bild, V.; Beschea Chiriac, S.I.; Solcan, C.; Bild, W.; Ababei, D.C. Alzheimer's Disease Pharmacotherapy in Relation to Cholinergic System Involvement. *Biomolecules* **2019**, *10*, 40. [CrossRef]
344. Ma, S.; Hangya, B.; Leonard, C.S.; Wisden, W.; Gundlach, A.L. Dual-transmitter systems regulating arousal, attention, learning and memory. *Neurosci. Biobehav. Rev.* **2018**, *85*, 21–33. [CrossRef]
345. Choong, C.J.; Sasaki, T.; Hayakawa, H.; Yasuda, T.; Baba, K.; Hirata, Y.; Uesato, S.; Mochizuki, H. A novel histone deacetylase 1 and 2 isoform-specific inhibitor alleviates experimental Parkinson's disease. *Neurobiol. Aging* **2016**, *37*, 103–116. [CrossRef]
346. D'Mello, S.R. Histone deacetylases as targets for the treatment of human neurodegenerative diseases. *Drug News Perspect.* **2009**, *22*, 513–524. [CrossRef]

347. Feng, H.L.; Leng, Y.; Ma, C.H.; Zhang, J.; Ren, M.; Chuang, D.M. Combined lithium and valproate treatment delays disease onset, reduces neurological deficits and prolongs survival in an amyotrophic lateral sclerosis mouse model. *Neuroscience* **2008**, *155*, 567–572. [CrossRef]
348. Lu, X.; Wang, L.; Yu, C.; Yu, D.; Yu, G. Histone Acetylation Modifiers in the Pathogenesis of Alzheimer's Disease. *Front. Cell. Neurosci.* **2015**, *9*, 226. [CrossRef] [PubMed]
349. Chuang, D.M.; Leng, Y.; Marinova, Z.; Kim, H.J.; Chiu, C.T. Multiple roles of HDAC inhibition in neurodegenerative conditions. *Trends Neurosci.* **2009**, *32*, 591–601. [CrossRef]
350. Kazantsev, A.G.; Thompson, L.M. Therapeutic application of histone deacetylase inhibitors for central nervous system disorders. *Nat. Rev. Drug Discov.* **2008**, *7*, 854–868. [CrossRef] [PubMed]
351. Peleg, S.; Sananbenesi, F.; Zovoilis, A.; Burkhardt, S.; Bahari-Javan, S.; Agis-Balboa, R.C.; Cota, P.; Wittnam, J.L.; Gogol-Doering, A.; Opitz, L.; et al. Altered histone acetylation is associated with age-dependent memory impairment in mice. *Science* **2010**, *328*, 753–756. [CrossRef] [PubMed]
352. Sharma, S.; Taliyan, R.; Ramagiri, S. Histone deacetylase inhibitor, trichostatin A, improves learning and memory in high-fat diet-induced cognitive deficits in mice. *J. Mol. Neurosci.* **2015**, *56*, 1–11. [CrossRef]
353. Peng, S.; Wuu, J.; Mufson, E.J.; Fahnestock, M. Precursor form of brain-derived neurotrophic factor and mature brain-derived neurotrophic factor are decreased in the pre-clinical stages of Alzheimer's disease. *J. Neurochem.* **2005**, *93*, 1412–1421. [CrossRef] [PubMed]
354. Qin, X.Y.; Cao, C.; Cawley, N.X.; Liu, T.T.; Yuan, J.; Loh, Y.P.; Cheng, Y. Decreased peripheral brain-derived neurotrophic factor levels in Alzheimer's disease: A meta-analysis study (N = 7277). *Mol. Psychiatry* **2017**, *22*, 312–320. [CrossRef]
355. Valenzuela, P.L.; Castillo-García, A.; Morales, J.S.; de la Villa, P.; Hampel, H.; Emanuele, E.; Lista, S.; Lucia, A. Exercise benefits on Alzheimer's disease: State-of-the-science. *Ageing Res. Rev.* **2020**, *62*, 101108. [CrossRef]
356. Glass, C.K.; Saijo, K.; Winner, B.; Marchetto, M.C.; Gage, F.H. Mechanisms underlying inflammation in neurodegeneration. *Cell* **2010**, *140*, 918–934. [CrossRef]
357. Swanton, T.; Cook, J.; Beswick, J.A.; Freeman, S.; Lawrence, C.B.; Brough, D. Is Targeting the Inflammasome a Way Forward for Neuroscience Drug Discovery? *SLAS Discov.* **2018**, *23*, 991–1017. [CrossRef]
358. Hyun, D.H.; Lee, M.; Halliwell, B.; Jenner, P. Proteasomal inhibition causes the formation of protein aggregates containing a wide range of proteins, including nitrated proteins. *J. Neurochem.* **2003**, *86*, 363–373. [CrossRef]
359. Lim, J.E.; Song, M.; Jin, J.; Kou, J.; Pattanayak, A.; Lalonde, R.; Fukuchi, K. The effects of MyD88 deficiency on exploratory activity, anxiety, motor coordination, and spatial learning in C57BL/6 and APPswe/PS1dE9 mice. *Behav. Brain Res.* **2012**, *227*, 36–42. [CrossRef]
360. Liu, X.; Wu, Z.; Hayashi, Y.; Nakanishi, H. Age-dependent neuroinflammatory responses and deficits in long-term potentiation in the hippocampus during systemic inflammation. *Neuroscience* **2012**, *216*, 133–142. [CrossRef] [PubMed]
361. Kim, D.Y.; Hao, J.; Liu, R.; Turner, G.; Shi, F.D.; Rho, J.M. Inflammation-mediated memory dysfunction and effects of a ketogenic diet in a murine model of multiple sclerosis. *PLoS ONE* **2012**, *7*, e35476. [CrossRef] [PubMed]
362. Pallàs, M.; Pizarro, J.G.; Gutierrez-Cuesta, J.; Crespo-Biel, N.; Alvira, D.; Tajes, M.; Yeste-Velasco, M.; Folch, J.; Canudas, A.M.; Sureda, F.X.; et al. Modulation of SIRT1 expression in different neurodegenerative models and human pathologies. *Neuroscience* **2008**, *154*, 1388–1397. [CrossRef]
363. Herskovits, A.Z.; Guarente, L. SIRT1 in neurodevelopment and brain senescence. *Neuron* **2014**, *81*, 471–483. [CrossRef]
364. Corpas, R.; Revilla, S.; Ursulet, S.; Castro-Freire, M.; Kaliman, P.; Petegnief, V.; Giménez-Llort, L.; Sarkis, C.; Pallàs, M.; Sanfeliu, C. SIRT1 Overexpression in Mouse Hippocampus Induces Cognitive Enhancement through Proteostatic and Neurotrophic Mechanisms. *Mol. Neurobiol.* **2017**, *54*, 5604–5619. [CrossRef]
365. Wang, R.; Zhang, Y.; Li, J.; Zhang, C. Resveratrol ameliorates spatial learning memory impairment induced by $A\beta_{1-42}$ in rats. *Neuroscience* **2017**, *344*, 39–47. [CrossRef]
366. Gao, J.; Wang, W.Y.; Mao, Y.W.; Gräff, J.; Guan, J.S.; Pan, L.; Mak, G.; Kim, D.; Su, S.C.; Tsai, L.H. A novel pathway regulates memory and plasticity via SIRT1 and miR-134. *Nature* **2010**, *466*, 1105–1109. [CrossRef]
367. Michán, S.; Li, Y.; Chou, M.M.; Parrella, E.; Ge, H.; Long, J.M.; Allard, J.S.; Lewis, K.; Miller, M.; Xu, W.; et al. SIRT1 is essential for normal cognitive function and synaptic plasticity. *J. Neurosci.* **2010**, *30*, 9695–9707. [CrossRef] [PubMed]
368. Han, S.; Choi, J.R.; Soon Shin, K.; Kang, S.J. Resveratrol upregulated heat shock proteins and extended the survival of G93A-SOD1 mice. *Brain Res.* **2012**, *1483*, 112–117. [CrossRef] [PubMed]
369. Wang, J.; Zhang, Y.; Tang, L.; Zhang, N.; Fan, D. Protective effects of resveratrol through the up-regulation of SIRT1 expression in the mutant hSOD1-G93A-bearing motor neuron-like cell culture model of amyotrophic lateral sclerosis. *Neurosci. Lett.* **2011**, *503*, 250–255. [CrossRef] [PubMed]
370. Mudò, G.; Mäkelä, J.; Di Liberto, V.; Tselykh, T.V.; Olivieri, M.; Piepponen, P.; Eriksson, O.; Mälkiä, A.; Bonomo, A.; Kairisalo, M.; et al. Transgenic expression and activation of PGC-1α protect dopaminergic neurons in the MPTP mouse model of Parkinson's disease. *Cell. Mol. Life Sci.* **2012**, *69*, 1153–1165. [CrossRef]
371. Karuppagounder, S.S.; Pinto, J.T.; Xu, H.; Chen, H.L.; Beal, M.F.; Gibson, G.E. Dietary supplementation with resveratrol reduces plaque pathology in a transgenic model of Alzheimer's disease. *Neurochem. Int.* **2009**, *54*, 111–118. [CrossRef]

372. St-Pierre, J.; Drori, S.; Uldry, M.; Silvaggi, J.M.; Rhee, J.; Jäger, S.; Handschin, C.; Zheng, K.; Lin, J.; Yang, W.; et al. Suppression of reactive oxygen species and neurodegeneration by the PGC-1 transcriptional coactivators. *Cell* **2006**, *127*, 397–408. [CrossRef] [PubMed]
373. Lin, J.; Wu, P.H.; Tarr, P.T.; Lindenberg, K.S.; St-Pierre, J.; Zhang, C.Y.; Mootha, V.K.; Jäger, S.; Vianna, C.R.; Reznick, R.M.; et al. Defects in adaptive energy metabolism with CNS-linked hyperactivity in PGC-1alpha null mice. *Cell* **2004**, *119*, 121–135. [CrossRef]
374. Wareski, P.; Vaarmann, A.; Choubey, V.; Safiulina, D.; Liiv, J.; Kuum, M.; Kaasik, A. PGC-1{alpha} and PGC-1{beta} regulate mitochondrial density in neurons. *J. Biol. Chem.* **2009**, *284*, 21379–21385. [CrossRef]
375. Zheng, B.; Liao, Z.; Locascio, J.J.; Lesniak, K.A.; Roderick, S.S.; Watt, M.L.; Eklund, A.C.; Zhang-James, Y.; Kim, P.D.; Hauser, M.A.; et al. PGC-1α, a potential therapeutic target for early intervention in Parkinson's disease. *Sci. Transl. Med.* **2010**, *2*, 52ra73. [CrossRef]
376. Gong, B.; Chen, F.; Pan, Y.; Arrieta-Cruz, I.; Yoshida, Y.; Haroutunian, V.; Pasinetti, G.M. SCFFbx2-E3-ligase-mediated degradation of BACE1 attenuates Alzheimer's disease amyloidosis and improves synaptic function. *Aging Cell* **2010**, *9*, 1018–1031. [CrossRef] [PubMed]
377. Kiaei, M.; Kipiani, K.; Chen, J.; Calingasan, N.Y.; Beal, M.F. Peroxisome proliferator-activated receptor-gamma agonist extends survival in transgenic mouse model of amyotrophic lateral sclerosis. *Exp. Neurol.* **2005**, *191*, 331–336. [CrossRef] [PubMed]
378. Zhao, W.; Varghese, M.; Yemul, S.; Pan, Y.; Cheng, A.; Marano, P.; Hassan, S.; Vempati, P.; Chen, F.; Qian, X.; et al. Peroxisome proliferator activator receptor gamma coactivator-1alpha (PGC-1α) improves motor performance and survival in a mouse model of amyotrophic lateral sclerosis. *Mol. Neurodegener.* **2011**, *6*, 51. [CrossRef] [PubMed]
379. Agarwal, S.; Yadav, A.; Chaturvedi, R.K. Peroxisome proliferator-activated receptors (PPARs) as therapeutic target in neurodegenerative disorders. *Biochem. Biophys. Res. Commun.* **2017**, *483*, 1166–1177. [CrossRef] [PubMed]
380. D'ANGELO, M.; Castelli, V.; Catanesi, M.; Antonosante, A.; Dominguez-Benot, R.; Ippoliti, R.; Benedetti, E.; Cimini, A. PPARγ and Cognitive Performance. *Int. J. Mol. Sci.* **2019**, *20*, 5068. [CrossRef] [PubMed]
381. Im, J.Y.; Lee, K.W.; Woo, J.M.; Junn, E.; Mouradian, M.M. DJ-1 induces thioredoxin 1 expression through the Nrf2 pathway. *Hum. Mol. Genet.* **2012**, *21*, 3013–3024. [CrossRef] [PubMed]
382. Kensler, T.W.; Wakabayashi, N.; Biswal, S. Cell survival responses to environmental stresses via the Keap1-Nrf2-ARE pathway. *Annu. Rev. Pharmacol. Toxicol.* **2007**, *47*, 89–116. [CrossRef]
383. Kincaid, B.; Bossy-Wetzel, E. Forever young: SIRT3 a shield against mitochondrial meltdown, aging, and neurodegeneration. *Front. Aging Neurosci.* **2013**, *5*, 48. [CrossRef] [PubMed]
384. Ramesh, S.; Govindarajulu, M.; Lynd, T.; Briggs, G.; Adamek, D.; Jones, E.; Heiner, J.; Majrashi, M.; Moore, T.; Amin, R.; et al. SIRT3 activator Honokiol attenuates β-Amyloid by modulating amyloidogenic pathway. *PLoS ONE* **2018**, *13*, e0190350. [CrossRef]
385. Song, W.; Song, Y.; Kincaid, B.; Bossy, B.; Bossy-Wetzel, E. Mutant SOD1G93A triggers mitochondrial fragmentation in spinal cord motor neurons: Neuroprotection by SIRT3 and PGC-1α. *Neurobiol. Dis.* **2013**, *51*, 72–81. [CrossRef] [PubMed]

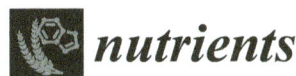

Article

Cognitive Outcomes and Relationships with Phenylalanine in Phenylketonuria: A Comparison between Italian and English Adult Samples

Cristina Romani [1,*], Filippo Manti [2], Francesca Nardecchia [2], Federica Valentini [3], Nicoletta Fallarino [3], Claudia Carducci [4], Sabrina De Leo [5], Anita MacDonald [6], Liana Palermo [7] and Vincenzo Leuzzi [2]

1. School of Life and Health Sciences, Aston University, Birmingham B4 7ET, UK
2. Department of Human Neuroscience—Unit of Child Neurology and Psychiatry, Sapienza University of Rome, 00185 Rome, Italy; filippo.manti@uniroma1.it (F.M.); francesca.nardecchia@uniroma1.it (F.N.); vincenzo.leuzzi@uniroma1.it (V.L.)
3. Department of Psychology, Sapienza University of Rome, 00185 Rome, Italy; valentini.fe@gmail.com (F.V.); fallarino.1707273@studenti.uniroma1.it (N.F.)
4. Department of Experimental Medicine, Sapienza University of Rome, 00185 Rome, Italy; claudia.carducci@uniroma1.it
5. Department of Clinical Medicine, Policlinico Umberto I, 00161 Rome, Italy; sabrina.deleo@libero.it
6. Birmingham Women's and Children's NHS Trust, Birmingham B15 2TG, UK; Anita.Macdonald@nhs.net
7. Department of Medical and Surgical Sciences, Magna Graecia University of Catanzaro, 88100 Catanzaro, Italy; liana.palermo@unicz.it
* Correspondence: C.Romani@Aston.ac.uk; Tel.: +44-(0)121-204-4081

Received: 26 August 2020; Accepted: 24 September 2020; Published: 3 October 2020

Abstract: We aimed to assess if the same cognitive batteries can be used cross-nationally to monitor the effect of Phenylketonuria (PKU). We assessed whether a battery, previously used with English adults with PKU (AwPKU), was also sensitive to impairments in Italian AwPKU. From our original battery, we selected a number of tasks that comprehensively assessed visual attention, visuo-motor coordination, executive functions (particularly, reasoning, planning, and monitoring), sustained attention, and verbal and visual memory and learning. When verbal stimuli/or responses were involved, stimuli were closely matched between the two languages for psycholinguistic variables. We administered the tasks to 19 Italian AwPKU and 19 Italian matched controls and compared results from with 19 English AwPKU and 19 English matched controls selected from a previously tested cohort. Participant election was blind to cognitive performance and metabolic control, but participants were closely matched for age and education. The Italian AwPKU group had slightly worse metabolic control but showed levels of performance and patterns of impairment similar to the English AwPKU group. The Italian results also showed extensive correlations between adult cognitive measures and metabolic measures across the life span, both in terms of Phenylalanine (Phe) levels and Phe fluctuations, replicating previous results in English. These results suggest that batteries with the same and/or matched tasks can be used to assess cognitive outcomes across countries allowing results to be compared and accrued. Future studies should explore potential differences in metabolic control across countries to understand what variables make metabolic control easier to achieve.

Keywords: PKU; cognitive outcomes; cross-cultural; cross-countries; Phe associations

1. Introduction

Phenylketonuria (PKU) is an inherited metabolic disease occurring in about 1/10,000 live births where an error in the gene coding for the enzyme phenylalanine hydroxylase (PAH) produces an inability to metabolize the amino acid phenylalanine (Phe) into tyrosine with serious consequences for brain health [1]. Tremendous advances have been made in our understanding and treatment of this disorder from the 1930s when it was first discovered by a Norwegian physician, Asbjørn Følling, who noticed high levels of phenylpyruvic acid in the urine of some patients with severe mental disability and established connections with high levels of Phe in the blood. Since the wide-spread introduction of new-born screening in the late seventies in most countries, infants with PKU follow a Phe-restricted diet which lowers blood Phe levels and eliminates mental disability. It is now recommended that a PKU diet is followed throughout life. Current European guidelines recommend Phe to be kept within the target range of 120–360 µmol/L till 12 years of age and within 120–600 µmol/L, above 12 years [2,3]. American guidelines recommend a target range of 120–360 µmol/L throughout life (American College of Medical Genetics and Genomics, ACMG) [4]. In classical PKU, without treatment, Phe could exceed >2000 µmol/L.

Maintaining a Phe-restricted diet allows people with PKU to lead normal lives. However, not all is well. The PKU diet is expensive, unpalatable, and unsociable. Thus, it is often self-relaxed in late childhood and abandoned during late adolescence [5–9]. Possibly because Phe levels remain suboptimal, on average, people with PKU do not reach their full cognitive potentials [7]. IQ is in the normal range, but lower than matched controls [10], and there are impairments in cognitive tasks, especially when speed of processing and higher cognitive functions are involved [11–16]. Moreover, this is the first generation of early treated adults with PKU (from now on AwPKU) to reach middle-age and we do not know the effects of prolonged high levels of Phe on aging brains.

Better management of PKU may be achieved with the wider use of existing pharmacological treatments [3,17,18] and the introduction of new ones [19–21], but it also depends on a better understanding of how the cognitive impairments experienced by this population relate to levels and variations in Phe levels across the life span. While Phe may be particularly toxic for developing brains, we need evidence of the safety of accumulating high Phe levels on aging brains. Finally, it is important to understand whether some individuals are less affected by high Phe since there is some evidence of individual variation [6,22–24]. For a few people with PKU, it may be less important to keep on a strict diet.

Establishing the efficacy of new treatments and the safety of existing ones relies on the comprehensive cognitive assessments of large samples of people with PKU and relative controls. Ideally, cognition should be tested across the board because the effects of Phe may vary for different cognitive functions. Moreover, it is important to use multiple measures to increase reliability since tasks do not tap cognitive function in a simple, univocal way. However, this is time-consuming and recruiting participants is challenging since PKU is a rare disease. These difficulties, compounded by resource limitations, mean that it is difficult for studies based on single clinical centres to achieve the desired breadth and depth of testing with enough power [15,16,25] making the ability to collate results across national and international centres particularly important. However, there is a lack of studies comparing results across national samples.

Similar negative effects of PKU on cognition have already been reported across countries (for example, deficits in executive functions have been reported in: Italy: Nardecchia et al. [26]; the Netherlands: Jahja et al. [27]; the UK: Palermo et al. [15]; the USA: Brumm et al. [25]; Christ, et al. [28]; Diamond et al. [2]; deficits of speed of processing have been reported in Australia: Moyle et al. [10]; Germany: Feldmann et al. [29]; the UK: Channon et al. [30]; Palermo et al. [15]; the USA: Janos et al. [31]). These results suggest that the effects of Phe on cognition are similar across countries, in spite of cultural and environmental differences in the approach to food and feeding. However, there is a lack of studies directly comparing results collected using the same tests and direct comparisons are important to give us confidence that results can be accrued.

The objectives of the present study are twofold: 1. we aim to replicate results previously obtained with a relatively large sample of English AwPKU ($N = 37$) [5,6,15,32] by administering a subset of tasks to a new sample of Italian patients; 2. we aim to demonstrate that the same tasks which are sensitive to blood Phe in English are also sensitive in Italian so that they also demonstrate impairments and relationships with blood Phe levels and Phe fluctuations throughout the lifespan. A comparison between English and Italian PKU samples is particularly relevant given differences in the approach to food and diet in the two countries. Note that there is no issue of validity and specificity in the cognitive assessment of PKU. We do not need to distinguish people with PKU from healthy people. Genetic tests reliably establish the presence/absence of PKU from birth and high-level of Phe are constant in people of PKU if the disease is untreated. What is important, instead, is test-sensitivity to variations in metabolic control so that cognitive outcomes can be properly monitored. This can be demonstrated by showing impairment compared to healthy controls and correlations with metabolic measures.

We assessed metabolic control and cognitive outcomes in 19 Italian early-treated AwPKU and 19 matched controls and compared performance with that of 19 English early-treated AwPKU and relative controls selected from our previously tested cohort [15]. All groups were matched for age and education. Comparisons between PKU groups were in terms of z scores which considered performance in terms of deviations from the relative control groups. In addition, we assessed the sensitivity of our cognitive battery in Italian by assessing correlations with current and historical blood Phe levels. The Italian and English testing batteries were matched as rigorously as possible. In most cases, our tests were exactly the same (the same materials and procedure); those with verbal stimuli were carefully matched for psycholinguistic variables such as word frequency and word length (e.g., Rey AVLT). Similar levels of impairments and similar correlations with Phe levels will demonstrate test reliability and sensitivity for different national PKU samples. It will also give us confidence that, when the same or matched tasks are used, results can be accrued, allowing more power for analyses.

2. Method

2.1. Participants

All PKU participants were adults diagnosed soon after birth (2–3 days in Italy and 5–7 days in the UK).

Nineteen Italian AwPKU were recruited from the Clinical Centre for Neurometabolic Diseases in the Department of Human Neuroscience, Child Neurology and Psychiatry Unit at the Sapienza University of Rome. Three participants were currently treated with sapropterin. Nineteen Italian control participants were recruited among students and friends of the researchers. They were matched to the Italian PKU participants for age and education. Among the Italian participants, 4 had a diagnostic blood Phe level > 600 µmol/L but <1200 µmol/L; 15 participants had Phe > 1200 µmol/L at birth.

To allow a direct comparison between an Italian and an English sample, 19 English AwPKU were selected from a larger sample of 37 AwPKU previously tested [15,16,32]. They were all tested at the Inherited Metabolic Disease Unit at the Queen Elizabeth Hospital in Birmingham. They all had Phe > 1200 µmol/L at birth. They were matched one-to-one with the Italian AwPKU for gender, age, and education. Matching was blind to cognitive performance and metabolic control as possible differences were assessed. Thirty English healthy controls were originally recruited through an advertising volunteering website. From this sample, we blindly selected 19 healthy controls matching the English PKU participants for age and education (in number of years).

Power calculations indicated that 20 participants were necessary in the clinical group and 20 participants in the control group for a one tail effect size of 0.8 (consistent with what we found in our previous studies) and =0.05, power (1-error probability) = 0.80. All AwPKU treated in the English and Italian centres were invited to participate and were accepted in the study on a first-come, first-served basis. Recruitment stopped when enough participants were tested. After the Italian PKU participants were contacted, one participant became unavailable and we were left with 19 participants, which still gave our study acceptable power (=0.78).

The English study received NHS ethical approval. The Italian study was approved by the local ethics committee. All participants provided informed consent to the study.

2.2. Ethical Approval

The study was conducted in accordance with the Declaration of Helsinki. All participants gave their informed consent for inclusion before they participated in the study. In the UK, the protocol was approved by the West Midlands NHS Ethics Committee (rec REC: 10/H1207/115). In Italy the protocol was approved by the Institutional Review Board of "Sapienza"—University of Rome (Project identification code 3629).

2.3. Metabolic Measures

For both the English and the Italian participants, metabolic measures were taken regularly since birth and extensive records were available. The number of measures did not differ between countries (see Table 1). Blood Phe monitoring was performed on dry blood spot collected after overnight fasting by High Performance Liquid Chromatography until 2010 and then via tandem mass spectroscopy. The laboratories of both centres have adhered and contributed to international quality control systems

Table 1. Demographic Variables in Terms of Age, Gender, Years of Education and Metabolic Control across Ages for the Two Matched Groups of Italian and English AwPKU. Blood Phe measured in μmol/L.

	Italian AwPKU		English AwPKU		English vs. Italian
	N = 19		N = 19		p Value
	Mean	SD	Mean	SD	
Age	25.4 (range: 19–33)	4.1	25.3 (range: 18–36)	6.1	n.s.
Education (in years)	14	1.8	14.6	1.9	n.s.
Gender (M/F)	8//11		8//11		
Verbal IQ	98.8	12.9	100.4	8.9	n.s.
Performance IQ	99.3	15	103.3	12.9	n.s.
Full IQ	98.9	14.5	102.1	10.4	n.s.
Childhood (0–10 years)					
Phe Average Median	499	149	386	168	$p = 0.04$
Phe Fluctuation	227	63	198	50	n.s.
Mean N observations per participant	208	79	259	156	n.s.
Adolescence (11–16 years)					
Phe Average Median	702	194	612	293	n.s.
Phe Fluctuation	170	51	165	34	n.s.
Mean N obs. per participant	77	54	98	74	n.s.
Adulthood (17 years +)					
Phe Average Median	970	239	733	344	$p = 0.02$
Phe Variation	217	65	122	41	$p < 0.001$
Mean N obs. per participant	58	49	62	58	n.s.
Lifetime					
Phe Average Median	695	198	516	233	$p = 0.02$
Phe Fluctuation (SD)	208	46	171	33	$p < 0.01$
Mean N observations. per participant	344	149	419	232	n.s.
Current Phe	1042	428	677	382	$p = 0.01$
Range	454–2081		65–1465		

AwPKU: adults with PKU, IQ: intelligence quotient, n.s.: not significant, Phe: Phenylalanine.

We averaged metabolic control in three age bands: childhood: 0–10 years old, adolescence: 11–16 years old, and adulthood: 17 years to present. We have also averaged measures throughout the life-time and considered current Phe levels. For the Italian group, current Phe has been measured immediately before the testing session/s or in the preceding few days; for the UK group, current Phe has been measured immediately before the two testing sessions and averaged. We considered two types of measures: Phe level and Phe fluctuation/variation (we will use the term fluctuation from now). Phe level in each band was calculated by taking the median values for each year and then averaging the year values; Phe fluctuation was calculated by taking the SD for each year and then averaging year values in the band.

2.4. Cognitive Assessment

Cognitive assessments were carried out in a quiet room at the clinical centres in Birmingham and Rome. The testing session for the Italian participants lasted between 2 and 3 h. The English participants carried out more tests and were tested in two separate sessions of similar length. Testing was carried out by a psychologist or a neuropsychiatrist with neuropsychological training.

IQ was measured, for the Italian participants, using the Wechsler Adult Intelligence Scale-Revised (WAIS-R) [33] and, for the English participants, the Wechsler abbreviated scale of intelligence (WASI) [34], which includes the following subtests: Vocabulary, Block Design, Similarities, and Matrix Reasoning. The WAIS-R and the WASI are strongly correlated providing similar validated measures of Full Scale IQ [35]. In addition, participants were given a set of tasks chosen from the larger set of tasks administered in our previous studies [15,16]. We chose tests which either showed a strong difference between PKU participants and controls and/or strong correlations with metabolic measures. We also prioritized tasks with non-linguistic stimuli which did not need adapting across languages. Therefore, we did not include tests of picture naming, reading, spelling, and orthographic knowledge (spoonerisms, phoneme deletions) where speed impairments could be due to a general reduction in speed of processing which was also tapped by visual search. In addition, we did not include tasks where relationship with metabolic measures are modest or absent [5]. Finally, to reduce the number of tasks tapping similar functions, we also did not administer the Tower of Hanoi, lexical learning task, the Stroop, and nonword repetition. Measures of short-term memory (digit span and Corsi span) and a baseline measure of peripheral speed of processing were included for completeness and to confirm or disprove impairments, given mixed results from the literature (for impairments in digit span and nonword repetition see Palermo et al. [15]; for contrasting results see Brumm et al. [25], and Moyle et al. [10]; see also Jahja et al. [27] for deficits with increasing working memory load).

The following cognitive areas were assessed:

2.4.1. Visual Attention

This was assessed with four tasks [15,16]: 1. Simple Detection: Press a response button as soon as a ladybird appears on the screen; 2. Detection with Distractors: Press a button whenever a ladybird appears on the screen alone or with a green bug, in the second part of the task the instruction was changed to press a button whenever a green bug appeared on the screen alone or with a ladybird; 3. Feature Search: Detect a target among distractors not sharing features by pressing a "yes" or "no" button (e.g., a red ladybird among green bugs); 4. Conjunction Search: Detect a target among distractors sharing features (e.g., red ladybird among red bugs and green bugs). Both reaction times (RT from now on) and accuracy measures (error rates) were taken.

2.4.2. Visuo-Motor Coordination

This was assessed with two tasks: 1. Grooved Pegboard Test [36]: Put pegs into the holes of a board using only one hand as quickly as possible (short version with two trials one with the dominant and one with the non-dominant hand for the Italian and English matched samples) and 2. Digit Symbol Task [33]: Fill as many boxes as possible with symbols corresponding to numbers (key with associations remains visible) in 90 s. Trail Making Test A (TMT A) [37,38]: connect circles containing numbers in ascending order of the numbers as quickly as possible.

2.4.3. Complex Executive Functions

This was assessed with four tasks tapping skills such as planning, flexibility, and abstract thinking: 1. The Wisconsin Card Sorting Test (WCST) 64 card version [39]: Discover the rules to match cards from a deck with four reference cards according to the shape, number or colour of the symbols on the card; feedback is provided to allow learning. Flexibility is required when the sorting rule is changed unknown to the participant and the new rule must be discovered. We used three different scores: total errors, number of perseverative responses and number of completed categories. 2. Difference in speed between Trail Making Test B-A (TMT B-A) [37,38]. A involves connecting circles containing numbers in ascending order; B also involves connecting circles in ascending order but alternating between the number and letters contained in the circles. Only time is considered in this test; when occasionally an error is made, it is corrected by the examiner and this affects the time to complete the task. 3 Fluency: For letter fluency: generate as many words as possible starting with a given letter in a minute of time (for Italian: P, F and L; Novelli et al. [40] for English: C, F and L; Benton et al. [41]); for semantic fluency [42,43]: generate as many names of animals as possible in 1 min of time. This requires planning an efficient search through the lexicon.

2.4.4. Short-term Memory/Working Memory

This was assessed with two tasks: 1. Digit Span: Repeat a sequence of digits spoken by the examiner soon after presentation; 2. Corsi Block Tapping Test [44]: The examiner taps a sequence of blocks and the participant must reproduce the sequence in the same order. Span was calculated as the longest sequence which could be repeated correctly (1 point was awarded for each length if all trials are correct; otherwise a corresponding fraction of point was awarded; for digit span where sequences started from length four, sequences of length 1–3 were assumed all correct, unless there were errors with sequences of four digits; in this case, sequences of shorter length were presented).

2.4.5. Sustained Attention

This was assessed with the Rapid Visual Information Processing task (RVP) [45]: detect three target sequences of three digits by pressing the response key when the last number of the sequence appears on the screen. Scores are percentage correct.

2.4.6. Verbal Memory and Learning

This was assessed with The Rey Auditory Verbal Learning Test [46,47] which asks for learning, immediate recall, and delayed recall of a list of 15 words. The list is presented five times and participants are asked to recall the words immediately after each presentation. After the 5th presentation (A5), an interfering list (B1) is presented and participants are asked to recall this list and then, once again, the original list (A6) without a further presentation. Finally, participants are asked to recall the original list after a 20-min filled interval. Our scores include total number of errors across the five learning trials (A1-5); errors in recalling the words after an interfering list (A6); and, again, errors in delayed recall of the original list.

2.4.7. Visual Memory and Learning

This was assessed with the Paired Associates Visual Learning [48]: Learn to associate objects with locations. Z scores for each participant for each task were computed using the relevant control group as a reference point. As well as considering performance in individual tasks, for each participant, we computed two indexes of overall cognitive performance: 1. We averaged z scores in all tasks and 2. We considered the rate of poor scores across all tasks (rate of Z scores => 1.5); this second index is important since an average Z score may mask significant areas of difficulties in a number of tasks (given a profile were some skills are good and others are impaired).

3. Data Analyses

We used two-tailed t-tests to compare the demographics and metabolic measures of the Italian and English AwPKU, as well as to compare the demographics and cognitive performance of each of these clinical groups with the corresponding control group. This allowed us to assess whether the Italian AwPKU demonstrated similar impairments to the English AwPKU [15]. Additionally, we computed Z scores for each PKU participant and each task, using the corresponding control group (subtracting each test value from the corresponding control mean and dividing by the control SD). Average Z scores for Italian and English AwPKU were analyzed using two-tailed t-tests to compare size of standardized effects. For this and all other analyses in the paper, we were more interested in comparing patterns across groups than in the significance of an individual measure. However, with the t-tests, we have indicated comparisons which remained significant after a Bonferroni correction.

To demonstrate that our battery is as sensitive to impairment in Italian as in English, we carried out Person r correlations between all our cognitive measures and measures of metabolic control, both current and historical. This resulted in a high overall number of correlations for each clinical group ($N = 144$). Individually, each correlation is not very reliable since correlations are notoriously unstable with a small N (19 participants). However, we were not interested in the significance of individual correlations, but, instead, in establishing the sensitive of our tasks to metabolic controls in Italian as in English, across measures. Considering patterns across a large number of cognitive tasks and metabolic measures will reduce error and boost power. We used a χ^2 s to assess the significance of a positive/negative correlations ratio against a chance 50/50 ratio, which is expected if no true relation exists between cognitive performance and metabolic control. In addition, we used a one-sample t-test to assess whether the average correlation was significantly different from 0 (see Romani et al., [6] for a similar methodology). We carried out these analyses on both Italian and English PKU samples.

4. Results

4.1. Demographics

Demographic and metabolic information for English and Italian PKU groups are shown in Table 1. The Italian and English groups were matched for age, education, and gender. They did not differ significantly for of any of these variables or for IQ. However, the average Phe level was higher in the Italian group, with differences reaching significance for all age bands but adolescence. In addition, Phe levels were more variable in the Italian than in the English group in adulthood and when measured throughout the lifetime.

4.2. Cognitive Performance

4.2.1. AwPKU vs. Controls

Table 2 shows the performance of the Italian and English PKU groups compared to matched samples of healthy controls. Results show that both Italian and English AwPKU were impaired in a similar range of tasks with good overlap with the English PKU group.

Both Italian and English AwPKU were impaired in IQ measures and showed a reduced speed in allocating visuo-spatial attention and good accuracy in visual search tasks. Both groups showed impairments in tasks tapping visuo-motor coordination (but for the Italian group differences reached significance only for the digit symbol test). The Italian group also showed impairments in the TMT b and a-b and in the fluency tasks and in the RVP task. Both groups showed no difference in the WCST. Finally, both groups performed well in verbal and visuo-spatial short-term memory tasks (digit span, Corsi Block tapping test) and in tasks tapping learning and memory with only a marginal impairment for the Italian AwPKU.

Table 2. Cognitive Performance of Italian and English PKU Participants and Healthy Controls Matched for Age and Educations to the Respective Clinical Groups.

| | ITALIAN PARTICIPANTS (N = 19 In Each Group) | | | | | ENGLISH PARTICIPANTS (N = 19 In Each Group) | | | | | |
| | AwPKU | | Controls | | Diff. | AwPKU | | Controls | | Diff. |
	Mean	SD	Mean	SD	p Value	Mean	SD	Mean	SD	p Value
Age	25.4	4.1	24.7	3.4	n.s.	25.3	6.1	24.4	5.35	n.s.
Education (in years)	14.0	1.8	13.9	1.7	n.s.	14.6	1.9	14.8	1.7	n.s.
Gender (M/F)	8/11		8/11			7/12		6/13		
VIQ	98.8	13	108.5	13.1	0.03	100.4	8.9	109.6	9.6	<0.001 #
PIQ	99.3	15	107.1	9.6	0.07	103.3	12.9	110.2	12.6	n.s.
FIQ	98.9	15	110.1	12.0	0.01	102.1	10.4	111.1	10.3	0.01
VISUAL ATTENTION										
Simple Detection (RT—ms)	325	46	315	44.6	n.s.	331	50.7	304.9	51.2	0.06
Detention with Distractors										
RT—ms	483	104	430	58	0.02	433	56.4	392	54.2	0.03
% errors	0.8	0.6	0.5	1.1	n.s.	0.8	0.8	0.5	0.6	n.s.
Feature Search										
RT—ms	752	262	586	113	0.02	581	111	492.3	70.5	0.01
% errors	1.6	4.7	0.6	1.2	n.s.	1.9	2.6	2.3	2.3	n.s.
Conjunction Search										
RT—ms	1152	237	938	203	<0.001 #	998	162	846	129.0	<0.001 #
% errors	3.2	4.7	2.8	4.7	n.s.	2	2.2	3.5	5.4	n.s.
VISUO-MOTOR COORDINATION										
Pegboard (Time-s)	76.7	11	70.6	9.0	0.06	71.9	9.9	66.0	6.1	0.03
Digit Symbol (%errors in 90 s)	41.6	12	39.4	9.1	<0.001 #	37.1	11.6	27.9	10.3	0.01
Trail-Making Test A (Time-s)	32.4	15	29.9	12.1	n.s.	24.0	7.0	20.2	3.7	0.04
EXECUTIVE FUNCTIONS										
WCST										

Table 2. *Cont.*

	ITALIAN PARTICIPANTS (N = 19 In Each Group)						ENGLISH PARTICIPANTS (N = 19 In Each Group)					
	AwPKU		Controls		Diff.		AwPKU		Controls		Diff.	
	Mean	SD	Mean	SD	*p* Value		Mean	SD	Mean	SD	*p* Value	
Total errors	13.6	6.9	13.6	5.3	n.s.		13.8	8.6	11.9	5.5	n.s.	
Perseverative responses	7.0	3.1	7.8	3.3	n.s.		7.9	5.1	7.5	5.3	n.s.	
N of Completed Categories	4.0	1.1	4.1	1.0	n.s.		3.9	1.2	4.3	0.9	n.s.	
Trail-Making Test												
B (sec)	79.8	34	54.4	19.7	0.01		42	10.8	43.2	16.0	n.s.	
B–A (sec)	47.5	29	24.4	13.1	<0.001 #		18	8.0	22.9	14.3	n.s.	
Verbal Fluency												
Letter (correct answers)	39.0	11	47.5	9.3	0.01		36.3	11.6	40.5	15.0	n.s.	
Semantic (correct answers)	20.1	4.8	23.5	3.6	0.02		21.6	5.8	25.1	5.0	0.06	
Rey Auditory Verbal Learning												
Retention after interference (% errors A6)	17.2	13	8.4	7.6	0.02		19.6	18.3	15.1	16.9	n.s.	
SUSTAINED ATTENTION												
RVP (% of errors)	24.2	12	15.9	9.6	0.03		16.8	9.5	13.2	9.4	n.s.	
SHORT-TERM MEMORY												
Digit span	5.9	0.9	5.9	1.1	n.s.		6.2	0.8	6.5	0.9	n.s.	
Corsi Block span	5.9	1.0	5.0	1.1	0.01 (opposite to expected)		5.3	0.8	5.6	0.9	n.s.	
MEMORY and LEARNING												
Rey Auditory Verbal Learning												
Trial A1–A5 (% errors)	20.8	8.8	19.7	6.1	n.s.		24.5	11.4	21.7	9.3	n.s.	
Delayed Recall (% errors)	10.2	11	4.9	7.0	0.08		18.6	18	14.7	14.8	n.s.	
Paired Associate Visual learning (% errors)	2.3	2.2	1.2	1.3	0.07		2.5	3	1.8	1.8	n.s.	

Italian and English PKU groups are also matched a-priori for age and education. Diff. = Difference. # = comparison which remains significant after Bonferroni correction. WCST: Wisconsin Card Sorting Test, RT: reaction Times, RVP: Rapid Visual Information Processing task, VIQ: verbal IQ, PIQ: performance IQ, FIQ: full IQ.

4.2.2. Italian AwPKU vs. English AwPKU

Table 3 compares standardized performance of Italian and English PKU groups. Despite their worse metabolic control, the Italian group performed significantly worse than the English PKU group in only a few tasks. They were worse on the TMT B and B-A and on letter-fluency, marginally worse on list recall after interference (retention A6), but better on the Corsi Block span. Overall, their performance was numerically worse in terms of average Z score, but this was not statistically significant. When we co-varied concurrent Phe, only the differences in trail making test B-A and Corsi span remained significant ($p = 0.009$ and $p < 0.001$); differences in Trail making B and letter fluency were only marginally significant ($p = 0.06$ and $p = 0.08$).

A detailed comparison of results in visual search tasks highlights the similarity of patterns in the Italian and English PKU groups. Figure 1 shows RTs in the different conditions. Errors were too few for analysis. Across groups, RTs in feature search do not increase with the number of distractors. This is because in this condition the target item "pops out" and a parallel search suffices for a correct answer (generating a flat profile). Instead, across groups, there is a steep increase in RTs with the number of distractors in conjunction search. This is consistent with the need to serially explore the distinct locations of the display in this condition. Moreover, all groups show slower RTs with "No" rather than "Yes" trials, especially in the conjunction search. This is also expected. To decide that an item is not present you need to check all locations in the display; instead to find a target item, only half of the locations need to be checked on average. The PKU groups show the same patterns of the controls, but they are slower in all conditions.

Trials (F (1, 36) = 43.9; $p < 0.001$; $\eta_p^2 = 0.550$). There were also a number of significant interactions: task x distracters (F (2, 72) = 77.7; $p < 0.001$; $\eta_p^2 = 0.683$), because responses were slower with more distracters in the conjunction search, but not in the feature search; distracters x trial (F (2, 72) = 16.0; $p < 0.001$; $\eta_p^2 = 0.307$) because the effect of the number of distracters was more marked in the "no" than the "yes" trials; task x trial (F (1, 36) = 64.8; $p < 0.001$; $\eta_p^2 = 0.643$) because slower responses in the "no" rather than the "yes" trials occurred in the conjunction search, but not in the feature search. Finally, there was a three-way interaction: task x distracters x trial (F (2, 72) = 12.6; $p < 0.001$; $\eta_p^2 = 0.259$) because responses were slower with the number of distracters more in the "no" than the "yes" trials, but only in the conjunction search. Crucially, however, there were no significant interactions within the group.

When PKU participants are compared to controls, differences are constant in all conditions, except in the conjoined task where the English PKU group shows increasing differences from controls with number of distractors: a fanning-out pattern (distracters x group: F (2, 72) = 3.8; $p = 0.03$; η_p^2). Instead, differences from controls always remained stable in the Italian group (F (2, 72) = 0.25; $p= 0.78$). We will comment on this difference in the General Discussion.

Finally, we want to highlight that, as reported for the English sample (Palermo et al., 2017), the variability in cognitive performance in Italian PKU participants is striking. Five PKU participants (26% of the sample) had a normal cognitive profile when compared to the control group (average Z score: −0.2; −0.7–0.1; % z score =>1.5: 5.0; 0–8.3; expected 6.7%; Full IQ = 114; 104–124). These participants had fast speed of processing while maintaining a good accuracy.

Table 3. Cognitive Performance of English and Italian PKU Groups in Term of Z Score Computed from Relative Control Groups Matched for Age, Gender, and Education.

DOMAIN/TASK	Italian AwPK Z Score		English AwPKU Z Score		Diff.
	Mean	SD	Mean	SD	p
IQ	1.0	1.0	0.9	1.0	n.s.
VISUO-SPATIAL ATTENTION RTs					
Simple Detection—ms	0.2	1.0	0.5	1.0	n.s.
Detention with Distractors—ms	1.3	2.1	0.8	1.0	n.s.
Feature Search—ms	1.5	2.3	1.3	1.6	n.s.
Conjunction Search ms	1.1	1.2	1.2	1.2	n.s.
VISUAL ATTENTION accuracy					
Detention with Distractors—% errors	0.2	0.6	0.5	1.3	n.s.
Feature Search—% errors	0.9	4.0	−0.2	1.1	n.s.
Conjunction Search—% errors	0.1	1.0	−0.3	0.4	n.s.
VISUO-MOTOR COORDINATION					
Pegboard—s	0.7	1.2	1.0	1.6	n.s.
Digit Symbol—% errors in 90 s	0.2	1.3	0.9	1.1	n.s.
Trail-Making Test A—s	0.2	1.2	1.0	1.9	n.s.
EXECUTIVE FUNCTIONS					
WCST					
Total errors	0.0	1.3	0.3	1.5	n.s.
Perseverative responses	−0.3	0.8	0.1	1.0	n.s.
N of Completed Categories	0.1	1.0	0.3	1.3	n.s.
Trail-Making Tests					
B (s)	1.3	1.7	−0.1	0.7	<0.001#
B−A (s)	1.8	2.2	−0.3	0.6	<0.001#
Verbal Fluency					
Letter (correct answers)	0.9	1.1	0.3	0.8	0.05
Semantic (correct answers)	1.0	1.3	0.7	1.2	n.s.
Rey Auditory Verbal Learning					
Retention after interference (% errors A6)	1.1	1.7	0.3	1.0	0.07
SUSTAINED ATTENTION					
RVP (% of errors)	0.9	1.3	0.4	1.0	n.s.
SHORT-TERM MEMORY					
Digit span	0.0	0.8	0.3	0.9	n.s.
Corsi Block span	−0.8	0.9	0.3	0.9	<0.001#
LEARNING					
Rey Auditory Verbal Learning Test					
Trial A1–A5—% errors	0.2	1.4	0.3	1.2	n.s.
Delayed Recall—% errors	0.8	1.5	0.3	1.2	n.s.
Paired Associate Visual learning—% err	0.9	1.7	0.4	1.7	n.s.
OVERALL Z SCORE excluding IQ					
mean	0.59		0.42		n.s.
SD	0.76		0.58		

Diff. = Difference. # = comparison which remains significant after Bonferroni correction.

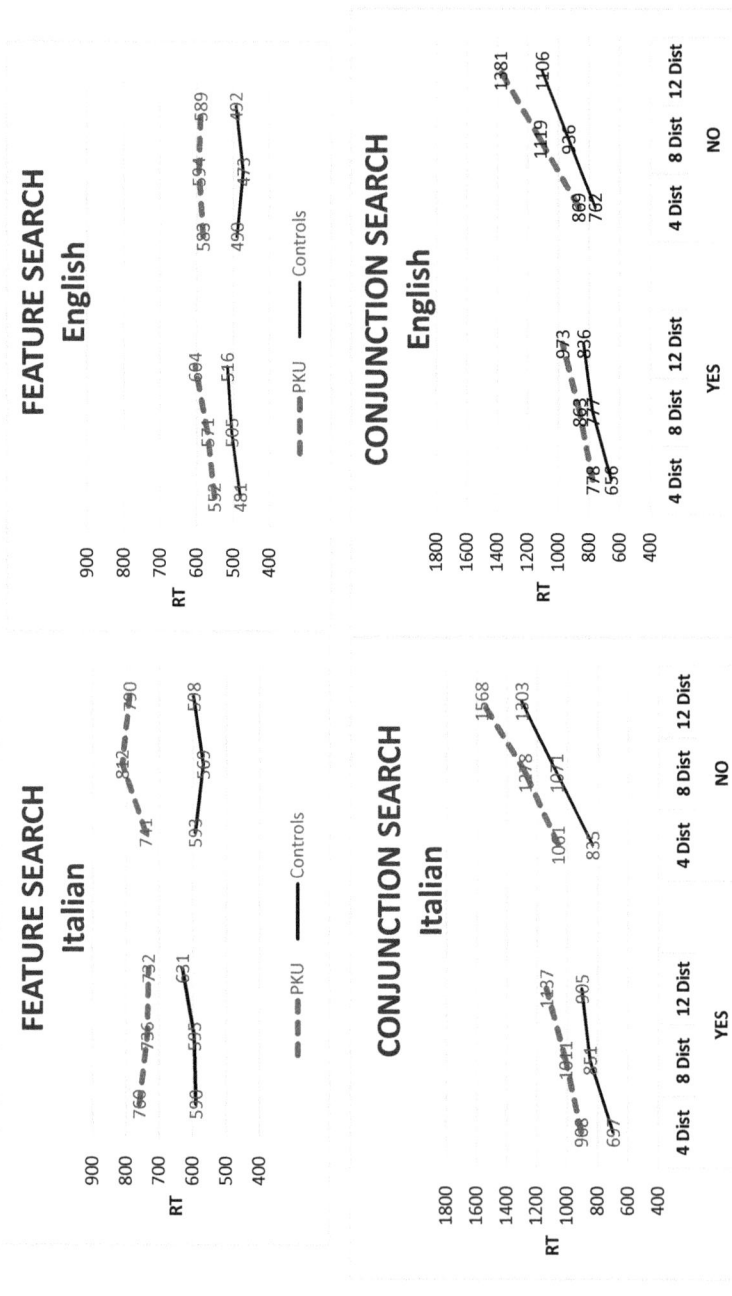

Figure 1. Performance of the UK and Italian PKU groups and relative control groups on the visual search tasks. Dist: distractors, PKU: Phenylketonuria, RT: reaction Times.

4.3. Cognitive Outcomes in Relation to Metabolic Control

We ran Bivariate Pearson r correlations between metabolic measures taken at different times during the life span and our adult cognitive measures. To reduce the number of variables per task, we only run correlations for search tasks, with RT measures; for TMT, with the B–A condition; for the WCST, with the total errors; and for the Rey, with total errors over 1–5 trials and with delay recall. Table 4 shows results for the Italian sample. Results for the larger sample of English AwPKU are reported in Romani et al. [5]. We do not report correlations with the English matched sub-sample because correlations with a small sample are notoriously unstable. Thus, results with a smaller sub-sample may differ from the results obtained with a larger sample in potentially misleading ways. However, to compare results for the two languages with samples of an equal size, we also report, with both PKU samples, the % of positive correlations and the average correlation.

The Italian sample had widespread significant correlations with only a few tasks failing to show any significant correlation with any metabolic measure (pegboard task, the semantic fluency task, and the Rey test). Almost all correlation (91%) were positive (132/144; $\chi^2 = 60.5$; $p < .001$). The average correlation across tasks was 0.29 (SD = 0.22), which was significantly different from 0 (one sample *t*-test (142) = 17.0; $p < 0.001$). In the English matched sample ($N = 19$), 69% of correlations were positive (99/144 = 69%; $\chi^2 = 10.5$; $p < 0.001$) and the average correlation was 0.12 (SD = 0.25; one sample *t*-test (142) = 5.7; $p < 0.001$). Taken together, these results indicate that our tests are sensitive to the level of metabolic control in both languages.

Considering the qualitative pattern of correlations in the Italian sample, a number of significant features can be noted which replicate findings from the larger English sample [5]: 1. Adult cognitive performance correlates with current Phe levels, but also with historical Phe records with significant correlations across the life-span; 2. Cognitive performance correlates with metabolic measures in terms of both average Phe levels and Phe fluctuations (average SD per year), this confirms the importance of maintaining not only low average Phe levels, but also of being constant and of avoid Phe peaks; 3. There are interactions between type of function an age when metabolic control is measured: some functions are more effected by childhood Phe measures than by current Phe levels (see visuo-attentional speed). Other functions, instead, show as much of an association with current levels as with historical measures (IQ, visuo-motor control, sustained attention, memory, and learning.

Table 4. Correlations Between Phe Measures Across the Life-Span and Cognitive Performance in Different Domains for the Italian PKU Sample ($N = 19$).

ITALIAN PKU			VISUAL ATTENTION SPEED					VISUO-MOTOR			EF-MONITORING				SUST. ATTENT	LEARNING AND MEMORY		
	FSIQ	Simple RT	Detection With distractors RT	Feature Search RT	Conj. Search RT	Peg-Board Sec.	Digit Symbol	WCST Total err	TMT b-a	Digit Span	Corsi Span	Sem Fluency	RVP %	Rey Words a1-a5	Rey Words Delayed	Paired Ass. Visual Learning
PHE																	
0-10 yrs																	
Average	0.38	0.43	0.42	0.15	0.30	0.05	0.28	0.19	0.55 *	0.57 *	0.37	0.03	0.43	0.17	0.08	0.30
SD	0.31	0.73 **	0.73 **	0.34	0.49 *	0.02	0.13	-0.10	0.55 *	0.66 **	0.42	0.08	0.57 *	0.34	0.25	0.36
11-16 yrs																	
Average	0.53 *	0.08	0.30	0.41	0.35	0.18	0.38	0.28	0.44	0.32	0.29	0.41	0.63 **	0.14	0.08	0.49 *
SD	0.02	0.29	0.32	0.37	0.20	-0.25	-0.10	-0.08	0.20	0.16	-0.04	0.38	0.37	-0.18	-0.29	0.30
17 yr to now																	
Average	0.58 **	0.03	0.37	0.38	0.41	0.32	0.60 **	0.59 **	0.56 *	0.60 **	0.60 **	0.24	0.48 *	0.11	0.09	0.30
SD	0.52 *	-0.06	0.06	0.16	0.22	0.29	0.43	0.46 *	0.52 *	0.38	0.28	0.21	0.33	0.05	-0.11	-0.20
Current	0.41	-0.10	0.05	0.03	0.01	0.12	0.61 **	0.58 **	0.54 *	0.60 **	0.37	0.00	0.30	0.21	0.16	0.11
Lifetime																	
Average	0.55 *	0.23	0.42	0.29	0.39	0.03	0.37	0.31	0.55 *	0.58 **	0.33	0.23	0.58 *	0.12	0.12	0.38
SD	0.47 *	0.45	0.54 *	0.40	0.45	0.05	0.24	0.16	0.60 *	0.55 *	0.35	0.28	0.58 *	0.13	0.00	0.26

Highlighted rows compare childhood Phe measures with current Phe. To facilitate interpretation, positive correlations always indicate that high Phe was associated with a worse performance. Thus, for IQ, digit span, Corsi span, and semantic fluency correlations were reversed. Significant measures are in bold. * = significant < 0.05; ** significant < 0.01. Phe SD: Phe fluctuations, FSIQ: full scale IQ, TMT: Trail Making Test, ATTENT: attention, PHE: Phenylalanine.

5. Discussion

There is a lack of studies which have assessed the behavioural effects of metabolic control in individuals with PKU across countries with the same testing materials, comparing sensitivity. This, instead, is important for establishing common PKU testing batteries and to accrue results across centers for a rare disease. In spite of tremendous advances in our knowledge of PKU, we lack a complete and reliable picture of cognitive outcomes in relation to metabolic controls at different ages, which is crucial to establish the efficacy of new therapeutic interventions and to track developmental trends which may demonstrate either cognitive improvements (by bridging developmental gaps) or cognitive deterioration with age (due to abandoning the diet and/or accelerated aging). Our study tested cognitive outcomes in two samples of Italian and English AwPKU closely matched for gender, age, and education, using the same or closely matched materials.

5.1. Metabolic Control

Our results showed better metabolic control in the English than the Italian PKU sample. This could be due to differences in clinical practice (the English group is one of the better controlled groups described in the literature so far, which is likely due to the strong clinical advice received) or to cultural differences in approaches to food across countries. While in Italy, the diet may be less protein-based than in England, the stronger centrality of food in Italian society may make following a separate diet more difficult. Our matched samples are small, and we do not have corroborative information indicating whether following a PKU diet may be easier in England than in Italy. Nonetheless, our results point to variability in metabolic control across groups, suggesting the need to explore possible, modulating socio-cultural factors which could affect clinical management.

5.2. Cognitive Impairments

Our results showed similar patterns of cognitive outcomes and associations with metabolic measures across the Italian and English groups. The Italian PKU participants performed worse than the matched English PKU participants in a few tasks, consistent with their worse metabolic control, but the overall level of impairment and the pattern of spared and impaired functions were similar across groups. The results with an Italian sample confirm patterns of impaired and spared functions previously reported with English participants [15]. They confirm substantial impairments in the following:

- Speed of processing, at least, with tasks tapping visual attention (no other RT tasks were used), confirming previous results [11,27], but good performance in the same tasks in terms of accuracy, confirming that AwPKU are slow, but accurate.
- Executive functions in terms of flexibility and planning (TMT B and B–A and verbal fluency), but no impairment in the WCST (see also Moyle et al. [49] for impairments in fluency, but no impairments in the TMT B; see also Brumm et al. [25]; Smith et al. [50], for impairments in the WCST; see Ris et al. [51], and Channon et al. [52], for impairments in a test similar to the WCST).
- Sustained attention (Rapid Visual Information Processing task; see also Channon et al. [52]; Bik-Multanowski et al., [53]; Jahja et al. [27]; Schmidt at al. [47]; Weglage et al. [9]).
- Visuo-motor coordination (marginal impairment in the peg-board task; see also Griffiths et al. [54]; Pietz et al. [55], but also Brumm et al. [25], for no impairment).

The Italian sample showed no impairments in verbal and visual short-term memory. Performance was in fact better than the controls in the Corsi task, confirming the lack of impairment found in Palermo et al., [15]. We have previously found a marginal impairment in digit span. The present results are also consistent with Moyle et al., [49], who found no impairment in the working memory index of the WAIS, and with Brumm et al. [25], who found no impairment in the forward digit span, but an impairment with the backwards span (see also Jahja et al. [27] for deficits with increasing working memory load).

Finally, our results confirm no or marginal impairments in verbal and visual learning (for no impairments in adults see also Channon et al. [52]; Moyle et al. [49]; for a review in children showing mixed results see Janzen and Nguyen, [14]). These results support the idea that AwPKU perform better when they can rely on learning and stored knowledge (see good performance in word spelling; better word than nonword reading speed; and better digit span than nonword repetition; [15,16]).

When we have analysed patterns in visual search tasks, the Italian and English PKU samples also showed similar results. Both groups were slower in conjunction than in feature search tasks and showed increased delays with a number of distractors, especially in conjoined search and target absent conditions. Compared to matched control, both Italian and English PKU samples showed delays across tasks and conditions. However, in conjunction search, the English PKU group showed increased delays with a number of distractors (a fanning out pattern), while the Italian PKU group showed stable differences. In Romani et al. [16], we argued that two different types of difficulties may contribute to a speed reduction in AwPKU: 1. Some specific processing difficulties such as a difficulty in allocating visual attention; this will result in increasing differences from the control with number of distractors; and 2. A general tendency to be more cautious/tentative in returning an answer which will result in a fixed delay across conditions (a flat profile across conditions; a pattern that we have seen with language tasks, see Romani et al., [16]). The Italian PKU sample is relatively small, and it is possible that noise may have obliterated a fanning-out pattern in conjunction search. With this caveat, a stable difference from controls, which is not affected by task difficulty, is more consistent with a delay in making decisions than with processing difficulties.

Taken together, our results highlight how PKU does not impact cognition homogeneously. Some functions are spared while others—like visuo-attentional speed—are severely impaired, showing average Z scores between 1.2 and 1.5 from the control mean (and Z score SDs between 1.2 and 2.3), which indicate that some people with PKU are at the extreme margin of the normal distribution. To consider this variability is important for an accurate evaluation of outcomes in relation to current and future treatment options. Our results also confirm the extreme variability in performance across individual participants. In the Italian sample, 5 participants (26% of sample) showed a completely normal cognitive performance.

Concerning the relationship between cognitive and metabolic measures, our Italian results confirm extensive correlations between current and historical Phe measures and performance in cognitive tasks. Previous studies have also found correlations between current and life-time Phe levels and cognitive functions (see Brumm et al. [25] for correlations with backwards span, fluency, WCST; Smith et al. [50] for a correlation with WCST; Moyle et al. [49] for correlations with TMT and visual memory; Jahja et al. [27] for correlation with visual search tasks with a memory load; see Romani et al. [5], and Hofman et al. [56], for a more detailed review of the literature). Other studies have found differences in cognitive abilities between AwPKU with better versus worse metabolic control. For example, Nardecchia et al. [26] found that patients with a worse metabolic control had a lower IQ and worse performance at the WCST and at the Elithorn's Perceptual Maze Test; Bik-Multanowski et al. [53] found that patients with a worse metabolic control performed worse in RVP, Spatial Span (SSP), Spatial Working Memory (SWM) and Stop Signal Task (SST; see also Brumm et al. [25] and Palermo et al. [15] for results on more comprehensive sets of cognitive tasks).

Our results also confirm that both measures in terms of average Phe and Phe fluctuations correlate with performance [57] and that there are interactions between type of function and age of metabolic control. Some functions are more affected by historical Phe and others by current Phe. Speed in visual attentional tasks is associated mainly with childhood Phe (both average and SD), while tasks tapping visuo-motor coordination (digit-symbol, TMT), sustained attention and memory and learning are also affected by current Phe [5,11].

Our results highlight the importance of using the right cognitive and metabolic measures to assess outcomes. For example, a recent study by Bartus et al. [58] found no correlations between Phe levels (current and life-time) and performance on three tasks of the computerized Cambridge

Cognition Test (CANTAB)—Motor screening test, Spatial Working Memory test, and The Stoking of Cambridge—in 47 AwPKU, nor any difference between groups with high vs. low Phe levels. However, we also found no correlations when we used similar tasks with our Italian/English samples (motor speed tapped by simple RT, visual WM tapped by Corsi span) or with larger English sample (the Tower of Hanoi was not tested here; see Romani et al., [5]). This example shows the importance of using both a comprehensive and an ad hoc set of tasks when assessing outcomes and their relationship with metabolic variables. Failing to do so runs the risk of reaching the wrong conclusions regarding the effects of relaxing metabolic control.

6. Conclusions

It is important to track the cognitive performance of people with PKU across the lifespan. This is the first generation of early-treated AwPKU to move towards middle-age and people with PKU show a tendency to progressively relax the diet with age [55,59–61]. However, we do not know what effects prolonged high-levels of Phe may have on aging brains. Our results suggest that the effect of Phe on the brain is different in childhood to early adulthood [6], but further interactions may be seen later in life. Knowing which functions and relative tasks are most affected and most sensitive to Phe in young adults with PKU provides an important base-line to compare outcomes across the life-span and evaluate the effectiveness of treatment. Our study has contributed to an identification of sensitive tasks by showing consistency across Italian and English samples in the patterns of impaired and spared functions and similar patterns of correlations with metabolic measures and by replicating previous findings. This provides preliminary evidence that common PKU batteries can be used across countries to detect impairments with similar sensitivity. The similarity of the results across the Italian and English PKU samples justified combining results in a single database in a follow-up study, giving us more power to assess the interactions between types of metabolic variable (Phe average vs. Phe fluctuation), age of metabolic control (childhood, adulthood, current) and type of cognitive functions, and more power to assess the relationships between cognitive scores and adherence to metabolic guidelines [6].

Limitations

The main limitation of our study lies in the small sample of AwPKU tested in Italian. Although this small sample is still sufficient to establish that our tasks are sensitive to metabolic control, larger samples are necessary to compare individual correlations and replicate our preliminary findings that qualitive patterns are the same across languages and nationalities. There was variability in the correlation patterns shown by the Italian and English PKU samples. This is not surprising. The two PKU samples were not matched for metabolic controls. More importantly, correlations are notoriously unstable and have small samples, and this is a major stumbling block for research trying to establish the relationship between metabolic controls and cognitive outcomes in people with PKU. However, it is precisely this limitation that makes it important to establish that tasks are equally sensitive across different nationalities so that results can be accrued. We hope that that our study will be followed by further research to assess the sensitivity of the same tasks across languages in people with PKU.

Author Contributions: The authors contributed to the studies as follows: conceptualization, C.R., F.M., F.N., A.M., L.P., V.L; methodology: C.R., F.M., F.N., A.M., L.P., V.L; software: C.R., L.P.; formal analysis: C.R., L.P.; investigation: F.V., N.F., C.C., S.D.L.; resources: V.L, C.R.; writing—original draft preparation: C.R.; writing—review and editing: C.R., F.M., F.N., A.M., L.P, V.L.; supervision: C.R., F.M., F.N., A.M., L.P., V.L. All authors have read and agreed to the published version of the manuscript.

Funding: This research received no external funding.

Acknowledgments: We would like to thank Tarekegn Gerberhiwot for having allowed access to the PKU participants, Cecilia Guariglia for having facilitated tested of the Italian control participants and Andrew Olson for helpful comments on a version of the manuscript. The original cohort of English patients was supported by a Marie Curie Intra European Fellowship within the 7th European Community Framework Programme granted to Liana Palermo under the supervision of Cristina Romani and by a grant of the University Hospital Birmingham Charity to Tarekegn Gerberhiwot.

Conflicts of Interest: The authors declare no conflict of interest.

References

1. Hardelid, P.; Cortina-Borja, M.; Munro, A.; Jones, H.; Cleary, M.; Champion, M.P.; Foo, Y.; Scriver, C.R.; Dezateux, C. The Birth Prevalence of PKU in Populations of European, South Asian and Sub-Saharan African Ancestry Living in South East England. *Ann. Hum. Genet.* **2007**, *72*, 65–71. [CrossRef] [PubMed]
2. Diamond, A.; Prevor, M.B.; Callender, G.; Druin, D.P. Prefrontal Cortex Cognitive Deficits in Children Treated Early and Continuously for PKU. *Monogr. Soc. Res. Child. Dev.* **1997**, *62*, 1–208. [CrossRef]
3. Douglas, T.D.; Ramakrishnan, U.; Kable, J.A.; Singh, R.H. Longitudinal quality of life analysis in a phenylketonuria cohort provided sapropterin dihydrochloride. *Heal. Qual. Life Outcomes* **2013**, *11*, 218. [CrossRef] [PubMed]
4. The American College of Medical Genetics and Genomics Therapeutic Committee; Vockley, J.; Andersson, H.C.; Antshel, K.M.; Braverman, N.E.; Burton, B.K.; Frazier, D.M.; Mitchell, J.J.; Smith, W.E.; Thompson, B.H.; et al. Phenylalanine hydroxylase deficiency: Diagnosis and management guideline. *Genet. Med.* **2013**, *16*, 188–200. [CrossRef]
5. Romani, C.; Palermo, L.; Macdonald, A.; Limback, E.; Hall, S.K.; Geberhiwot, T. The impact of phenylalanine levels on cognitive outcomes in adults with phenylketonuria: Effects across tasks and developmental stages. *Neuropsychology* **2017**, *31*, 242–254. [CrossRef]
6. Romani, C.; Manti, F.; Nardecchia, F.; Valentini, F.; Fallarino, N.; Carducci, C.; De Leo, S.; Macdonald, A.; Palermo, L.; Leuzzi, V. Adult cognitive outcomes in phenylketonuria: Explaining causes of variability beyond average Phe levels. *Orphanet J. Rare Dis.* **2019**, *14*, 1–17. [CrossRef]
7. Blau, N.; Bélanger-Quintana, A.; Demirkol, M.; Feillet, F.; Giovannini, M.; Macdonald, A.; Trefz, F.K.; Van Spronsen, F. Management of phenylketonuria in Europe: Survey results from 19 countries. *Mol. Genet. Metab.* **2010**, *99*, 109–115. [CrossRef]
8. Walter, J.; White, F.; Hall, S.; Macdonald, A.; Rylance, G.; Boneh, A.; Francis, D.; Shortland, G.; Schmidt, M.; Vail, A. How practical are recommendations for dietary control in phenylketonuria? *Lancet* **2002**, *360*, 55–57. [CrossRef]
9. Weglage, J.; Fromm, J.; Van Teeffelen-Heithoff, A.; Möller, H.E.; Koletzko, B.; Marquardt, T.; Rutsch, F.; Feldmann, R. Neurocognitive functioning in adults with phenylketonuria: Results of a long term study. *Mol. Genet. Metab.* **2013**, *110*, S44–S48. [CrossRef]
10. Moyle, J.; Fox, A.M.; Bynevelt, M.; Arthur, M.; Burnett, J.R. A neuropsychological profile of off-diet adults with phenylketonuria. *J. Clin. Exp. Neuropsychol.* **2007**, *29*, 436–441. [CrossRef]
11. Albrecht, J.; Garbade, S.F.; Burgard, P. Neuropsychological speed tests and blood phenylalanine levels in patients with phenylketonuria: A meta-analysis. *Neurosci. Biobehav. Rev.* **2009**, *33*, 414–421. [CrossRef] [PubMed]
12. Christ, S.E.; Huijbregts, S.C.; De Sonneville, L.M.; White, D.A. Executive function in early-treated phenylketonuria: Profile and underlying mechanisms. *Mol. Genet. Metab.* **2010**, *99*, S22–S32. [CrossRef] [PubMed]
13. Deroche, K.; Welsh, M. Twenty-Five Years of Research on Neurocognitive Outcomes in Early-Treated Phenylketonuria: Intelligence and Executive Function. *Dev. Neuropsychol.* **2008**, *33*, 474–504. [CrossRef] [PubMed]
14. Janzen, D.; Nguyen, M. Beyond executive function: Non-executive cognitive abilities in individuals with PKU. *Mol. Genet. Metab.* **2010**, *99*, S47–S51. [CrossRef] [PubMed]
15. Palermo, L.; Geberhiwot, T.; Macdonald, A.; Limback, E.; Hall, S.K.; Romani, C. Cognitive outcomes in early-treated adults with phenylketonuria (PKU): A comprehensive picture across domains. *Neuropsychology* **2017**, *31*, 255–267. [CrossRef]
16. Romani, C.; Macdonald, A.; De Felice, S.; Palermo, L. Speed of processing and executive functions in adults with phenylketonuria: Quick in finding the word, but not the ladybird. *Cogn. Neuropsychol.* **2017**, *35*, 171–198. [CrossRef]
17. Koch, R.; Moseley, K. Phenylketonuria: Newborn identification through to adulthood. In *Amino Acids in Human Nutrition and Health*; CABI Publishing: Wallingford, UK, 2011; pp. 406–417.

18. Rohr, F.J.; Wessel, A.; Brown, M.; Charette, K.; Levy, H.L. Adherence to tetrahydrobiopterin therapy in patients with phenylketonuria. *Mol. Genet. Metab.* **2015**, *114*, 25–28. [CrossRef]
19. Thomas, J.; Levy, H.; Amato, S.; Vockley, J.; Zori, R.; Dimmock, D.; Harding, C.O.; Bilder, D.A.; Weng, H.H.; Olbertz, J.; et al. Pegvaliase for the treatment of phenylketonuria: Results of a long-term phase 3 clinical trial program (PRISM). *Mol. Genet. Metab.* **2018**, *124*, 27–38. [CrossRef]
20. Harding, C.O.; Amato, R.S.; Stuy, M.; Longo, N.; Burton, B.K.; Posner, J.; Weng, H.H.; Meriläinen, M.; Gu, Z.; Jiang, J.; et al. Pegvaliase for the treatment of phenylketonuria: A pivotal, double-blind randomized discontinuation Phase 3 clinical trial. *Mol. Genet. Metab.* **2018**, *124*, 20–26. [CrossRef]
21. Pascucci, T.; Rossi, L.; Colamartino, M.; Gabucci, C.; Carducci, C.; Valzania, A.; Sasso, V.; Bigini, N.; Pierigè, F.; Viscomi, M.T.; et al. A new therapy prevents intellectual disability in mouse with phenylketonuria. *Mol. Genet. Metab.* **2018**, *124*, 39–49. [CrossRef]
22. Manti, F.; Nardecchia, F.; Paci, S.; Chiarotti, F.; Carducci, C.; Carducci, C.; Dalmazzone, S.; Cefalo, G.; Salvatici, E.; Banderali, G.; et al. Predictability and inconsistencies in the cognitive outcome of early treated PKU patients. *J. Inherit. Metab. Dis.* **2017**, *40*, 793–799. [CrossRef] [PubMed]
23. Van Spronsen, F.; Huijbregts, S.; Bosch, A.; Leuzzi, V. Cognitive, neurophysiological, neurological and psychosocial outcomes in early-treated PKU-patients: A start toward standardized outcome measurement across development. *Mol. Genet. Metab.* **2011**, *104*, S45–S51. [CrossRef] [PubMed]
24. Van Vliet, D.; Van Wegberg, A.M.; Ahring, K.; Bik-Multanowski, M.; Blau, N.; Bulut, F.D.; Casas, K.; Didycz, B.; Djordjevic, M.; Federico, A.; et al. Can untreated PKU patients escape from intellectual disability? A systematic review. *Orphanet J. Rare Dis.* **2018**, *13*, 149. [CrossRef]
25. Brumm, V.L.; Azen, C.; Moats, R.A.; Stern, A.M.; Broomand, C.; Nelson, M.D.; Koch, R. Neuropsychological outcome of subjects participating in the PKU Adult Collaborative Study: A preliminary review. *J. Inherit. Metab. Dis.* **2004**, *27*, 549–566. [CrossRef] [PubMed]
26. Nardecchia, F.; Manti, F.; Chiarotti, F.; Carducci, C.; Carducci, C.; Leuzzi, V. Neurocognitive and neuroimaging outcome of early treated young adult PKU patients: A longitudinal study. *Mol. Genet. Metab.* **2015**, *115*, 84–90. [CrossRef]
27. Jahja, R.; Huijbregts, S.; De Sonneville, L.M.J.; Van Der Meere, J.J.; Legemaat, A.M.; Bosch, A.M.; Hollak, C.E.; Rubio-Gozalbo, M.E.; Brouwers, M.C.G.J.; Hofstede, F.C.; et al. Cognitive profile and mental health in adult phenylketonuria: A PKU-COBESO study. *Neuropsychology* **2017**, *31*, 437–447. [CrossRef]
28. Christ, S.E.; Steiner, R.; Grange, D.K.; Abrams, R.A.; White, D.A. Inhibitory Control in Children With Phenylketonuria. *Dev. Neuropsychol.* **2006**, *30*, 845–864. [CrossRef] [PubMed]
29. Feldmann, R.; Denecke, J.; Grenzebach, M.; Weglage, J. Frontal lobe-dependent functions in treated phenylketonuria: Blood phenylalanine concentrations and long-term deficits in adolescents young adults. *J. Inherit. Metab. Dis.* **2005**, *28*, 445–455. [CrossRef]
30. Channon, S.; Mockler, C.; Lee, P. Executive Functioning and Speed of Processing in Phenylketonuria. *Neuropsychology* **2005**, *19*, 679–686. [CrossRef]
31. Janos, A.L.; Grange, D.K.; Steiner, R.D.; White, D.A. Processing speed and executive abilities in children with phenylketonuria. *Neuropsychology* **2012**, *26*, 735–743. [CrossRef]
32. De Felice, S.; Romani, C.; Geberhiwot, T.; Macdonald, A.; Palermo, L. Language processing and executive functions in early treated adults with phenylketonuria (PKU). *Cogn. Neuropsychol.* **2018**, *35*, 148–170. [CrossRef] [PubMed]
33. Wechsler, D. *Wechsler Adult Intelligence Scale*, 3rd ed.; The Psychological Corporation: San Antonio, TX, USA, 1997.
34. Wechsler, D. *Wechsler Abbreviated Scale of Intelligence (WASI)*; Harcourt Assessment: San Antonio, TX, USA, 1999.
35. Schrimsher, G.W.; O'Bryant, S.E.; O'Jile, J.R.; Sutker, P.B. Comparison of Tetradic WAIS-III Short Forms in Predicting Full Scale IQ Scores in Neuropsychiatric Clinic Settings. *J. Psychopathol. Behav. Assess.* **2007**, *30*, 235–240. [CrossRef]
36. Trites, R. *Grooved Pegboard Test*; Lafayette Instrument: Lafayette, IN, USA, 1977.
37. AITB. *Army Individual Test. Battery. Manual of Directions and Scoring*; War Department, Adjutant General's Office: Washington, DC, USA, 1944.

38. Sánchez-Cubillo, I.; A Periañez, J.; Adrover-Roig, D.; Rodríguez-Sánchez, J.; Rios-Lago, M.; Tirapu, J.; Barcelo, F. Construct validity of the Trail Making Test: Role of task-switching, working memory, inhibition/interference control, and visuomotor abilities. *J. Int. Neuropsychol. Soc.* **2009**, *15*, 438–450. [CrossRef] [PubMed]
39. Kongs, S.K.; Thompson, L.L.; Iverson, G.L.; Heaton, R.K. *WCST-64: Wisconsin Card Sorting Test.-64 Card Version, Professional Manual*; Psychological Assessment Resources: Odessa, FL, USA, 2000.
40. Novelli, G.; Papagno, C.; Capitani, E.; Laiacona, M.; Vallar, G.; Cappa, S.F. Tre test clinici di ricerca e produzione lessicale. Taratura su soggetti normali. *Arch. Neurol. Psychiatry* **1986**, *47*, 477–506.
41. Benton, A.L.; deS, K.; Sivan, A.B. *Multilingual Aphasia Examination*; AJA Associates: Iowa City, IA, USA, 1994.
42. Rosen, W.G. Verbal fluency in aging and dementia. *J. Clin. Neuropsychol.* **1980**, *2*, 135–146. [CrossRef]
43. Costa, A.; Bagoj, E.; Monaco, M.; Zabberoni, S.; De Rosa, S.; Papantonio, A.M.; Mundi, C.; Caltagirone, C.; Carlesimo, G.A. Standardization and normative data obtained in the Italian population for a new verbal fluency instrument, the phonemic/semantic alternate fluency test. *Neurol. Sci.* **2013**, *35*, 365–372. [CrossRef]
44. Corsi, P.M. Human Memory and the Medial Temporal Region of the Brain. Unpublished Doctoral Dissertation, McGill University, Montreal, QC, Canada, 1972.
45. Sahakian, B.J.; Jones, G.; Levy, R.; Gray, J.; Warburton, D. The Effects of Nicotine on Attention, Information Processing, and Short-Term Memory in Patients with Dementia of the Alzheimer Type. *Br. J. Psychiatry* **1989**, *154*, 797–800. [CrossRef]
46. Rey, A. *L'Examen Clinique en Psychologie (Clinical Examination in Psychology)*; Presses Universitaires de France: Paris, France, 1964.
47. Schmidt, E.; Rupp, A.; Burgard, P.; Pietz, J.; Weglage, J.; De Sonneville, L.M.J. Sustained attention in adult phenylketonuria: The influence of the concurrent phenylalanine-blood-level. *J. Clin. Exp. Neuropsychol.* **1994**, *16*, 681–688. [CrossRef]
48. Sahakian, B.J.; Morris, R.G.; Evenden, J.L.; Heald, A.; Levy, R.; Philpot, M.; Robbins, T. A Comparative Study of Visuospatial Memory and Learning in Alzheimer-Type Dementia and Parkinson's Disease. *Brain* **1988**, *111*, 695–718. [CrossRef]
49. Moyle, J.J.; Fox, A.M.; Arthur, M.; Bynevelt, M.; Burnett, J.R. Meta-Analysis of Neuropsychological Symptoms of Adolescents and Adults with PKU. *Neuropsychol. Rev.* **2007**, *17*, 91–101. [CrossRef]
50. Smith, M.L.; Klim, P.; Mallozzi, E.; Hanley, W.B. A test of the frontal-specificity hypothesis in the cognitive performance of adults with phenylketonuria. *Dev. Neuropsychol.* **1996**, *12*, 327–341. [CrossRef]
51. Ris, M.; Williams, S.E.; Hunt, M.M.; Berry, H.K.; Leslie, N. Early-treated phenylketonuria: Adult neuropsychologic outcome. *J. Pediatr.* **1994**, *124*, 388–392. [CrossRef]
52. Channon, S.; German, E.; Cassina, C.; Lee, P. Executive Functioning, Memory, and Learning in Phenylketonuria. *Neuropsychology* **2004**, *18*, 613–620. [CrossRef] [PubMed]
53. Bik-Multanowski, M.; Pietrzyk, J.J.; Mozrzymas, R. Routine use of CANTAB system for detection of neuropsychological deficits in patients with PKU. *Mol. Genet. Metab.* **2011**, *102*, 210–213. [CrossRef]
54. Griffiths, P.; Paterson, L.; Harvie, A. Neuropsychological effects of subsequent exposure to phenylalanine in adolescents and young adults with early-treated phenylketonuria. *J. Intellect. Disabil. Res.* **1995**, *39*, 365–372. [CrossRef]
55. Pietz, J.; Dunckelmann, R.; Rupp, A.; Rating, D.; Meinck, H.-M.; Schmidt, H.; Bremer, H.J. Neurological outcome in adult patients with early-treated phenylketonuria. *Eur. J. Nucl. Med. Mol. Imaging* **1998**, *157*, 824–830. [CrossRef]
56. Hofman, D.L.; Champ, C.L.; Lawton, C.L.; Henderson, M.; Dye, L. A systematic review of cognitive functioning in early treated adults with phenylketonuria. *Orphanet J. Rare Dis.* **2018**, *13*, 150. [CrossRef]
57. Cleary, M.; Trefz, F.; Muntau, A.C.; Feillet, F.; Van Spronsen, F.J.; Burlina, A.; Bélanger-Quintana, A.; Gizewska, M.; Gasteyger, C.; Bettiol, E.; et al. Fluctuations in phenylalanine concentrations in phenylketonuria: A review of possible relationships with outcomes. *Mol. Genet. Metab.* **2013**, *110*, 418–423. [CrossRef]
58. Bartus, A.; Palasti, F.; Juhasz, E.; Kiss, E.; Simonova, E.; Sumanszki, C.; Reismann, P. The influence of blood phenylalanine levels on neurocognitive function in adult PKU patients. *Metab. Brain Dis.* **2018**, *33*, 1609–1615. [CrossRef]
59. Vilaseca, M.A.; Campistol, J.; Cambra, F.J.; Lambruschini, N. Index of dietary control of PKU patients. *Quím. Clín.* **1995**, *14*, 271.

60. Vilaseca, M.A.; Lambruschini, N.; Gómez-López, L.; Gutiérrez, A.; Fusté, E.; Gassió, R.; Artuch, R.; Campistol, J. Quality of dietary control in phenylketonuric patients and its relationship with general intelligence. *Nutr. Hosp.* **2010**, *25*, 60–66. [PubMed]
61. Feldmann, R.; Osterloh, J.; Onon, S.; Fromm, J.; Rutsch, F.; Weglage, J. Neurocognitive functioning in adults with phenylketonuria: Report of a 10-year follow-up. *Mol. Genet. Metab.* **2019**, *126*, 246–249. [CrossRef] [PubMed]

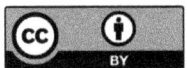

© 2020 by the authors. Licensee MDPI, Basel, Switzerland. This article is an open access article distributed under the terms and conditions of the Creative Commons Attribution (CC BY) license (http://creativecommons.org/licenses/by/4.0/).

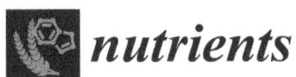

Review

The Potential Roles of Blood–Brain Barrier and Blood–Cerebrospinal Fluid Barrier in Maintaining Brain Manganese Homeostasis

Shannon Morgan McCabe and Ningning Zhao *

Department of Nutritional Sciences, The University of Arizona, Tucson, AZ 85721, USA; morgans3@email.arizona.edu
* Correspondence: zhaonn@email.arizona.edu

Abstract: Manganese (Mn) is a trace nutrient necessary for life but becomes neurotoxic at high concentrations in the brain. The brain is a "privileged" organ that is separated from systemic blood circulation mainly by two barriers. Endothelial cells within the brain form tight junctions and act as the blood–brain barrier (BBB), which physically separates circulating blood from the brain parenchyma. Between the blood and the cerebrospinal fluid (CSF) is the choroid plexus (CP), which is a tissue that acts as the blood–CSF barrier (BCB). Pharmaceuticals, proteins, and metals in the systemic circulation are unable to reach the brain and spinal cord unless transported through either of the two brain barriers. The BBB and the BCB consist of tightly connected cells that fulfill the critical role of neuroprotection and control the exchange of materials between the brain environment and blood circulation. Many recent publications provide insights into Mn transport in vivo or in cell models. In this review, we will focus on the current research regarding Mn metabolism in the brain and discuss the potential roles of the BBB and BCB in maintaining brain Mn homeostasis.

Keywords: manganese; blood–brain barrier; blood–cerebrospinal fluid barrier; choroid plexus

1. Manganese Dyshomeostasis and Neuropathological Consequences

Manganese (Mn) is essential for life as it is necessary for the normal function of several enzymes, including the antioxidant enzyme Mn superoxide dismutase (MnSOD) [1] and the neurotransmitter synthesis enzyme glutamine synthetase [2]. Since adequate Mn is easily obtained through a healthy diet, Mn deficiency is uncommon. However, Mn overload occurs more frequently and becomes a public health concern. Exposure to high levels of Mn in occupational environments such as mining, welding, and dry cell battery production can lead to manganism, which is a disorder characterized by serious and irreversible neurological symptoms similar to those seen in Parkinson's disease. Early symptoms of manganism caused by occupational hazards include neurobehavioral changes such as impulsiveness and irritability, followed by changes in gait and difficulty with speech as the disease progresses [3]. High Mn levels in local drinking water, along with elevated Mn in blood and hair samples, reveals a correlation between higher Mn levels and decreased memory, verbal, and overall IQ scores [4]. Elevated environmental Mn exposure in children is also correlated with poorer academic achievement [5], altered performance on visual perception and memory tasks [6], and reduced Full Scale IQ [7].

In patients with mutations in Mn-transport proteins, excess Mn accumulates in the blood and brain, causing neurological symptoms. Blood Mn levels in healthy individuals is <320 nmol/L, while patients experiencing neurological symptoms of Mn overload have levels exceeding 2500 nmol/L [8,9]. Additional data from patients with inherited disorders of Mn homeostasis have been recently summarized [10]. Individuals can also receive excess Mn from environmental sources. A group of people living in an area with high Mn in drinking water (1.8–2.3 µg/mL) experienced many of the neurological symptoms related

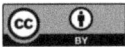

to manganism, such as tremors, gait disturbances, and memory dysfunction [11], thus highlighting the dangers of excess Mn to neurological health.

Older adults are also at risk of the neurological effects of excess Mn in the brain. Alzheimer's disease (AD) and related dementias are a group of neurological disorders that first present as cognitive impairment in aging individuals. There is no known cause for late-onset AD, but environmental pollutants such as heavy metals are thought to be a contributor [12]. In the brain, reactive oxygen and nitrogen species (ROS/NOS) are normally produced at manageable levels during oxidative phosphorylation. MnSOD is an antioxidant enzyme that requires Mn, but excess Mn reduces its antioxidant activity. In the brain of a patient with AD, there is a decrease of MnSOD activity and increased oxidative stress [13,14]. In non-human primates, chronic Mn exposure induced amyloid-beta precursor-like protein 1 expression and increased the formation of amyloid plaques, which is one of the main neuropathological hallmarks of AD [15,16]. A recent study used a transgenic mouse model of AD and exposed subjects to additional Mn via drinking water (0.36 mg/mL) over five months [17]. At the end of the study, mice consuming Mn-treated water had more beta amyloid deposition in the cortex and hippocampus than untreated transgenic mice. This result shows that Mn consumption may contribute to the severity of AD. In another study, mice were administered daily $MnCl_2$ doses of either 15 mg/kg or 60 mg/kg intraperitoneally. The study concludes that increased Mn exposure is correlated with increased amyloid-beta in the blood and decreased cognitive test scores in mice [18]. These results suggest that brain Mn dyshomeostasis may be a factor in the development of AD.

2. Structure of the Brain Barriers

The brain has developed physiological barriers to selectively restrict the exchange of ions and solutes between the blood and brain, allowing a tight regulation of the brain microenvironment for proper neuronal function. In order to enter the brain microenvironment, Mn from the systemic circulation has to cross either of the two strictly controlled blood–brain interfaces: the blood–brain barrier (BBB) and the blood–cerebrospinal fluid (CSF) barrier (BCB). Therefore, the BBB and BCB are the points of restriction for Mn entering the brain from systemic circulation (Figure 1). The accumulation of Mn within the brain and the export of excess Mn back into blood circulation occurs mainly across these two barriers.

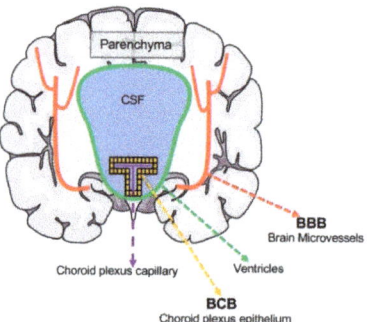

Figure 1. Localizations of the brain barrier interfaces. The blood–brain barrier (BBB) is localized to the microvasculature of the central nervous system and separates the lumen of cerebral blood vessels and brain parenchyma. Neurons and glia are found in the CNS parenchyma and thus protected from the periphery by the BBB. The blood–CSF barrier (BCB) is formed mainly by the choroid plexus epithelium located between choroid plexus capillaries and the CSF. Materials transported through the choroid plexus epithelium reach the CSF, where they can diffuse into the brain parenchyma.

The unique structures of the brain barriers provide insights into which cell types might express metal transporters. Further, cell models of the BBB and BCB may reflect the physiological structure and features of each barrier. Brain vasculature delivers oxygen and nutrients throughout the brain and shuttles toxins and unneeded materials away from the central nervous system. Unlike other organs, the exchange of molecules between the blood vessel and the brain environment is tightly regulated to prevent the infiltration of harmful pathogens, toxins, and immune factors. The BCB also restricts the movement of molecules between the blood and CSF. In essence, the brain environment beyond the blood vessel or CP epithelium is separated from general blood circulation.

2.1. Structure of the BBB

Regulatory control of the BBB is provided by specialized barrier cells and their unique structures and junction proteins. The BBB primarily consists of three unique cell types (Figure 2A): endothelial cells of the brain blood vessels, astrocytic end feet encasing the endothelium, and pericytes that form a basement membrane between the blood vessel and astrocyte [19,20]. Endothelial cells of the BBB are polarized, with the abluminal surface toward the brain environment, and the luminal surface facing the blood vessel lumen (Figure 2A). These endothelial cells are linked by tight junctions and adherens junctions to prevent the paracellular movement of water-soluble molecules.

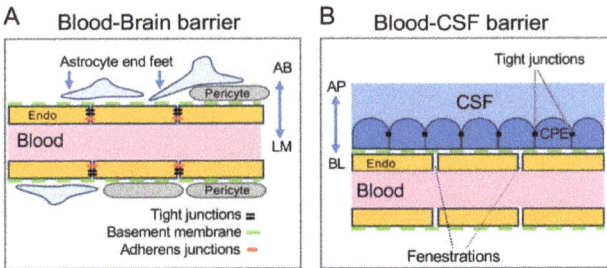

Figure 2. Cellular structures of the brain barriers. (**A**) The BBB is composed of endothelial cells (endo) of the brain blood vessel, and it is supported by pericytes, basement membrane proteins (green dashed line), and astrocytic end feet. The luminal (LM) side of BBB endothelial cells faces the inside of the blood vessel. It is also referred to as the apical side. The abluminal (AB) side faces the brain parenchyma and can exchange between the endothelial cell and the astrocytic end foot or brain extracellular space. It can be considered the basolateral side of BBB endothelium. (**B**) The BCB is made up of choroid plexus epithelial (CPE) cells connected to each other by tight junctions and attached to the blood vessel via basement membrane proteins (green dashed line). The apical (AP), or CSF-facing side of the CPE expresses transporters necessary for the secretion of CSF. On the basolateral (BL), or blood-facing side, CPE cells exchange materials with circulating blood, since endothelial cells in the CP lack tight junctions and permit larger molecules to diffuse.

Tight junction proteins exist almost entirely on the interior, protoplasmic face of the endothelial cell membrane. One group of these proteins are zonula occludens-1 and -2 (ZO-1, ZO-2). Both ZO proteins are required for the formation of tight junction strands between endothelial cells in the BBB [21,22]. Junctional adhesion molecule (JAM) proteins are another group of tight junction proteins [23]. Of the three JAM proteins found in the BBB, no individuals appear to be necessary for BBB integrity [23]. However, JAM proteins are highly enriched in BBB tight junctions and are responsible for the apical–basal polarity of endothelial cells, and therefore contribute to BBB formation [24]. Other components of BBB tight junctions are the claudins and occludin. Claudin-5 is the only protein of its family that appears to be localized to the BBB and contributes to barrier integrity [23]. It is also particularly enriched in the brain endothelium over other peripheral blood vessels, indicating the importance of claudin-5 in the formation of the BBB. Similar to claudin, occludin is an endothelial transmembrane protein. Mice with occludin deficiency had increased calcium precipitation in the brain despite normal serum calcium concentration, suggesting that occludin may be necessary for BBB tight junction integrity [25].

Adherens junctions between endothelial cells of the BBB help maintain the integrity of this barrier by regulating the adhesion between cells and controlling the flow of molecules between the blood and brain [26]. Adherens junctions are primarily composed of vascular endothelial cadherins, catenins, and nectins. Cadherins interact with catenins to facilitate their linkage to the actin cytoskeleton, forming the cadherin-based adhesions between the BBB endothelial cells [23], while nectins promote the establishment of endothelial apical–basal polarity and contribute to adherens junction integrity [27].

Each of these junctions exist between endothelial cells of the BBB, but other cell types are necessary for the barrier structure and function. Pericytes are found in the basement membrane of capillaries and surround the vessel. Differences in pericyte population sizes suggest that pericytes are directly involved in BBB permeability but do not alter tight junction formation [28]. Contractile smooth muscle cells fully surround arterioles to provide blood flow control [29]. Both pericytes and smooth muscle cells assist in the structural development of the brain blood vessels [23]. Surrounding the majority of the abluminal blood vessel are astrocytic end feet. Astrocytes associated with BBB endothelial cells increase the integrity of the BBB by decreasing the permeability of tight junctions [19,30]. Astrocytes function as an extensive network and interact with each other via gap junctions to coordinate ion changes [31], while their end feet are specifically responsible for the exchange of ions and molecules with the blood vessel in order to maintain ion homeostasis [32]. A basement membrane layer fills the gap between the endothelial cells and astrocytes, with pericytes and smooth muscle cells embedded within. Pericytes and endothelial cells form a 3D structure of laminins, nidogens, collagens, and heparan sulfate proteoglycans [33,34]. Communication and transport between the blood and astrocytes occurs through this matrix.

In most other tissues, blood vessels have small gaps, or fenestrations, between endothelial cells to allow larger molecules to cross from blood to tissue. The BBB is considered a physical barrier due to its lack of fenestrations [20], presence of tight junctions, and lack of permeability to large molecules [35]. Transport of hydrophilic molecules, such as glucose and metal ions, requires specific transporters to cross the endothelial membrane, while large molecules can cross via receptor-mediated endocytosis [20].

This highly selective barrier exists in all brain blood vessels, with the exception of the vessels in the meninges and those near the circumventricular organs. The pituitary and pineal glands, as well as the median eminence, paraphysis, and area postrema, possess a less restrictive barrier in order to allow signaling molecules and hormones to reach specific brain areas, without crossing the BBB into off-target areas [36].

2.2. Structure of the BCB

The other major brain barrier is the BCB, which is localized to the choroid plexus (CP) within the four brain ventricles (Figure 2B). CP tissues in the left and right lateral, and third ventricles are made up of epithelial cells surrounding the anterior choroidal and posterior choroidal arteries, while the fourth ventricle epithelium receives blood flow from the anterior and posterior inferior cerebellar arteries [37]. A thin endothelial basement membrane lies on the abluminal side of the blood vessel [38]. In contrast to the blood vessels forming the BBB, the capillaries of the CP are highly fenestrated and lack tight junctions to connect the endothelial cells, allowing the movement of larger molecules from the blood vessel to the CP tissue. These molecules first reach the stroma, which is a layer of fibroblastic mesenchymal-like cells that surround the CP blood vessels [37,39,40]. Leukocytes, macrophage, and dendritic cells are known to migrate to this cell layer from the blood vessel before being transported across the epithelial layer into the brain [40–42].

The outermost layer consists of polarized CP epithelial cells that are connected to the basement membrane and stromal layer on their basolateral side, allowing the cells to interact with systemic blood circulation while the apical, CSF-facing side is responsible for producing CSF and exchanging materials with the ventricles [40,43]. The presence of microvilli on the apical brush border of the epithelial cells increases the surface area and facilitates the transport of molecules into the ventricle [44].

CP epithelial cells are connected by tight junctions, thus restricting free passage of large or hydrophilic molecules into and out of the brain. While knowledge of CP tight junction proteins is less complete than that of the BBB, it is currently understood that many tight junction proteins of the BBB are also expressed in CP epithelial cells. The decreased occludin level induces epithelial permeability to larger molecules, suggesting that occludin may be a necessary component for the formation of CP tight junctions to block the transfer of large molecules across this barrier [45]. The expression of various claudins in the CP epithelium may be specific to developmental stages and species [46,47]; however, consistent reports of human and murine tight junctions show that claudin-1, -2, and -3 can be detected in CP epithelial tight junctions [48,49]. As in the BBB, the epithelial cells of the BCB express intracellular accessory protein ZO-1 [50] that seems to be required for tight junction integrity, since decreases in ZO-1 expression by inflammation cause an increase in the BCB permeability [51]. Lining all other surfaces of the ventricular walls are ependymal cells—cuboidal epithelial cells that lack tight junctions and are permeable to macromolecules [52]. Since the only structure between the CSF and brain parenchyma is this permeable ependymal cell barrier, molecules in the CSF could enter brain parenchyma by diffusion. Thus, the BCB function is carried out mainly by the single layer of CP epithelial cells and the tight junctions that link them [53,54].

3. Mn Homeostasis at the Brain Barriers: Evidence of Involved Metal Transporters

3.1. Potential Roles of Iron Transport Pathway Proteins in Mediating Mn Delivery at the Brain Barriers

3.1.1. Transferrin (Tf)

Many divalent metals share the same set of transporters. Studies of iron transport and absorption led to the first understandings of Mn homeostasis, particularly in studies of transferrin/transferrin receptor 1 (Tf/TfR1) and divalent metal transporter-1 (DMT1). The Tf cycle is the primary pathway for cells to take up iron. In this pathway, the circulating Tf carries Fe^{3+}, followed by binding to the cell surface TfR1 and subsequent invagination into intracellular vesicles. The acidic pH inside the vesicles causes the release of Fe^{3+} from Tf. Then, Fe^{3+} is reduced to Fe^{2+} and transported into the cytoplasm via DMT1 [55,56]. In addition to Fe^{3+}, Tf can bind to trivalent Mn (Mn^{3+}) [57,58] because Mn^{3+} is very similar in structure to Fe^{3+} [59]. Moreover, Mn and Fe accumulate in many of the same brain areas during overload conditions [60]. Therefore, the transport of Mn is presumably tied to the proteins involved in iron transport, including Tf. However, it has been shown that mice with Tf deficiency had similar levels of Mn in the brain compared to the wild-type animals, indicating that Tf is not necessary for the delivery of Mn to the brain [58].

3.1.2. DMT1

As mentioned above, DMT1 is a metal transporter that mediates the efflux of divalent metals from a vesicle to the cytoplasm. DMT1 functions optimally at pH 5.5, but its functionality in cells at pH 7.4 has also been observed [61]. DMT1 can localize to the plasma membranes of enterocytes or hepatocytes in high- or low-Fe conditions, respectively; whereas in regular dietary conditions, DMT1 remained primarily in the cytoplasm [62]. While DMT1 can adapt to changing substrate availability and subcellularly localize accordingly, its expression in the brain barriers is low. DMT1 mRNA expression is very low in isolated rat brain capillaries [63] and brain endothelial cells in culture [55]. In addition, protein expression is not detectable in brain endothelial cells of adult or early postnatal mice [64]. In a developmental study carried out in rats, the expression of DMT1 was detected by immunohistochemistry in the choroid plexus during early postnatal days, with increased expression at postnatal day 15. DMT1 was detected when staining cerebral blood vessels, but it aligned very closely with astrocyte localization; therefore, the transporter could be present on either the endothelial or glial cells [65]. In contrast, adult rats appear to express DMT1 protein in the CP epithelial cells, but not in microvascular endothelial cells [66], and the expression of DMT1 in CP epithelial cells was observed primarily in the cytoplasm.

A study of brain microvascular endothelial cells of human origin (hBMVEC) provides an analysis of time-dependent uptake of $^{54}Mn^{2+}$ that increased in the presence of a clathrin-dependent endocytosis inhibitor [67], demonstrating that the receptor-mediated endocytosis in the Tf/TfR1 and DMT1 pathway is not involved in Mn transport in this BBB cell model. Moreover, in Belgrade rats that lack functional DMT1, brain Mn levels remained normal in the olfactory bulb, cortex, striatum, hippocampus, and cerebellum, while Fe levels decreased in all brain areas tested [68], suggesting that DMT1 is not required for Mn delivery into the brain.

3.2. ZIP- and ZnT-Family Transporters

3.2.1. ZIP8 and ZIP14

ZIP14 and ZIP8 are two recently identified members of the Zrt- and Irt-like protein family of metal transporters. Both proteins have been investigated for their roles in brain Mn homeostasis [10,69–72].

In polarized HIBCPP cells, a cell model for the BCB epithelium, ZIP14, was enriched on the basolateral membrane, while ZIP8 was enriched on the apical membrane [73]. The knockdown of ZIP14 or ZIP8 using siRNA-mediated technology led to a decrease in ^{54}Mn accumulation in HIBCPP cells, although the decrease in ^{54}Mn accumulation was much greater with ZIP14 knockdown [73]. These results suggest that both ZIP14 and ZIP8 are involved in Mn uptake in this CP epithelial cell model, which is consistent with previous studies on epithelial cell models of intestine [70], lung [74], and liver [75].

In human primary brain microvessel endothelial cells (hBMVEC), a cell model for the BBB endothelium, the expression of both ZIP14 and ZIP8 were identified [67]. The uptake of ^{54}Mn was dependent on both ZIP8 or ZIP14, with significantly decreased ^{54}Mn accumulation when one or both proteins were knocked down. In contrast to the expression pattern observed in HIBCPP cells, ZIP14 and ZIP8 were localized to both sides of the polarized hBMVEC cells, where both proteins seem to be involved in apical-to-basolateral and basolateral-to-apical transport of Mn. Flux in the basolateral-to-apical direction was more prominent, modeling the movement of Mn from the brain to the blood through the BBB.

These studies using cell models of the BCB and BBB may provide insights into how Mn is transported within these two barriers. By identifying the polarized localization of ZIP14 and ZIP8 in CP-derived cells, we can begin to understand how Mn is transported at the BCB. Apical ZIP8 expression in HIBCPP cells suggests that Mn could be transported from the CSF into the epithelial cells to facilitate apical-to-basolateral movement of Mn out of the brain. In the same way, basolateral ZIP14 expression in CP-derived epithelial cells indicates that ZIP14 could be involved in the blood-to-brain movement of Mn via import of Mn from the blood to the epithelial cell of the BCB. The uptake experiments in hBMVEC endothelial cells suggest that both ZIP8 and ZIP14 play a significant role in Mn uptake into endothelial cells of the BBB. The basolateral-to-apical flux of Mn in these cells translates to a brain-to-blood movement of Mn in vivo. Thus, the BBB could have a considerable role in Mn clearance from the brain, dependent on coordinated transport by ZIP8 and ZIP14. A future study in the CP-derived HIBCPP cells could be useful to indicate the direction of Mn transport in cells with polarized expression of Mn transporters.

3.2.2. ZnT10

ZnT10 is a member of the Zinc Transporter family proteins. Patients with an inherited homozygous *ZnT10* mutation resulting in a non-functional ZnT10 protein exhibit high Mn levels in the blood and brain, as well as Mn toxicity-induced dystonia [76–78]. In cell culture studies, ZnT10 appears to be a Mn efflux transporter [79] expressed on the surfaces of enterocytes [78] and neuronal cells [80]. In both humans and mice, ZnT10 was highly expressed in the brain, liver, and intestine [78,80,81].

There is evidence showing that ZnT10 mRNA is expressed in the CP in rats [82], but there is no evidence to show that ZnT10 is expressed in the brain microvessels at either the gene or protein level. A recent study used pan-neuronal/glial *Znt10* knockout mice and detected no difference in brain Mn levels with standard dietary conditions [78]. In this study, *Znt10* knockout mice lack the protein in the vast majority of brain cells, including all neurons, astrocytes, and oligodendrocytes. As an efflux transporter, ZnT10 would likely protect neurons and glia from high Mn levels when overloaded, but a lack of increased Mn in the knockout mice indicates that these brain cells are not accumulating Mn, at least in normal conditions. Thus, a normal amount of Mn was circulating in the interstitial fluid and CSF, regardless of ZnT10 expression. This finding provides key information about Mn balance within the brain parenchyma, but the brain environment is controlled by the BCB and BBB. Therefore, Mn levels within the brain may not change without a change in transporter expression in either of the brain barriers. Interestingly, *Znt10* neuronal/glial knockout mice exposed to high dietary Mn experienced a greater increase of Mn in specific brain areas compared to exposed wild-type littermates. This result suggests that there is less Mn transported out of the brains lacking ZnT10, which could indicate that the efflux transporter is normally localized to either the brain endothelium or CP epithelium.

The expression pattern of ZnT10 in the BBB or BCB is unknown. As an efflux transporter, cell type localization of ZnT10 is necessary to understand which barrier is responsible for Mn efflux. Additionally, ZnT10 is likely polarized to either the basolateral or apical surfaces of the epithelial or endothelial cells. If polarized, its location would indicate whether ZnT10 is responsible for brain Mn accumulation or clearance. In addition, cell culture models of BBB and BCB are ideal to elucidate Mn transport mechanisms at the cellular level. Uptake and transport studies, such as those completed in previous studies of ZIP8 and ZIP14, would indicate if ZnT10 is necessary for normal Mn accumulation or efflux. Additionally, transport studies in polarized epithelial or endothelial monolayers would confirm the direction of Mn transport to which ZnT10 contributes.

3.3. ATP13A2

Another transporter associated with brain Mn homeostasis is ATP13A2. Mice with *Atp13a2* knockout accumulated more Mn in the brain compared to wild-type mice after intraperitoneal administration of $MnCl_2$ [83]. Since brain Mn levels tend to rise when the blood levels of Mn increase, a future investigation should report blood or serum levels in order to further understand the location of accumulated Mn in *Atp13a2* knockout mice. While knockout of *Atp13a2* causes brain Mn accumulation, overexpression of ATP13A2 in HeLa cells and nematode dopamine neurons had a protective effect against high Mn exposure [84]. Taken together, ATP13A2 appears to have a role in Mn homeostasis within the brain, but it is unclear how it could act as a Mn transporter at the BBB or BCB. To date, there are no publications showing evidence of ATP13A2 in human or mouse brain endothelium or choroid plexus tissue. Future studies of ATP13A2 should identify the transporter's tissue and membrane localization within the brain barriers to determine if the protective effect of this transporter against high Mn exposure is applicable to CP epithelial cells and brain endothelial cells. Major evidence of the metal transporters' involvement in Mn homeostasis at the BBB and BCB is summarized in Table 1.

Table 1. Evidence of metal transporters involved in Mn homeostasis at the brain barriers.

Protein	Experimental Model	Major Results and Conclusions	Reference
Transferrin (Tf)	Hypotransferrinemic (Hpx) mice as a model for Tf deficiency	▪ Hpx mice had normal brain Mn accumulation. ▪ Suggests that Tf is not required for brain Mn loading.	[58]
DMT1	Human brain endothelial cells (hBMVEC) as a model for the BBB	▪ Increased Mn uptake despite inhibition of clathrin-mediated endocytosis. ▪ Suggests that DMT1 and Tf/TfR1 pathway is not necessary for Mn uptake in brain endothelial cells.	[67]
	Belgrade rats as a model for DMT1 deficiency	▪ Belgrade rats have normal brain Mn levels. ▪ Indicates that DMT1 is not necessary for brain Mn accumulation.	[68]
ZIP8	Choroid plexus epithelial cells (HIBCPP) as a model for the BCB	▪ ZIP8 knockdown reduces Mn uptake. ▪ ZIP8 is primarily localized to the apical membrane. ▪ Suggests that ZIP8 may mediate apical Mn uptake into CP epithelial cells.	[73]
	hBMVEC cell model of BBB	▪ ZIP8 is expressed on both apical and basolateral membrane. ▪ ZIP8 is involved in both apical-to-basolateral and basolateral-to-apical Mn transport.	[67]
ZIP14	HIBCPP cell model of BCB	▪ ZIP14 knockdown reduces Mn uptake. ▪ ZIP14 is expressed on the basolateral membrane. ▪ Suggests that ZIP14 may mediate basolateral Mn transport into CP epithelial cells.	[73]
	hBMVEC cell model of BBB	▪ ZIP14 is expressed at both apical and basolateral membrane. ▪ ZIP14 is involved in both apical-to-basolateral and basolateral-to-apical Mn transport.	[67]
ZnT10	Pan-neuronal/glial *Znt10* knockout (KO) mice as a model for brain ZnT10 deficiency	▪ Pan-neuronal/glial Znt10 KO mice have increased Mn accumulation in certain brain areas under Mn overload conditions induced by subcutaneous Mn injection. ▪ Suggests reduced Mn efflux from the brain with ZnT10 deficiency when body Mn levels increase.	[78]
ATP13A2	*Atp13a2*$^{-/-}$ mice as a model for ATP13A2 deficiency	▪ Atp13a2$^{-/-}$ mice accumulate more Mn in the brain compared to the control mice after intraperitoneal administration of MnCl$_2$.	[83]
	HeLa cells and *C. elegans* with ATP13A2 overexpression	▪ Overexpression of ATP13A2 protects HeLa cells from Mn-induced cytotoxicity. ▪ *C. elegans* overexpressing ATP13A2 in dopamine neurons are more resistant to Mn-induced neurotoxicity. ▪ Suggests that ATP13A2 may have a role in maintaining brain Mn homeostasis.	[84]

4. Brain Mn Accumulation Is Likely to Occur via the BCB

The BBB and BCB are required to maintain the normal physiological conditions of the central nervous system. These two barriers have distinct but overlapping roles in the exchange of material from the blood to brain, as demonstrated by the difference in transporter expression and transport activity in each barrier. For example, both the CP and the brain endothelium express glucose transporters that deliver energy to the brain via facilitated diffusion [85]. Glucose is transported into the brain through both barriers, although it is estimated that the BCB imports only about 1/100th of the glucose that the BBB transports [86,87]. This pattern of uneven transport may also be applicable to Mn distribution into the brain.

A cell culture study of Mn transport across porcine BCB and BBB models indicated that the BCB is likely the primary route for brain Mn uptake. First, uptake studies indicated that CP epithelial cells accumulate nearly three times more Mn than endothelial cells when exposed to the same amount of $MnCl_2$ in media. Second, in a Transwell model of polarized cells with $MnCl_2$ added to each side, it was found that epithelial cells accumulated significantly more Mn in the apical chamber, suggesting that CP epithelial cells predominantly transport Mn in the basolateral-to-apical direction. In the BBB model, endothelial cells did not accumulate more Mn in one chamber than the other, indicating that the BBB transports Mn in both directions equally [88]. A future study might compare these findings with lower Mn concentrations that could be more relevant to physiological or Mn-overload conditions. Nevertheless, the results from this study provide valuable information about the activity of Mn transport across the brain barriers. Importantly, if these results reflect the in vivo behavior of the BCB, increased blood Mn would cause higher basolateral-to-apical Mn transport through the CP epithelium.

In vivo studies also provide evidence for the primary role of the BCB in brain Mn uptake. Brain Mn-mapping studies carried out in animals using peripheral Mn^{2+} administration followed by enhanced magnetic resonance imaging suggest that the entry of Mn into the CNS occurs predominantly through BCB. First, in mice, 2 h after intraperitoneal $MnCl_2$ injection, the Mn signal was first enhanced in the CSF-containing ventricles. This ventricular signal cleared over the next 24 h accompanied by a gradual increase of parenchymal Mn intensity. A close examination of different brain regions revealed that the Mn signal was highest in areas immediately adjacent to the CSF-containing ventricles, while the signal intensity steadily decreased with increasing distance from the ventricles [89]. Second, in rats, within 5 min of $MnCl_2$ injection through the tail vein, the Mn signal was first enhanced in the choroid plexus. At 10 min, the signal diffused to the entire CSF-containing ventricles, and by 100 min post injection, the Mn signal spread into the periventricular tissues that are in contact with the CSF [90]. Third, in marmosets, 1.5 h after the start of $MnCl_2$ infusion through the tail vein, the Mn signal was initially enhanced in the CP, and at the 2.5 h time point, the signal was detected in the parenchyma surrounding the ventricles. In contrast, throughout the entire 6 h infusion course, no Mn signal was detected in brain regions that are not adjacent to the ventricles [91].

These findings in cell models and animals suggest that a main route for Mn uptake into the brain is from the CP, through the CSF, and then to the brain parenchyma. The cell culture studies suggest that the BBB has a role in Mn transport, but it does not cause the accumulation of Mn in the brain from the blood. Meanwhile, the BCB preferentially transports Mn from the blood into the brain, potentially contributing to brain Mn overload. Since the brain endothelial cells appear to transport Mn in both directions, and CP epithelial cells transport more Mn into the brain than into the blood, future studies in cell models or in vivo could investigate transporters involved in unidirectional or bidirectional transport of manganese across endothelial or epithelial cells.

5. Future Directions

To further understand Mn homeostasis across the brain barriers, more in vitro models of the BBB and BCB that reflect the barrier qualities of each cell layer need to be developed. Cells modeling the BBB or BCB must polarize, form tight junctions, and prevent the diffusion of large or hydrophilic molecules. Such models are necessary to identify the efflux and influx of Mn through the cells of the brain barriers at different Mn concentrations. For example, Mn accumulation studies in animals indicated that Mn crosses the choroid plexus and quickly travels into the CSF, suggesting a major role for the BCB in Mn uptake. Cellular transport experiments in CP epithelial cells could distinguish how Mn is transported across the basolateral and apical membranes and would bolster the conclusion that the BCB is the primary site of Mn absorption into the brain. Due to the growing knowledge of Mn metabolism, modulators of Mn transport may be developed in the near future, but no such technology exists at this time. Fundamental research of brain Mn homeostasis may eventually facilitate the development of methods to control the balance of metals in the brain to limit the negative effects of excess Mn.

In vivo research is a necessary step to establish Mn transport mechanisms, but there are a few limitations of animal research in this area. To study Mn transport, there is the difficulty of identifying where Mn is concentrated within the brain parenchyma. In Mn overload conditions, it is unknown whether Mn accumulates in neurons and glia of specific brain regions or within the interstitial fluid and CSF. Most publications report brain Mn levels as the level of Mn in the whole brain homogenate, making it difficult to distinguish between Mn accumulating in brain cells or CSF and interstitial fluid. Future studies are needed to understand this important distinction. To function and fire quickly, neurons rely on steep ionic gradients between their intracellular environment and the surrounding interstitial fluid. Since the concentrations of Ca^{2+}, Na^+, K^+, and Cl^- would be vastly different when sampling either neurons or the extracellular fluid, we could logically understand that levels of other charged ions such as Mn^{2+} would be different within the neuron or out in the interstitial fluid. Additionally, astrocytes are known to release and take up ions and nutrients, while the brain has changing demands for these materials. Astrocytes may sequester Mn intracellularly or release it back into the interstitial fluid, leaving the total brain Mn concentration unchanged. When using a whole brain homogenate to measure metal levels, the extracellular environment around the BCB cannot be sampled separately. To accurately reflect the Mn concentrations on each side of the BCB, Mn levels in both CSF and blood can be measured. In addition, knowledge of Mn accumulation in separate brain compartments, as well as improved understanding of transporter expression in human and animal tissues, will help make significant advances in the field of Mn homeostasis within the brain barriers.

Author Contributions: Conceptualization, S.M.M., N.Z.; writing—original draft preparation, S.M.M.; writing—review and editing, S.M.M., N.Z.; supervision, N.Z.; project administration, N.Z.; funding acquisition, N.Z. All authors have read and agreed to the published version of the manuscript.

Funding: Research reported in this publication was supported by the National Institute of Diabetes and Digestive and Kidney Diseases (NIDDK) and the Office of Dietary Supplements (ODS) of the National Institutes of Health (NIH) (R01DK123113). The content is solely the responsibility of the authors and does not necessarily represent the official views of the National Institutes of Health.

Conflicts of Interest: The authors declare no conflict of interest.

References

1. Borgstahl, G.E.; Parge, H.E.; Hickey, M.J.; Beyer, W.F., Jr.; Hallewell, R.A.; Tainer, J.A. The structure of human mitochondrial manganese superoxide dismutase reveals a novel tetrameric interface of two 4-helix bundles. *Cell* **1992**, *71*, 107–118. [CrossRef]
2. Wedler, F.C.; Denman, R.B. Glutamine synthetase: The major Mn(II) enzyme in mammalian brain. *Curr. Top. Cell Regul.* **1984**, *24*, 153–169. [CrossRef] [PubMed]
3. Cersosimo, M.G.; Koller, W.C. The diagnosis of manganese-induced parkinsonism. *Neurotoxicology* **2006**, *27*, 340–346. [CrossRef]
4. Iyare, P.U. The effects of manganese exposure from drinking water on school-age children: A systematic review. *Neurotoxicology* **2019**, *73*, 1–7. [CrossRef]
5. Khan, K.; Wasserman, G.A.; Liu, X.; Ahmed, E.; Parvez, F.; Slavkovich, V.; Levy, D.; Mey, J.; van Geen, A.; Graziano, J.H.; et al. Manganese exposure from drinking water and children's academic achievement. *Neurotoxicology* **2012**, *33*, 91–97. [CrossRef] [PubMed]
6. Hernandez-Bonilla, D.; Escamilla-Nunez, C.; Mergler, D.; Rodriguez-Dozal, S.; Cortez-Lugo, M.; Montes, S.; Tristan-Lopez, L.A.; Catalan-Vazquez, M.; Schilmann, A.; Riojas-Rodriguez, H. Effects of manganese exposure on visuoperception and visual memory in schoolchildren. *Neurotoxicology* **2016**, *57*, 230–240. [CrossRef] [PubMed]
7. Bouchard, M.F.; Sauve, S.; Barbeau, B.; Legrand, M.; Brodeur, M.E.; Bouffard, T.; Limoges, E.; Bellinger, D.C.; Mergler, D. Intellectual impairment in school-age children exposed to manganese from drinking water. *Environ. Health Perspect.* **2011**, *119*, 138–143. [CrossRef]
8. Tuschl, K.; Mills, P.B.; Parsons, H.; Malone, M.; Fowler, D.; Bitner-Glindzicz, M.; Clayton, P.T. Hepatic cirrhosis, dystonia, polycythaemia and hypermanganesaemia—A new metabolic disorder. *J. Inherit. Metab. Dis.* **2008**, *31*, 151–163. [CrossRef]

9. Ribeiro, R.T.; dos Santos-Neto, D.; Braga-Neto, P.; Barsottini, O.G. Inherited manganism. *Clin. Neurol. Neurosurg.* **2013**, *115*, 1536–1538. [CrossRef]
10. Winslow, J.W.W.; Limesand, K.H.; Zhao, N. The Functions of ZIP8, ZIP14, and ZnT10 in the Regulation of Systemic Manganese Homeostasis. *Int. J. Mol. Sci.* **2020**, *21*, 3304. [CrossRef]
11. Kondakis, X.G.; Makris, N.; Leotsinidis, M.; Prinou, M.; Papapetropoulos, T. Possible health effects of high manganese concentration in drinking water. *Arch. Environ. Health* **1989**, *44*, 175–178. [CrossRef] [PubMed]
12. Bakulski, K.M.; Seo, Y.A.; Hickman, R.C.; Brandt, D.; Vadari, H.S.; Hu, H.; Park, S.K. Heavy Metals Exposure and Alzheimer's Disease and Related Dementias. *J. Alzheimers Dis.* **2020**, *76*, 1215–1242. [CrossRef] [PubMed]
13. Zhao, Y.; Zhao, B. Oxidative stress and the pathogenesis of Alzheimer's disease. *Oxid. Med. Cell. Longev.* **2013**, *2013*, 316523. [CrossRef]
14. Leuner, K.; Schutt, T.; Kurz, C.; Eckert, S.H.; Schiller, C.; Occhipinti, A.; Mai, S.; Jendrach, M.; Eckert, G.P.; Kruse, S.E.; et al. Mitochondrion-derived reactive oxygen species lead to enhanced amyloid beta formation. *Antioxid. Redox Signal.* **2012**, *16*, 1421–1433. [CrossRef] [PubMed]
15. Guilarte, T.R. APLP1, Alzheimer's-like pathology and neurodegeneration in the frontal cortex of manganese-exposed non-human primates. *Neurotoxicology* **2010**, *31*, 572–574. [CrossRef]
16. Guilarte, T.R.; Burton, N.C.; Verina, T.; Prabhu, V.V.; Becker, K.G.; Syversen, T.; Schneider, J.S. Increased APLP1 expression and neurodegeneration in the frontal cortex of manganese-exposed non-human primates. *J. Neurochem.* **2008**, *105*, 1948–1959. [CrossRef]
17. Lin, G.; Li, X.; Cheng, X.; Zhao, N.; Zheng, W. Manganese Exposure Aggravates beta-Amyloid Pathology by Microglial Activation. *Front. Aging Neurosci.* **2020**, *12*, 556008. [CrossRef]
18. Tong, Y.; Yang, H.; Tian, X.; Wang, H.; Zhou, T.; Zhang, S.; Yu, J.; Zhang, T.; Fan, D.; Guo, X.; et al. High manganese, a risk for Alzheimer's disease: High manganese induces amyloid-beta related cognitive impairment. *J. Alzheimers Dis.* **2014**, *42*, 865–878. [CrossRef]
19. Abbott, N.J.; Ronnback, L.; Hansson, E. Astrocyte-endothelial interactions at the blood-brain barrier. *Nat. Rev. Neurosci.* **2006**, *7*, 41–53. [CrossRef]
20. Ballabh, P.; Braun, A.; Nedergaard, M. The blood-brain barrier: An overview: Structure, regulation, and clinical implications. *Neurobiol. Dis.* **2004**, *16*, 1–13. [CrossRef]
21. Vermette, D.; Hu, P.; Canarie, M.F.; Funaro, M.; Glover, J.; Pierce, R.W. Tight junction structure, function, and assessment in the critically ill: A systematic review. *Intensive Care Med. Exp.* **2018**, *6*, 37. [CrossRef] [PubMed]
22. Umeda, K.; Ikenouchi, J.; Katahira-Tayama, S.; Furuse, K.; Sasaki, H.; Nakayama, M.; Matsui, T.; Tsukita, S.; Furuse, M.; Tsukita, S. ZO-1 and ZO-2 independently determine where claudins are polymerized in tight-junction strand formation. *Cell* **2006**, *126*, 741–754. [CrossRef]
23. Castro Dias, M.; Mapunda, J.A.; Vladymyrov, M.; Engelhardt, B. Structure and Junctional Complexes of Endothelial, Epithelial and Glial Brain Barriers. *Int. J. Mol. Sci.* **2019**, *20*, 5372. [CrossRef]
24. Ebnet, K.; Aurrand-Lions, M.; Kuhn, A.; Kiefer, F.; Butz, S.; Zander, K.; Meyer zu Brickwedde, M.K.; Suzuki, A.; Imhof, B.A.; Vestweber, D. The junctional adhesion molecule (JAM) family members JAM-2 and JAM-3 associate with the cell polarity protein PAR-3: A possible role for JAMs in endothelial cell polarity. *J. Cell Sci.* **2003**, *116*, 3879–3891. [CrossRef]
25. Saitou, M.; Furuse, M.; Sasaki, H.; Schulzke, J.D.; Fromm, M.; Takano, H.; Noda, T.; Tsukita, S. Complex phenotype of mice lacking occludin, a component of tight junction strands. *Mol. Biol. Cell* **2000**, *11*, 4131–4142. [CrossRef]
26. Lampugnani, M.G. Endothelial adherens junctions and the actin cytoskeleton: An 'infinity net'? *J. Biol.* **2010**, *9*, 16. [CrossRef] [PubMed]
27. Indra, I.; Hong, S.; Troyanovsky, R.; Kormos, B.; Troyanovsky, S. The adherens junction: A mosaic of cadherin and nectin clusters bundled by actin filaments. *J. Investig. Dermatol.* **2013**, *133*, 2546–2554. [CrossRef]
28. Armulik, A.; Genove, G.; Mae, M.; Nisancioglu, M.H.; Wallgard, E.; Niaudet, C.; He, L.; Norlin, J.; Lindblom, P.; Strittmatter, K.; et al. Pericytes regulate the blood-brain barrier. *Nature* **2010**, *468*, 557–561. [CrossRef] [PubMed]
29. Hill, R.A.; Tong, L.; Yuan, P.; Murikinati, S.; Gupta, S.; Grutzendler, J. Regional Blood Flow in the Normal and Ischemic Brain Is Controlled by Arteriolar Smooth Muscle Cell Contractility and Not by Capillary Pericytes. *Neuron* **2015**, *87*, 95–110. [CrossRef]
30. Dehouck, M.P.; Meresse, S.; Delorme, P.; Fruchart, J.C.; Cecchelli, R. An easier, reproducible, and mass-production method to study the blood-brain barrier in vitro. *J. Neurochem.* **1990**, *54*, 1798–1801. [CrossRef] [PubMed]
31. Ma, B.; Buckalew, R.; Du, Y.; Kiyoshi, C.M.; Alford, C.C.; Wang, W.; McTigue, D.M.; Enyeart, J.J.; Terman, D.; Zhou, M. Gap junction coupling confers isopotentiality on astrocyte syncytium. *Glia* **2016**, *64*, 214–226. [CrossRef]
32. Simard, M.; Nedergaard, M. The neurobiology of glia in the context of water and ion homeostasis. *Neuroscience* **2004**, *129*, 877–896. [CrossRef] [PubMed]
33. Motallebnejad, P.; Azarin, S.M. Chemically defined human vascular laminins for biologically relevant culture of hiPSC-derived brain microvascular endothelial cells. *Fluids Barriers CNS* **2020**, *17*, 54. [CrossRef] [PubMed]
34. Thomsen, M.S.; Routhe, L.J.; Moos, T. The vascular basement membrane in the healthy and pathological brain. *J. Cereb. Blood Flow Metab.* **2017**, *37*, 3300–3317. [CrossRef] [PubMed]

35. Van Itallie, C.M.; Holmes, J.; Bridges, A.; Gookin, J.L.; Coccaro, M.R.; Proctor, W.; Colegio, O.R.; Anderson, J.M. The density of small tight junction pores varies among cell types and is increased by expression of claudin-2. *J. Cell Sci.* **2008**, *121*, 298–305. [CrossRef] [PubMed]
36. Ganong, W.F. Circumventricular organs: Definition and role in the regulation of endocrine and autonomic function. *Clin. Exp. Pharmacol. Physiol.* **2000**, *27*, 422–427. [CrossRef]
37. Damkier, H.H.; Brown, P.D.; Praetorius, J. Cerebrospinal fluid secretion by the choroid plexus. *Physiol. Rev.* **2013**, *93*, 1847–1892. [CrossRef]
38. Serot, J.M.; Bene, M.C.; Faure, G.C. Choroid plexus, aging of the brain, and Alzheimer's disease. *Front. Biosci.* **2003**, *8*, s515–s521. [CrossRef]
39. Lun, M.P.; Monuki, E.S.; Lehtinen, M.K. Development and functions of the choroid plexus-cerebrospinal fluid system. *Nat. Rev. Neurosci.* **2015**, *16*, 445–457. [CrossRef]
40. Hofman, F.M.; Chen, T.C. Choroid Plexus: Structure and Function. In *The Choroid Plexus and Cerebrospinal Fluid*; Neman, J., Chen, T.C., Eds.; Academic Press: Cambridge, MA, USA, 2016; pp. 29–40.
41. Wojcik, E.; Carrithers, L.M.; Carrithers, M.D. Characterization of epithelial V-like antigen in human choroid plexus epithelial cells: Potential role in CNS immune surveillance. *Neurosci. Lett.* **2011**, *495*, 115–120. [CrossRef]
42. Strominger, I.; Elyahu, Y.; Berner, O.; Reckhow, J.; Mittal, K.; Nemirovsky, A.; Monsonego, A. The Choroid Plexus Functions as a Niche for T-Cell Stimulation Within the Central Nervous System. *Front. Immunol.* **2018**, *9*, 1066. [CrossRef]
43. Ransohoff, R.M.; Engelhardt, B. The anatomical and cellular basis of immune surveillance in the central nervous system. *Nat. Rev. Immunol.* **2012**, *12*, 623–635. [CrossRef] [PubMed]
44. Brown, P.D.; Davies, S.L.; Speake, T.; Millar, I.D. Molecular mechanisms of cerebrospinal fluid production. *Neuroscience* **2004**, *129*, 957–970. [CrossRef]
45. Wong, V.; Gumbiner, B.M. A synthetic peptide corresponding to the extracellular domain of occludin perturbs the tight junction permeability barrier. *J. Cell Biol.* **1997**, *136*, 399–409. [CrossRef]
46. Kominsky, S.L.; Tyler, B.; Sosnowski, J.; Brady, K.; Doucet, M.; Nell, D.; Smedley, J.G., 3rd; McClane, B.; Brem, H.; Sukumar, S. Clostridium perfringens enterotoxin as a novel-targeted therapeutic for brain metastasis. *Cancer Res.* **2007**, *67*, 7977–7982. [CrossRef]
47. Szczepkowska, A.; Kowalewska, M.; Skipor, J. Melatonin from slow-release implants upregulates claudin-2 in the ovine choroid plexus. *J. Physiol. Pharmacol.* **2019**, *70*, 249–254. [CrossRef]
48. Steinemann, A.; Galm, I.; Chip, S.; Nitsch, C.; Maly, I.P. Claudin-1, -2 and -3 Are Selectively Expressed in the Epithelia of the Choroid Plexus of the Mouse from Early Development and into Adulthood While Claudin-5 is Restricted to Endothelial Cells. *Front. Neuroanat.* **2016**, *10*, 16. [CrossRef] [PubMed]
49. Kratzer, I.; Vasiljevic, A.; Rey, C.; Fevre-Montange, M.; Saunders, N.; Strazielle, N.; Ghersi-Egea, J.F. Complexity and developmental changes in the expression pattern of claudins at the blood-CSF barrier. *Histochem. Cell Biol.* **2012**, *138*, 861–879. [CrossRef] [PubMed]
50. Solar, P.; Zamani, A.; Kubickova, L.; Dubovy, P.; Joukal, M. Choroid plexus and the blood-cerebrospinal fluid barrier in disease. *Fluids Barriers CNS* **2020**, *17*, 35. [CrossRef]
51. Shrestha, B.; Paul, D.; Pachter, J.S. Alterations in tight junction protein and IgG permeability accompany leukocyte extravasation across the choroid plexus during neuroinflammation. *J. Neuropathol. Exp. Neurol.* **2014**, *73*, 1047–1061. [CrossRef]
52. Johansson, C.; Stopa, E.; McMillan, P.; Roth, D.; Funk, J.; Krinke, G. The distributional nexus of choroid plexus to cerebrospinal fluid, ependyma and brain: Toxicologic/pathologic phenomena, periventricular destabilization, and lesion spread. *Toxicol. Pathol.* **2011**, *39*, 186–212. [CrossRef] [PubMed]
53. Spector, R.; Keep, R.F.; Robert Snodgrass, S.; Smith, Q.R.; Johanson, C.E. A balanced view of choroid plexus structure and function: Focus on adult humans. *Exp. Neurol.* **2015**, *267*, 78–86. [CrossRef] [PubMed]
54. Erickson, M.A.; Banks, W.A. Neuroimmune Axes of the Blood-Brain Barriers and Blood-Brain Interfaces: Bases for Physiological Regulation, Disease States, and Pharmacological Interventions. *Pharmacol. Rev.* **2018**, *70*, 278–314. [CrossRef]
55. Skjorringe, T.; Burkhart, A.; Johnsen, K.B.; Moos, T. Divalent metal transporter 1 (DMT1) in the brain: Implications for a role in iron transport at the blood-brain barrier, and neuronal and glial pathology. *Front. Mol. Neurosci.* **2015**, *8*, 19. [CrossRef] [PubMed]
56. Andrews, N.C. Forging a field: The golden age of iron biology. *Blood* **2008**, *112*, 219–230. [CrossRef]
57. Vincent, J.B.; Love, S. The binding and transport of alternative metals by transferrin. *Biochim. Biophys. Acta* **2012**, *1820*, 362–378. [CrossRef] [PubMed]
58. Herrera, C.; Pettiglio, M.A.; Bartnikas, T.B. Investigating the role of transferrin in the distribution of iron, manganese, copper, and zinc. *J. Biol. Inorg. Chem.* **2014**, *19*, 869–877. [CrossRef]
59. Neilands, J.B. Microbial iron compounds. *Annu. Rev. Biochem.* **1981**, *50*, 715–731. [CrossRef] [PubMed]
60. Bradbury, M.W. The developing experimental approach to the idea of a blood-brain barrier. *Ann. N. Y. Acad. Sci.* **1986**, *481*, 137–141. [CrossRef]
61. Garrick, M.D.; Kuo, H.C.; Vargas, F.; Singleton, S.; Zhao, L.; Smith, J.J.; Paradkar, P.; Roth, J.A.; Garrick, L.M. Comparison of mammalian cell lines expressing distinct isoforms of divalent metal transporter 1 in a tetracycline-regulated fashion. *Biochem. J.* **2006**, *398*, 539–546. [CrossRef] [PubMed]

62. Trinder, D.; Oates, P.S.; Thomas, C.; Sadleir, J.; Morgan, E.H. Localisation of divalent metal transporter 1 (DMT1) to the microvillus membrane of rat duodenal enterocytes in iron deficiency, but to hepatocytes in iron overload. *Gut* **2000**, *46*, 270–276. [CrossRef]
63. Enerson, B.E.; Drewes, L.R. The rat blood-brain barrier transcriptome. *J. Cereb. Blood Flow Metab.* **2006**, *26*, 959–973. [CrossRef]
64. Moos, T.; Skjoerringe, T.; Gosk, S.; Morgan, E.H. Brain capillary endothelial cells mediate iron transport into the brain by segregating iron from transferrin without the involvement of divalent metal transporter 1. *J. Neurochem.* **2006**, *98*, 1946–1958. [CrossRef] [PubMed]
65. Siddappa, A.J.; Rao, R.B.; Wobken, J.D.; Casperson, K.; Leibold, E.A.; Connor, J.R.; Georgieff, M.K. Iron deficiency alters iron regulatory protein and iron transport protein expression in the perinatal rat brain. *Pediatr. Res.* **2003**, *53*, 800–807. [CrossRef]
66. Moos, T.; Morgan, E.H. The significance of the mutated divalent metal transporter (DMT1) on iron transport into the Belgrade rat brain. *J. Neurochem.* **2004**, *88*, 233–245. [CrossRef]
67. Steimle, B.L.; Smith, F.M.; Kosman, D.J. The solute carriers ZIP8 and ZIP14 regulate manganese accumulation in brain microvascular endothelial cells and control brain manganese levels. *J. Biol. Chem.* **2019**, *294*, 19197–19208. [CrossRef] [PubMed]
68. Han, M.; Chang, J.; Kim, J. Loss of divalent metal transporter 1 function promotes brain copper accumulation and increases impulsivity. *J. Neurochem.* **2016**, *138*, 918–928. [CrossRef] [PubMed]
69. Aydemir, T.B.; Cousins, R.J. The Multiple Faces of the Metal Transporter ZIP14 (SLC39A14). *J. Nutr.* **2018**, *148*, 174–184. [CrossRef]
70. Scheiber, I.F.; Wu, Y.; Morgan, S.E.; Zhao, N. The intestinal metal transporter ZIP14 maintains systemic manganese homeostasis. *J. Biol. Chem.* **2019**, *294*, 9147–9160. [CrossRef] [PubMed]
71. Aydemir, T.B.; Thorn, T.L.; Ruggiero, C.H.; Pompilus, M.; Febo, M.; Cousins, R.J. Intestine-specific deletion of metal transporter Zip14 (Slc39a14) causes brain manganese overload and locomotor defects of manganism. *Am. J. Physiol. Gastrointest. Liver Physiol.* **2020**, *318*, G673–G681. [CrossRef] [PubMed]
72. Felber, D.M.; Wu, Y.; Zhao, N. Regulation of the Metal Transporters ZIP14 and ZnT10 by Manganese Intake in Mice. *Nutrients* **2019**, *11*, 2099. [CrossRef] [PubMed]
73. Morgan, S.E.; Schroten, H.; Ishikawa, H.; Zhao, N. Localization of ZIP14 and ZIP8 in HIBCPP Cells. *Brain Sci.* **2020**, *10*, 534. [CrossRef]
74. Scheiber, I.F.; Alarcon, N.O.; Zhao, N. Manganese Uptake by A549 Cells is Mediated by Both ZIP8 and ZIP14. *Nutrients* **2019**, *11*, 1473. [CrossRef] [PubMed]
75. Thompson, K.J.; Wessling-Resnick, M. ZIP14 is degraded in response to manganese exposure. *Biometals* **2019**, *32*, 829–843. [CrossRef]
76. Quadri, M.; Federico, A.; Zhao, T.; Breedveld, G.J.; Battisti, C.; Delnooz, C.; Severijnen, L.A.; Di Toro Mammarella, L.; Mignarri, A.; Monti, L.; et al. Mutations in SLC30A10 cause parkinsonism and dystonia with hypermanganesemia, polycythemia, and chronic liver disease. *Am. J. Hum. Genet.* **2012**, *90*, 467–477. [CrossRef] [PubMed]
77. Tuschl, K.; Clayton, P.T.; Gospe, S.M., Jr.; Gulab, S.; Ibrahim, S.; Singhi, P.; Aulakh, R.; Ribeiro, R.T.; Barsottini, O.G.; Zaki, M.S.; et al. Syndrome of hepatic cirrhosis, dystonia, polycythemia, and hypermanganesemia caused by mutations in SLC30A10, a manganese transporter in man. *Am. J. Hum. Genet.* **2012**, *90*, 457–466. [CrossRef] [PubMed]
78. Taylor, C.A.; Hutchens, S.; Liu, C.; Jursa, T.; Shawlot, W.; Aschner, M.; Smith, D.R.; Mukhopadhyay, S. SLC30A10 transporter in the digestive system regulates brain manganese under basal conditions while brain SLC30A10 protects against neurotoxicity. *J. Biol. Chem.* **2019**, *294*, 1860–1876. [CrossRef]
79. Leyva-Illades, D.; Chen, P.; Zogzas, C.E.; Hutchens, S.; Mercado, J.M.; Swaim, C.D.; Morrisett, R.A.; Bowman, A.B.; Aschner, M.; Mukhopadhyay, S. SLC30A10 is a cell surface-localized manganese efflux transporter, and parkinsonism-causing mutations block its intracellular trafficking and efflux activity. *J. Neurosci.* **2014**, *34*, 14079–14095. [CrossRef]
80. Bosomworth, H.J.; Thornton, J.K.; Coneyworth, L.J.; Ford, D.; Valentine, R.A. Efflux function, tissue-specific expression and intracellular trafficking of the Zn transporter ZnT10 indicate roles in adult Zn homeostasis. *Metallomics* **2012**, *4*, 771–779. [CrossRef]
81. Bosomworth, H.J.; Adlard, P.A.; Ford, D.; Valentine, R.A. Altered expression of ZnT10 in Alzheimer's disease brain. *PLoS ONE* **2013**, *8*, e65475. [CrossRef]
82. Saunders, N.R.; Dziegielewska, K.M.; Mollgard, K.; Habgood, M.D.; Wakefield, M.J.; Lindsay, H.; Stratzielle, N.; Ghersi-Egea, J.F.; Liddelow, S.A. Influx mechanisms in the embryonic and adult rat choroid plexus: A transcriptome study. *Front. Neurosci.* **2015**, *9*, 123. [CrossRef]
83. Fleming, S.M.; Santiago, N.A.; Mullin, E.J.; Pamphile, S.; Karkare, S.; Lemkuhl, A.; Ekhator, O.R.; Linn, S.C.; Holden, J.G.; Aga, D.S.; et al. The effect of manganese exposure in Atp13a2-deficient mice. *Neurotoxicology* **2018**, *64*, 256–266. [CrossRef]
84. Ugolino, J.; Dziki, K.M.; Kim, A.; Wu, J.J.; Vogel, B.E.; Monteiro, M.J. Overexpression of human Atp13a2Isoform-1 protein protects cells against manganese and starvation-induced toxicity. *PLoS ONE* **2019**, *14*, e0220849. [CrossRef]
85. Chiba, Y.; Murakami, R.; Matsumoto, K.; Wakamatsu, K.; Nonaka, W.; Uemura, N.; Yanase, K.; Kamada, M.; Ueno, M. Glucose, Fructose, and Urate Transporters in the Choroid Plexus Epithelium. *Int. J. Mol. Sci.* **2020**, *21*, 7230. [CrossRef] [PubMed]
86. Hladky, S.B.; Barrand, M.A. Fluid and ion transfer across the blood-brain and blood-cerebrospinal fluid barriers; a comparative account of mechanisms and roles. *Fluids Barriers CNS* **2016**, *13*, 19. [CrossRef]
87. Deane, R.; Segal, M.B. The transport of sugars across the perfused choroid plexus of the sheep. *J. Physiol.* **1985**, *362*, 245–260. [CrossRef] [PubMed]

88. Bornhorst, J.; Wehe, C.A.; Huwel, S.; Karst, U.; Galla, H.J.; Schwerdtle, T. Impact of manganese on and transfer across blood-brain and blood-cerebrospinal fluid barrier in vitro. *J. Biol. Chem.* **2012**, *287*, 17140–17151. [CrossRef]
89. Yu, X.; Wadghiri, Y.Z.; Sanes, D.H.; Turnbull, D.H. In vivo auditory brain mapping in mice with Mn-enhanced MRI. *Nat. Neurosci.* **2005**, *8*, 961–968. [CrossRef]
90. Aoki, I.; Wu, Y.J.; Silva, A.C.; Lynch, R.M.; Koretsky, A.P. In vivo detection of neuroarchitecture in the rodent brain using manganese-enhanced MRI. *Neuroimage* **2004**, *22*, 1046–1059. [CrossRef] [PubMed]
91. Bock, N.A.; Paiva, F.F.; Nascimento, G.C.; Newman, J.D.; Silva, A.C. Cerebrospinal fluid to brain transport of manganese in a non-human primate revealed by MRI. *Brain Res.* **2008**, *1198*, 160–170. [CrossRef] [PubMed]

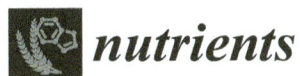

Review

The Protective and Long-Lasting Effects of Human Milk Oligosaccharides on Cognition in Mammals

Sylvia Docq [1], Marcia Spoelder [1], Wendan Wang [2] and Judith R. Homberg [1,*]

[1] Department of Cognitive Neuroscience, Donders Institute for Brain, Cognition and Behaviour, Radboud University Medical Center, 6525 EN Nijmegen, The Netherlands; Sylvia.Docq@radboudumc.nl (S.D.); Marcia.Spoelder-Merkens@radboudumc.nl (M.S.)
[2] Inner Mongolia Yili Industrial Group, Co., Ltd., Jinshan road 1, Hohhot 010110, China; wangwendan@yili.com
* Correspondence: Judith.homberg@radboudumc.nl; Tel.: +31-24-3610906

Received: 30 September 2020; Accepted: 19 November 2020; Published: 21 November 2020

Abstract: Over the last few years, research indicated that Human Milk Oligosaccharides (HMOs) may serve to enhance cognition during development. HMOs hereby provide an exciting avenue in the understanding of the molecular mechanisms that contribute to cognitive development. Therefore, this review aims to summarize the reported observations regarding the effects of HMOs on memory and cognition in rats, mice and piglets. Our main findings illustrate that the administration of fucosylated (single or combined with Lacto-N-neoTetraose (LNnT) and other oligosaccharides) and sialylated HMOs results in marked improvements in spatial memory and an accelerated learning rate in operant tasks. Such beneficial effects of HMOs on cognition already become apparent during infancy, especially when the behavioural tasks are cognitively more demanding. When animals age, its effects become increasingly more apparent in simpler tasks as well. Furthermore, the combination of HMOs with other oligosaccharides yields different effects on memory performance as opposed to single HMO administration. In addition, an enhanced hippocampal long-term potentiation (LTP) response both at a young and at a mature age are reported as well. These results point towards the possibility that HMOs administered either in singular or combination forms have long-lasting, beneficial effects on memory and cognition in mammals.

Keywords: human milk oligosaccharides; cognition; brain development; animal behaviour; fucosyllactose; sialyllactose; long term potentiation

1. Introduction

The natural composition of breast milk is well recognized as the golden standard of infant nutrition [1] and is associated with long-term health benefits [2–10]. Studies have shown that exclusive breastfeeding is accompanied by a reduced risk for developing medical conditions during childhood such as gastrointestinal infections (e.g., necrotizing enterocolitis) [5,6]. Indications that breastfeeding confers protective effects in the onset and course of allergic diseases such as atopic dermatitis, food allergy and asthma have also emerged over the recent years [7–9]. Such protective effects of breastfeeding have been attributed to multiple factors related to the gut, as it is found that breastfeeding can improve immune functioning, promoting a healthy gut microflora [11]. Apart from the gut, bioactive components within breast milk such as the adipokines (e.g., leptin, ghrelin) help regulate appetite control and energy intake. Breast milk also contains growth factors, such as neuronal growth factors (NGF) and epidermal growth factors (EGF), which exert trophic effects on the neonatal nervous system and enhance gastrointestinal mucosal maturation respectively [11–13]. In recent years, the mental health benefits that breastfeeding provides have garnered much more attention in neuroscientific research. Notably, breastfeeding is associated with improved cognitive development, as demonstrated by improved IQ scores [14] and a reduced risk of childhood behavioural disorders [15,16]. These findings also coincide with studies showing enhanced brain development parameters, such as white matter development in frontal and temporal regions [17] and maturation of the basal ganglia and thalamus [18]. On the whole, these studies indicate that there are clear developmental and cognitive benefits related to breastfeeding and breast milk, which raises the question: which breast milk factors facilitate cognitive development?

Breast milk is a complex liquid which contains many different lipids (such as the Milk Fat Globule rich in phospholipids and long chain fatty acids), an assortment of vitamins (Vitamin A, B, C, D K), sialic acid (both in free form and bound to oligosaccharides, glycoproteins and glycolipids) and other biologically active components, some of which affect neurodevelopment [19–22]. Of particular interest to infant nutrition and development are the Human Milk Oligosaccharides (HMOs). These non-digestible carbohydrates are the third most abundant class of breast milk components, and over 200 HMOs, comprised out of 5 monosaccharides (glucose, galactose, N-Acetyl-Glucosamine, fucose and sialic acid) have thus far been identified [23]. HMOs have recently moved into the spotlight of cognitive research due to its widespread effects on infant development and cognition [4,11,20]. There are three main families of HMOs; the non-fucosylated neutral HMOs, (e.g., Lacto-N-neoTetraose (LNnT)), the fucosylated HMOs (e.g., 2′Fucosyllactose (2′-FL)) and the sialylated (SL) HMOs (e.g., 3′Sialyllactose (3-SL) and 6′-Sialyllactose (6-SL)) [23,24]. Oligosaccharides are present in all mammalian milk [25]. However, what makes human milk unique compared to other mammalian milk is that it contains the largest diversity of complex oligosaccharides [25,26] and high concentrations of 2′-FL. It should be noted that the presence of 2′-FL is subject to large inter individual variation depending on the Lewis antigen blood group system of the mother, which encompasses two genes; the Lewis gene (Le gene or FUT-3 gene) and the Secretor gene (Se gene or FUT-2 gene) [27]. Depending on genetic expression, women are either defined as "secretors" (Se+), or "non secretors" (Se-), and Lewis positive (Le+) or Lewis negative (Le-) [23,27]. Both Secretor and Lewis genes are responsible for yielding fucosyltransferase-2 (FUT-2) and fucosyltransferase-3 (FUT-2) respectively, which append fucose to the core oligosaccharides. Depending on which of these FUT enzymes are active, different oligosaccharides will be created; as FUT2 expression results in the synthesis of 2′-FL, while FUT3 expression has been associated with the formation of LNFP-II instead [28–30]. These polymorphisms essentially give rise to four major milk groups within the human population, as both genes can be active, inactive or either one of the two is active, hereby resulting in a variable HMO content in breast milk [29]. Around 60–72% of the maternal population are secretors, and the milk of these "secretor mothers" contains an overall higher concentration of HMOs in breastmilk as compared to non-secretors [23,27,31,32]. All in all, a large variability exists within the human population concerning the exact proportions of different HMOs [28]. Moreover, HMOs are also subject to dynamic changes within the same breastfeeding female, depending on factors such as circadian rhythm, lactation stage, maternal diet, and maternal genetic background [4,11,20,28–34].

Supplementation of infant formula with HMOs renders the composition and downstream effects of infant formula to become closer to those of breastmilk. One of the well-documented advantages of HMOs is its prebiotic role and the capacity to regulate the immune system in the periphery. HMOs can exert antimicrobial and antiviral effects by binding to pathogens which reach the mucosal surfaces in the gut or by directly binding to the gut epithelial receptors, effectively blocking the access of pathogens [11,20]. Experimental studies in infants showed enhancing effects on the immune response of additional 2′-FL supplementation. Goehring and colleagues [35] observed that infants who were fed breastmilk or a 2′-FL enriched formula had lower concentrations of plasma inflammatory cytokines (IL-1α, IL-1ß, IL-6, TNF-α) when compared to children fed the ordinary (non-enriched) infant formula [35]. Furthermore, ex vivo stimulation of peripheral blood mononuclear cells (PBMCs) yielded lower levels of TNF-α and IL-6 when infants were breastfed or were on a 2-′FL enriched diet. Enriching infant formula with 2′-FL and LNnT also renders the gut microbiome composition and its metabolites (propionate, butyrate and lactate) of formula-fed infants closer to that of breastfed infants [36]. It stands to reason that, if the supplementation of HMOs to infant formula produces immunological and health responses similar to those of breastfed infants, this may also partly account for cognitive outcomes [14]. Indeed, apart from HMOs involvement in immune functioning, a recent study by Berger and colleagues [37] reported that the amount of 2′-FL, measured in mother's breast milk one month after birth, predicted improved cognitive outcomes in two-year-old children. Since it is known that alterations in the immune system impacts brain development and later life cognitive functioning [38], it is possible that the HMO mediated immune response provides a route via which HMOs could contribute to cognition. Thus, investigating how HMOs impact underlying neural mechanisms of their associated cognitive outcomes will provide valuable insight in HMOs' role in brain development and functioning.

While there have been correlational studies exploring the role of HMOs on development in humans, no direct human study has thus far investigated both immune and cognitive outcomes with HMO analysis in breast milk or upon HMO supplementation in infant formula. However, direct studies on the effects of HMOs and cognition have been undertaken in murine models and piglets. While there are obvious differences between species, several animal models have been used extensively in behavioural research due to their translational value in brain development and behaviour. The behavioural tasks used in animal models in probing various cognitive functions are well validated [39]. Moreover, since the life span of rodents in particular is relatively short, animal models allow the investigation of the most sensitive developmental period to HMO supplementation. In addition, behavioural studies in animals can be corroborated by more invasive measures in vivo, granting a live view on the underlying neurobiological processes. One method commonly used in rodent memory studies is electrophysiology. Long Term Potentiation (LTP) involves the strengthening of synapses in response to prior stimulation during memory formation and retrieval. This produces a long-lasting shift in synaptic strength and is therefore an important underlying mechanism of synaptic plasticity and memory [40]. Findings derived from preclinical work could prove to be informative and may serve as input to future longitudinal studies on the contribution of HMOs to the cognitive development of humans.

This review's aim is twofold. Firstly, it aims to summarize the effects of HMOs in animal research and their subsequent cognitive and electrophysiological outcomes. Special consideration is given to the type of HMO used (e.g., fucosylated (2′-FL), neutral (LNnT) and sialylated (3′-SL, 6′-SL)), the age of the animals upon HMO administration, the used cognitive task complexity and the age of the animals during testing. Its second purpose is to provide additional interesting avenues for future research to explore. The search for relevant articles was conducted in Pubmed in the period of 1979 until August 2020, using a specialized search string comprised of both Mesh terms and key words in the title and abstract (Appendix A). This resulted in the inclusion of nine articles that contained (1) an animal model, (2) HMOs and (3) cognitive behavioural tests.

2. Assessing the Effects of HMOs on Cognitive Measures in Animal Models

Rodents and piglets are naturally curious and intelligent animals, which results in their frequent use as animal models for the assessment of cognition in a wide variety of behavioural tasks [41–45]. Behavioural tests are considered to be a valid, minimally invasive way to expose underlying cognitive processes, under the condition that the animal is capable of, and facilitated in, expressing such processes externally. In the context of HMO research, the focus has mainly been on memory and learning behaviour as cognitive capabilities. In the following sections, we will first graphically present an overview of the animal tests which investigated the consequences of HMOs on cognition. Subsequently, we present the main findings of the selected nine articles, grouped by the type of HMO (fucosylated or sialylated), in Table 1. Thereafter, the main results will be described, which is then followed by a discussion about the implications of the findings reported in the investigations.

The type of behavioural tests used to study the effects of HMOs on cognition make use of either the intrinsic rewarding value of an animal's natural curiosity in new exposures (Figure 1A,B,E) [41,42], the aversion to uncontrolled swimming without a platform to rest on (Figure 1D) [43] or the willingness to obtain an extrinsic reward like food or water (Figure 1C,F,G) [44,45]. Since animals prefer to be exposed to new items or environments to explore, the time spent to explore this new item or environment can be used as a measure for spatial or recognition memory. The willingness to obtain a food or water reward is commonly measured in operant conditioning tasks in either a skinner box or an Intellicage [44,45]. Operant conditioning tasks encompass associative learning paradigms, in which certain behaviour is reinforced via a reward or a punishment. In operant conditioning, different reinforcement schedules exist, such as the Fixed Ratio (FR) schedule, in which animals have to reach a certain criterion before they receive a reward. For example, an FR(4) schedule requires 4 correct responses from the animal in order for it to obtain a reward.

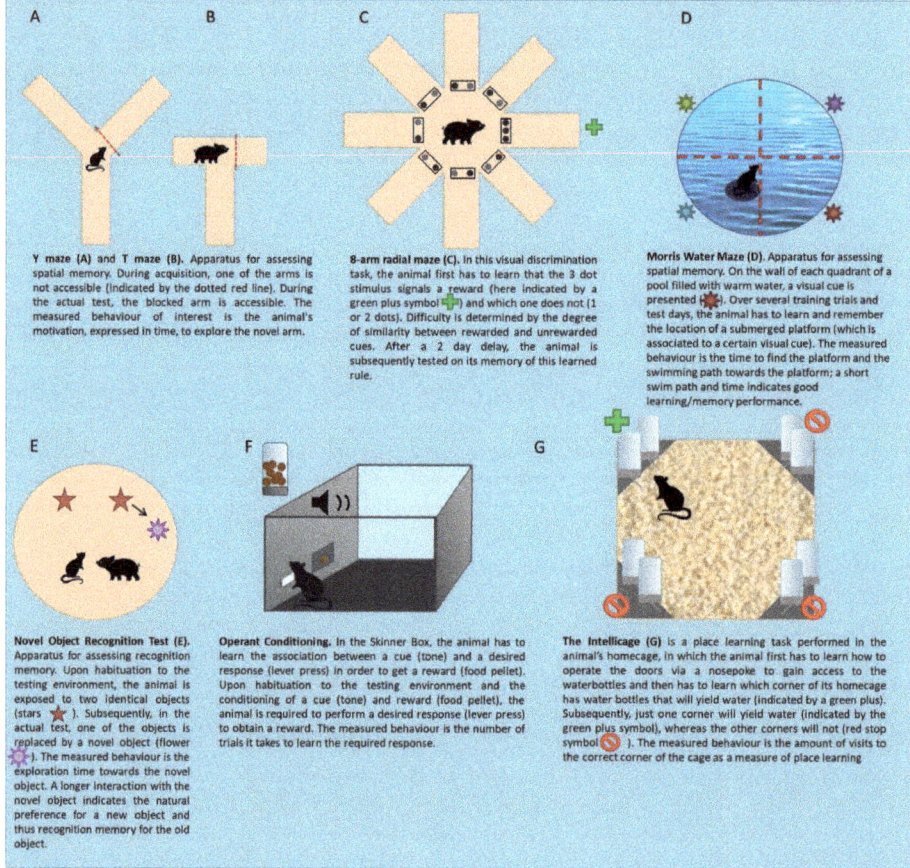

Figure 1. Summary of the behavioural tests used in the HMO studies. The type of animal placed inside the test (rodent or piglet) corresponds to the animal model used in the behavioural paradigms included in this review.

Overall, these cognitive tasks can be grouped by the level of complexity, as tasks that require a few trials are considered to be easier to perform than a task that requires weeks of training. In light of this, we have grouped the Y maze, T maze, Morris Water Maze (MWM) and the Novel Object Recognition

Test (NORT) as simple cognitive tests and the 8-arm radial maze and the operant tasks (Skinner box and Intellicage) as the complex cognitive tasks.

3. Effects of HMOs on Cognition in Mammals

3.1. Main Behavioural Findings

Supplementing mammals with additional HMOs leads to beneficial cognitive outcomes under certain specific circumstances (Table 1, Figure 2). In general, both fucosylated and sialylated HMOs contribute to an improved memory performance and faster learning speed (tests described in Figure 1A–G) when tested in mature adulthood, irrespective of the age of administration of these HMOs (e.g., during infancy or adulthood) [46–54].

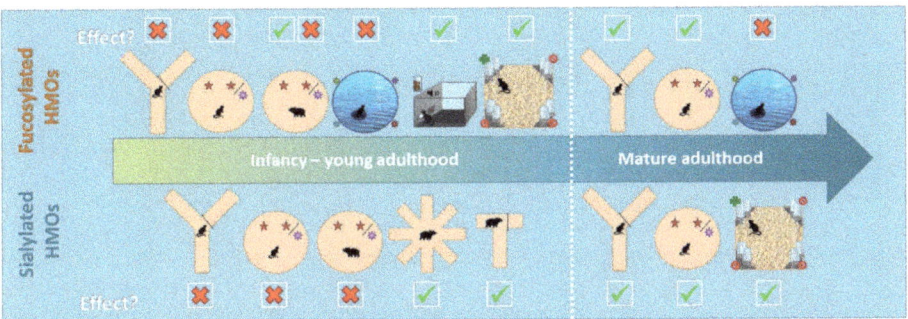

Figure 2. Graphical summary of behavioural tests results. The results have been grouped based on the type of HMO (Fucosylated versus Sialylated), animal model (rodents versus piglets) and the age of when the behavioural test has been performed. Infancy–young adulthood has been defined as the period ranging from PND1–6 months of age, while mature adulthood encompasses animals of 1 year old. Red crosses indicate that no significant differences were observed between the HMO and the control group, while green check marks indicate that positive effects due to HMO supplementation were reported. Details on the nature of such effects are summarized in Table 1.

3.1.1. Simple Cognitive Tasks

When rodents performed spatial and recognition memory tests during adolescence and early adulthood, no effects of either fucosylated or sialylated HMOs, as assessed by the NORT (when tested 24 h after the acquisition phase), MWM and the Y maze, were reported. Contrary to the rodent studies, three piglet studies showed that supplementing HMOs during the lactation period resulted in improved spatial memory (T maze) in infancy [51] and object recognition (NORT) [52,53]. Supplementing only oligofructose or the combination of 2′FL and LNnT increased object recognition when piglets were tested one hour after the acquisition phase. When tested 48 h later, only the piglets who received a combination of either Bovine Milk Oligosaccharides (mostly neutral non fucosylated oligosaccharides) and 2′FL and LNnT [52] or Oligofructose and 2′-FL [53] displayed long-term recognition memory. In mature adulthood (older than 1 year), rodent studies also found significant differences in both the Y maze and the NORT for both sialylated and fucosylated HMOs. However, the sialyllactose piglet study performed by Fleming and colleagues [54] yielded no results. In this study, they found no differences between the sialyllactose group and control group on the NORT performed during infancy.

Table 1. Summary behavioural studies.

Study	Species	HMO Component and Dose	Age and Duration Administration	Age Test	Tests	Key Results
		Fucosylated HMOs				
Oliveros et al., 2016 [46]	Lister Hooded Rats	2′-FL (1 g/KG/BW)	From PND 3–weaning	Long Term study: (1) 4–6 weeks (2) 1 year old	NORT Y maze MWM LTP (only at 1 year)	At 6 weeks of age no differences in behaviour ($n = 12$) were found. At 1 year of age, 2′-FL rats showed improved performance in the NORT and Y-maze paradigms. No effect was observed in the MWM. LTP was more intense and long lasting in the 2′-FL supplemented groups ($n = 10$)
	Sprague Dawley Rats	2′-FL (1 g/KG/BW)	From PND3 until week 6	Short Term study: 6 weeks	LTP	LTP was more intense and long lasting in the 2′-FL supplemented groups ($n = 10$).
Vazquez et al., 2016 [48]	Sprague Dawley Rats	2′FL (350 mg/kg/BW via AIN-93M diet) L-Fucose (Fuc) (equimolar amounts of fuc and 2′-FL via AIN-93M diet)	3–4.5 months old for 5 weeks	Started at 2.5–4 months old	Operant conditioning (FR1) LTP	2′-FL but not fuc displayed enhanced LTP. Vagotomy inhibited the effects of oral 2′-FL on LTP ($n = 10$) and operant learning paradigms ($n = 10$).
Fleming et al., 2020a [52]	Pigs (1050 Cambro genetics)	Three groups: Oligofructose (OF) 5 g/L OF + 2′-FL 5 g/L OF + 1 g/L 2′-FL Control. Nothing	PND 2-33	PND 22	NORT	Pigs ($n = 12$) who received Oligofructose (OF) displayed enhanced object recognition when tested 1 h after being habituated to the two objects. When pigs consumed both 2′-FL and OF, they showed improved recognition memory after a 48-h delay.
Fleming et al., 2020b [53]	Pigs (1050 Cambro genetics)	Four groups: HMOs (2′FL + LNnT) 1 g/L 2′-FL + 0.5 g/L LNnT BMOs 12.4 g/L HMOs + BMOs 1 g/L 2′-FL + 0.5 g/L LNnT + 12.4 g/L BMOs Control. Nothing	PND 2-33	PND 22	NORT	Pigs ($n = 12$) who received only HMOs displayed enhanced object recognition when tested 1 h after being habituated to the two objects. When pigs consumed both HMOs and BMOs, they showed improved recognition memory after a 48-h delay.

Table 1. Cont.

Study	Species	HMO Component and Dose	Age and Duration Administration	Age Test	Tests	Key Results
Fucosylated HMOs						
Vazquez et al., 2015 [46]	Sprague Dawley Rats	2′FL (1 g/Kg/BW) via oral gavage during acute administration and 2′-FL (350 mg/Kg/BW) via AIN-93G diet, during short time feeding	Acute administration: when rats were 3 months old. Short-time feeding from 2.5–4 months, for 5 weeks	Operant tests started when administration started. LTP was performed after administration period.	Operant conditioning (FR1) LTP	2′-FL groups performed better in operant learning paradigms (rats $n = 10$, mice $n = 28$) and showed an enhanced LTP response (rats and mice $n = 8$). The long-time supplementation of 2′FL also increased the expression of molecules involved in storage newly acquired memories (BDNF, PSD-95 phosphorylated CamKII, etc.)
	C57BL/6 mice	2′FL (350 mg/Kg/BW via AIN-93G diet)	Long-time feeding from 2–3.5 months old, for 12 weeks		Intellicage (FR1, FR4, FR8) LTP	
Sialylated HMOs						
Oliveros et al., 2018 [47]	Sprague Dawley Rats	Neu5Ac 6′-SL (Dose ranged from 400 mg/Kg/BW to 2600 mg/Kg/BW based on theoretical model)	From PND 3 until weaning	After weaning 1 year old	NORT Y maze NORT Y maze Intellicage LTP	No effects detected after weaning ($n = 10$). At 1 year old, sia (Neu5Ac and 6′-SL) exposed rats ($n = 8$?) showed improved performance on all the behavioural tests (NORT, Y-maze, Intellicage) and showed enhanced LTP ($n = 10$) when compared to the control group. Of the SL supplemented animals, the 6′-SL group performed better than the Neu5AC group
Wang et al., 2007 [50]	Piglets Landrace/Large White cross	Sialic Acid (ingredient of Casein glycomacropeptide cGMP) (4 groups of animals with their own dose each; 0 mg/L (control), 140 mg/L; 300 mg/L, 635 mg/L and 830 mg/L)	From PND 3 until end of experiment	PND 21–PND 35	8-arm Radial maze	Supplemented groups ($n = 12$–14 per group) required less trials to learn the required response, with a dose–response correlation for the difficult task.
Obelitz-Ryom et al., 2019 [51]	Pre-term delivered (experimental groups) Piglets Landrace x Yorkshire x Duroc	Sialyllactose (6′-SL + 3′-SL) (380 mg/L) Lactose (control) (6000 mg/L)	PND1–PND19	PND13–PND18	Spatial T-maze	Four experimental groups were included in the study; PRE-SAL ($n = 10$ ♀, 10 ♂), PRE-CON ($n = 9$ ♀, 11 ♂), TERM-CON ($n = 9$ ♀, 5 ♂) and TERM-SAL ($n = 6$ ♀, 6 ♂). TERM CON piglets reached learning criteria of 80% correct choices on day 3, PRE-SAL on day 4 and PRE-CON on day 5. More PRE-SAL piglets reached the T maze learning criteria compared to PRE-CON piglets. Upregulation of genes for sialic acid metabolism, myelination and ganglioside biosynthesis were present in the hippocampus of SL supplemented preterm piglets.
	Term delivered piglets (reference groups) Landrace x Yorkshire x Duroc	Lactose (control) (6000 mg/L) Pig's milk (under natural rearing conditions)				
Fleming et al., 2018 [54]	Piglets (no breed specified)	Sialyllactose (380 mg/L)	PND2–PND22	PND15–PND22	NORT	No effects ($n = 17$) were observed.

NORT: Novel Object Recognition Test, MWM: Morris Water Maze, LTP: Long-Term Potentiation. BMO: Bovine Milk Oligosaccharide. When provided, strains of species have been included in the table. In all studies presented here, the HMOs were administered orally. All animals used in the studies were male, unless otherwise specified. When the experimental groups have not been detailed in the key results column, the reported n indicates the number of animals per experimental group of that study.

3.1.2. Complex Cognitive Tasks

When considering the tasks that probe conditioning and learning capabilities and in which the cognitive difficulty could be varied, such as the 8-arm radial maze [50] and operant tasks [47–49], beneficial effects of HMO already surface at a young age in rats, mice and piglets alike. These effects also persist throughout adulthood. Perhaps the beneficial effects of HMOs become especially apparent upon increments on the cognitive load to meet the task demands.

3.2. Effects of HMOs on Long Term Potentiation (LTP)

The method of in vivo LTP induction in the studies listed here involved the implanting of stimulating electrodes on the Schaffer's collateral of the dorsal hippocampus and 2 to 4 recording electrodes in the stratum radiatum underneath CA1 [46–49]. A high frequency stimulation (200-Hz trains of pulses, 100 ms each and presented repeatedly with 1-min intervals) was delivered to the Schaffer's collateral and 30 min later the field excitatory post-synaptic potentials (fEPSPs) were recorded. Enhanced LTP responses are reported in all these studies [46–49], both after weaning and during adulthood, when animals were supplemented with fucosylated or sialylated HMOs.

4. Discussion

To the best of our knowledge, this review is the first to summarise the effects of fucosylated and sialylated HMOs on cognition and electrophysiological brain recordings in rodents and piglets. The effects of both types of HMOs uncovered in the reported investigations unequivocally point towards long lasting beneficial effects on cognition and memory, which is further supported by changes in the underlying physiological mechanisms as measured by LTP [46–49].

The majority of the reported animal studies, included in Table 1, revealed that HMOs enhance learning and memory. For the simple cognitive tasks, the effects of HMOs are not unequivocal, as differences are observed between the animal model used, task parameters, the dosage used and age of administration and testing. It should be noted that in the majority of the studies, the HMO dosage was comparable to concentrations found in human milk [28–31,33], and effects of HMO supplementation were already visible at these physiological relevant dosages.

In rodents, no significant effects on spatial memory or long-term recognition memory are reported when the animals' age ranges from juvenile to young adulthood. In piglets, HMOs are found to affect spatial memory and intermediate recognition memory but not long-term recognition memory when they were fed only HMOs during infancy. Inter species differences between rodents and piglets may help to explain why effects of HMO administration are visible in piglets but not in rodents when tested at a very young age. The third trimester in human gestation coincides with the first ten postnatal days of rat pups, while the neurodevelopmental trajectory and morphological properties of piglet brains are much more comparable to humans [41,55–57]. This complicates the comparison of the effects of oral delivery of HMOs between piglets and rodents. Differences reside in the immediate environment upon birth and the extent to which the brain and body have developed at that point, as neonatal rat pups would be more comparable to prenatal piglets in the final days before parturition, and there are no studies performed on the cognitive effects of HMOs on piglets in young adulthood. This interspecies difference in developmental stage upon birth and subsequent postnatal period might contribute to the heterogeneity in the findings between species on simple behavioural tests such as the NORT and the T maze.

Nevertheless, one cannot exclude the possibility that other factors than mere species differences may be at play, for example, the test parameters used in the studies. In the NORT of the rodent studies, the retention interval (time between acquisition phase and test phase) was 24 h, which is considered to be fairly long and is considered to be a measure of long-term recognition memory [42]. In the piglet studies, different retention intervals, ranging from 1 h (intermediate) to 48 h (long-term), were used. It is possible that similar enhancing effects of HMO administration on recognition memory (NORT) reported by Fleming and colleagues [52,53] would have been found in juvenile rodents if the retention interval was 1 h instead of 24 h and if the rodents had been fed a similar combination of oligosaccharides as the piglets received. However, when probing such a long-term recognition memory of one-year old rodents, an improved recognition memory is observed in the HMO supplemented animals, together with improved spatial memory as measured by the Y maze. As long-term recognition memory was not observed in juvenile piglets and rodents when supplied with only one HMO but was observed in piglets when they were given a combination of oligosaccharides, this may not be a simple matter of species differences. Another explanation could be that within the developing brain, there are different processes at play when retrieving a newly consolidated memory (one hour later) versus an older memory (24–48 h later), which may require more resources, such as the combination of various types of oligosaccharides. Interestingly, when piglets were supplemented with a complex mixture of oligosaccharides (HMOs and BMOs or Oligofructose), they displayed an improved long-term recognition memory. Perhaps the effects when HMOs form combinations or are provided with other oligosaccharides are more potent and thus easier to discern than the effects of singular HMOs on memory.

Other factors such as gender and sample size could also contribute to the heterogeneity of the simple behavioural test findings, but it is uncertain to what extent these factors may have influenced the results. Only two sialyllactose studies (and no fucosyllactose study) used both males and females, one rodent study by Oliveros and colleagues [47] and one piglet study by Obelitz-Ryom and colleagues [51]. However, no separation based on gender was performed in the analysis. As studies on postnatal administration of compounds, such as the study by Shumake and colleagues [58] have demonstrated gender specific effects in rats, it stands to reason that early life HMO supplementation could produce gender specific outcomes. Nonetheless, when comparing the findings generated by Oliveros et al. [47] and Obelitz-Ryom et al. [51] with the exclusively male studies of the same species and HMO administered, the behavioural results remained very similar. Furthermore, the majority of the studies employed comparable sample sizes ($n = 10$–12 on average), and effects of HMOs on cognition were already reported in studies with the lower sample sizes. While potential effects of variation in sample size cannot be completely excluded, HMO supplementation already produces beneficial results in experiments with lower sample sizes. Therefore, the heterogeneity in findings between studies is more likely due to a combination of factors such as species and task parameters, as previously discussed.

When both piglets and rodents were tested on complex cognitive tasks from a young age onwards, HMOs exerted a beneficial effect on learning and memory. Therefore, it is possible that the HMOs effects become more apparent when cognitive load is increased, either due to task difficulty or due to aging. This may explain why the beneficial effects of HMOs are especially visible when the tasks are cognitively more strenuous, such is the case with the 8-arm radial maze or the operant tests, as increases in cognitive load make brain limitations more discernible.

While behavioural tests on learning and memory at a young age in general yielded mixed results, HMO supplementation did significantly improve LTP from a young age onwards. Interestingly, while in both young adult (2.5 months old) and mature adult (1 year old) just one HFS application was sufficient to induce LTP, very young rodents (6 weeks old) required a second high-frequency stimulation (HFS) to induce LTP. Nonetheless, HMO administration resulted in an enhanced LTP response in both younger and older rodents alike. It is possible that LTP might be a more sensitive measure to investigate the beneficial effects of HMOs on cognitive outcomes at a young age. Furthermore, under normal circumstances, the LTP response is reduced in older rats as a natural result of aging [46]. This natural reduction in LTP response was not encountered when the animals were supplemented with HMOs. On the contrary, supplementation with HMOs facilitated an enhanced LTP response. Because LTP is a measure of synaptic plasticity, it stands to reason that synaptic plasticity benefits from HMOs both in the short-term as in the long-term. Therefore, supplementation of HMOs, both sialylated and fucosylated, in infancy could have long-lasting protective effects on the molecular underpinnings of learning and memory.

It should be noted that these results have been gathered from only nine articles, which is the main limitation of the present review. Nevertheless, while there are a limited number of studies on the cognitive effects of HMO supplementation, the studies currently available show promising results of how HMOs could contribute to cognitive development. These findings call for further in-depth research on the cognitive effects of HMOs and to delineate their underlying mechanisms.

Potential Underlying Mechanisms

There are a few possible factors which could account for the cognition enhancing effects of HMOs in mammals.

In the case of sialylated HMOs, Polysialylated Neural Cell Adhesion Molecules (PSA-NCAM) could be upregulated. The PSA-NCAM complex is upregulated in newborn, immature neurons and growing fibre tracts during embryogenesis and has been linked to increased synaptic plasticity [59–62]. Within the adult brain, PSA-NCAM is expressed in brain regions with high rates of neural plasticity and neurogenesis, such as the olfactory bulb and the hippocampus [61]. Improved neural plasticity and the survival of newborn neurons contribute to cognition and memory [62]. Therefore, it is possible that sialylated HMOs are capable of influencing neurogenesis via upregulation of PSA-NCAM, which in turn contributes to the reported improvement in cognition. This suggestion is further supported by Oliveros and colleagues [47]. These authors found an increase in PSA-NCAM in 6-SL supplemented animals. However, the role of fucosylated HMOs in plasticity and neurogenesis is currently not well understood and requires further investigation.

A second possible factor is the improved immune functioning due to the supplementation of HMOs and their well-established role in the immune system. As mentioned in the introduction, immune factors also contribute to cognitive functioning [38], though there are multiple hypotheses on how this may occur. One hypothesis states that perinatal immune activation directly affects neurodevelopmental pathways necessary for learning and memory, which leads to reduced neurotransmitter function, a reduction in hippocampal presynaptic proteins and impaired LTP [38]. A second hypothesis postulates that early life immune activation indirectly determines the adult response to an infection with a pathogen, either via exaggerated pro-inflammatory cytokines or via a decrease in anti-inflammatory cytokines. This in turn could lead to downstream changes in cognition and neural function [38]. As HMOs are capable of regulating the neonatal cytokine response in the periphery [11,33,35,63], it is possible that they also exert their enhancing effects on cognition via the immune system.

A last possible factor through which HMOs may improve cognition involves the microbiome. HMOs contribute to the microbiome composition within the gut and therefore could interact with the brain via the resulting bacterial metabolites such as the Short Chain Fatty Acids [64]. As certain gut bacteria are specific for the utilization of sialylated HMOs and other bacteria for the fucosylated HMOs, a larger variety of HMOs may go hand in hand with a larger yield of specific gut bacteria capable of metabolizing these HMOs, and thus determining their subsequent metabolites [65]. Interactions between single HMOs and the microbiome have been previously reported by Tarr and colleagues [66]. They demonstrated that the administration of sialylated HMOs changed the microbial composition in the gut of mice, which in turn led to a reduction in anxiety-related behaviour and a maintenance of neurogenesis. The influence of the gut–brain axis has also been touched upon by Vazquez and colleagues [48], as they found that ablating the vagal nerve, which is part of the gut–brain axis, diminished the beneficial effects of orally supplied 2′-FL on LTP. Similar to these results, Kuntz and colleagues examined the metabolic fate of 2′-FL and found that 2′-FL was not directly incorporated in the brain but required an intact gut microbiome for the generation of fucose metabolites, which are subsequently taken up into the systemic circulation and organs [67]. In addition, it is possible that combinational HMOs may generate better effects than alone. This idea has already been demonstrated at the level of the growth and function of gut bacteria [68,69]. Different HMOs are processed by different bacteria, which contain either sialidases or fucosidases to cleave sia and fuc of the carbohydrates [65]. In turn, another group of bacteria can feed on the HMOs once the fuc and sia moieties are removed.

These bacterial interactions, which depend on the HMOs present in the gut, may exert downstream effects on memory and cognition via the gut–brain axis. In light of potential downstream effects of the microbiome on behaviour, environmental housing conditions which affect the microbiome should also be considered [70] in this context, although it is uncertain to what extent the microbiotic variations due to husbandry may have influenced the effects of HMO supplementation on subsequent behaviour. Finally, another important factor to consider in the context of the microbiome is gender specific effects. While infant sex is reported to be largely unrelated to the HMO composition within human breastmilk [31], another study by Moossavi and colleagues [71] found that the milk microbiota vary depending on infant sex. This could potentially be attributed to cross interactions with the gut microbiome of the infant, as gender differences have been reported there [71]. As HMOs interact with both the milk and the gut microbiome [72,73], it is therefore possible that sex-dependent variations could lead to differential cognitive outcomes of HMO supplementation.

5. Conclusions

The observation that HMOs are capable of enhancing cognition has initiated the search for a better mechanistic understanding of its functioning. Nonetheless, there are still several outstanding questions on the relationship between HMO and neonatal brain development, which warrant further investigation. An important aspect that needs to be addressed is the apparent age-related differences when assessing various cognitive tests. This point illustrates one of the current issues on HMO research in animals, as the tools currently used may not be sensitive enough to fully explore the range to which HMOs may affect brain development and cognition. Thus, one of the more complex tools could be the use of challenging operant tasks, such as the Trial Unique Delayed Non-Matching to Location (TUNL) measuring spatial memory and pattern separation [74], the 5-Choice Serial Reaction Time Task measuring attention and motor impulsivity [75], or delayed reinforcement tasks measuring choice impulsivity [76], ideally performed in the animal's home cage. The difficulty of such tasks can be varied and may thus be more suited to test cognitive functioning in young animals, as at a young age, only effects of HMOs were found in difficult tasks.

Another important issue is that due to the large variability between the experimental design and methods used across studies, comparing the effects of different HMOs between studies is difficult. Such variability includes the age of testing, the tests and experimental parameters, the HMO components used, the gender of the animals, variation in sample sizes, the environmental conditions and the variation in (neuro)developmental stage during which the animals were supplemented the HMOs. These limitations call for a larger, unified study in which the effects of different HMOs on complex cognitive functioning are systematically compared, when administered both independently and as in conjunction. In such a unified study, all these factors can be accounted for, enabling a systematic comparison.

A last important issue is that most HMO studies so far have focused on singular HMOs, with the exception of the two most recent studies performed by Fleming in 2020. The focus on singular HMOs is a limitation because it does not reflect a naturalistic situation where maternal milk provides a combination of different HMOs [77]. Therefore, considering the interactions of HMOs when supplemented in combination would provide valuable insights on the influence of the gut microbiome and its downstream effects on cognition and development.

While research on the cognitive implications of HMOs is still in its infancy, the early findings reporting its long-lasting beneficial effects on memory and cognition are promising. Further studies on the exact molecular mechanisms, ranging from immune functioning to neuroplasticity and the microbiome will prove to be useful in deepening our understanding of how HMOs and their interactions contribute to cognition and development.

Author Contributions: Conceptualization, S.D., and J.R.H.; writing—original draft preparation, S.D.; re-writing, S.D., review and editing, S.D., J.R.H., M.S. and W.W.; Table and Figure creation, S.D.; supervision, J.R.H. and M.S. All authors have read and agreed to the published version of the manuscript.

Funding: This research received no external funding.

Conflicts of Interest: W.W. is an employee of Inner Mongolia Yili Industrial Group, Co., Ltd. The other authors declare no conflicts of interest.

Appendix A

The following search string, comprised of both Mesh terms and key words in the title and abstract was composed and entered in Pubmed:

(Oligosaccharides[MeSH Terms] AND milk, human[MeSH Terms] OR oligosaccharide*[Title/Abstract] OR HMO*[Title/Abstract]) AND (learning[MeSH Terms] OR cognition[MeSH Terms] OR memory[Title/Abstract] OR cognition[Title/Abstract] OR behavior[Title/Abstract] OR behaviour[Title/Abstract]) AND ("sialic acids" [MeSH Terms] OR sialyl*[Title/Abstract] OR fucosyl*[Title/Abstract] OR fucose[MeSH Terms] OR lacto-N-*[Title/Abstract] OR LNnT[Title/Abstract])

This search string enables the detection of articles that contain information regarding HMOs, their cognitive outcomes and specific HMO components. Using the above search strategy, 108 articles were found. Further exclusion criteria were articles that did not pertain to cognition or its associated processes (learning and memory) and that did not make use of administered HMOs. This finally resulted in 9 articles.

References

1. World Health Organization. Available online: https://www.who.int/health-topics/breastfeeding#tab=tab_1 (accessed on 6 May 2020).
2. Feldman, R.; Eidelman, A.I. Direct and indirect effects of breast milk on the neurobehavioral and cognitive development of premature infants. *Dev. Psychobiol.* **2003**, *43*, 109–119. [CrossRef] [PubMed]
3. Boquien, C.-Y. Human Milk: An Ideal Food for Nutrition of Preterm Newborn. *Front. Pediatr.* **2018**, *6*, 1–9. [CrossRef] [PubMed]
4. Vandenplas, Y.; Berger, B.; Carnielli, V.P.; Ksiazyk, J.; Lagström, H.; Luna, M.S.; Migacheva, N.; Mosselmans, J.M.; Picaud, J.C.; Possner, M.; et al. Human milk oligosaccharides: 2′-fucosyllactose (2′-FL) and lacto-n-neotetraose (LNnT) in infant formula. *Nutrients* **2018**, *10*, 1161. [CrossRef]
5. Bar, S.; Milanaik, R.; Adesman, A. Long-term neurodevelopmental benefits of breastfeeding. *Curr. Opin. Pediatr.* **2016**, *28*, 559–566. [CrossRef] [PubMed]
6. Nolan, L.S.; Parks, O.B.; Good, M. A review of the immunomodulating components of maternal breast milk and protection against necrotizing enterocolitis. *Nutrients* **2019**, *12*, 14. [CrossRef]
7. Carucci, L.; Nocerino, R.; Paparo, L.; Di Scala, C.; Canani, R.B. Dietary Prevention of Atopic March in Pediatric Subjects With Cow's Milk Allergy. *Front. Pediatr.* **2020**, *8*, 1–9. [CrossRef]
8. Munblit, D.; Peroni, D.G.; Boix-Amoros, A.; Hsu, P.S.; Van't Land, B.; Gay, M.C.L.; Kolotilina, A.; Skevaki, C.; Boyle, R.J.; Collado, M.C.; et al. Human Milk and Allergic Diseases: An Unsolved Puzzle. *Nutrients* **2017**, *9*, 894. [CrossRef]
9. Rajani, P.S.; Seppo, A.E.; Järvinen, K.M. Immunologically Active Components in Human Milk and Development of Atopic Disease, With Emphasis on Food Allergy, in the Pediatric Population. *Front. Pediatr.* **2018**, *6*, 1–13. [CrossRef]
10. Den Dekker, H.T.; Sonnenschein-van der Voort, A.M.M.; Jaddoe, V.W.V.; Reiss, I.K.; de Jongste, J.C.; Duijts, L. Breastfeeding and asthma outcomes at the age of 6 years: The Generation R Study. *Pediatr. Allergy Immunol.* **2016**, *27*, 486–492. [CrossRef]
11. Le Doare, K.; Holder, B.; Bassett, A.; Pannaraj, P.S. Mother's Milk: A purposeful contribution to the development of the infant microbiota and immunity. *Front. Immunol.* **2018**, *9*, 1–10. [CrossRef]
12. Çatli, G.; Dündar, N.O.; Dündar, B.N. Adipokines in Breast Milk: An Update. *J. Clin. Res. Pediatr. Endocrinol.* **2014**, *6*, 192–201. [CrossRef] [PubMed]
13. Gila-Diaz, A.; Arribas, S.M.; Algara, A.; Martín-Cabrejas, M.A.; López de Pablo, Á.L.; Sáenz de Pipaón, M.; Ramiro-Cortijo, D. A Review of Bioactive Factors in Human Breastmilk: A Focus on Prematurity. *Nutrients* **2019**, *11*, 1307. [CrossRef] [PubMed]

14. Kramer, M.S.; Aboud, F.; Mironova, E.; Vanilovich, I.; Platt, R.W.; Matush, L.; Igumnov, S.; Fombonne, E.; Bogdanovich, N.; Ducruet, T.; et al. Breastfeeding and child cognitive development: New evidence from a large randomized trial. *Arch. Gen. Psychiatry* **2008**, *65*, 578–584. [CrossRef] [PubMed]
15. Poton, W.L.; Soares, A.L.G.; de Oliveira, E.R.A.; Gonçalves, H. Breastfeeding and behavior disorders among children and adolescents: A systematic review. *Rev. Saude Publica* **2018**, *52*, 1–17. [CrossRef] [PubMed]
16. Horta, B.L.; Loret De Mola, C.; Victora, C.G. Breastfeeding and intelligence: A systematic review and meta-analysis. *Acta Paediatr. Int. J. Paediatr.* **2015**, *104*, 14–19. [CrossRef] [PubMed]
17. Deoni, S.C.L.; Dean, D.C.; Piryatinsky, I.; O'Muircheartaigh, J.; Waskiewicz, N.; Lehman, K.; Han, M.; Dirks, H. Breastfeeding and early white matter development: A cross-sectional study. *Neuroimage* **2013**, *82*, 77–86. [CrossRef] [PubMed]
18. Herba, C.M.; Roza, S.; Govaert, P.; Hofman, A.; Jaddoe, V.; Verhulst, F.C.; Tiemeier, H. Breastfeeding and early brain development: The Generation R study. *Matern. Child Nutr.* **2013**, *9*, 332–349. [CrossRef]
19. Allen-Blevins, C.R.; You, X.; Hinde, K.; Sela, D.A. Handling stress may confound murine gut microbiota studies. *PeerJ* **2017**, *5*, 1–21. [CrossRef]
20. Andreas, N.J.; Kampmann, B.; Mehring Le-Doare, K. Human breast milk: A review on its composition and bioactivity. *Early Hum. Dev.* **2015**, *91*, 629–635. [CrossRef]
21. Mudd, A.T.; Dilger, R.N. Early-Life Nutrition and Neurodevelopment: Use of the Piglet as a Translational Model. *Adv. Nutr. Int. Rev. J.* **2017**, *8*, 92–104. [CrossRef]
22. Wang, H.J.; Hua, C.Z.; Ruan, L.L.; Hong, L.Q.; Sheng, S.Q.; Shang, S.Q. Sialic Acid and Iron Content in Breastmilk of Chinese Lactating Women. *Indian Pediatr.* **2017**, *54*, 1029–1031. [CrossRef] [PubMed]
23. Ayechu-Muruzabal, V.; van Stigt, A.H.; Mank, M.; Willemsen, L.E.M.; Stahl, B.; Garssen, J.; van't Land, B. Diversity of human milk oligosaccharides and effects on early life immune development. *Front. Pediatr.* **2018**, *6*, 1–9. [CrossRef] [PubMed]
24. Hegar, B.; Wibowo, Y.; Basrowi, R.W.; Ranuh, R.G.; Sudarmo, S.M.; Munasir, Z.; Atthiyah, A.F.; Widodo, A.D.; Supriatmo Kadim, M.; Suryawan, A.; et al. The Role of Two Human Milk Oligosaccharides, 2'-Fucosyllactose and Lacto-N-Neotetraose, in Infant Nutrition. *Pediatr. Gastroenterol. Hepatol. Nutr.* **2019**, *22*, 330–340. [CrossRef] [PubMed]
25. Urashima, T.; Saito, T.; Nakamura, T.; Messer, M. Oligosaccharides of milk and colostrum in non-human mammals. *Glycoconj. J.* **2001**, *18*, 357–371. [CrossRef]
26. Ten Bruggencate, S.J.; Bovee-Oudenhoven, I.M.; Feitsma, A.L.; van Hoffen, E.; Schoterman, M.H. Functional role and mechanisms of sialyllactose and other sialylated milk oligosaccharides. *Nutr. Rev.* **2014**, *72*, 377–389. [CrossRef]
27. Kunz, C.; Meyer, C.; Collado, M.C.; Geiger, L.; Garcia-Mantrana, I.; Bertua-Rios, B.; Martinez-Costa, C.; Borsch, C.; Rudloff, S. Influence of Gestational Age, Secretor, and Lewis Blood Group Status on the Oligosaccharide Content of Human Milk. *J. Pediatr. Gastroenterol. Nutr.* **2017**, *64*, 789–798. [CrossRef]
28. Austin, S.; de Castro, C.A.; Bénet, T.; Hou, Y.; Sun, H.; Thakkar, S.K.; Vinyes-Pares, G.; Zhang, Y.; Wang, P. Temporal change of the content of 10 oligosaccharides in the milk of Chinese urban mothers. *Nutrients* **2016**, *8*, 346. [CrossRef]
29. Thurl, S.; Munzert, M.; Henker, J.; Boehm, G.; Müller-Werner, B.; Jelinek, J.; Stahl, B. Variation of human milk oligosaccharides in relation to milk groups and lactational periods. *Br. J. Nutr.* **2010**, *104*, 1261–1271. [CrossRef]
30. Austin, S.; De Castro, C.A.; Sprenger, N.; Binia, A.; Affolter, M.; Garcia-Rodenas, C.L.; Beauport, L.; Tolsa, J.F.; Fischer Fumeaux, C.J. Human milk oligosaccharides in the milk of mothers delivering term versus preterm infants. *Nutrients* **2019**, *11*, 1282. [CrossRef]
31. Azad, M.B.; Robertson, B.; Atakora, F.; Becker, A.B.; Subbarao, P.; Moraes, T.J.; Mandhane, P.J.; Turvey, S.E.; Lefebvre, D.L.; Sears, M.R.; et al. Human Milk Oligosaccharide Concentrations Are Associated with Multiple Fixed and Modifiable Maternal Characteristics, Environmental Factors, and Feeding Practices. *J. Nutr.* **2018**, *148*, 1733–1742. [CrossRef]
32. Paganini, D.; Uyoga, M.; Kortman, G.A.M.; Boekhorst, J.; Schneeberger, S.; Karanja, S.; Hennet, T.; Zimmerman, M.B. Maternal Human Milk Oligosaccharide Profile Modulates the Impact of an Intervention with Iron and galacto-Oligosaccharides in Kenyan Infants. *Nutrients* **2019**, *11*, 2596. [CrossRef] [PubMed]

33. Lis-Kuberka, J.; Orczyk-Pawilowicz, M. Sialylated Oligosaccharides and Glycoconjugates of Human Milk. The Impact on Infant and Newborn Protection, Development and Well-Being. *Nutrients* **2019**, *11*, 306. [CrossRef] [PubMed]
34. Sánchez, C.L.; Cubero, J.; Sánchez, J.; Franco, L.; Rodriguez, A.B.; Rivero, M. Evolution of the circadian profile of human milk amino acids during breastfeeding. *J. Appl. Biomed.* **2013**, *11*, 59–70. [CrossRef]
35. Goehring, K.C.; Marriage, B.J.; Oliver, J.S.; Wilder, J.A.; Barrett, E.G.; Buck, R.H. Similar to Those Who Are Breastfed, Infants Fed a Formula Containing 2′-Fucosyllactose Have Lower Inflammatory Cytokines in a Randomized Controlled Trial. *J. Nutr.* **2016**, *146*, 2559–2566. [CrossRef] [PubMed]
36. Steenhout, P.; Sperisen, P.; Martin, F.P.; Sprenger, N.; Wernimont, S.; Pecquet, S.; Berger, B. Term infant formula supplemented with human milk oligosaccharides (2′fucosyllactose and lacto-N-neotetraose) shifts stool microbiota and metabolic signatures closer to that of breastfed infants. *FASEB J.* **2016**, *30*, 275–277. [CrossRef]
37. Berger, P.K.; Plows, J.F.; Jones, R.B.; Alderete, T.L.; Yonemitsu, C.; Poulsen, M.; Ryoo, J.H.; Peterson, B.S.; Bode, L.; Goran, M.I. Human milk oligosaccharide 2′-fucosyllactose links feedings at 1 month to cognitive development at 24 months in infants of normal and overweight mothers. *PLoS ONE* **2020**, *15*, e228323. [CrossRef]
38. Bilbo, S.D.; Schwarz, J.M. The Immune System and Developmental Programming of Brain Front Neuroendocrinol Author Manuscript and Behavior. *NIH Public Access* **2012**, *33*, 267–286. [CrossRef]
39. Wallace, T.L.; Ballard, T.M.; Glavis-Bloom, C. Animal Paradigms to Assess Cognition with Translation to Humans. *Handb. Exp. Pharmacol.* **2015**, *228*, 27–57. [CrossRef]
40. Wiera, G.; Nowak, D.; van Hove, I.; Dziegiel, P.; Moons, L.; Mozrzymas, J.W. Mechanisms of NMDA receptor- and voltage-gated L-type calcium channel-dependent hippocampal LTP critically rely on proteolysis that is mediated by distinct metalloproteinases. *J. Neurosci.* **2017**, *37*, 1240–1256. [CrossRef]
41. Gieling, E.T.; Nordquist, R.E.; van der Staay, F.J. Assessing learning and memory in pigs. *Anim. Cogn.* **2011**, *14*, 151–173. [CrossRef]
42. Antunes, M.; Biala, G. The novel object recognition memory: Neurobiology, test procedure, and its modifications. *Cogn. Process.* **2012**, *13*, 93–110. [CrossRef] [PubMed]
43. Vorhees, C.V.; Williams, M.T. Assessing Spatial Learning and Memory in Rodents. *ILAR J.* **2014**, *55*, 310–332. [CrossRef] [PubMed]
44. Song, K.; Takahashi, S.; Sakurai, Y. Reinforcement schedules differentially affect learning in neuronal operant conditioning in rats. *Neurosci. Res.* **2020**, *153*, 62–67. [CrossRef] [PubMed]
45. Kiryk, A.; Janusz, A.; Zglinicki, B.; Turkes, E.; Knapska, E.; Konopka, W.; Lipp, H.P.; Kaczmarek, L. IntelliCage as a tool for measuring mouse behaviour—20 years perspective. *Behav. Brain Res.* **2020**, *388*, 1–17. [CrossRef]
46. Oliveros, E.; Ramirez, M.; Vazquez, E.; Barranco, A.; Gruart, A.; Delgado-Garcia, J.M.; Buck, R.; Rueda, R.; Martin, M.J. Oral supplementation of 2′-fucosyllactose during lactation improves memory and learning in rats. *J. Nutr. Biochem.* **2015**, *31*, 20–27. [CrossRef] [PubMed]
47. Oliveros, E.; Vázquez, E.; Barranco, A.; Ramírez, M.; Gruart, A.; Delgado-Garcia, J.M.; Buck, R.; Rueda, R.; Martín, M.J. Sialic acid and sialylated oligosaccharide supplementation during lactation improves learning and memory in rats. *Nutrients* **2018**, *10*, 1519. [CrossRef]
48. Vazquez, E.; Barranco, A.; Ramirez, M.; Gruart, A.; Delgado-Garcia, J.M.; Jimenez, M.L.; Buck, R.; Rueda, R. Dietary 2′-fucosyllactose enhances operant conditioning and long-term potentiation via gut-brain communication through the vagus nerve in rodents. *PLoS ONE* **2016**, *11*, e166070. [CrossRef]
49. Vázquez, E.; Barranco, A.; Ramírez, M.; Delgado-Garcia, J.M.; Martínez-Lara, E.; Blanco, S.; Martín, M.J.; Castanys, E.; Buck, R.; Prieto, P.; et al. Effects of a human milk oligosaccharide, 2′-fucosyllactose, on hippocampal long-term potentiation and learning capabilities in rodents. *J. Nutr. Biochem.* **2015**, *26*, 455–465. [CrossRef]
50. Wang, B.; Yu, B.; Karim, M.; Hu, H.; Sun, Y.; McGreevy, P.; Petocz, P.; Held, S.; Brand-Miller, J. Dietary sialic acid supplementation improves learning and memory in piglets. *Am. J. Clin. Nutr.* **2007**, *85*, 561–569. [CrossRef]
51. Obelitz-Ryom, K.; Bering, S.B.; Overgaard, S.H.; Eskildsen, S.F.; Ringgaard, S.; Olesen, J.L.; Skovgaard, K.; Pankratova, S.; Wang, B.; Brunse, A.; et al. Bovine Milk Oligosaccharides with Sialyllactose Improves Cognition in Preterm Pigs. *Nutrients* **2019**, *11*, 1335. [CrossRef]

52. Fleming, S.A.; Mudd, A.T.; Hauser, J.; Yan, J.; Metairon, S.; Steiner, P.; Donovan, S.M.; Dilger, R.N. Human and Bovine Milk Oligosaccharides Elicit Improved Recognition Memory Concurrent With Alterations in Regional Brain Volumes and Hippocampal mRNA Expression. *Front. Neurosci.* **2020**, *14*, 1–14. [CrossRef] [PubMed]
53. Fleming, S.A.; Mudd, A.T.; Hauser, J.; Yan, J.; Metairon, S.; Steiner, P.; Donovan, S.M.; Dilger, R.N. Dietary Oligofructose Alone or in Combination with 2′-Fucosyllactose Differentially Improves Recognition Memory and Hippocampal mRNA Expression. *Nutrients* **2020**, *12*, 2131. [CrossRef] [PubMed]
54. Fleming, S.A.; Chichlowski, M.; Berg, B.M.; Donovan, S.M.; Dilger, R.N. Dietary sialyllactose does not influence measures of recognition memory or diurnal activity in the young pig. *Nutrients* **2018**, *10*, 395. [CrossRef] [PubMed]
55. Pressler, R.; Auvin, S. Comparison of brain maturation among species: An example in translational research suggesting the possible use of bumetanide in newborn. *Front. Neurol.* **2013**, *4*, 1–4. [CrossRef] [PubMed]
56. Semple, B.D.; Blomgren, K.; Gimlin, K.; Ferriero, D.M.; Noble-Haeusslein, L.J. Brain development in rodents and humans: Identifying benchmarks of maturation and vulnerability to injury across species. *Prog. Neurobiol.* **2013**, *106–107*, 1–16. [CrossRef] [PubMed]
57. Radlowski, E.C.; Conrad, M.S.; Lezmi, S.; Dilger, R.N.; Sutton, B.; Larsen, R.; Johnson, R.W. A Neonatal Piglet Model for Investigating Brain and Cognitive Development in Small for Gestational Age Human Infants. *PLoS ONE* **2014**, *9*, e91951. [CrossRef]
58. Shumake, J.; Barrett, D.W.; Lane, M.A.; Wittke, A.J. Behavioral effects of bovine lactoferrin administration during postnatal development of rats. *BioMetals* **2014**, *27*, 1039–1055. [CrossRef]
59. Bonfanti, L. PSA-NCAM in mammalian structural plasticity and neurogenesis. *Prog. Neurobiol.* **2006**, *80*, 129–164. [CrossRef]
60. Weledji, E.P.; Assob, J.C. The ubiquitous neural cell adhesion molecule (N-CAM). *Ann. Med. Surg.* **2014**, *3*, 77–81. [CrossRef]
61. Murrey, H.E.; Hsieh-Wilson, L.C. The chemical neurobiology of carbohydrates. *Chem Rev.* **2008**, *108*, 1708–1731. [CrossRef]
62. Sahay, A.; Scobie, K.N.; Hill, A.S.; O'Carroll, C.M.; Kheirbek, M.A.; Burghardt, N.S.; Fenton, A.A.; Dranovsky, A.; Hen, R. Increasing adult hippocampal neurogenesis is sufficient to improve pattern separation. *Nature* **2011**, *472*, 466–470. [CrossRef] [PubMed]
63. Yu, Z.T.; Nanthakumar, N.N.; Newburg, D.S. The human milk oligosaccharide 2′-fucosyllactose quenches Campylobacter jejuni-induced inflammation in human epithelial cells HEp-2 and HT-29 and in mouse intestinal Mucosa1-3. *J. Nutr.* **2016**, *146*, 1980–1990. [CrossRef] [PubMed]
64. Dalile, B.; Van Oudenhove, L.; Vervliet, B.; Verbeke, K. The role of short-chain fatty acids in microbiota–gut–brain communication. *Nat. Rev. Gastroenterol. Hepatol.* **2019**, *16*, 461–478. [CrossRef]
65. Bode, L. The functional biology of human milk oligosaccharides. *Early Hum. Dev.* **2015**, *91*, 619–622. [CrossRef] [PubMed]
66. Tarr, A.J.; Galley, J.D.; Fisher, S.; Chichlowski, M.; Berg, B.M.; Bailey, M.T. The prebiotics 3′Sialyllactose and 6′Sialyllactose diminish stressor-induced anxiety-like behavior and colonic microbiota alterations: Evidence for effects on the gut-brain axis. *Brain Behav. Immun.* **2016**, *50*, 166–177. [CrossRef]
67. Kuntz, S.; Kunz, C.; Borsch, C.; Vazquez, E.; Buck, R.; Reutzel, M.; Eckert, G.P.; Rudloff, S. Metabolic Fate and Distribution of 2′-Fucosyllactose: Direct Influence on Gut Microbial Activity but not on Brain. *Mol. Nutr. Food Res.* **2019**, *63*, 1–8. [CrossRef]
68. Thongaram, T.; Hoeflinger, J.L.; Chow, J.M.; Miller, M.J. Human milk oligosaccharide consumption by probiotic and human-associated bifidobacteria and lactobacilli. *J. Dairy Sci.* **2017**, *100*, 7825–7833. [CrossRef]
69. Lawson, M.; O'Neill, I.J.; Kujawska, M.; Javvadi, S.G.; Wijeyesekera, A.; Flegg, Z.; Chalklen, L.; Hall, L.J. Breast milk-derived human milk oligosaccharides promote Bifidobacterium interactions within a single ecosystem. *ISME J.* **2020**, *14*, 635–648. [CrossRef]
70. Lees, H.; Swann, J.; Poucher, S.M.; Nicholson, J.K.; Holmes, E.; Wilson, I.D.; Marchesi, J.R. Age and microenvironment outweigh genetic influence on the Zucker rat microbiome. *PLoS ONE* **2014**, *9*, e100916. [CrossRef]
71. Moossavi, S.; Sepehri, S.; Robertson, B.; Bode, L.; Goruk, S.; Field, C.J.; Lix, L.M.; de Souza, R.J.; Becker, A.B.; Mandhane, P.J.; et al. Composition and Variation of the Human Milk Microbiota Are Influenced by Maternal Early-Life Factors. *Cell Host Microbe* **2019**, *25*, 324–335.e4. [CrossRef]

72. Ramani, S.; Stewart, C.J.; Laucirica, D.R.; Ajami, N.J.; Robertson, B.; Autran, C.A.; Shinge, D.; Rani, S.; Anandan, S.; Hu, L.; et al. Human milk oligosaccharides, milk microbiome and infant gut microbiome modulate neonatal rotavirus infection. *Nature* **2018**, *9*, 1–12. [CrossRef] [PubMed]
73. Borewicz, K.; Gu, F.; Saccenti, E.; Hechler, C.; Beijers, R.; de Weerth, C.; van Leeuwen, S.S.; Schols, H.A.; Smidt, H. The association between breastmilk oligosaccharides and faecal microbiota in healthy breastfed infants at two, six and twelve weeks of age. *Sci Rep* **2020**, *10*, 4270. [CrossRef] [PubMed]
74. Oomen, C.A.; Hvoslef-Eide, M.; Heath, C.J.; Mar, A.C.; Horner, A.E.; Bussey, T.J.; Saksida, L.M. The touchscreen operant platform for testing working memory and pattern separation in rats and mice. *Nat. Protoc.* **2013**, *8*, 2006–2021. [CrossRef] [PubMed]
75. Higgins, G.A.; Silenieks, L.B. Rodent test of attention and impulsivity: The 5-choice serial reaction time task. *Curr. Protoc. Pharmacol.* **2017**, *78*, 5.49.1–5.49.34. [CrossRef] [PubMed]
76. Dunnett, S.B.; Heuer, A.; Lelos, M.; Brooks, S.P.; Rosser, A.E. Bilateral striatal lesions disrupt performance in an operant delayed reinforcement task in rats. *Brain Res. Bull.* **2012**, *88*, 251–260. [CrossRef] [PubMed]
77. Bode, L. Human milk oligosaccharides: Every baby needs a sugar mama. *Glycobiology* **2012**, *22*, 1147–1162. [CrossRef] [PubMed]

Publisher's Note: MDPI stays neutral with regard to jurisdictional claims in published maps and institutional affiliations.

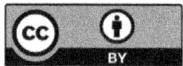

© 2020 by the authors. Licensee MDPI, Basel, Switzerland. This article is an open access article distributed under the terms and conditions of the Creative Commons Attribution (CC BY) license (http://creativecommons.org/licenses/by/4.0/).

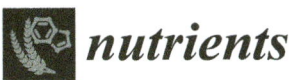

Review

The Role of the Gut Microbiota in the Development and Progression of Major Depressive and Bipolar Disorder

Tom Knuesel and M. Hasan Mohajeri *

Department of Anatomy, University of Zurich, Winterthurerstrasse 190, 8057 Zürich, Switzerland; tom.knuesel@uzh.ch
* Correspondence: mhasan.mohajeri@uzh.ch; Tel.: +41-79-938-1203

Abstract: A growing number of studies in rodents indicate a connection between the intestinal microbiota and the brain, but comprehensive human data is scarce. Here, we systematically reviewed human studies examining the connection between the intestinal microbiota and major depressive and bipolar disorder. In this review we discuss various changes in bacterial abundance, particularly on low taxonomic levels, in terms of a connection with the pathophysiology of major depressive and bipolar disorder, their use as a diagnostic and treatment response parameter, their health-promoting potential, as well as novel adjunctive treatment options. The diversity of the intestinal microbiota is mostly decreased in depressed subjects. A consistent elevation of phylum Actinobacteria, family Bifidobacteriaceae, and genus *Bacteroides*, and a reduction of family Ruminococcaceae, genus *Faecalibacterium*, and genus *Roseburia* was reported. Probiotics containing *Bifidobacterium* and/or *Lactobacillus* spp. seemed to improve depressive symptoms, and novel approaches with different probiotics and synbiotics showed promising results. Comparing twin studies, we report here that already with an elevated risk of developing depression, microbial changes towards a "depression-like" microbiota were found. Overall, these findings highlight the importance of the microbiota and the necessity for a better understanding of its changes contributing to depressive symptoms, potentially leading to new approaches to alleviate depressive symptoms via alterations of the gut microbiota.

Keywords: depression; affective disorder; gut-brain-axis; bacteria; probiotics; therapy; treatment

Citation: Knuesel, T.; Mohajeri, M.H. The Role of the Gut Microbiota in the Development and Progression of Major Depressive and Bipolar Disorder. *Nutrients* 2022, 14, 37. https://doi.org/10.3390/nu14010037

Academic Editor: Giovanna Muscogiuri

Received: 30 November 2021
Accepted: 20 December 2021
Published: 23 December 2021

Publisher's Note: MDPI stays neutral with regard to jurisdictional claims in published maps and institutional affiliations.

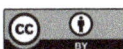

Copyright: © 2021 by the authors. Licensee MDPI, Basel, Switzerland. This article is an open access article distributed under the terms and conditions of the Creative Commons Attribution (CC BY) license (https://creativecommons.org/licenses/by/4.0/).

1. Introduction

Psychiatric disorders belong to the world's most disabling diseases, particularly major depressive disorder (MDD, unipolar disorder) and bipolar disorder (BD). Approximately 4.4% of the world's population is affected by depression. According to the World Health Organization, depression is the largest contributor to global disability and "non-fatal health loss", as well as the major contributor to suicide deaths [1]. Patients with MDD show typical symptoms of sadness, loss of interest and pleasure, feelings of low self-worth, guilt and tiredness, disturbed sleep, and poor concentration. BD is characterized by episodes of depression and mania, separated by episodes of normal mood. Mania includes elevated mood, increased energy and activity, pressure to speech, and decreased need to sleep [1].

In twin and family studies, heritability rates, defined as genetic factors contributing to the occurrence of a certain disease, were found to be moderate in MDD [2], and high in BD [3,4]. Despite significant advances, the pathogenesis of MDD and BD is still not fully understood. The diagnosis is based only on clinical symptoms, and a high rate of treatment resistance is observed [5]. Poverty, unemployment, severe life events, physical illness, and the consumption of alcohol and drugs are risk factors, but anyone can be affected by depression [1]. Especially functional gastrointestinal disorders (FGID) like irritable bowel syndrome (IBS) are often associated with depression, with the co-occurrence estimated at 30% [6]. Altered neurotransmission, changes in the hypothalamic-pituitary-adrenal axis (HPA axis), chronic low-grade inflammation, reduced neuroplasticity, and neuronal network dysfunction probably contribute to the pathogenesis of depression [7]. IBS pathogenesis shares several of these changes, indicating a multifactorial association between both diseases [8]. Additional evidence suggests a connection between depression, increased gut wall permeability, and bacterial translocation, resulting in increased immune activation and inflammation, with the intestinal microbiota being an important contributor [9,10].

The human gut microbiota consists of an estimated number of 3.8×10^{13} (38 trillion) bacteria, containing slightly more bacteria than cells of the human body (approximately 3.0×10^{13}), and by far more genes than its human host [11]. In addition, after the brain, the human gut contains the second greatest number of neurons. Heritability rates of the gut microbiota in humans were estimated between 1.9% and 8.1% [12]. A disturbed intestinal microbiota, often associated with reduced diversity, was found in a variety of diseases, including hypertension [13], obesity [14], gastrointestinal disorders (such as inflammatory bowel disease (IBD) [15,16], and IBS [17]), brain disorders (such as Alzheimer's disease [18], Parkinson's disease [19], autism spectrum disorder [20], and attention-deficit/hyperactivity disorder [21]), autoimmune diseases [22], as well as some types of cancer (for example colorectal cancer [23]). It was even suggested that a disturbed intestinal microbiota in obese patients may be a further reason for increased coronavirus disease 2019 (COVID-19) severity [24].

The intestinal microbiota can interfere with the HPA axis. Stress-induced stimulation of the HPA axis leads to elevated adrenocorticotrophin (ACTH) release and therefore results in a higher glucocorticoid excretion. In restraint-stressed germ-free mice, elevated ACTH and corticosterone (a glucocorticoid) levels were found, compared to specific pathogen-free mice [25], showing a direct connection between the HPA axis and the microbiota. The HPA axis can also be influenced through metabolites produced by the intestinal bacteria, like cytokines and prostaglandins, leading to exaggerated or attenuated stress response [26]. The gut microbiota can break down otherwise indigestible food substances and produce micronutrients [27], short-chain fatty acids (SCFAs) [28], neurotransmitters such as gamma-aminobutyric acid (GABA) [29], and brain active non-SCFA metabolites [18]. Acetate, propionate, and butyrate are the most abundant SCFAs in the human intestine [30]. They can influence emotion, cognition, and the immune system. In particular, a correlation between higher depression scores and lower levels of acetate and propionate was found in women, while sodium butyrate reversed depressive and manic symptoms in mice and was suggested as a mood stabilizer in humans [31,32]. Bacterial metabolites can translocate out of the gut and interact with the HPA axis, with the immune system, and with vagal afferents, leading to an exaggerated (or attenuated) HPA response and consequently to a modulation of the immune system [26,33,34]. Further research reported a systemic chronic low-grade inflammation in mice models, as well as in a significant proportion of depressed subjects, suggesting the presence of a mucosal dysfunction in depressed individuals, leading to an elevated translocation of intestinal bacteria into the circulation [35–37]. Consequently, an increased antibody response against lipopolysaccharides (LPS) from gram-negative bacteria is induced in diseased individuals [9]. In mice, intraperitoneally injected LPS caused a depressive-like behavior, and a following treatment with sodium butyrate ameliorated these changes, underlining the negative influence of translocated bacteria and LPS, as well as the positive influence of butyrate on the depression pathophysiology [35].

Several possible connections between the intestinal microbiota and depression are currently being discussed. The gut microbiota is considered to be under-explored, and its detailed investigation is needed for revealing specific associations. Most studies examining a possible connection between the gut microbiota and depression are conducted in rodents, while human research is still lagging. Hence, we systematically reviewed the connection between the human intestinal microbiota and major depressive and bipolar disorder, intending to analyze which bacteria could possibly influence depression or vice versa, and which bacteria future studies should primarily focus on.

2. Materials and Methods

The main question of this review was whether there is a connection between the intestinal microbiota and major depressive and bipolar disorder in human subjects. Does the intestinal microbiota influence the development, severity, and remission of affective disorder? The databases Scopus and PubMed were searched until 1 May 2020, with the following MeSH and search terms: "microbiota", "microbiome", "depression", "depressive", "bipolar disorder".

Additional inclusion criteria were as follows:
- Studies were written in English
- Studies were conducted with human subjects
- Studies at least partly focused on depression or depressive symptoms, and their correlation with the intestinal microbiota
- Diseased and healthy subjects were analyzed in the study

We focused on bacterial taxa and therefore excluded results regarding fungi, archaea, and viruses. Studies investigating microbiomes other than the intestinal microbiota were also excluded. We included all studies related to MDD, BD, and the intestinal microbiota, leading to the high heterogeneity of the reports, but providing a comprehensive overview of published data on this topic.

Twelve articles were excluded after full-text assessment due to not focusing on depression, depressive symptoms ($n = 9$) or the intestinal microbiota ($n = 3$).

A total of 57 studies were included in this review (Figure 1), most of which were published between 2016 and 2020, demonstrating a rapidly growing interest in this topic in recent years.

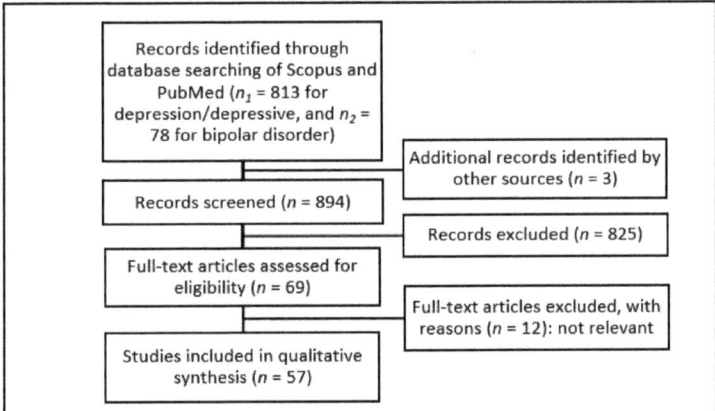

Figure 1. Methodical approach of our review due to PRISMA criteria [38].

3. Results

3.1. Diversity

Microbial diversity can be specified as alpha-diversity and beta-diversity. Alpha-diversity describes the species richness and evenness (inequality of the relative abundance) within a sample. In the reviewed studies it was most often determined by using the Shannon index, but several measures are common for richness and evenness estimation, as the ACE-, Chao1-, and Simpson index, phylogenetic diversity, and the number of observed species [39]. Beta-diversity describes the difference between multiple samples and is mostly analyzed by using unweighted/weighted UniFrac distances and Bray-Curtis dissimilarity [40]. Additionally, PLS-DA (partial least squares discriminant analysis) was used to detect microbial patterns that separate depressed subjects from healthy controls (HC) [41].

Apart from Jiang et al. [42] who reported an increased alpha-diversity in active-MDD subjects, all alpha-diversity indices, and other measures were consistently reported to be equal or reduced in depressed subjects among the other studies. For example, four studies reported a negative correlation between the Shannon index and depression, while 13 reported no correlation. Similar results were found concerning the other above-mentioned indices and measures for "within-sample" alpha-diversity (Table 1).

Regarding "between-samples" beta-diversity changes, a correlation with depression could be found in most studies. Both studies comparing MDD and BD subjects to HC using Bray-Curtis dissimilarity found a significant difference [43,44]. Regarding unweighted and weighted UniFrac distances, studies reported contradictory results, and no final statement can be made as to whether depressed subjects show different UniFrac distances compared to HC (Table 1).

Using PLS-DA, all four studies found significant differences between the depressed and the HC group. In addition, with a PLS-DA model, Li et al. found significant correlations between microbial and mood changes in healthy adults over time [45].

Table 1. A selection of the most used diversity indices and measures, showing an unchanged or lower microbial diversity in depressed individuals.

Source	Shannon	Ace	Chao1	Nr. OTUs	UniFrac	PLS-DA
[41]				D =		D sign.
[42]	aMDD ↑, rMDD =	MDD =	MDD =		MDD =	
[43]	MDD =					
[44]	MDD =				MDD =	
[46]		BD ↓, MDD =	BD ↓, MDD =			BD, MDD, C sign.
[47]	P =				P =	
[48]	P ↓			P ↓		
[49]		MDD =	MDD =			MDD sign.
[50]	MDD =, BD =		MDD ↓, BD =			
[51]	MDD =		MDD =	MDD =		MDD sign.
[52]	BD =		BD =	BD =	BD =	
[53]	D =			D ↓	D =	
[54]		BD ↓ *	BD ↓ *			BD sign.
[55]			D = IBS	D = IBS	D, IBS sign.	
[56]	IBS ↓				IBS sign.	
[57]	MDD =			MDD =		MDD sign.
[58]	MDD ↓	MDD ↓	MDD ↓		MDD sign.	
[59]	pm =					
[60]	D ↓, IBS ↓					
[61]	D ↓			D ↓		
[62]					MDD sign.	
[63]	MDD =				MDD sign.	
[64]	BD =			BD =	BD sign.	
[65]	BD =				BD sign.	

"UniFrac" includes weighted and/or unweighted UniFrac distances. "↓" shows a significantly reduced diversity in diseased subjects compared to controls or an inverse correlation with more severe symptoms, while "↑" indicates a significantly increased diversity or a positive correlation with more severe symptoms. "=" demonstrates no significant difference, while "sign." shows a significant difference. Empty cells symbolize that no results were reported. Abbreviations: MDD, major depressive disorder; BD, bipolar disorder; C, control group; P, psychiatric subjects; D, depression in general; IBS, irritable bowel syndrome; a, active disease group; r, response group; pm, psychiatric measures; OTU, operational taxonomic unit; *, only showing a trend, due to small sample size.

Overall, the microbial diversity of depressed individuals was reported unchanged or reduced, compared to the general population. These findings support the hypothesis that the intestinal microbiota is connected with the development, preservation, and remission of depression. With a better understanding of this link, depressive symptoms could potentially be positively influenced by specific alterations of the microbiota. Our analysis also shows that a reduced diversity is not present in all depressed subjects, and therefore cannot be used as a reliable diagnosis parameter. However, using the diversity change over time as a treatment response and prognosis parameter could be possible, but whether this is clinically feasible remains to be proven.

3.2. Phylum

On the phylum level, Bacteroidetes phylum was reported to be reduced in depressed subjects in multiple studies, but other studies reported opposite results (Table 2). Important to mention is that Chen et al. reported an elevation of Bacteroidetes in young MDD individuals, while in middle-aged MDD individuals Bacteroidetes were reduced, compared to age-matched controls [49]. On the one hand, comparing the studies which reported an elevation of Bacteroidetes in depressed patients, Liu et al. [44] only included MDD subjects between age 18 and 25, Hu et al. [66] used a young BD group (mean age 24 years), with an older, not age-matched control group, and Jiang et al. [42] only included MDD patients aged 40 or younger. On the other hand, studies reporting a reduction of Bacteroidetes correlating with depression were mostly conducted with older subjects. For example, in the study by Lai et al. [43], MDD individuals were between 32 and 52 years old, in Rong et al. [50] the mean age of all groups was between 38 and 42 years, and in Chen et al. [67] MDD subjects were 44 years old on average. Summarized, strong evidence was found that in young patients suffering from affective disorder, phylum Bacteroidetes is elevated, while in middle-aged patients these bacteria are reduced, compared to age-matched HC. This could point towards different causes of depression or a different manifestation of depressive behavior with age, leading to a different microbiota in depressed subjects.

The phylum Firmicutes was reported to alter in both directions (Table 2). However, most studies reporting an increase of Firmicutes also found a reduction of Bacteroidetes, or vice versa. Above mentioned changes due to different age ranges can also be applied to the phylum Firmicutes. Chen et al. [49] found lower Firmicutes mainly in the young MDD group, and Jiang et al. [42], Liu et al. [44], and Hu et al. [66] all studied young MDD or BD subjects and reported a reduced abundance of Firmicutes in the depressed group. Studies with older (middle-aged) subjects rather reported an elevation of Firmicutes abundance (Table 2).

Concerning the phylum Proteobacteria, results were highly controversial. Zheng et al. [46] and Rong et al. [50] both reported an elevation in BD, but not in MDD subjects, suggesting a potential difference between BD and MDD. In contrast, Hu et al. [66] found reduced Proteobacteria in untreated, compared to treated BD subjects, but not compared to HC. A recent review reported a lower abundance of phylum Proteobacteria in healthy subjects, while an elevated abundance was associated with a variety of diseases, including IBD, metabolic disorder, or malnutrition [68]. However, a link between phylum Proteobacteria and depression could not be shown, and neither age-dependent changes nor a difference between BD and MDD subjects could be further supported in this review.

The phylum Actinobacteria was consistently found to be elevated in MDD or BD individuals. Nine studies reported an elevation, while none found a decrease of Actinobacteria in patients with affective disorder (Table 2). Therefore, strong evidence for a close connection between an elevation of phylum Actinobacteria and depression was found, and more attention should be paid towards this phylum, looking for possible causes and consequences of an increase in Actinobacteria abundance.

Summarized, age seemed to firmly influence bacterial abundance. While in young-aged patients Bacteroidetes were elevated and Firmicutes reduced, in middle-aged subjects a reduction of Bacteroidetes and an elevation of Firmicutes was reported, compared to age-matched HC, whereas Actinobacteria was consistently elevated regardless of age. However, on lower taxonomic levels correlations could show opposite directions even for closely related bacteria, suggesting that the abundance of a specific phylum is not as decisive as the abundance of certain bacteria on lower taxonomic levels, i.e., on the genus or species level.

Table 2. Different abundance on phylum level, with the studies sorted by age of the diseased subjects.

Source	Mean Age (Years)	Bacteroidetes	Firmicutes	Proteobacteria	Actinobacteria
[44]	MDD 21.9; C 22.1	MDD ↑	MDD ↓		
[49]	MDD 24.0; C 25.0	MDD ↑	MDD ↓		
[66]	BD 24.2; C 36.3	BD ↑	BD ↓	BD ↓ *	
[42]	aMDD 25.3; rMDD 27.1; C 26.8	MDD ↑	MDD ↓	MDD ↑	MDD ↑
[46]	MDD 26.5; BD 25.6; C 26.9	MDD ↑ BD ↓		BD ↑	
[69]	non-D 33.4			↓	
[48]	P 35.7		↓		
[62]	MDD 36.2; C 38.1	MDD ↓	M ↑		MDD ↑ *
[63]	MDD 40.6; C 41.8	MDD ↓			MDD ↑
[52]	BD 41.3; C 31.4				BD ↑
[57]	MDD 41.5; C 44.0	MDD ↓			MDD ↑
[50]	MDD 41.6; BD 38.4; C 39.5	MDD ↓; BD ↓	MDD ↑; BD ↑	BD ↑	MDD ↑; BD ↑
[43]	MDD 43.7; C 39.4	MDD ↓			MDD ↑
[67]	MDD 43.9; C 39.6	MDD ↓	M ↑	MDD ↓	MDD ↑
[60]	D 44.8; IBS 38.5; D + IBS 39.0; C 43.9	D ↑	D ↓		
[55]	IBS + Di 45.0; IBS (non-Di) 33.0			↑	
[49]	MDD 45.0; C 47.2	MDD ↓			MDD ↑
[51]	MDD 45.8; C 41.2	MDD ↓	MDD ↑	MDD ↓	MDD ↑
[58]	MDD 48.7; C 42.3		MDD ↓		
[41]	D 49.2; C 46.1	D ↓			

Elevated Bacteroidetes and reduced Firmicutes were found in young-aged, depressed subjects, while in middle-aged those phyla showed opposite correlations. Actinobacteria was consistently increased. "↓" and green symbolizes a significant reduction in diseased subjects or inverse correlation with more severe symptoms, while "↑" and orange shows a significant elevation or positive correlation with more severe symptoms. Grey symbolizes only a trend, while empty cells symbolize that no significant results were reported. Abbreviations: MDD, major depressive disorder; BD, bipolar disorder; C, control group; D, depression in general; non-D, non-depressed subjects; Di, distressed subjects; IBS, irritable bowel syndrome; P, psychiatric subjects; a, active disorder group; r, response group; *, only showing an insignificant trend.

3.3. Bacteroidetes

The phylum Bacteroidetes is the most dominant in the human gut [70]. It contains four important families, namely Bacteroidaceae, Tannerellaceae, Prevotellaceae, and Rikenellaceae.

Most studies reported a correlation between depressive symptoms and the family Bacteroidaceae or genus *Bacteroides*, the most abundant family and genus of the intestinal microbiota [70]. Especially genus *Bacteroides* was repeatedly associated with affective disorder, high anhedonia, and negative mood (Table 3). In general, *Bacteroides* were found to be negatively associated with inflammation [50,71], to contribute to the gut colonization resistance (the resistance against colonization of enteric pathogens), and to produce SCFAs, mostly acetate and propionate, which are important for gut homeostasis [72,73]. *Bacteroides* are known as starch degraders and they potentially cross-feed other species, like *Eubacterium ramulus*, which in turn can produce beneficial molecules like butyrate, and therefore reduce gut hyperpermeability by increased expression of tight-junctions [72]. Even though genus *Bacteroides* was found to provide beneficial effects on the human host, the family Bacteroidaceae and genus *Bacteroides* were repeatedly found to be elevated in depressed subjects. While some of the reviewed studies were conducted only with few individuals, Cheng et al. included thousands of subjects, strongly supporting this correlation [74]. These findings may hint at a compensatory mechanism and suggest that the alteration in the abundance of a certain bacteria may not necessarily have negative health effects. A higher taxonomic resolution could lead to more precise information about these correlations.

Table 3. Different abundance of genus Bacteroides.

Source	Genus *Bacteroides*	
[42]	aMDD ↓	rMDD ↑
[45]	negative mood ↑	
[46]	BD ↑ (1 OTU)	
	MDD ↑/↓ (OTUs)	
[47]	anhedonia ↑	
	anxiety ↓	
[50]	MDD ↓, BD ↓	
[55]	anxiety ↑	
[57]	MDD ↑ (m)	
[60]	D ↑; IBS ↑; D + IBS ↑	
[66]	BD ↑	
[74]	MDD ↑	
[75]	BD ↑ (B-P group)	

Most studies reported an elevation correlating with affective disorder and depressive symptoms. "↓" and green symbolizes a significant reduction in diseased subjects or inverse correlation with more severe symptoms, while "↑" and orange shows a significant elevation or positive correlation with more severe symptoms, and grey symbolizes alterations in both directions or not evaluable. Brackets include additional information about the reported correlation (which bacteria showed a correlation or in which subgroup of subjects a correlation was found). Abbreviations: MDD, major depressive disorder; BD, bipolar disorder; D, depression in general; IBS, irritable bowel syndrome; B-P group, Bacteroides-Prevotella group; m, a correlation only in male subjects; a, active disease group; r, response group; OTU, operational taxonomic unit within genus Bacteroides.

Genus *Parabacteroides* of the Tannerellaceae family tended to be elevated in depressed subjects, but two studies reported contrary results [60,69]. These two studies used a small sample size of depressed subjects (*n* = 15), and reported a reduction in non-depressed participants to correlate with anxiety and DASS-42 (depression anxiety and stress scales) scores, but not directly with depression, respectively [60,69]. Investigating the three studies which compared MDD or BD subjects with HC, all three reported an elevation of *Parabacteroides* correlating with depression [42,51,66]. *Parabacteroides* produce SCFAs, especially acetate, and can reduce neutrophils in the blood [76]. Even though they have health-promoting effects, they tended to be more abundant in individuals with affective disorders. Therefore, as with the family Bacteroidaceae, an elevation of *Parabacteroides* could be a compensatory mechanism, rather than unfavorably influencing the host's mood.

The abundance of the Prevotellaceae family altered in both directions in depressed subjects, with no tendency overall. Worth mentioning is that Chen et al. found a reduction of Prevotellaceae in middle-aged MDD, compared to young-aged MDD individuals [49]. This goes in line with our general findings, with two studies reporting a reduced Prevotellaceae abundance in middle-aged MDD subjects (mean age 45.8 and 43.9 years, respectively) [51,67]. On genus level, *Prevotella* inversely correlated with depression, lower mood, or lower quality of life in four studies [42,45,51,77], while others reported a positive correlation [60,62]. Therefore, the suggestion of Lin et al. [62], to use changes of *Prevotella* and *Klebsiella* for laboratory diagnosis and treatment evaluation in MDD, could not be further supported regarding *Prevotella* changes, because the results showed no clear tendency and additional studies even found an opposite correlation. Concerning *Klebsiella* changes, more research is needed to be able to draw a conclusion (further information in the paragraph "Proteobacteria"). Interestingly, two studies conducted with IBS subjects reported an elevation of Prevotellaceae, as well as an elevation of *Prevotella* and *Paraprevotella* to correlate with depressive symptoms, indicating a potential correlation with IBS and comorbid depression [55,60]. However, due to small sample sizes and different study designs of these two studies, additional research focusing on bacterial alterations in IBS subjects is required.

Within the family Rikenellaceae, results showed an elevation of genus *Alistipes* or operational taxonomic units (OTUs) within this genus to correlate with depression [41,42,63]. While *Alistipes* seemed to attenuate the severity of colitis via attenuating the expression of anti-inflammatory cytokines in mice, this genus was found to be increased in stressed mice, as well as in patients suffering from chronic fatigue syndrome. It is proposed to decrease serotonin concentration and therefore negatively influence the gut-brain axis, which is in line with our conclusion that an elevated *Alistipes* abundance is associated with unfavorable health effects and potentially promotes the pathogenesis of depression [78]. More studies are needed to further investigate the influence of the Rikenellaceae family on depression.

3.4. Firmicutes

The phylum Firmicutes is the second most abundant phylum in the human intestinal microbiome [70]. It was also the most changed, as well as the most discussed phylum within the reviewed studies.

Class Bacilli includes two important families, the families of Lactobacillaceae and Streptococcaceae. *Lactobacillus* bacteria are widely known for their beneficial health effects and their use as probiotics. Despite several studies reporting a higher abundance of *Lactobacillus* to be associated with diverse positive factors like sleep and self-judgment, no direct correlation of *Lactobacillus* abundance and affective disorder could be identified [79,80]. Family Streptococcaceae and genus *Streptococcus* showed a positive correlation with depression and lower quality of life scores. For example, beta-hemolytic Streptococcus Group A infections are known to potentially cause Pediatric Autoimmune Neuropsychiatric Disorders (Associated with Streptococcal Infections, "PANDAS"), which are associated with alterations in the gut microbiome and the nervous system [81]. Although not fully understood, it demonstrates that *Streptococcus* infections can lead to an autoimmune response, severe brain alterations, disturbed neurotransmitters, and can cause psychiatric symptoms like obsessive-compulsive disorder, tics, anxiety, and sometimes even depression [82]. Of the included studies, four reported an elevation of Streptococcaceae (or OTUs within this family) and *Streptococcus* in MDD and BD [50,51,62,63]. Additionally, investigating a large cohort, Valles-Colomer et al. found a negative association between *Streptococcus* and body pain, but no direct association with depression, maybe due to the cohort representing the general population and not being limited to specifically MDD or BD subjects [77]. Hence, there is a need for more studies on the Streptococcaceae family and *Streptococcus* genus regarding their influence on mental health, with potential for novel therapeutic approaches.

Concerning the class Clostridia, a reduction of class Clostridia or order Clostridiales seemed to correlate with worse health and depressive symptoms. However, on lower taxonomic levels, probably due to the diversity of the family Clostridiaceae [83] and an insufficient number of well-controlled studies, no clear association could be identified between Clostridiaceae or *Clostridium* and depression, and studies reported ambiguous findings. There is a need for in-depth studies at high taxonomic resolution to further investigate a potential connection between certain genera or species within the family Clostridiaceae and affective disorder. In addition, an antidepressant therapy with adjunctive probiotic *Clostridium butyricum MIYAIRI 588* showed a high response rate with significant improvement of depressive symptoms in treatment-resistant MDD subjects (further information in the paragraph "human interventional trials in depression") [84]. Family Christensenellaceae and Christensenellaceae R-7 group were reported to be less abundant in subjects with affective disorder and to inversely correlate with more severe symptoms and higher anhedonia in three studies, while none reported opposite results [44,47,53]. Family Christensenellaceae has been shown to produce acetate and butyrate, and was negatively associated with visceral fat mass [85,86]. Even though, to our knowledge, not much is known about this family so far, a higher abundance of family Christensenellaceae is related to beneficial health effects, while depression correlates with a reduction of this family.

Family Peptostreptococcaceae or genus *Peptostreptococcus* were associated with depression [51,58] and anxiety [69] in three studies. In general, while some studies found a connection between *Peptostreptococcus* species and colorectal cancer [87], others proposed a beneficial effect via the production of indoleacrylic acid (a metabolite of tryptophan), improving the intestinal epithelial barrier function, as well as suppressing inflammatory response [88]. Despite these potentially beneficial effects, a rather negative correlation between *Peptostreptococcus* and depression was reported in the reviewed studies. But with only two studies finding a significantly altered abundance in small cohorts of depressed individuals, while none of the studies with more subjects reported similar results, an important association with depression is unlikely.

Family Eubacteriaceae and especially species *E. rectale* tended to be more abundant in healthy subjects and increased after antipsychotic BD treatment with quetiapine [44,47,57,75]. *Eubacterium* spp. can produce propionate and butyrate, and therefore suppress inflammation, enhance the intestinal barrier integrity, and thereby benefit the host's health [89]. This is in line with our findings, where Eubacteriaceae correlated with better general health. But the evidence in terms of an association with depression remains scarce.

Family Lachnospiraceae is the second most abundant family in the human gut [70]. On the family level, studies did not show a clear connection between Lachnospiraceae and depression, with Lachnospiraceae being altered in both directions in depressed individuals. However, on the genus level, several inverse correlations with depression were found. Genus *Coprococcus* and OTUs within this genus were found to be less abundant in depressed subjects and to correlate with higher quality of life [46,48,58,60,63,66,77]. One study found specifically *C. catus* to be less abundant in subjects with more severe depressive symptoms and to positively correlate with remission [48]. Genus *Coprococcus* is known for its butyrate production [90], and previous research found a reduced *Coprococcus* abundance in several diseases, like inflammatory bowel disease [16], colorectal cancer [91], and preeclampsia [90]. According to Zhang et al., *Coprococcus* abundance can be increased by omega-3 polyunsaturated fatty acids (PUFAs), while lower levels of omega-3 PUFAs were found in depressed subjects [92,93]. Therefore, a connection between genus *Coprococcus*, PUFAs (especially omega-3 PUFAs), and depression is imaginable, emphasizing the importance of a healthy diet and its influence on the intestinal microbiota and depression. The abundance of genus *Fusicatenibacter* or unclassified species within this genus were reduced in depressed subjects and associated with a higher quality of life in three studies, indicating a slightly beneficial effect of these bacteria [44,55,77]. Due to contradictory results concerning genus *Blautia*, no final statement could be made regarding a link of genus *Blautia* with depression. Genus *Roseburia* or OTUs within this genus were mostly reported to be reduced in subjects with depressive symptoms and correlated with remission and positive mood (Table 4). Research showed that *R. intestinalis* suppressed inflammation and promoted anti-inflammatory cytokines in a colitis mouse model, and found *Roseburia*, together with *Faecalibacterium*, to be one of the most abundant known butyrate-producing bacteria in the human gut [94,95]. This is in line with our findings of *Roseburia* being reduced in depressed individuals. Therefore, an increase of bacteria belonging to the genera *Roseburia* or *Coprococcus* may provide beneficial physical and mental health effects, and further investigation is needed as to whether this effect can be used in the treatment of affective disorder.

Concerning the family Ruminococcaceae, most studies found a higher abundance in healthier subjects (Table 5). Interestingly, the abundance of family Ruminococcaceae was associated with remission, but several taxa within Ruminococcaceae positively correlated with symptom severity of psychiatric subjects [48]. Additionally, both increased and decreased OTUs within this family were found in MDD patients, underlining the differences of bacterial abundance on low taxonomic levels [49,57]. On genus and species level, on the one hand, multiple studies reported a higher abundance of genus *Oscillibacter* in depressed subjects [41–43,50]. Genus *Oscillibacter* is suggested to be elevated rather as a result of depression, due to its potential to metabolize proteins [96]. Underlining this, in MDD subjects, disturbed bacterial proteins were found, which are involved especially in metabolic pathways related to amino acid metabolism [67]. On the other hand, genus *Ruminococcus*, *Gemmiger*, and especially *Faecalibacterium* were more abundant in healthier subjects in the majority of the reviewed studies (Table 5). *Faecalibacterium* is known for its butyrate production, anti-inflammatory potential, and intestinal barrier function improvement, and was suggested as a probiotic for IBD, gut dysfunction, and low-grade inflammation treatment [95,97,98]. In the reviewed studies, a negative correlation with depressive symptoms and a positive correlation with remission and higher quality of life was reported, highlighting the potential of probiotic *Faecalibacterium* as a novel treatment option, and their abundance as a parameter for diagnosis or treatment response. Even though several studies reported opposite correlations, contradictory results can mostly be explained by very small sample sizes, age and sex differences, and by not unexceptionally used false discovery rate. In conclusion, the family Ruminococcaceae is a perfect example that even closely related bacteria can show an altered abundance in opposite directions. Even though on the family level, most of the studies reported a higher abundance in healthier subjects, on lower taxonomic levels bacterial alterations were found in both directions. Similar to other families, a higher taxonomic resolution of this family and its genera is needed for a more specific examination of these bacteria and their interaction with the host, with especially genus *Faecalibacterium* showing a close negative association with depression.

Table 4. Different abundance of genus Roseburia.

Source	Genus *Roseburia*
[42]	aMDD ↑
[45]	↓ positive mood
[46]	BD ↓ (1 OTU)
[47]	anhedonia ↓
[48]	P ↓ remission (*R. inuliniforans*)
[52]	BD ↓ *
[55]	D ↓ (unclassified species)
[57]	MDD ↑ (f)
[60]	D ↓
[63]	MDD ↓ (OTUs)
[66]	BD ↓

Most studies reported a reduction correlating with affective disorder and negative mood. "↓" and green symbolizes a significant reduction in diseased subjects or inverse correlation with more severe symptoms, while "↑" and orange shows a significant elevation or positive correlation with more severe symptoms, and grey symbolizes only a trend. Brackets include additional information about the reported correlation (which bacteria showed a correlation or in which subgroup of patients a correlation was found). Abbreviations: MDD, major depressive disorder; BD, bipolar disorder; D, depression in general; f, a correlation only in female subjects; a, active disorder; OTU, operational taxonomic unit within genus Roseburia; *, only negatively correlating with symptom severity, but not significantly correlating with BD compared to healthy controls.

Table 5. Different abundance of family Ruminococcaceae and two of its members, genus Ruminococcus and Faecalibacterium.

Source	Family Ruminococcaceae	Genus *Ruminococcus*	Genus *Faecalibacterium*
[42]	MDD ↓	aMDD ↓	MDD ↓
[44]	MDD ↓	MDD ↓ (*Ruminococcus 1*)	MDD ↓
[45]			negative mood ↑
[46]	MDD ↓ (OTUs) BD ↑/↓ (OTUs)		
[47]	anhedonia ↓		
[48]	P ↓ remission	P ↑ (*Ruminococcus 1*)	P ↓ remission (*F. prausnitzii*)
[49]	MDD ↑/↓ (OTUs)		
[51]		MDD ↑	
[52]	BD ↓		BD ↓
[54]	BD ↓		BD ↓
[55]			D ↑ (unclassified species)
[57]	MDD ↑/↓ (OTUs)		MDD ↑ (f)
[58]	MDD ↓		
[60]		D ↓	
[63]	MDD ↑ (OTUs)		MDD ↓ (OTUs)
[66]		BD ↓	BD ↓
[67]	MDD ↑		MDD ↓
[75]			BD ↑ (*F. prausnitzii*)
[77]			lower QoL ↓

Table 5. *Cont.*

Source	Family Ruminococcaceae	Genus *Ruminococcus*	Genus *Faecalibacterium*
[99]		DASS ↑ (*R. gnavus*)	
[100]	BD ↓ (1 OTU)		BD ↓

Most studies reported an elevation of these bacteria correlating with better health. "↓" and green symbolizes a significant reduction in diseased subjects or inverse correlation with more severe symptoms, while "↑" and orange shows a significant elevation or positive correlation with more severe symptoms, and grey symbolizes alterations in both directions. Brackets include additional information about the reported correlation (which bacteria showed a correlation or in which subgroup of patients a correlation was found). Empty cells symbolize that no significant results were reported. Abbreviations: MDD, major depressive disorder; BD, bipolar disorder; D, depression in general; P, psychiatric subjects; DASS, depression anxiety stress scales; QoL, quality of life; f, a correlation only in female subjects; a, active disorder; OTU, operational taxonomic unit.

Additionally, an elevation of genus *Flavonifractor* was associated with depression, symptom severity, or worse physical functioning, with no contradictory results [42,44,48,64,77]. Even though *Flavonifractor plautii* was recently found to suppress the immune response in mice in multiple studies conducted by the same research group [101–103], it was repeatedly associated with several diseases, including ulcerative colitis, autoimmune diseases, obesity, and even with a poor diet [104,105]. Our findings of elevated *Flavonifractor*, with no study finding opposite results, strongly support its negative influence on the host's health, including affective disorder.

3.5. Proteobacteria

Within the phylum Proteobacteria, most differences between depressed individuals and HC were found within order Burkholderiales of class Betaproteobacteria. Five studies reported a reduction of family Sutterellaceae, OTUs within this family, or genus *Sutterella* in depressed subjects [51,57,60,63,67]. Additionally, Peter et al. [55] reported an association between order Burkholderiales abundance and perceived stress, which is inconsistent with the other results on lower taxonomic levels, demonstrating that a high taxonomic resolution should be striven for. No study found elevated Sutterellaceae or *Sutterella* in patients with affective disorder. Hence, a negative association with depression is conceivable on these taxonomic levels. Even though not very much is known about this family, it seems to be associated with diseases like autism spectrum disorder, down syndrome, and IBD. Furthermore, a mild pro-inflammatory capacity of certain species within genus *Sutterella* was proposed [106]. Therefore, the origin and consequence of reduced Sutterellaceae and *Sutterella* in depressed individuals remain unclear.

Within class Gammaproteobacteria, family Enterobacteriaceae tended to be elevated in subjects with affective disorder, but with controversial results. At the genus level, few studies reported a higher abundance of *Enterobacter* and *Klebsiella* to correlate with worse health [54,62,75]. The family Enterobacteriaceae, with its well-known genera *Enterobacter*, *Escherichia*, *Klebsiella*, *Salmonella*, and *Shigella*, is associated with many different clinical syndromes and diseases, including foodborne infectious diarrhea, enteritis, colitis, hemolytic uremic syndrome, as well as extraintestinal diseases [107]. Maes et al. found increased serum immune globulin M (IgM) against LPS of Gammaproteobacteria in depressed individuals, highlighting the link between intestinal mucosal dysfunction, increased bacterial translocation, immune response, and depression [9]. Family Pseudomonadaceae and genus *Pseudomonas* were elevated in depressed subjects in two studies, but with controversial results regarding only MDD subjects [46,58]. Maes et al. also found increased IgM against *Pseudomonas* in MDD subjects, compared to HC [33]. Here too, as concluded for other families, more detailed information on lower taxonomic levels is needed for a clear-cut statement.

Genus *Desulfovibrio* of class Deltaproteobacteria seemed to positively correlate with MDD and BD, but only three of all reviewed studies found a different abundance [44,57,74]. Cheng et al. analyzed published genome-wide association study data sets with high numbers of cases and controls [74]. They reported an association of genus *Desulfovibrio* with MDD, BD, and other mental disorders, suggesting a crucial role of this genus in mental disorders. However, these findings are not consistent with the results of the other two studies, which found *Desulfovibrio* to be elevated only in female but not in male MDD subjects, and even reported an inverse correlation with MDD, respectively [44,57]. Age could be an important confounding factor, due to young participants in Liu et al. [44] and middle-aged in Chen et al. [57]. Therefore, genus *Desulfovibrio* could be reduced in young-aged, depressed subjects, while in middle-aged these bacteria could be elevated, but further investigation is needed.

3.6. Actinobacteria

Within the phylum Actinobacteria, study results tended towards an increase of class Coriobacteria, order Coriobacteriales, family Coriobacteriaceae, or OTUs within this family correlating with depression, but with inconsistent results [47,49,52,57,63]. However, on the genus level, a higher abundance of genus *Collinsella* was associated with lower anhedonia, BD treatment, and remission [47,48,66]. Only one study reported an association of elevated *Collinsella* with depression scores, suggesting that there is little evidence for a positive correlation with depression [57]. Other research found a stress-induced increase of an unspecified genus of Coriobacteriaceae in mice, a reduction of genus *Collinsella* after weight loss in obese type 2 diabetics, and a positive correlation of *Collinsella* with circulating insulin levels and low dietary fiber intake, while a high fiber intake supports SCFA-promoting gut bacteria [108–110]. Therefore, *Collinsella* is generally associated with worse health, and consequently, it remains unclear why especially genus *Collinsella* tended to be associated with ameliorated depressive symptoms. Even though closely related, genus *Eggerthella* was shown to be associated with MDD and higher depression and perceived stress scores in the reviewed research [43,51,57]. An elevated *Eggerthella* abundance was also found in immune-mediated inflammatory diseases like Crohn's disease and ulcerative colitis [111]. In conclusion, while on a higher taxonomic level an increase of these bacteria was found in depressed subjects, on lower taxonomic levels this consistent increase could not be seen, due to a reduction of genus *Collinsella* correlating with depression.

Within the order Bifidobacteriales, genus *Bifidobacterium* is known for its beneficial effects on the host's health and a lower abundance is associated with several diseases [112]. Counterintuitively, most studies found a positive association with depression and negative mood, while only three studies reported an elevation correlating with better health or depression treatment (Table 6). While in depressed subjects *Bifidobacterium* abundance seemed to be elevated, most studies reported a significant improvement in depressive symptoms with probiotics containing *Bifidobacterium* spp. (Table 7). The reason for those seemingly contradicting results remains unclear and needs further research.

Table 6. Different abundances of family Bifidobacteriaceae and genus Bifidobacterium.

Source	Family Bifidobacteriaceae	Genus *Bifidobacterium*
[43]		MDD ↑
[45]		negative mood ↑
[46]	MDD ↑	BD =
[47]	anhedonia ↓	anhedonia ↓
[50]		MDD ↑, BD ↑
[51]	MDD ↑	MDD ↑
[56]		HDRS ↑ (*B. longum*)
[57]		MDD ↑ (f)
[67]	MDD ↑	
[79]		BD =
[113]		MDD ↓

Results tended to show a negative effect of an elevation of these bacteria. "↓" and green symbolizes a significant reduction in diseased subjects or inverse correlation with more severe symptoms, while "↑" and orange shows a significant elevation or positive correlation with more severe symptoms, and "=" and grey symbolizes no correlation. Brackets include additional information about the reported correlation (which bacteria showed a correlation or in which subgroup of patients a correlation was found). Empty cells symbolize that no significant results were reported. Abbreviations: MDD, major depressive disorder; BD, bipolar disorder; HDRS, Hamilton depression rating scale; f, a correlation only in female subjects.

In general, most of the investigated bacteria belonging to phylum Actinobacteria tended to correlate with worse health and depression, which is again contrary to the general finding of Actinobacteria having a positive influence on human health and its beneficial effects as probiotics [112]. Microbial bacteria are firmly influenced by diet [112], but only few studies included dietary data. Therefore, different eating habits could be a possible factor leading to elevated Actinobacteria in depressed individuals, but a satisfactory explanation is not possible to date.

3.7. Human Interventional Trials in Depression

A total 13 studies investigated the influence of probiotic *Lactobacillus* and/or *Bifidobacterium* on depression. While six studies found no significant improvement in depressive scores, seven reported a significant amelioration of depression (Table 7). Three of them were conducted by the same research group, focusing specifically on the species *Lactobacillus gasseri* [114–116]. These three studies reported the most positive and most diverse results. According to them, *L. gasseri* ameliorated depression and anxiety, shortened sleep latency and awake time, lightened fatigue, improved global sleep quality, but also lowered salivary cortisol levels, and even suppressed unfavorable intestinal bacteria. However, to our knowledge, no other studies investigated the effect of *L. gasseri* supplementation on depressive symptoms to date. It might be essential to verify these highly encouraging results with *L. gasseri* probiotics by additional independent research groups. Supporting these beneficial findings of *Lactobacillus* and *Bifidobacterium* probiotics, Heym et al. reported a strong correlation between *Lactobacillus* spp. abundance and positive self-judgment, but only an indirect relationship between *Lactobacillus* spp. and depression, while *Bifidobacterium* spp. showed no association with any psychometric measures [80]. However, all but one of the compared studies reported a beneficial effect of these probiotics, and despite often not reaching significance level, depression scores mostly showed a slight reduction. This indicates that probiotic *Lactobacillus* and *Bifidobacterium* have a modest beneficial effect on depressive symptoms. Whether the effect size is large enough to be of clinical importance needs further investigation, but with none of these 13 studies reporting a worsening of depression or other serious side effects in the probiotic groups, probiotic *Lactobacillus* and *Bifidobacterium* should be considered as an adjunctive treatment in the therapy of affective disorder and depressive symptoms.

Additional studies investigated the use of prebiotics, synbiotics, and different probiotics on depression (Table 7). While in the probiotic group depressive scores only tended to ameliorate, in the synbiotic group a significant difference was found by Haghighat et al. [117]. Therefore, an additional supplementation containing fructo-oligosaccharides, galacto-oligosaccharides, and inulin could further support the beneficial effects of probiotic *Lactobacillus* and *Bifidobacterium*. In treatment-resistant MDD subjects, probiotic *Clostridium butyricum MIYAIRI 588*, a butyrate, acetate, and propionate producing bacteria, showed in combination with antidepressant medication not only an improvement of depressive symptoms but also a response rate as high as 70%, with 35% reaching complete remission [84]. These results are very promising and as mentioned before, further studies may pave the way for the use of probiotic *C. butyricum MIYAIRI 588* in depressive patients. The use of no probiotic food or supplementation was associated with higher odds of depression in a large cross-sectional study. However, individuals consuming probiotics were wealthier and showed a healthier lifestyle on average, resulting in a lower risk of developing depression [118]. These data indicate only an indirect link of probiotics and depression and emphasize that not all probiotic bacteria result in lower rates of depression.

3.8. Studies Involving Twins and Their Relatives

As genetics and environmental factors have a huge influence not only on the development of depression but also on the microbiome, three studies examined whether there is a correlation between the intestinal microbiota and depression in twins and relatives. Two studies investigated the difference of the microbiota in twins [53,54], and one study examined the difference between the microbiota of patients with newly diagnosed BD and their first-degree relatives [64].

Table 7. Effect of prebiotics, probiotics, and synbiotics on depression.

Source	Subjects; Pre-/Syn-/Probiotics	Influence on Depression/Depressive Symptoms
[84]	MDD; *C. butyricum*	+(treatment response, remission)
[99]	D; Lactobacilli, Bifidobacteria	=(BDI, BAI, DASS)
[114]	H; *L. gasseri*	+(depression, anxiety, sleep)
[115]	H; *L. gasseri*	+(HADS, fatigue, mental state)
[116]	H; *L. gasseri*	+(depressive mood, anxiety, sleep, stress)
[118]	C; any probiotics/supplementation	=(PHQ-9)
[117]	Dialysis; *L. acidophilus*, Bifidobacteria; fiber	+with synbiotics (HADS, BDNF)=with probiotics (HADS, BDNF)
[119]	MDD; galacto-oligosaccaride; *L. helveticus*, *B. longum*	=with prebiotics (BDI)+with probiotics (BDI)
[120]	MDD; *L. plantarum*	=(HDRS, PSS)+(attention, perceptivity, verbal learning)
[121]	D; *L. helveticus*, *B. longum*	=(MADRS, DASS)
[122]	H; *L. rhamnosus*	+(depression, anxiety)
[123]	IBS with anx. or depr.; *B. longum*	+(HADS, QoL, brain activity)
[124]	H; Lactobacilli, Bifidobacteria	=(BDI, BAI)+(cognitive reactivity to sad mood)
[125]	MDD; Lactobacilli, *B. bifidum*	+(BDI, serum hs-CPR)
[126]	BD; *L. acidophilus*, Bifidobacteria	=(YMRS, HDRS)

Results mostly showed positive effects, but several studies could not find significant differences. "+" symbolizes a significantly positive health effect, while "=" indicates no significant difference. In brackets a selection of the investigated measures is given. Abbreviations: MDD, major depressive disorder; BD, bipolar disorder; D, participants with depressive symptoms; H, healthy participants; C, cross-sectional study; IBS, irritable bowel syndrome; BDI, Beck depression inventory; BAI, Beck anxiety inventory; DASS, depression anxiety stress scales; HADS, hospital anxiety and depression scale; PHQ-9, patient health questionnaire; HDRS, Hamilton depression rating scale; PSS, perceived stress scale; MADRS, Montgomery-Åsberg depression rating scale; BDNF, brain-derived neurotrophic factor; QoL, quality of life; hs-CPR, high-sensitivity C-reactive protein; YMRS, young mania rating scale.

The two twin studies investigated 128 monozygotic twins and one pair of monozygotic twins, respectively [53,54]. Vinberg et al. distinguished between affected twins (with a diagnosis of MDD or BD in remission), unaffected high-risk twins (with a co-twin history of depression), and low-risk twins (without any histories of depression in the family) [53]. They found a lower diversity and richness of the microbiota of affected twins, while high-risk twins showed the same pattern, but with the lower diversity only being a trend. Affected and high-risk twins also showed an absence of an OTU belonging to the family Christensenellaceae. However, no correlation of the microbiota with illness severity was found. Jiang et al. reported a less similar microbiota between the pair of discordant twins (one twin with a history of depression and one without) than the microbiota of two healthy spouses [54]. Moreover, the similarity of the microbiota reached its maximum after achieving full remission of the affected twin, with the level of Ruminococcaceae and *Faecalibacterium* increasing and *Enterobacter* decreasing during the responsive and remission periods. Several SCFA-producing genera, mainly belonging to the families Lachnospiraceae and Ruminococcaceae, were reduced in the active-BD state compared to the healthy spouses [54]. Further, an over-representation of LPS biosynthesis genes in the gut microbiota during the active depressive period was found, whereas in the remissive state these genes decreased, indicating a potential recovery of the microbiota during the responsive and remissive period. But with only one pair of monozygotic twins, these results must be taken with caution.

According to Coello et al., newly diagnosed BD subjects had a different microbiota, while the microbiota of unaffected first-degree relatives did not differ significantly from the microbiota of HC [64]. Especially the presence of *Flavonifractor* was associated with an increased odds ratio for having BD. After adjusting for smoking, this association attenuated, indicating an additional correlation of *Flavonifractor* with smoking, as well as with the female gender. It is hypothesized that the microbiota of BD patients is characterized by the different presence or absence of bacteria, especially of *Flavonifractor*, rather than the difference of bacterial abundance.

In summary, these studies support the hypothesis of a close connection between the intestinal microbiota and depression, and significant differences in the microbiota composition of depressed subjects were found. They even showed that a higher risk of developing depression is already associated with minor changes of the microbiota, and that with remission of depression, the intestinal bacteria change back towards a more "normal" composition. Comparing the reported bacterial alterations with our general findings, a beneficial effect of Christensenellaceae, Ruminococcaceae, and *Faecalibacterium*, and a negative effect of *Flavonifractor* show most experimental evidence.

4. Discussion

Our data show that the intestinal microbiota is closely linked with major depressive and bipolar disorder. The complexity of the microbiota makes it challenging to find clear causative associations, and a higher taxonomic resolution for determining the intestinal bacteria would be of importance for a more accurate analysis. Further studies with more participants are needed to verify specific bacterial alterations since the reviewed studies were mostly conducted with small sample sizes of up to 150 participants (with few exceptions). Study designs, inclusion criteria, analysis methods, and confounding factors varied widely, making a comparison difficult and may explain the contradicting results for certain bacteria. Therefore, a review of such heterogeneous studies is also associated with major limitations, and more standardized studies would facilitate a comparison.

Despite these limitations, this review demonstrated that certain bacteria consistently correlate with depression. The strongest and most consistent correlations are demonstrated in Table 8.

Table 8. Bacteria (with taxonomic level) that correlated most with depression.

More Abundant in Depressive Subjects	Less Abundant in Depressive Subjects
Actinobacteria (phylum)	Christensenellaceae and *Christensenella* (family and genus)
Alistipes (genus)	*Coprococcus* (genus)
Bacteroides (genus)	*Eubacterium* and *E. rectale* (genus and species)
Bifidobacteriaceae and *Bifidobacterium* (family and genus)	*Faecalibacterium* and *F. prausnitzii* (genus and species)
Flavonifractor (genus)	*Roseburia* (genus)
Parabacteroides (genus)	Ruminococcaceae (family)
Streptococcus (genus)	Sutterellaceae and *Sutterella* (family and genus)

Additionally, phylum Bacteroidetes consistently positively correlated with depression in young individuals, whereas in middle-aged individuals a strong inverse correlation with depression was found, while phylum Firmicutes showed opposite correlations.

Noticeably, apart from phylum Bacteroidetes, Firmicutes, and Actinobacteria, the strongest correlations with depression were found on low taxonomic levels (particularly on genus level), underlining the importance of high taxonomic resolution to identify bacterial alterations in depressed subjects. Further studies specifically focusing on these altered bacteria and their interactions with the host could provide a better insight into the connection between depression and the human gut microbiota. SCFA-producing bacteria were mostly found to be reduced in depressed individuals, emphasizing the beneficial influence on their host. With a better understanding of the intestinal microbiota, new therapeutic strategies for the treatment of affective disorder could be found, which is crucial considering the high therapy resistance and relapse rates [5]. However, considering the complexity of the intestinal microbiota and the diversity of the bacterial changes found in this review, it is conceivable that bacterial clusters would show better correlations with depression. Consequently, studies with more participants are needed to identify depression-like bacterial clusters, as well as novel potential treatment approaches.

Changing the intestinal microbiota (for instance through specific diets, supplementations, probiotics, synbiotics, or fecal microbiota transplantation (FMT)) could potentially support the host's health and mitigate depressive symptoms. While multiple clinical studies found probiotics and synbiotics to have a positive impact on mood and behavior, clinical FMT studies in depressed subjects remain scarce. FMT has repeatedly been shown to ameliorate depression [127]. After receiving fecal transplants of depressive patients, a depression-like behavior of germ-free mice was observed, compared to mice receiving fecal transplants of healthy individuals [63,128]. In a clinical study, patients with gastrointestinal complaints reported an improvement in depression scores after FMT, and in a case report, a treatment-resistant BD patient achieved full remission after FMT [56,129]. Further studies exploring the effect of probiotics, synbiotics and FMT with more individuals are required to strengthen these positive findings. In addition, since diet significantly influences the intestinal microtioba composition [112] and only few studies included dietary questionnaires, it is essential to adjust for dietary changes between depressed subjects and HC. Thereby bacterial alterations only due to different eating habits could be excluded in future studies.

Stevens et al. were able to differentiate depressed and non-depressed subjects using a machine learning approach [130]. Additional similar studies could offer the potential of finding specific bacterial clusters and changes in metabolic pathways associated with affective disorder. Moreover, it is suggested by these authors that this novel approach may be used as a reliable diagnostic tool to identify different depression phenotypes in the future, potentially even leading to personalized treatment of depression [130]. Even though reliably distinguishing between depressed and non-depressed individuals, it remains doubtful whether similar approaches would be of clinical importance as a diagnostic tool.

Another key question is how depressed subjects develop different abundances of certain intestinal bacteria. Does it depend on the diet, with depressed individuals showing different eating habits, do they have a special intestinal milieu that secondarily favors the colonization of certain bacteria, or are there other factors influencing the intestinal microbiota towards a depressive-like composition? Answering this question, which is the scope of another dedicated report, would help to prevent unfavorable microbiota changes and would provide further information about the bidirectional connection of the microbiota and depression.

While most of the studies only investigated MDD subjects, research with BD subjects is lagging, but an increasing number of studies including BD individuals in recent years shows a growing interest. In this review, we could not identify unequivocal differences between the microbiota abundance of MDD and BD subjects. Three studies juxtaposed MDD and BD individuals and found a distinct microbiota, but the results were controversial and inconsistent with the other studies including only MDD or BD subjects [46,50,74]. Therefore, a distinguishable microbiota is conceivable, but major differences could not be found.

In conclusion, strong correlations between the intestinal microbiota and affective disorder were found. Specifically investigating only MDD or BD individuals would decrease the heterogeneity of the disease manifestation, but other factors such as the analysis methods, subject heterogeneity, medication, nutrition, and lifestyle factors essentially confound the results. Additional standardized research is needed to elucidate the connection between the intestinal microbiota and depression and to further examine their interdependencies to eventually find novel therapeutic approaches and lower the rates of treatment-resistant affective disorder.

Author Contributions: Conceptualization, T.K. and M.H.M.; methodology, T.K. and M.H.M.; validation, M.H.M.; formal analysis, T.K. and M.H.M.; investigation, T.K.; resources, T.K.; data curation, T.K.; writing—original draft preparation, T.K.; writing—review and editing, T.K. and M.H.M.; visualization, T.K.; supervision, M.H.M.; project administration, M.H.M. and T.K. All authors have read and agreed to the published version of the manuscript.

Funding: This research received no external funding.

Acknowledgments: We would like to thank David Wolfer for useful comments and the review of this paper.

Conflicts of Interest: The authors declare no conflict of interest.

Abbreviations

ACTH	Adrenocorticotrophin
BAI	Beck anxiety inventory
BD	Bipolar disorder
BDI	Beck depression inventory
BDNF	Brain-derived neurotrophic factor
BMI	Body mass index
COVID-19	Coronavirus disease 2019
CRP	C-reactive protein
DASS	Depression anxiety stress scales
FMT	Fecal microbiota transplantation
FGID	Functional gastrointestinal disorders
GABA	Gamma-aminobutyric acid
HADS	Hospital anxiety and depression scale
HC	Healthy controls
HDRS	Hamilton depression rating scale
HPA axis	Hypothalamic-pituitary-adrenal axis
IBD	Inflammatory bowel disease
IBS	Irritable bowel syndrome
IgM	Immune globulin M
LPS	Lipopolysaccharides
MADRS	Montgomery-Åsberg depression rating scale
MDD	Major depressive disorder
OTU	Operational taxonomic unit
PANDAS	Pediatric autoimmune neuropsychiatric disorders associated with streptococcal infections
PHQ-9	Patient health questionnaire
PLS-DA	Partial least squares discriminant analysis
PSS	Perceived stress scale
PUFA	Polyunsaturated fatty acids
QoL	Quality of life
SCFA	Short-chain fatty acids
spp.	Species
YMRS	Young mania rating scale

References

1. *Depression and Other Common Mental Disorders: Global Health Estimates*; World Health Organization: Geneva, Switzerland, 2017; Licence: CC BY-NC-SA 3.0 IGO.
2. Klengel, T.; Binder, E.B. Gene—Environment Interactions in Major Depressive Disorder. *Can. J. Psychiatry* **2013**, *58*, 76–83. [CrossRef] [PubMed]
3. Craddock, N.; Jones, I. Genetics of bipolar disorder. *J. Med. Genet.* **1999**, *36*, 585–594. [CrossRef] [PubMed]
4. Goes, F.S. Genetics of Bipolar Disorder. *Psychiatr. Clin. N. Am.* **2016**, *39*, 139–155. [CrossRef]
5. McIntyre, R.S.; Filteau, M.-J.; Martin, L.; Patry, S.; Carvalho, A.; Cha, D.S.; Barakat, M.; Miguelez, M. Treatment-resistant depression: Definitions, review of the evidence, and algorithmic approach. *J. Affect. Disord.* **2014**, *156*, 1–7. [CrossRef] [PubMed]

6. Lee, C.; Doo, E.; Choi, J.M.; Jang, S.; Ryu, H.-S.; Lee, J.Y.; Oh, J.H.; Park, J.H.; Kim, Y.S. Brain-Gut Axis Research Group of Korean Society of Neurogastroenterology and Motility The Increased Level of Depression and Anxiety in Irritable Bowel Syndrome Patients Compared with Healthy Controls: Systematic Review and Meta-analysis. *J. Neurogastroenterol. Motil.* **2017**, *23*, 349–362. [CrossRef]
7. Dean, J.; Keshavan, M. The neurobiology of depression: An integrated view. *Asian J. Psychiatry* **2017**, *27*, 101–111. [CrossRef]
8. Mudyanadzo, T.A.; Hauzaree, C.; Yerokhina, O.; Architha, N.N.; Ashqar, H.M. Irritable Bowel Syndrome and Depression: A Shared Pathogenesis. *Cureus* **2018**, *10*, e3178. [CrossRef] [PubMed]
9. Maes, M.; Kubera, M.; Leunis, J.-C.; Berk, M. Increased IgA and IgM responses against gut commensals in chronic depression: Further evidence for increased bacterial translocation or leaky gut. *J. Affect. Disord.* **2012**, *141*, 55–62. [CrossRef]
10. Maes, M. Depression is an inflammatory disease, but cell-mediated immune activation is the key component of depression. *Prog. Neuro-Psychopharmacol. Biol. Psychiatry* **2011**, *35*, 664–675. [CrossRef] [PubMed]
11. Sender, R.; Fuchs, S.; Milo, R. Revised Estimates for the Number of Human and Bacteria Cells in the Body. *PLoS Biol.* **2016**, *14*, e1002533. [CrossRef]
12. Rothschild, D.; Weissbrod, O.; Barkan, E.; Kurilshikov, A.; Korem, T.; Zeevi, D.; Costea, P.I.; Godneva, A.; Kalka, I.N.; Bar, N.; et al. Environment dominates over host genetics in shaping human gut microbiota. *Nature* **2018**, *555*, 210–215. [CrossRef]
13. Yang, T.; Santisteban, M.M.; Rodriguez, V.; Li, E.; Ahmari, N.; Carvajal, J.M.; Zadeh, M.; Gong, M.; Qi, Y.; Zubcevic, J.; et al. Gut Dysbiosis Is Linked to Hypertension. *Hypertension* **2015**, *65*, 1331–1340. [CrossRef] [PubMed]
14. Aron-Wisnewsky, J.; Prifti, E.; Belda, E.; Ichou, F.; Kayser, B.D.; Dao, M.C.; Verger, E.O.; Hedjazi, L.; Bouillot, J.-L.; Chevallier, J.-M.; et al. Major microbiota dysbiosis in severe obesity: Fate after bariatric surgery. *Gut* **2019**, *68*, 70–82. [CrossRef] [PubMed]
15. Machiels, K.; Joossens, M.; Sabino, J.; Preter, V.D.; Arijs, I.; Eeckhaut, V.; Ballet, V.; Claes, K.; Immerseel, F.V.; Verbeke, K.; et al. A decrease of the butyrate-producing species *Roseburia hominis* and *Faecalibacterium prausnitzii* defines dysbiosis in patients with ulcerative colitis. *Gut* **2014**, *63*, 1275–1283. [CrossRef] [PubMed]
16. Gevers, D.; Kugathasan, S.; Denson, L.A.; Vázquez-Baeza, Y.; Van Treuren, W.; Ren, B.; Schwager, E.; Knights, D.; Song, S.J.; Yassour, M.; et al. The Treatment-Naive Microbiome in New-Onset Crohn's Disease. *Cell Host Microbe* **2014**, *15*, 382–392. [CrossRef] [PubMed]
17. Hong, S.N. Unraveling the ties between irritable bowel syndrome and intestinal microbiota. *World J. Gastroenterol.* **2014**, *20*, 2470–2481. [CrossRef] [PubMed]
18. Tran, S.M.-S.; Mohajeri, M.H. The Role of Gut Bacterial Metabolites in Brain Development, Aging and Disease. *Nutrients* **2021**, *13*, 732. [CrossRef]
19. Gerhardt, S.; Mohajeri, M. Changes of Colonic Bacterial Composition in Parkinson's Disease and Other Neurodegenerative Diseases. *Nutrients* **2018**, *10*, 708. [CrossRef]
20. Srikantha, P.; Mohajeri, M.H. The Possible Role of the Microbiota-Gut-Brain-Axis in Autism Spectrum Disorder. *Int. J. Mol. Sci.* **2019**, *20*, 2115. [CrossRef]
21. Bull-Larsen, S.; Mohajeri, M.H. The Potential Influence of the Bacterial Microbiome on the Development and Progression of ADHD. *Nutrients* **2019**, *11*, 2805. [CrossRef]
22. Lerner, A.; Aminov, R.; Matthias, T. Dysbiosis May Trigger Autoimmune Diseases via Inappropriate Post-Translational Modification of Host Proteins. *Front. Microbiol.* **2016**, *7*, 84. [CrossRef] [PubMed]
23. Sobhani, I.; Tap, J.; Roudot-Thoraval, F.; Roperch, J.P.; Letulle, S.; Langella, P.; Corthier, G.; Van Nhieu, J.T.; Furet, J.P. Microbial Dysbiosis in Colorectal Cancer (CRC) Patients. *PLoS ONE* **2011**, *6*, e16393. [CrossRef]
24. Belančić, A. Gut microbiome dysbiosis and endotoxemia—Additional pathophysiological explanation for increased COVID-19 severity in obesity. *Obes. Med.* **2020**, *20*, 100302. [CrossRef]
25. Sudo, N.; Chida, Y.; Aiba, Y.; Sonoda, J.; Oyama, N.; Yu, X.-N.; Kubo, C.; Koga, Y. Postnatal microbial colonization programs the hypothalamic-pituitary-adrenal system for stress response in mice: Commensal microbiota and stress response. *J. Physiol.* **2004**, *558*, 263–275. [CrossRef]
26. Misiak, B.; Łoniewski, I.; Marlicz, W.; Frydecka, D.; Szulc, A.; Rudzki, L.; Samochowiec, J. The HPA axis dysregulation in severe mental illness: Can we shift the blame to gut microbiota? *Prog. Neuro-Psychopharmacol. Biol. Psychiatry* **2020**, *102*, 109951. [CrossRef]
27. LeBlanc, J.G.; Milani, C.; de Giori, G.S.; Sesma, F.; van Sinderen, D.; Ventura, M. Bacteria as vitamin suppliers to their host: A gut microbiota perspective. *Curr. Opin. Biotechnol.* **2013**, *24*, 160–168. [CrossRef]
28. D'Argenio, G.; Mazzacca, G. Short-Chain Fatty Acid in the Human Colon. In *Advances in Nutrition and Cancer 2*; Zappia, V., Della Ragione, F., Barbarisi, A., Russo, G.L., Iacovo, R.D., Eds.; Advances in Experimental Medicine and Biology; Springer: Boston, MA, USA, 1999; Volume 472, pp. 149–158. ISBN 978-1-4419-3331-7.
29. Barrett, E.; Ross, R.P.; O'Toole, P.W. γ-Aminobutyric acid production by culturable bacteria from the human intestine. *J. Appl. Microbiol.* **2012**, *113*, 411–417. [CrossRef]
30. den Besten, G.; van Eunen, K.; Groen, A.K.; Venema, K.; Reijngoud, D.-J.; Bakker, B.M. The role of short-chain fatty acids in the interplay between diet, gut microbiota, and host energy metabolism. *J. Lipid Res.* **2013**, *54*, 2325–2340. [CrossRef]
31. Skonieczna-Żydecka, K.; Grochans, E.; Maciejewska, D. Faecal Short Chain Fatty Acids Profile is Changed in Polish Depressive Women. *Nutrients* **2018**, *10*, 1937. [CrossRef] [PubMed]
32. Resende, W.R.; Valvassori, S.S.; Réus, G.Z.; Varela, R.B.; Arent, C.O.; Ribeiro, K.F.; Bavaresco, D.V.; Andersen, M.L.; Zugno, A.I.; Quevedo, J. Effects of sodium butyrate in animal models of mania and depression: Implications as a new mood stabilizer. *Behav. Pharmacol.* **2013**, *24*, 569–579. [CrossRef] [PubMed]

33. Maes, M.; Kubera, M.; Leunis, J.-C. The gut-brain barrier in major depression: Intestinal mucosal dysfunction with an increased translocation of LPS from gram negative enterobacteria (leaky gut) plays a role in the inflammatory pathophysiology of depression. *Neuro Endocrinol. Lett.* **2008**, *29*, 117–124. [PubMed]
34. Vagnerová, K.; Vodička, M.; Hermanová, P.; Ergang, P.; Šrůtková, D.; Klusoňová, P.; Balounová, K.; Hudcovic, T.; Pácha, J. Interactions Between Gut Microbiota and Acute Restraint Stress in Peripheral Structures of the Hypothalamic–Pituitary–Adrenal Axis and the Intestine of Male Mice. *Front. Immunol.* **2019**, *10*, 2655. [CrossRef] [PubMed]
35. Yamawaki, Y.; Yoshioka, N.; Nozaki, K.; Ito, H.; Oda, K.; Harada, K.; Shirawachi, S.; Asano, S.; Aizawa, H.; Yamawaki, S.; et al. Sodium butyrate abolishes lipopolysaccharide-induced depression-like behaviors and hippocampal microglial activation in mice. *Brain Res.* **2018**, *1680*, 13–38. [CrossRef]
36. Miller, A.H.; Raison, C.L. The role of inflammation in depression: From evolutionary imperative to modern treatment target. *Nat. Rev. Immunol.* **2016**, *16*, 22–34. [CrossRef]
37. Maes, M.; Mihaylova, I.; Kubera, M.; Ringel, K. Activation of cell-mediated immunity in depression: Association with inflammation, melancholia, clinical staging and the fatigue and somatic symptom cluster of depression. *Prog. Neuro-Psychopharmacol. Biol. Psychiatry* **2012**, *36*, 169–175. [CrossRef]
38. Moher, D.; Liberati, A.; Tetzlaff, J. Preferred Reporting Items for Systematic Reviews and Meta-Analyses: The PRISMA Statement. *Phys. Ther.* **2009**, *89*, 873–880. [CrossRef]
39. Koh, H.; Tuddenham, S.; Sears, C.L.; Zhao, N. Meta-analysis methods for multiple related markers: Applications to microbiome studies with the results on multiple α-diversity indices. *Stat. Med.* **2021**, *40*, 2859–2876. [CrossRef]
40. Su, X. Elucidating the Beta-Diversity of the Microbiome: From Global Alignment to Local Alignment. *mSystems* **2021**, *6*, e00363-21. [CrossRef]
41. Naseribafrouei, A.; Hestad, K.; Avershina, E.; Sekelja, M.; Linløkken, A.; Wilson, R.; Rudi, K. Correlation between the human fecal microbiota and depression. *Neurogastroenterol. Motil.* **2014**, *26*, 1155–1162. [CrossRef]
42. Jiang, H.; Ling, Z.; Zhang, Y.; Mao, H.; Ma, Z.; Yin, Y.; Wang, W.; Tang, W.; Tan, Z.; Shi, J.; et al. Altered fecal microbiota composition in patients with major depressive disorder. *Brain Behav. Immun.* **2015**, *48*, 186–194. [CrossRef] [PubMed]
43. Lai, W.; Deng, W.; Xu, S.; Zhao, J.; Xu, D.; Liu, Y.; Guo, Y.; Wang, M.; He, F.; Ye, S.; et al. Shotgun metagenomics reveals both taxonomic and tryptophan pathway differences of gut microbiota in major depressive disorder patients. *Psychol. Med.* **2019**, *51*, 90–101. [CrossRef]
44. Liu, R.T.; Rowan-Nash, A.; Sheehan, A. Reductions in anti-inflammatory gut bacteria are associated with depression in a sample of young adults. *Brain, Behav. Immun.* **2020**, *88*, 308–324. [CrossRef] [PubMed]
45. Li, L.; Su, Q.; Xie, B.; Duan, L.; Zhao, W.; Hu, D.; Wu, R.; Liu, H. Gut microbes in correlation with mood: Case study in a closed experimental human life support system. *Neurogastroenterol. Motil.* **2016**, *28*, 1233–1240. [CrossRef]
46. Zheng, P.; Yang, J.; Li, Y.; Wu, J.; Liang, W.; Yin, B.; Tan, X.; Huang, Y.; Chai, T.; Zhang, H.; et al. Gut Microbial Signatures Can Discriminate Unipolar from Bipolar Depression. *Adv. Sci.* **2020**, *7*, 1902862. [CrossRef]
47. Mason, B.L.; Li, Q.; Minhajuddin, A.; Czysz, A.H.; Coughlin, L.A.; Hussain, S.K.; Koh, A.Y.; Trivedi, M.H. Reduced anti-inflammatory gut microbiota are associated with depression and anhedonia. *J. Affect. Disord.* **2020**, *266*, 394–401. [CrossRef] [PubMed]
48. Madan, A.; Thompson, D.; Fowler, J.C. The gut microbiota is associated with psychiatric symptom severity and treatment outcome among individuals with serious mental illness. *J. Affect. Disord.* **2020**, *264*, 98–106. [CrossRef] [PubMed]
49. Chen, J.-J.; He, S.; Fang, L.; Wang, B.; Bai, S.-J.; Xie, J.; Zhou, C.-J.; Wang, W.; Xie, P. Age-specific differential changes on gut microbiota composition in patients with major depressive disorder. *Aging* **2020**, *12*, 2764–2776. [CrossRef]
50. Rong, H.; Xie, X.; Zhao, J. Similarly in depression, nuances of gut microbiota_ Evidences from a shotgun metagenomics sequencing study on major depressive disorder versus bipolar disorder with current major depressive episode patients. *J. Psychiatr. Res.* **2019**, *113*, 90–99. [CrossRef] [PubMed]
51. Chung, Y.-C.E.; Chen, H.-C.; Chou, H.-C.L.; Chen, I.-M.; Lee, M.-S.; Chuang, L.-C.; Liu, Y.-W.; Lu, M.-L.; Chen, C.-H.; Wu, C.-S.; et al. Exploration of microbiota targets for major depressive disorder and mood related traits. *J. Psychiatr. Res.* **2019**, *111*, 74–82. [CrossRef]
52. Painold, A.; Mörkl, S.; Kashofer, K.; Halwachs, B.; Dalkner, N.; Bengesser, S.; Birner, A.; Fellendorf, F.; Platzer, M.; Queissner, R.; et al. A step ahead: Exploring the gut microbiota in inpatients with bipolar disorder during a depressive episode. *Bipolar Disord.* **2019**, *21*, 40–49. [CrossRef]
53. Vinberg, M.; Ottesen, N.M.; Meluken, I.; Sørensen, N.; Pedersen, O.; Kessing, L.V.; Miskowiak, K.W. Remitted affective disorders and high familial risk of affective disorders associate with aberrant intestinal microbiota. *Acta Psychiatr. Scand.* **2019**, *139*, 174–184. [CrossRef]
54. Jiang, H.; Xu, L.; Zhang, X.; Zhang, Z.; Ruan, B. The Microbiome in Bipolar Depression: A Longitudinal Study of One Pair of Monozygotic Twins. *Bipolar Disord.* **2018**, *21*, 93–97. [CrossRef] [PubMed]
55. Peter, J.; Fournier, C.; Durdevic, M.; Knoblich, L.; Keip, B.; Dejaco, C.; Trauner, M.; Moser, G. A Microbial Signature of Psychological Distress in Irritable Bowel Syndrome. *Psychosom. Med.* **2018**, *80*, 698–709. [CrossRef]
56. Kurokawa, S.; Kishimoto, T.; Mizuno, S.; Masaoka, T.; Naganuma, M.; Liang, K.; Kitazawa, M.; Nakashima, M.; Shindo, C.; Suda, W.; et al. The effect of fecal microbiota transplantation on psychiatric symptoms among patients with irritable bowel syndrome, functional diarrhea and functional constipation: An open-label observational study. *J. Affect. Disord.* **2018**, *235*, 506–512. [CrossRef] [PubMed]
57. Chen, J.; Zheng, P.; Liu, Y.; Zhong, X.; Wang, H.; Guo, Y.; Xie, P. Sex differences in gut microbiota in patients with major depressive disorder. *Neuropsychiatr. Dis. Treat.* **2018**, *14*, 647–655. [CrossRef] [PubMed]
58. Huang, Y.; Shi, X.; Li, Z.; Shen, Y.; Shi, X.; Wang, L.; Li, G.; Yuan, Y.; Wang, J.; Zhang, Y.; et al. Possible association of Firmicutes in the gut microbiota of patients with major depressive disorder. *Neuropsychiatr. Dis. Treat.* **2018**, *14*, 3329–3337. [CrossRef] [PubMed]

59. Kleiman, S.C.; Bulik-Sullivan, E.C.; Glenny, E.M.; Zerwas, S.C.; Huh, E.Y.; Tsilimigras, M.C.B.; Fodor, A.A.; Bulik, C.M.; Carroll, I.M. The Gut-Brain Axis in Healthy Females: Lack of Significant Association between Microbial Composition and Diversity with Psychiatric Measures. *PLoS ONE* **2017**, *12*, e0170208. [CrossRef]
60. Liu, Y.; Zhang, L.; Wang, X.; Wang, Z.; Zhang, J.; Jiang, R.; Wang, X.; Wang, K.; Liu, Z.; Xia, Z.; et al. Similar Fecal Microbiota Signatures in Patients With Diarrhea-Predominant Irritable Bowel Syndrome and Patients With Depression. *Clin. Gastroenterol. Hepatol.* **2016**, *14*, 1602–1611.e5. [CrossRef]
61. Kleiman, S.C.; Watson, H.J.; Bulik-Sullivan, E.C.; Huh, E.Y.; Tarantino, L.M.; Bulik, C.M.; Carroll, I.M. The Intestinal Microbiota in Acute Anorexia Nervosa and During Renourishment: Relationship to Depression, Anxiety, and Eating Disorder Psychopathology. *Psychosom. Med.* **2015**, *77*, 969–981. [CrossRef]
62. Lin, P.; Ding, B.; Feng, C.; Yin, S.; Zhang, T.; Qi, X.; Lv, H.; Guo, X.; Dong, K.; Zhu, Y.; et al. Prevotella and Klebsiella proportions in fecal microbial communities are potential characteristic parameters for patients with major depressive disorder. *J. Affect. Disord.* **2017**, *207*, 300–304. [CrossRef]
63. Zheng, P.; Zeng, B.; Zhou, C.; Liu, M.; Fang, Z.; Xu, X.; Zeng, L.; Chen, J.; Fan, S.; Du, X.; et al. Gut microbiome remodeling induces depressive-like behaviors through a pathway mediated by the host's metabolism. *Mol. Psychiatry* **2016**, *11*. [CrossRef] [PubMed]
64. Coello, K.; Hansen, T.H.; Sørensen, N.; Munkholm, K.; Kessing, L.V.; Pedersen, O.; Vinberg, M. Gut microbiota composition in patients with newly diagnosed bipolar disorder and their unaffected first-degree relatives. *Brain Behav. Immun.* **2019**, *75*, 112–118. [CrossRef]
65. McIntyre, R.S.; Subramaniapillai, M.; Shekotikhina, M.; Carmona, N.E.; Lee, Y.; Mansur, R.B.; Brietzke, E.; Fus, D.; Coles, A.S.; Iacobucci, M.; et al. Characterizing the gut microbiota in adults with bipolar disorder: A pilot study. *Nutr. Neurosci.* **2019**, *24*, 173–180. [CrossRef]
66. Hu, S.; Li, A.; Huang, T.; Lai, J.; Li, J.; Sublette, M.E.; Lu, H.; Lu, Q.; Du, Y.; Hu, Z.; et al. Gut Microbiota Changes in Patients with Bipolar Depression. *Adv. Sci.* **2019**, *6*, 1900752. [CrossRef] [PubMed]
67. Chen, Z.; Li, J.; Gui, S.; Zhou, C.; Chen, J.; Yang, C.; Hu, Z.; Wang, H.; Zhong, X.; Zeng, L.; et al. Comparative metaproteomics analysis shows altered fecal microbiota signatures in patients with major depressive disorder. *NeuroReport* **2018**, *29*, 417–425. [CrossRef]
68. Shin, N.-R.; Whon, T.W.; Bae, J.-W. Proteobacteria: Microbial signature of dysbiosis in gut microbiota. *Trends Biotechnol.* **2015**, *33*, 496–503. [CrossRef]
69. Taylor, A.M.; Thompson, S.V.; Edwards, C.G.; Musaad, S.M.A.; Khan, N.A.; Holscher, H.D. Associations among diet, the gastrointestinal microbiota, and negative emotional states in adults. *Nutr. Neurosci.* **2020**, *23*, 983–992. [CrossRef]
70. King, C.H.; Desai, H.; Sylvetsky, A.C.; LoTempio, J.; Ayanyan, S.; Carrie, J.; Crandall, K.A.; Fochtman, B.C.; Gasparyan, L.; Gulzar, N.; et al. Baseline human gut microbiota profile in healthy people and standard reporting template. *PLoS ONE* **2019**, *14*, e0206484. [CrossRef]
71. Zhou, Y.; Zhi, F. Lower Level of *Bacteroides* in the Gut Microbiota Is Associated with Inflammatory Bowel Disease: A Meta-Analysis. *BioMed Res. Int.* **2016**, *2016*, 5828959. [CrossRef]
72. Zafar, H.; Saier, M.H. Gut *Bacteroides* species in health and disease. *Gut Microbes* **2021**, *13*, 1848158. [CrossRef] [PubMed]
73. Kim, S.; Covington, A.; Pamer, E.G. The intestinal microbiota: Antibiotics, colonization resistance, and enteric pathogens. *Immunol. Rev.* **2017**, *279*, 90–105. [CrossRef]
74. Cheng, S.; Han, B.; Ding, M.; Wen, Y.; Ma, M.; Zhang, L.; Qi, X.; Cheng, B.; Li, P.; Kafle, O.P.; et al. Identifying psychiatric disorder-associated gut microbiota using microbiota-related gene set enrichment analysis. *Brief. Bioinform.* **2020**, *21*, 1016–1022. [CrossRef] [PubMed]
75. Lu, Q.; Lai, J.; Lu, H.; Ng, C.; Huang, T.; Zhang, H.; Ding, K.; Wang, Z.; Jiang, J.; Hu, J.; et al. Gut Microbiota in Bipolar Depression and Its Relationship to Brain Function: An Advanced Exploration. *Front. Psychiatry* **2019**, *10*, 784. [CrossRef]
76. Lei, Y.; Tang, L.; Liu, S.; Hu, S.; Wu, L.; Liu, Y.; Yang, M.; Huang, S.; Tang, X.; Tang, T.; et al. Parabacteroides produces acetate to alleviate heparanase-exacerbated acute pancreatitis through reducing neutrophil infiltration. *Microbiome* **2021**, *9*, 115. [CrossRef]
77. Valles-Colomer, M.; Falony, G.; Darzi, Y.; Tigchelaar, E.F.; Wang, J.; Tito, R.Y.; Schiweck, C.; Kurilshikov, A.; Joossens, M.; Wijmenga, C.; et al. The neuroactive potential of the human gut microbiota in quality of life and depression. *Nat. Microbiol.* **2019**, *4*, 623–632. [CrossRef] [PubMed]
78. Parker, B.J.; Wearsch, P.A.; Veloo, A.C.M.; Rodriguez-Palacios, A. The Genus Alistipes: Gut Bacteria With Emerging Implications to Inflammation, Cancer, and Mental Health. *Front. Immunol.* **2020**, *11*, 906. [CrossRef] [PubMed]
79. Aizawa, E.; Tsuji, H.; Asahara, T.; Takahashi, T.; Teraishi, T.; Yoshida, S.; Koga, N.; Hattori, K.; Ota, M.; Kunugi, H. Bifidobacterium and Lactobacillus Counts in the Gut Microbiota of Patients With Bipolar Disorder and Healthy Controls. *Front. Psychiatry* **2019**, *9*, 730. [CrossRef]
80. Heym, N.; Heasman, B.C.; Hunter, K. The role of microbiota and inflammation in self-judgement and empathy: Implications for understanding the brain-gut-microbiome axis in depression. *Psychopharmacology* **2019**, *12*, 1459–1470. [CrossRef]
81. Baj, J.; Sitarz, E.; Forma, A.; Wróblewska, K.; Karakuła-Juchnowicz, H. Alterations in the Nervous System and Gut Microbiota after β-Hemolytic Streptococcus Group A Infection—Characteristics and Diagnostic Criteria of PANDAS Recognition. *Int. J. Mol. Sci.* **2020**, *21*, 1476. [CrossRef] [PubMed]
82. Pabst, C.; Subasic, K. PANDAS Pediatric Autoimmune Neuropsychiatric Disorders Associated with Streptococcal Infection. *AJN Am. J. Nurs.* **2020**, *120*, 32–37. [CrossRef] [PubMed]
83. *The Prokaryotes*; Rosenberg, E.; DeLong, E.F.; Lory, S.; Stackebrandt, E.; Thompson, F. (Eds.) Springer: Berlin, Germany, 2014; ISBN 978-3-642-30119-3.
84. Miyaoka, T.; Kanayama, M.; Wake, R.; Hashioka, S.; Hayashida, M.; Nagahama, M.; Okazaki, S.; Yamashita, S.; Miura, S.; Miki, H.; et al. Clostridium butyricum MIYAIRI 588 as Adjunctive Therapy for Treatment-Resistant Major Depressive Disorder: A Prospective Open-Label Trial. *Clin. Neuropharmacol.* **2018**, *41*, 151–155. [CrossRef]

85. Morotomi, M.; Nagai, F.; Watanabe, Y. Description of *Christensenella minuta* gen. nov., sp. nov., isolated from human faeces, which forms a distinct branch in the order *Clostridiales*, and proposal of *Christensenellaceae* fam. nov. *Int. J. Syst. Evol. Microbiol.* **2012**, *62*, 144–149. [CrossRef]
86. Tavella, T.; Rampelli, S.; Guidarelli, G.; Bazzocchi, A.; Gasperini, C.; Pujos-Guillot, E.; Comte, B.; Barone, M.; Biagi, E.; Candela, M.; et al. Elevated gut microbiome abundance of *Christensenellaceae, Porphyromonadaceae and Rikenellaceae* is associated with reduced visceral adipose tissue and healthier metabolic profile in Italian elderly. *Gut Microbes* **2021**, *13*, 1880221. [CrossRef] [PubMed]
87. Long, X.; Wong, C.C.; Tong, L. Peptostreptococcus anaerobius promotes colorectal carcinogenesis and modulates tumour immunity. *Nat. Microbiol.* **2019**, *4*, 2319–2330. [CrossRef] [PubMed]
88. Wlodarska, M.; Luo, C.; Kolde, R.; d'Hennezel, E.; Annand, J.W.; Heim, C.E.; Krastel, P.; Schmitt, E.K.; Omar, A.S.; Creasey, E.A.; et al. Indoleacrylic Acid Produced by Commensal Peptostreptococcus Species Suppresses Inflammation. *Cell Host Microbe* **2017**, *22*, 25–37.e6. [CrossRef] [PubMed]
89. Mukherjee, A.; Lordan, C.; Ross, R.P.; Cotter, P.D. Gut microbes from the phylogenetically diverse genus *Eubacterium* and their various contributions to gut health. *Gut Microbes* **2020**, *12*, 1802866. [CrossRef]
90. Altemani, F.; Barrett, H.L.; Gomez-Arango, L.; Josh, P.; David McIntyre, H.; Callaway, L.K.; Morrison, M.; Tyson, G.W.; Dekker Nitert, M. Pregnant women who develop preeclampsia have lower abundance of the butyrate-producer Coprococcus in their gut microbiota. *Pregnancy Hypertens.* **2021**, *23*, 211–219. [CrossRef]
91. Ai, D.; Pan, H.; Li, X.; Gao, Y.; Liu, G.; Xia, L.C. Identifying Gut Microbiota Associated With Colorectal Cancer Using a Zero-Inflated Lognormal Model. *Front. Microbiol.* **2019**, *10*, 826. [CrossRef]
92. Zhang, Y.; Zhang, B.; Dong, L.; Chang, P. Potential of Omega-3 Polyunsaturated Fatty Acids in Managing Chemotherapy- or Radiotherapy-Related Intestinal Microbial Dysbiosis. *Adv. Nutr.* **2019**, *10*, 133–147. [CrossRef]
93. Lin, P.-Y.; Huang, S.-Y.; Su, K.-P. A Meta-Analytic Review of Polyunsaturated Fatty Acid Compositions in Patients with Depression. *Biol. Psychiatry* **2010**, *68*, 140–147. [CrossRef] [PubMed]
94. Shen, Z.; Zhu, C.; Quan, Y.; Yang, J.; Yuan, W.; Yang, Z.; Wu, S.; Luo, W.; Tan, B.; Wang, X. Insights into *Roseburia intestinalis* which alleviates experimental colitis pathology by inducing anti-inflammatory responses: *Roseburia intestinalis* reduces colitis. *J. Gastroenterol. Hepatol.* **2018**, *33*, 1751–1760. [CrossRef] [PubMed]
95. Hold, G.L.; Schwiertz, A.; Aminov, R.I.; Blaut, M.; Flint, H.J. Oligonucleotide Probes That Detect Quantitatively Significant Groups of Butyrate-Producing Bacteria in Human Feces. *Appl. Environ. Microbiol.* **2003**, *69*, 4320–4324. [CrossRef]
96. Cheung, S.G.; Goldenthal, A.R.; Uhlemann, A.-C.; Mann, J.J.; Miller, J.M.; Sublette, M.E. Systematic Review of Gut Microbiota and Major Depression. *Front. Psychiatry* **2019**, *10*, 34. [CrossRef]
97. Sokol, H.; Pigneur, B.; Watterlot, L.; Lakhdari, O.; Bermudez-Humaran, L.G.; Gratadoux, J.-J.; Blugeon, S.; Bridonneau, C.; Furet, J.-P.; Corthier, G.; et al. Faecalibacterium prausnitzii is an anti-inflammatory commensal bacterium identified by gut microbiota analysis of Crohn disease patients. *Proc. Natl. Acad. Sci. USA* **2008**, *105*, 16731–16736. [CrossRef]
98. Martín, R.; Miquel, S.; Chain, F.; Natividad, J.M.; Jury, J.; Lu, J.; Sokol, H.; Theodorou, V.; Bercik, P.; Verdu, E.F.; et al. Faecalibacterium prausnitzii prevents physiological damages in a chronic low-grade inflammation murine model. *BMC Microbiol.* **2015**, *15*, 67. [CrossRef] [PubMed]
99. Chahwan, B.; Kwan, S.; Isik, A.; van Hemert, S.; Burke, C.; Roberts, L. Gut feelings: A randomised, triple-blind, placebo-controlled trial of probiotics for depressive symptoms. *J. Affect. Disord.* **2019**, *253*, 317–326. [CrossRef]
100. Evans, S.J.; Bassis, C.M.; Hein, R.; Assari, S.; Flowers, S.A.; Kelly, M.B.; Young, V.B.; Ellingrod, V.E.; McInnis, M.G. The gut microbiome composition associates with bipolar disorder and illness severity. *J. Psychiatr. Res.* **2017**, *87*, 23–29. [CrossRef] [PubMed]
101. Mikami, A.; Ogita, T.; Namai, F.; Shigemori, S.; Sato, T.; Shimosato, T. Oral administration of Flavonifractor plautii attenuates inflammatory responses in obese adipose tissue. *Mol. Biol. Rep.* **2020**, *47*, 6717–6725. [CrossRef] [PubMed]
102. Ogita, T.; Yamamoto, Y.; Mikami, A.; Shigemori, S.; Sato, T.; Shimosato, T. Oral Administration of Flavonifractor plautii Strongly Suppresses Th2 Immune Responses in Mice. *Front. Immunol.* **2020**, *11*, 379. [CrossRef]
103. Mikami, A.; Ogita, T.; Namai, F.; Shigemori, S.; Sato, T.; Shimosato, T. Oral Administration of Flavonifractor plautii, a Bacteria Increased With Green Tea Consumption, Promotes Recovery From Acute Colitis in Mice via Suppression of IL-17. *Front. Nutr.* **2021**, *7*, 610946. [CrossRef]
104. Li, W.; Sun, Y.; Dai, L.; Chen, H.; Yi, B.; Niu, J.; Wang, L.; Zhang, F.; Luo, J.; Wang, K.; et al. Ecological and network analyses identify four microbial species with potential significance for the diagnosis/treatment of ulcerative colitis (UC). *BMC Microbiol.* **2021**, *21*, 138. [CrossRef] [PubMed]
105. Straub, T.J.; Chou, W.-C.; Manson, A.L.; Schreiber, H.L.; Walker, B.J.; Desjardins, C.A.; Chapman, S.B.; Kaspar, K.L.; Kahsai, O.J.; Traylor, E.; et al. Limited effects of long-term daily cranberry consumption on the gut microbiome in a placebo-controlled study of women with recurrent urinary tract infections. *BMC Microbiol.* **2021**, *21*, 53. [CrossRef]
106. Hiippala, K.; Kainulainen, V.; Kalliomäki, M.; Arkkila, P.; Satokari, R. Mucosal Prevalence and Interactions with the Epithelium Indicate Commensalism of *Sutterella* spp. *Front. Microbiol.* **2016**, *7*, 1706. [CrossRef] [PubMed]
107. Janda, J.M.; Abbott, S.L. The Changing Face of the Family Enterobacteriaceae (Order: "Enterobacterales"): New Members, Taxonomic Issues, Geographic Expansion, and New Diseases and Disease Syndromes. *Clin. Microbiol. Rev.* **2021**, *34*, 45. [CrossRef]
108. Bangsgaard Bendtsen, K.M.; Krych, L.; Sørensen, D.B.; Pang, W.; Nielsen, D.S.; Josefsen, K.; Hansen, L.H.; Sørensen, S.J.; Hansen, A.K. Gut Microbiota Composition Is Correlated to Grid Floor Induced Stress and Behavior in the BALB/c Mouse. *PLoS ONE* **2012**, *7*, e46231. [CrossRef]

109. Frost, F.; Storck, L.J.; Kacprowski, T.; Gärtner, S.; Rühlemann, M.; Bang, C.; Franke, A.; Völker, U.; Aghdassi, A.A.; Steveling, A.; et al. A structured weight loss program increases gut microbiota phylogenetic diversity and reduces levels of Collinsella in obese type 2 diabetics: A pilot study. *PLoS ONE* **2019**, *14*, e0219489. [CrossRef] [PubMed]
110. Gomez-Arango, L.F.; Barrett, H.L.; Wilkinson, S.A.; Callaway, L.K.; McIntyre, H.D.; Morrison, M.; Dekker Nitert, M. Low dietary fiber intake increases *Collinsella* abundance in the gut microbiota of overweight and obese pregnant women. *Gut Microbes* **2018**, *9*, 189–201. [CrossRef]
111. Forbes, J.D.; Chen, C.; Knox, N.C.; Marrie, R.-A.; El-Gabalawy, H.; de Kievit, T.; Alfa, M.; Bernstein, C.N.; Van Domselaar, G. A comparative study of the gut microbiota in immune-mediated inflammatory diseases—does a common dysbiosis exist? *Microbiome* **2018**, *6*, 221. [CrossRef]
112. Binda, C.; Lopetuso, L.R.; Rizzatti, G.; Gibiino, G.; Cennamo, V.; Gasbarrini, A. Actinobacteria: A relevant minority for the maintenance of gut homeostasis. *Dig. Liver Dis.* **2018**, *50*, 421–428. [CrossRef]
113. Aizawa, E.; Tsuji, H.; Asahara, T.; Takahashi, T.; Teraishi, T.; Yoshida, S.; Ota, M.; Koga, N.; Hattori, K.; Kunugi, H. Possible association of Bifidobacterium and Lactobacillus in the gut microbiota of patients with major depressive disorder. *J. Affect. Disord.* **2016**, *202*, 254–257. [CrossRef]
114. Nishida, K.; Sawada, D.; Kuwano, Y. Health benefits of lactobacillus gasseri cp2305 tablets in young adults exposed to chronic stress: A randomized, double-blind, placebo-controlled study. *Nutrients* **2019**, *11*, 1859. [CrossRef] [PubMed]
115. Sawada, D.; Kuwano, Y.; Tanaka, H.; Hara, S.; Uchiyama, Y.; Sugawara, T.; Fujiwara, S.; Rokutan, K.; Nishida, K. Daily intake of Lactobacillus gasseri CP2305 relieves fatigue and stress-related symptoms in male university Ekiden runners: A double-blind, randomized, and placebo-controlled clinical trial. *J. Funct. Foods* **2019**, *57*, 465–476. [CrossRef]
116. Sawada, D.; Kawai, T.; Nishida, K.; Kuwano, Y.; Fujiwara, S.; Rokutan, K. Daily intake of Lactobacillus gasseri CP2305 improves mental, physical, and sleep quality among Japanese medical students enrolled in a cadaver dissection course. *J. Funct. Foods* **2017**, *31*, 188–197. [CrossRef]
117. Haghighat, N.; Rajabi, S.; Mohammadshahi, M. Effect of synbiotic and probiotic supplementation on serum brain-derived neurotrophic factor level, depression and anxiety symptoms in hemodialysis patients: A randomized, double-blinded, clinical trial. *Nutr. Neurosci.* **2019**, *24*, 490–499. [CrossRef]
118. Cepeda, M.S.; Katz, E.G.; Blacketer, C. Microbiome-Gut-Brain Axis: Probiotics and Their Association With Depression. *J. Neuropsychiatry Clin. Neurosci.* **2017**, *29*, 39–44. [CrossRef]
119. Kazemi, A.; Noorbala, A.A.; Azam, K.; Eskandari, M.H.; Djafarian, K. Effect of probiotic and prebiotic vs placebo on psychological outcomes in patients with major depressive disorder: A randomized clinical trial. *Clin. Nutr.* **2019**, *38*, 522–528. [CrossRef] [PubMed]
120. Rudzki, L.; Ostrowska, L.; Pawlak, D.; Małus, A.; Pawlak, K.; Waszkiewicz, N.; Szulc, A. Probiotic Lactobacillus Plantarum 299v decreases kynurenine concentration and improves cognitive functions in patients with major depression: A double-blind, randomized, placebo controlled study. *Psychoneuroendocrinology* **2019**, *100*, 213–222. [CrossRef]
121. Romijn, A.R.; Rucklidge, J.J.; Kuijer, R.G.; Frampton, C. A double-blind, randomized, placebo-controlled trial of *Lactobacillus helveticus* and *Bifidobacterium longum* for the symptoms of depression. *Aust. N. Z. J. Psychiatry* **2017**, *51*, 810–821. [CrossRef] [PubMed]
122. Slykerman, R.F.; Hood, F.; Wickens, K.; Thompson, J.M.D.; Barthow, C.; Murphy, R.; Kang, J.; Rowden, J.; Stone, P.; Crane, J.; et al. Effect of Lactobacillus rhamnosus HN001 in Pregnancy on Postpartum Symptoms of Depression and Anxiety: A Randomised Double-blind Placebo-controlled Trial. *EBioMedicine* **2017**, *24*, 159–165. [CrossRef] [PubMed]
123. Pinto-Sanchez, M.I.; Hall, G.B.; Ghajar, K.; Nardelli, A.; Bolino, C.; Lau, J.T.; Martin, F.-P.; Cominetti, O.; Welsh, C.; Rieder, A.; et al. Probiotic Bifidobacterium longum NCC3001 Reduces Depression Scores and Alters Brain Activity: A Pilot Study in Patients With Irritable Bowel Syndrome. *Gastroenterology* **2017**, *153*, 448–459.e8. [CrossRef]
124. Steenbergen, L.; Sellaro, R.; van Hemert, S.; Bosch, J.A.; Colzato, L.S. A randomized controlled trial to test the effect of multispecies probiotics on cognitive reactivity to sad mood. *Brain Behav. Immun.* **2015**, *48*, 258–264. [CrossRef] [PubMed]
125. Akkasheh, G.; Kashani-Poor, Z.; Tajabadi-Ebrahimi, M. Clinical and metabolic response to probiotic administration in patients with major depressive disorder: A randomized, double-blind, placebo-controlled trial. *Nutrition* **2016**, *32*, 315–320. [CrossRef] [PubMed]
126. Eslami Shahrbabaki, M.; Sabouri, S.; Sabahi, A.; Barfeh, D.; Divsalar, P.; Divsalar, P.; Esmailzadeh, M.; Ahmadi, A. The Efficacy of Probiotics for Treatment of Bipolar Disorder- Type 1: A Randomized, Double-Blind, Placebo-Controlled Trial. *Iran. J. Psychiatry* **2020**, *15*, 10–16. [CrossRef] [PubMed]
127. Rao, J.; Xie, R.; Lin, L.; Jiang, J.; Du, L.; Zeng, X.; Li, G.; Wang, C.; Qiao, Y. Fecal microbiota transplantation ameliorates gut microbiota imbalance and intestinal barrier damage in rats with stress-induced depressive-like behavior. *Eur. J. Neurosci.* **2021**, *53*, 3598–3611. [CrossRef] [PubMed]
128. Kelly, J.R.; Borre, Y.; O' Brien, C.; Patterson, E.; El Aidy, S.; Deane, J.; Kennedy, P.J.; Beers, S.; Scott, K.; Moloney, G.; et al. Transferring the blues: Depression-associated gut microbiota induces neurobehavioural changes in the rat. *J. Psychiatr. Res.* **2016**, *82*, 109–118. [CrossRef] [PubMed]
129. Hinton, R. A case report looking at the effects of faecal microbiota transplantation in a patient with bipolar disorder. *Aust. N. Z. J. Psychiatry* **2020**, *54*, 649–650. [CrossRef] [PubMed]
130. Stevens, B.R.; Roesch, L.; Thiago, P.; Russell, J.T.; Pepine, C.J.; Holbert, R.C.; Raizada, M.K.; Triplett, E.W. Depression phenotype identified by using single nucleotide exact amplicon sequence variants of the human gut microbiome. *Mol. Psychiatry* **2020**, *26*, 4277–4287. [CrossRef]

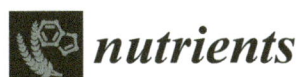

Review

The Role of Gut Bacterial Metabolites in Brain Development, Aging and Disease

Shirley Mei-Sin Tran and M. Hasan Mohajeri *

Department of Medicine, Institute of Anatomy, University of Zurich, Winterthurerstrasse 190, 8057 Zürich, Switzerland; tran.shirleymeisin@gmail.com
* Correspondence: mhasan.mohajeri@uzh.ch; Tel.: +41-79-938-1203

Abstract: In the last decade, emerging evidence has reported correlations between the gut microbiome and human health and disease, including those affecting the brain. We performed a systematic assessment of the available literature focusing on gut bacterial metabolites and their associations with diseases of the central nervous system (CNS). The bacterial metabolites short-chain fatty acids (SCFAs) as well as non-SCFAs like amino acid metabolites (AAMs) and bacterial amyloids are described in particular. We found significantly altered SCFA levels in patients with autism spectrum disorder (ASD), affective disorders, multiple sclerosis (MS) and Parkinson's disease (PD). Non-SCFAs yielded less significantly distinct changes in faecal levels of patients and healthy controls, with the majority of findings were derived from urinary and blood samples. Preclinical studies have implicated different bacterial metabolites with potentially beneficial as well as detrimental mechanisms in brain diseases. Examples include immunomodulation and changes in catecholamine production by histone deacetylase inhibition, anti-inflammatory effects through activity on the aryl hydrocarbon receptor and involvement in protein misfolding. Overall, our findings highlight the existence of altered bacterial metabolites in patients across various brain diseases, as well as potential neuroactive effects by which gut-derived SCFAs, p-cresol, indole derivatives and bacterial amyloids could impact disease development and progression. The findings summarized in this review could lead to further insights into the gut–brain–axis and thus into potential diagnostic, therapeutic or preventive strategies in brain diseases.

Keywords: gut–brain–axis; gut microbiome; short-chain fatty acids; bacterial metabolites; SCFA

1. Introduction

We are exposed to bacterial organisms from the beginning of our existence to the end of it. Even before birth, bacteria have been detected in the meconium of newborns, thus discrediting the pre-existing idea of a sterile foetal stage [1]. Later on, the early postnatal exposure to either the mother's vaginal flora or microbes from the environment, depending on delivery, impacts microbial colonization patterns, overall health and the neurodevelopment of the individual [2]. Although the microbial residents in our gastrointestinal tract (GIT) have already been known to impact the state of human health, the theory of a bidirectional gut–brain–axis (GBA) has taken the spotlight of global researchers mostly after the turn of the millennium.

Individuals are globally affected by increasing morbidity and mortality of psychiatric, neurodegenerative and neurodevelopmental disorders. The aetiology and pathophysiology of these brain diseases remain to this day to be fully elucidated and treatment options are largely of symptomatic nature. Therefore, researchers have unsurprisingly been looking at novel perspectives of disease, such as the GBA. Emerging findings on gut microbial influence on our nervous system were reported, involving bacterial-derived toxins, vitamins and neurotransmitters, yet the precise mechanisms, the "language of the GBA" [3], remain to be fully elucidated. Some newly examined neuroactive bacterial metabolites have nevertheless shown potential to play a role in this communication (Figure 1).

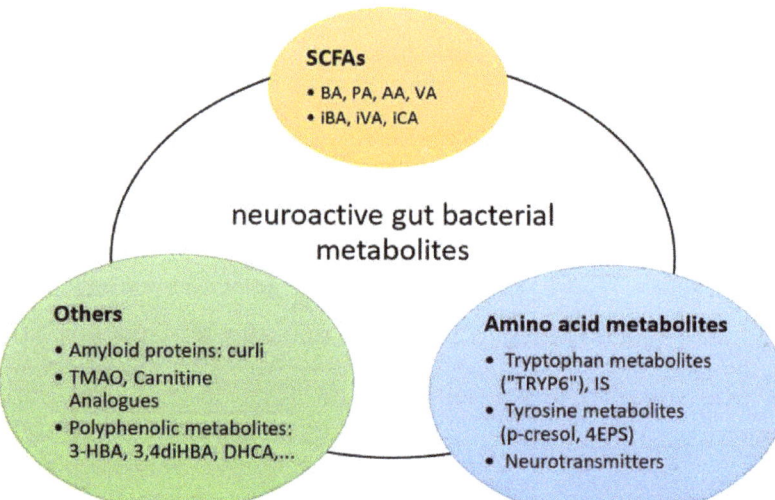

Figure 1. Non-exhaustive overview of neuroactive gut bacterial metabolites. SCFAs = short-chain fatty acids; BA = butyric acid; PA = propionic acid; AA = acetic acid; VA = valeric acid; iBA = isobutyric acid; iVA = isovaleric acid; iCA = isocaproic acid; TMAO = trimethylamine N-oxide; 3-HBA = 3-hydroxybenzoic acid; 3,4-diHBA = 3,4-dihydroxybenzoic acid; DHCA = dihydrocaffeic acid; IS = indoxyl sulphate; 4EPS = 4-ethylphenylsulfate.

This systematic review intends to summarize the research on various families of neuroactive bacterial metabolites as probable key players in the GBA. The focus is their effects on disorders of the brain, ranging from neurodevelopmental stages in childhood to neurodegenerative diseases in advanced age. Although intriguing evidence has emerged about the GBA's role in brain tumorigenesis via the modulation of the immune system, we refer the reader to a recent extensive study [4], as a detailed examination of this subject is beyond the scope of this review. Considering the magnitude of various influences from bacterial metabolites on the human organism, we will focus mostly on direct neuroactive effects on the brain. Most papers have largely emphasized taxonomic shifts in gut microbiota in specific diseases, or short-chain fatty acids (SCFAs) to date. One of our objectives is to provide a summary of findings between SCFAs and brain diseases, while in the second part of this review, reports of less explored non-SCFAs will take centre stage.

2. Materials and Methods

This systematic review was conducted according to the Preferred Reporting Items for Systematic Reviews and Meta-Analyses (PRISMA) guidelines [5]. The main objective was to explore and summarize the available data on influences of gut bacterial metabolites on the brain, with a focus on neurodevelopmental, autoimmune-mediated neuroinflammatory, and neurodegenerative diseases.

The first PubMed and SCOPUS databank searches were conducted on 20 November 2019. A second search was performed on the 8 July 2020 with the objective to include additional recently published data. The following search parameters and MeSH (Medical Subject Headings) terms "bacterial metabolites" combined with "brain development", "brain aging", "brain ageing", "brain disorders", "brain diseases", "neurodegenerative", "neuroprotective", "gut brain axis" and "gut-brain-axis" delivered 216 hits after removing duplicates (Figure 2). The second search with the same search parameters delivered 76 new hits. One hundred and forty-seven additional records with relevant information were individually selected from the list of references of the initially identified papers. Our focus on gut bacterial metabolites warranted the exclusion of data on viruses, archaea, and fungi

as well as data on bacteria not related to the gut microbiome. Original papers as well as reviews were included, while no restriction on publication year was applied. The inclusion criteria were the following:
- Published in a peer-reviewed article;
- Paper available in full-text PDF;
- Paper available in English;
- Paper discussing metabolites from bacteria found in gastrointestinal tracts of animals.

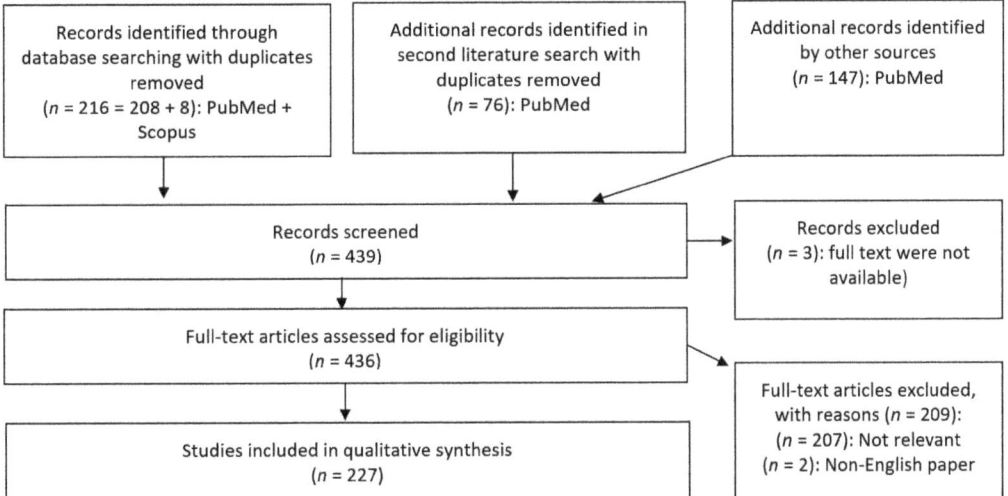

Figure 2. Methodical approach of our systematic review adhering to Preferred Reporting Items for Systematic Reviews and Meta-Analyses (PRISMA) criteria (PRISMA criteria [5]).

Most of the papers were dated from 2013 to 2019. Three papers lacking full texts, as well as two non-English publications, were excluded (Figure 2). Two hundred and seven papers were further excluded based on the lack of relevance to the topic. Finally, 227 studies were inspected for the qualitative synthesis. As to our knowledge, no other review to date has undertaken an analysis to this extent of links between several categories of gut bacterial metabolites and brain diseases.

3. Short-Chain Fatty Acids

Short-chain fatty acids (SCFAs) are saturated fatty acids produced by the bacterial fermentation of dietary fibre [6]. The majority of SCFAs consist of acetic (AA), propionic (PA) and butyric acid (BA), which are mostly deprotonated in the intestine (acetate, propionate, butyrate) [7]. Some gut bacterial species capable of generating SCFAs are *Bacteroides*, *Bifidobacterium*, *Propionibacterium*, *Eubacterium*, *Lactobacillus*, *Clostridium*, *Roseburia* and *Prevotella*. Among them, *Roseburia*, *Eubacterium* and Lachnospiraceae (Firmicutes phylum, Clostridia class) are strong BA producers, while AA producers belong to the *Bifidobacteria spp.* [8]. Considering their production site, the initial point of contact with the human organism are colonocytes and other intestinal cells. This naturally leads to discussions of local impacts from SCFAs on overall gut health, predominantly in the context of diseases like irritable bowel syndrome (IBS) [9–11] and the inflammatory bowel diseases Morbus Crohn and Colitis Ulcerosa [12,13]. Local effects facilitated by SCFAs have previously been discussed in detail and will not be further elaborated in this review [12,14,15].

It is known that SCFAs are able to modulate gut permeability by upregulating tight junction proteins [16,17], which are also part of the blood–brain barrier (BBB). This conceivably raises the idea that barrier integrity of gut and brain could be similarly affected by

SCFAs [18]. Indeed, studies in germ-free (GF) mice demonstrated that SCFAs are capable of modulating BBB permeability, which consequently impacts the extent to which beneficial or harmful molecules in circulation can reach brain tissue [19,20]. For example, physiological amounts of PA have been recently shown to protect the BBB from oxidative stress [21] and to decrease paracellular permeability [22]. Similarly, BA and BA-producing *Clostridium butyricum* can lower BBB permeability through enhancing tight-junction expression in mice [22]. In addition to directly affecting the BBB, SCFAs might actually reduce systemic inflammation by decreasing gut permeability, thereby decreasing circulating gut-derived bacterial components that trigger neuroinflammation by injuring the BBB or by affecting immune cells and cytokines in the brain [15]. SCFAs also act upon various gut–brain–pathways including immune, endocrine, vagal and direct humoral pathways (extensively reviewed by Dalile et al. [15]) and some effects in cellular systems, namely:

1. Histone deacetylase inhibition (HDACI) through BA, PA and AA, resulting in up-regulated gene transcriptions in the context of epigenetic modulation [23,24]. As extensively reviewed by Stilling et al. [24] with a focus on BA, studies on this subject are mainly conducted in animal models and in supraphysiological concentrations, thus the validity of any conclusions drawn from the current evidence is promising, yet limited for human application as of now.
2. Agonistic effects on G-protein-coupled receptors (GPCRs), namely free fatty acid receptors FFAR2 (GPR43), FFAR3 (GPR41) and the niacin receptor 1 (NIACR1, also known as hydroxycarboxylic acid receptor 2 (HCAR2) or GPR109A) [15,25]. Whether these effects are relevant in humans is to be determined, since current findings on these GPCRs are mostly based on rodent or cell models. FFAR3 for example, was found in the CNS and sympathetic ganglia of rats, and in the peripheral nervous system of mice [15]. Moreover, results linking these GPCRs with microglia cell morphology and growth hormone secretion in pituitary cells [25,26] call for further research with a focus on SCFAs as potential bacterial mediators of brain function.
3. Modifications of cellular metabolism and activity in immune cells [27,28]. Similar to points 1 and 2, findings on these SCFA-mediated mechanisms are currently derived from animal and cell-based models. Nevertheless, studies have demonstrated striking results on BA promoting cell metabolism and differentiation in memory T cells [27,28], which underlines the importance of this mechanism.
4. Regulatory effects on transcription factors like peroxisome proliferator-activated receptor γ (PPAR-y) and hypoxia inducible factor-1 (HIF-1) [23,25,29] involved in inflammatory processes were also registered, though studies beyond rodents and cell models are currently lacking.

These studies have demonstrated SCFAs to be capable of regulating neuroinflammatory processes involving immune cell recruitment and cytokine secretion [29]. Microglia, immune cells residing in the CNS, were observed to be dysregulated in various psychiatric disorders like depression, schizophrenia, autism spectrum disorder (ASD) and obsessive–compulsive disorder [15] as well as in germ-free animals [28]. Interestingly, Toll-like receptors (TLRs) known to recognize bacterial compounds and to regulate inflammatory responses in our gastrointestinal tract (GIT) were found on various cell-types of the CNS, thus further supporting a link between gut and brain immune processes [30]. SCFAs also seem to directly impact neuronal function, as reported by studies showing PA and BA affecting intracellular potassium concentrations [31] and findings on influences on neurotransmitter metabolism [15]. Furthermore, beneficial effects on preserving memory function in experimental meningitis and protection from ouabain-induced hyperlocomotion were reported through a modulatory effect on the expression and activity of neurotrophic factors like brain-derived neurotrophic factor (BDNF), nerve growth factor (NGF) and glial cell line-derived neurotrophic factor (GDNF) in rats [32,33]. Interesting to note are the effects on synaptic plasticity by HDACI, since this process involves protein synthesis and therefore, gut-derived SCFAs might be potential epigenetic modulators of learning, memory formation and storage [34,35]. In light of these findings, altered SCFA production in the presence of gut microbiome disturbances, also known as dysbiosis, has been postulated as a potential risk for brain developmental and neurodegenerative diseases. Currently, CNS pathologies are often associated with changes in taxonomical gut microbiome and bacterial metabolites, as will be elaborated on in the following chapters.

3.1. SCFA and Autism Spectrum Disorder

Autism spectrum disorder (ASD), a neurodevelopmental disorder characterized by behavioural abnormalities including repetitive behaviour, communication deficits and sensitivity to environmental changes, is often linked to gastrointestinal problems and alterations in the gut microbial community [36–39]. This was shown in a cohort of human infants, that distinct gut bacterial composition variations, at times called enterotypes, might correlate with cognitive performance [40]. Recent studies indeed reported the gut microbiome compositions of children with ASD to be significantly distinct from their neurotypical (NT) developing peers, and furthermore detected overall lower alpha diversity in ASD gut microbiomes [41].

Only a handful of human studies have measured faecal metabolites in ASD, with some of them reporting elevated [42] and others decreased total SCFA levels [39,43] in children with ASD (Table 1). Contrarily, Kang et al. [41] reported no significant differences in SCFAs levels between ASD and NT control group. Adams et al. [43] reported lower faecal levels across all SCFAs (AA, BA, PA, valeric acid (VA)) in children with ASD. Others observed lower levels of AA and BA, but no significant alterations in PA-levels [44]. Conversely, significantly increased faecal levels across all SCFAs (AA, BA, PA, VA, isobutyric and isovaleric acid) in one study [42], and significantly elevated AA and PA in another study were detected in ASD faecal samples [39,43]. In support of the findings on decreased BA in two of the studies mentioned, a metagenomic analysis on faecal samples resulted in a lower abundance of microbial genes involved in the production of BA [38], which also parallels a prior reported decrease in BA-producing *Faecalium prausnitzii* in autistic patients [41].

Supporting the idea of gut microbial influence on ASD development, Sharon et al. [45] demonstrated that faecal microbiome transplants (FMT) from human ASD donors were able to invoke ASD-like behavioural traits in mice. Moreover, El-Ansary et al. [46] reported neuronal DNA damage induced by PA oral administration in a hamster model. These suggested that PA could play a role in neurotoxicity by damaging mitochondrial DNA by ATP-depletion, thus leading to mitochondrial dysfunction and oxidative stress in neurons. This postulated pathway in autism has been underscored by earlier findings in rat pups exposed to PA, exhibiting various immune, mitochondrial and ASD-like behaviour changes similar to ASD in humans [46–49]. PA-induced ASD in rodents is a validated model for ASD research that has presented with abnormal neural cell organization and hippocampal histology, increased microglia activity, neurotoxic cytokine secretion, and typical ASD-like behaviour traits [50]. Moreover, perturbed microbiota with increased PA-producers and decreased BA producers correlated with the severity of disease burden in ASD [26,43], even if studies of PA faecal levels in children with ASD compared to healthy controls (HCs) have produced conflicting data [39,41].

Contrarily to PA, BA has shown overall beneficial effects in ASD. BA administration alleviated ASD-like behaviour and normalized changes in gene transcription related to inhibitory/excitatory balance in the frontal cortex of the T+tf/J strain of the black and tan brachyury (BTBR) mouse autism model [51]. Nankova et al. [23] reported that SCFA as epigenetic regulators might affect genes assumed to be involved in ASD. BA and PA were able to increase catecholamine production as HDACI by regulating the tyrosine hydroxylase (TH) gene in an in vitro neuronal cell line (PC12 cells). PA and BA also modulated lipid homeostasis and inflammatory processes [23]. Moreover, SCFAs' influence on various genes of the dopaminergic pathway were detected, specifically on dopamine beta-hydroxylase (DBH) which, when dysregulated, shows associations with ASD in humans [23]. Interestingly, the serotonin system has been shown to only be affected by the administration of PA [52]. Furthermore, the study presented downregulating effects by PA or BA in the expression of fragile X mental retardation 1 (FMR1), neurexin and neuroligin, genes previously reported to relate to ASD [53–56]. BA, among all SCFAs, is the most important HDACI to modulate brain function through epigenetic processes [57] and thus, altered BA levels might potentially modify neuronal function.

In addition to the potential role of BA and PA in ASD, it is worth noting that the structurally related valproic acid (VPA), a branched SCFA, effectively creates a frequently used ASD mouse model that mimics both behavioural as well as gut microbiome traits in ASD patients [58]. In addition, prenatal exposure to VPA significantly increases the risk of ASD and showed epigenetic effects on neurotransmitter homeostasis via HDACI, similarly to BA and PA [59–62]. Additionally, VPA invokes dysfunctions in glutamate and GABA-neurotransmission and is thus likely to produce an altered balance between excitation and inhibition in the cerebral cortex [63].

These studies have shown that alterations of SCFAs can intricately influence neurodevelopmental processes via epigenetic modulation as HDACI. In support of a connection to ASD, Stilling et al. [64] detected upregulated cAMP response element-binding protein (CREB)-dependent gene expression in amygdala of GF mice, a limbic structure involved in emotion, memory and behaviour. It is thus understandable that a dysfunctional amygdala has been associated with neuropsychiatric disorders like anxiety disorder, post-traumatic stress disorder (PTSD) and ASD [65].

In contradiction with the above data, no significant changes in SCFA production were found in GF mice inoculated with microbiota from poor growth and good growth preterm infants, even though the administered microbiota was associated with pathologic developmental changes in neurons and oligodendrocytes of the receiving mice [66]. This might point to a different and/or additional pathway than SCFA, by which gut microbiota may affect early neurodevelopment.

Overall, support for SCFAs as putative influencers on ASD are present in a handful of clinical and mainly preclinical studies, though the research is still in its infancy. Therefore, further investigation to bring light into this emerging theory is strongly recommended.

3.2. SCFAs and Affective Disorders

Pathophysiological factors in affective disorders are multifaceted and gut microbial involvement has gradually become a potential contributing factor. Faecal SCFA levels from humans [67,68] and primates [67,68] with major depressive disorder (MDD) showed an overall decrease and altered composition compared to HCs (Table 1). AA, PA and isovaleric acid significantly decreased while only isocaproic acid increased in faecal samples of depressed individuals [67,68]. In contrast, one study reported no significant changes in faecal SCFAs in depressed patients [69]. Nevertheless, researchers previously showed distinct differences between faecal microbial compositions of HCs and MDD through taxonomic association studies [70]. Further links between affective disorders and a disturbed gut environment might be provided through observations in functional gut disorders like irritable bowel syndrome (IBS), exemplified by the results of a recent meta-analysis with significantly increased anxiety and depression in IBS patients [71].

A mentionable study by Kelly et al. [69] presented that depressive behaviour can be transferred from humans to germ-free rats by FMT, suggesting a strong connection between gut bacteria and affective disorders like major depressive disorder (MDD). Interestingly, there were discrepant findings regarding the role of SCFAs: faecal AA and total SCFA levels were higher in rats receiving FMT from patients than from HCs. However, depressed and healthy human donors showed no significant differences in their faecal SCFA levels. This calls for further investigations in clinical studies since interspecies differences might be a contributing factor in this case. Recently, rats bred for high anxiety-like behaviour (HAB), an animal model for anxiety and depression, displayed lower microglia numbers in distinct brain regions (infralimbic and prelimbic prefrontal cortex) and gut microbial shifts toward decreased counts of the BA-producing Lachnospiraceae family [72]. Treatment with antibiotic minocycline alleviated male HAB rats of depressive symptoms, further decreased circulating inflammatory cytokines and microglial count, as well as enriched their microbiota with known BA and 3-OH-butyrate producers Lachnospiraceae and Clostridiales family XIII. In fact, Clostridia are considered as the main BA-producing class of the human gut microbiome [73] (Table 2). These findings, together with previous propositions for immunomodulatory effects of BA and 3-OH-butyrate on inflammation, T-cell and microglial activity [13,28,29,74,75] point towards an intricate relationship between microbial derived SCFAs and affective disorders, that might benefit from their anti-inflammatory effects. In support of this theory, increased markers of inflammation such as pro-inflammatory cytokines in circulation and the brain are correlated with MDD [76]. Moreover, studies have successfully demonstrated SCFA-mediated anxiolytic and antidepressant effects in mice undergoing induced psychosocial stress [77]. In particular, the administration of sodium butyrate (NaB, the sodium salt of BA) has been reported to alleviate pathologic affective behaviours in rat models, including hyperactivity, depressive and manic symptoms [26]. Future work on this subject, especially through metabolomic studies in humans, might enlighten the intricate gut bacterial metabolite–brain axis interplay in affective disorders, as the current state of research provides only few clinical studies on this particular subject.

3.3. SCFAs and Autoimmune Diseases of the Brain: Multiple Sclerosis (MS)

Multiple sclerosis (MS) is an autoimmune disease of the CNS that mainly damages the myelin sheaths of motor neurons. An imbalance between anti-inflammatory Treg cells and proinflammatory Th1 and Th17 cells are widely understood to take part in the MS pathophysiology [78].

Individuals with MS have been reported to harbour microbiomes that are significantly different from HCs [79,80]. Indeed, one recent study reported increased *Streptococcus*, decreased *Prevotella_9* and overall decreased faecal SCFAs (AA, PA and BA) in a Chinese cohort of MS patients [81]. *Streptococcus* is known to produce all SCFAs [44,82] and *Prevotella_9* is able to generate AA and PA [81] (Table 2). MS patients displayed higher abundance of inflammatory Th17 cells, as anti-inflammatory Treg cells were decreased. Interestingly, faecal SCFA concentrations positively correlated with levels of circulating Treg cells in this study, thus suggesting that SCFAs exert anti-inflammatory effects due to elevated Treg/Th17–cell ratios. Similarly, significantly decreased SCFAs—were detected in blood samples of patients with active secondary progressive MS [29]. These two human studies might suggest an overall decrease in faecal and consecutively depleted circulating SCFA levels in MS patients (Table 1), that might shift the immune system towards proinflammatory processes due to lower Treg/Th17 cell ratios.

Autoimmune processes in the CNS were affected by the gut through SCFAs and long-chain fatty acids (LCFAs) in the experimental autoimmune encephalomyelitis (EAE) mouse model of MS. The differentiation of pro-inflammatory Th1 and Th17 cells were increased by LCFAs, while anti-inflammatory Treg cell differentiation was boosted by SCFAs through the downregulation of the JNK1 and p38 pathway. Therefore, LCFAs exacerbated, while SCFAs alleviated disease and subdued axonal damage. Additionally, PA demonstrated the most stimulating effect on Treg cell differentiation, which improved histopathological outcomes of the spinal cord in EAE mice [13]. Melbye et al. [83] reviewed two other studies in EAE mice, who supported the ameliorating role of SCFAs in disease activity by modulating an increase in anti-inflammatory Treg cells and a decrease in pro-inflammatory Th1 and Th17 cells. BA too, was able to ameliorate demyelination in rats and importantly, exposing an organotypic slice culture to BA resulted in suppressed lysolecithin-induced demyelination and enhanced remyelination, represented by higher counts of mature oligodendrocytes [84]. In congruence with these studies, a recent review concluded that PA and BA ameliorated the clinical symptoms of EAE by inducing immune tolerance epigenetically as HDACIs. The proposed mechanism involves an upregulation of the transcription factor Foxp3 leading to increased Foxp3+ T regulatory lymphocytes, also known as Treg cells that inhibit proinflammatory Th1 and Th17 cells [85]. In addition to these findings that support an overall anti-inflammatory effect through SCFAs, Park et al. [29] recently demonstrated that SCFA administration to EAE mice models increased anti-inflammatory IL10+Tcells and IL-10, as well as pro-inflammatory Th1, Th17 and Tc cells. Moreover, SCFA receptors GPR41 and GPR43 have demonstrated proinflammatory effects in EAE pathogenesis [29]. These results underline the importance of SCFAs to protect from inflammatory processes in the CNS. Their uncovered pro-inflammatory effects, however, indicate a complex system in immunomodulation, which calls for further work in this subject in order to evaluate potential interventions involving SCFAs in neuroinflammatory diseases.

3.4. SCFAs and Neurodegenerative Diseases of the Brain

Neurodegenerative diseases are becoming increasingly prevalent as the population gradually grows older. Researchers are trying to elucidate the pathomechanisms of the various brain diseases including Alzheimer's disease (AD), Parkinson's disease (PD), dementia with Lewy bodies (DLB), multiple system atrophy (MSA) and Huntington's disease (HD) [86]. This chapter will first briefly list some findings on SCFAs and neurodegenerative processes in general before focusing on AD and PD.

3.4.1. General Findings on Neurodegenerative Processes

A recent in vitro study investigated the direct influences of the SCFAs NaB, sodium valerate and hexanoic acid on neuroinflammation and found that high concentrations of NaB were able to decrease the basal levels of the proinflammatory cytokine IL-6 in human glioblastoma–astrocytoma U373 cells [87]. However, further findings showed no neuroprotection from induced oxidative stress in differentiated SH-SY5Y cells (human-derived neuroblastoma cells) by any SCFAs. Interestingly, exposure to BA and valerate was able to induce neuronal maturation through MAP2-gene expression in undifferentiated neuroblastoma cells, thus hinting towards a beneficial effect on neurogenesis [87]. BA's effects in animal models include the potential to alleviate impaired cognition, enhancing neuronal plasticity, improve learning and memory performance, as well as neuroprotection, all beneficial processes regarding neurodegenerative diseases [57].

Overall, direct impacts on brain cells by SCFAs seem to be complex as well as dose-dependent, which supports a hypothesis that anti-inflammatory processes in the brain, neuroplasticity and neurogenesis could be positively modulated through the manipulation of gut bacterial production and/or external supplementation of SCFAs. Recent research further provided evidence for an ameliorating role of SCFAs in inflammatory hippocampal neurodegeneration in mice through the reduced impairment of the intestinal barrier, which was induced by a high-fructose diet. It was suggested that SCFAs could amend the faulty colonic NLRP6 inflammasome responsible for epithelial impairment to alleviate hippocampal neuroinflammation, thus possibly reducing the likelihood of neurodegenerative processes associated with a typically high-fructose Western-style diet [88]. This might be an indirect mechanism by which SCFAs could exert neuroprotective effects.

3.4.2. SCFAs and Alzheimer's Disease

Gut microbiome of Alzheimer's disease (AD) patients were observed to be altered, with decreased overall richness and diversity as well as some shifts within taxonomical compositions [89,90]. Some studies presented AD progression to associate with dysbiosis and that a healthy gut microbiome provides beneficial effects in AD patients and rodent models [90,91]. Recent studies further showed significant changes in gut microbiome compositions between AD patients and HCs at the genetic level, suggesting some bacterial AD-associated PCR products to be a potential marker of AD risk [92]. As Franceschi et al. described in their review in 2019, disturbances in the gut microbiome might influence processes involved in AD pathogenesis, such as chronic inflammation, molecular mimicry and Aβ accumulation. Furthermore, the presence of microbiome enterotype III (low *Bacteroides* and *Prevotella*) and the absence of enterotype I (>30% *Bacteroides*) were reported with stronger associations to the presence of dementia than classic markers (Table 3) [93]. This highlights the potential of the GBA to impact pathogenesis in dementia, though unfortunately, no human studies that measured SCFA faecal levels have been reported as to our literature search.

The GF condition in transgenic AD mice models were observed to slow the progression of disease symptoms [94], underlining an important role for the presence of the gut microbiome, including bacteria and their metabolites in AD pathogenesis. A study with the APP/PS1 mouse model of AD reported disturbed microbiota composition and diversity, as well as overall lower SCFAs levels compared to wild-type (WT) controls. Additionally, over 30 metabolic pathways possibly related to amyloid deposition and ultrastructural anomalies were detected in intestine samples of the AD group [95]. Zheng et al. [96] have introduced a method of stable isotope labelling and liquid chromatography–tandem mass spectrometry to sensitively detect 21 SCFAs in mice faecal samples of AD and WT mice. In an AD mouse model, decreased levels of PA, isobutyric acid, 3-hydroxybutyric acid, and 3-hydroxyisovaleric acid were detected while increased levels of lactic acid, 2-hydroxybutyric acid, 2-hydroxyisobutyric acid, levulinic acid and valproic acid were found. In contrast to these findings, faecal PA was enriched in mice receiving FMT from an AD donor in comparison to a healthy one [97]. However, two faecal donor samples selected out of groups of 14 healthy and 13 AD volunteers might limit that study's evidential impact due to putative inter-individual variations.

The prevention of Aβ accumulation and the removal of accumulated amyloid plaque have been at the core of anti-AD therapeutic undertakings for more than two decades [98]. It is important to highlight an in vitro study reporting that valeric acid (VA), BA and PA, but not isobutyric acid, isovaleric acid and AA, to be capable of stopping the misfolding of Aβ40 peptides to neurotoxic Aβ40 aggregates in a dose-dependent manner [99]. Additionally, the same experiment on Aβ42 aggregation showed that only VA could inhibit the process dose-dependently. A third experiment determined that VA and BA successfully halted Aβ fibril formation in a dose-dependent manner. These results demonstrate a mechanism by which gut microbial-derived SCFAs may benefit AD patients and that a gut microbiome depleted of SCFA producers might promote neurotoxic amyloid build up in the CNS. In support of this theory, Sun et al. [100] reported that FMT from WT-mice to the APP/PS1 mice model of AD resulted in the alleviated brain deposition of Aβ as well as levels of neurotoxic Aβ40 and Aβ42, tau protein phosphorylation, synaptic dysfunction, neuroinflammation and cognitive deficits, accompanied with restored alterations in gut microbiota and faecal SCFA levels. The AD mice harboured a perturbed microbiome enriched with Proteobacteria, Verrucomicrobio (phylum level), and *Akkermansia*, *Desulfovibrio* (genus level), with depleted Bacteroidetes phyla. All these conditions were reversed through FMT treatment. However, these microbial changes were lacking consistency in the relative abundance of bacterial species, for example a relative increase in Bacteroidetes or BA-producing Firmicutes has been previously observed in animal and human studies of AD [91]. Therefore, definite conclusions about distinct AD gut microbiome compositions and their capacity of SCFA production cannot be made at this point in time, which further warrants our focus on disease correlations with bacterial metabolites instead.

Impaired epigenetic gene expression has been discussed as a key factor in AD pathogenesis [101], which conceivably led to a study of BA's role as HDACI in an AD mouse model. Treatment with BA was able to improve associative memory function at an advanced stage of disease [102]. Other studies mentioned the neuroprotective capacity of BA to manipulate regulatory regions of the Forkhead box gene locus as HDACI. This provides a preventative and/or therapeutic potential to affect the balance between life-promoting and apoptotic cell processes critical in neurodegenerative diseases [8]. BA as NaB has shown neuroprotective benefits as HDACI in studies of PD, AD and HD, particularly leading to improved learning and memory in dementia, the prevention of oxidative stress and neuronal cell death in HD and PD, as well as overall upregulated transcription of neurotrophic factors involved in plasticity, survival and regeneration [103]. These results might indicate that decreased or overall altered gut microbial SCFAs and thus, dysregulated histone-acetylation, might indeed be connected to AD and related brain diseases. We therefore suggest future studies to look for putative impacts of altered SCFA-producing gut microbiota on AD-related epigenetic processes in the brain. SCFAs might also impact AD indirectly through additional pathways via the regulation of intestinal gluconeogenesis by FFAR3 signalling, which affects the activity of the dorsal motor nucleus of the vagus, a structure with altered activity in PD and AD [8]. BA especially has also been hypothesized to positively impact cognition in AD patients via the stimulation of vagal afferents [8].

In a study with rats fed a high-fat diet, it was shown that the administration of two valeric acid esters (monovalerin and trivalerin) led to higher levels of AA in the brain, serum and liver, while caecal levels decreased. These data suggest that AA can actually be increased in the brain by oral supplementation and uptake in the gut [104]. This might be of interest, since AA administration to lipopolysaccharide (LPS)-stimulated astrocyte cultures was successful in producing anti-inflammatory effects [105]. BA exposure invoked anti-inflammatory effects as well, as shown by the reduced microglial activation and decreased secretion of inflammatory cytokines. BA inhibits the secretion of HDAC gut microbe-derived circulating inflammatory cytokines and thus limits their effects on neuroinflammatory processes that have been postulated to be involved in AD pathology [91]. Pro-inflammatory cytokines derived from dysbiosis might invoke the formation of Aβ aggregates as well as cause the dysfunctional maturation of microglia, thus leading to increased amyloid accumulation in the CNS [91]. Taken together, healthy gut flora with undisturbed SCFA production might benefit AD patients with decreased neuroinflammation and amyloid accumulation.

3.4.3. SCFAs and Parkinson's Disease

PD is, after AD, the second-most prevalent neurodegenerative disease in the world [106] and is part of a cluster of neurodegenerative disorders associated with aggregated amyloid proteins. Misfolded alpha-synuclein proteins (αSyn) are specifically implicated in PD, DLB and MSA, also jointly known as "Synucleopathies" [107]. In PD, the dopaminergic neurons residing in the substantia nigra pars compacta are lost, subsequently leading to impaired motor functions [108]. Gut dysbiosis and GI dysfunction have been repeatedly mentioned as a hallmark of PD [108–114], thus investigations of mechanistic processes involving the GBA have emerged in recent years. This conceivably led to questions about gut microbial participation in pathophysiological processes of PD, such as the spreading of αSyn aggregates from gut to brain via the vagal nerve [115] as well as probable connections between gut dysbiosis, neuroinflammation and misfolding of αSyn [116].

Overall decreased SCFA levels with relatively low BA and a microbiome with reduced Bacteroidetes, Prevotellaceae as well as enriched Enterobacteriaceae were reported in PD [117] (Table 1). Underlining these findings, a recent review reported trends of reduction in SCFA producers in a PD patient's microbiomes, specifically reduced Lachnospiraceae (*Blautia, Dorea, Coprococcus, Rosburia, Clostridium XIV*), *Faecalibacterium* and *Bacteroides* [109]. Interesting to mention is the overall increased abundance of Enterobacteriacea, a phylum that is known to produce SCFAs (Table 2) and to also associate with the severity of motor symptoms in PD patients [112]. This finding might at the first glance appear counterintuitive under the assumption that SCFAs and their producers are beneficial to PD. On the other hand, the relative abundance in Enterobacteriaceae might further indicate the production of other metabolites involved in PD, as will be elaborated on later in the chapter discussing bacterial amyloids.

Two studies in rodents reported further contradicting results regarding SCFA levels in PD. Sampson et al. [118] used a transgenic αSyn-overexpressing mouse model of PD, that presented ameliorated PD pathologies when in a germ-free (GF) state or treated with antibiotics (AT). These GF/AT mice were then inoculated with human PD-donor microbiota. This treatment significantly altered faecal microbial communities and SCFA composition, displaying lower AA, but higher PA and BA, as well as worsened motor dysfunction compared to those receiving healthy FMT. Thus, the administration of a mixture of SCFAs to GF/AT mice was effective in inducing motor deficits, as well as αSyn aggregation and microglial activation in the brain. This suggested a relevant role for SCFAs as mediators of PD in a genetically susceptible animal model [118]. Supporting these findings, the 1-methyl-4-phenyl-1,2,3,6-tetrahydropyridine(MPTP) – induced PD mice model presented an increased abundance of faecal SCFAs. The gut microbiome of this PD model was administrated to normal mice, which resulted in motor impairment and decreased striatal neurotransmitters, while FMT from healthy donors alleviated those symptoms [119]. The inconsistencies within the previously mentioned studies in human subjects, regarding beneficial or detrimental effects of SCFAs in PD, might point towards inter-species differences of mice and humans and the GF state of acutely inoculated mice. This could further suggest that even though the presence of SCFAs seems necessary to trigger pathological changes in genetically vulnerable organisms, shifts towards depleted SCFA levels and their bacterial producers might play a role in already established PD.

Several lines of evidence suggest that SCFAs, BA in particular, may exert possible beneficial effects in PD. First, BA might play a role in PD as a neuroprotective agent due to its agonistic effect on the receptor GPR109A, which promotes anti-inflammatory processes [120]. In addition, BA might also benefit PD patients with reduced neuroinflammation, indirectly enhanced dopamine synthesis through increased free niacin levels, as well as improved energy homeostasis and mitochondrial function [103,121]. Lastly, SCFAs ameliorated dysfunctional microglia in GF mice, which was represented by improved microglial maturation, morphology and function [28]. Proper mature microglial function includes decreased inflammatory activity and phagocytosis for amyloid proteins like tau, Aβ, and αSyn. Therefore, the state of the gut microbiome and its production power for SCFAs might positively influence several aspects of neurodegenerative diseases [91]. It might be of interest that mice lacking the SCFA receptor FFAR2 have shown dysfunctional microglia similar to GF animals, however, that particular study suggested alternative pathways by which SCFAs directly exert their effects on microglia due to a lack of evidence for FFAR2-expression on CNS cells [28]. Definite mechanisms involved in receptor-mediated processes of SCFAs remain to be determined.

As previously mentioned, SCFAs can upregulate gene-expression as HDACI. This process was shown to facilitate neuroplasticity and long-term memory, involving CREB-dependent gene regulation [122,123]. In vitro studies also discovered PA and BA to modulate transcription of the tyrosine hydroxylase gene in brain cells and thus to influence catecholaminergic biosynthesis [23]. Catecholamines like DOPA, dopamine (DA), noradrenaline and adrenaline are essential neurotransmitters with important roles in brain diseases, exemplified by the depletion of DA being a key factor in PD [52,106,124]. Especially relevant to PD is that the enzyme tyrosine hydroxylase catalyses the rate-limiting step of DA synthesis [8]. Further research on BA's role as HDACI revealed protective effects for dopaminergic cells, namely rescuing them from αSyn-mediated DNA damage [125] or MPP+-induced toxicity [126] through an enhanced expression of DNA damage response genes. Supporting evidence come from a study in a drosophila model of PD in which BA has been reported to alleviate motor dysfunction and mortality [127]. Moreover, altered gut levels of SCFAs and neurotransmitters were associated with the surface area of the insula [9], a brain region that is understood to be dysfunctional in neurological and psychiatric disorders [128].

The influence of gut microbiota on PD might further impact the conventional therapy of levodopa administration, since the abundance of the gene for tyrosine decarboxylase, an enzyme converting levodopa to DA, in the microbiome of PD patients correlates with higher dosage needs for levodopa/carbidopa. Furthermore, it was shown in rats, serum levels of the aforementioned drug negatively correlated with the host's microbiome tyrosine decarboxylase gene levels [129]. These findings might provide the base for further clinical studies on gut microbial modulations in PD patients with increased levodopa/carbidopa dosages.

Taken together, SCFAs seem to exert overall beneficial effects on the CNS regarding autoimmune brain diseases and neurodegenerative diseases. However, preclinical findings on probable detrimental effects upon SCFA exposure in rodents suggests that these bacterial metabolites might function as double-edged swords when it comes to brain health. Thus, the thorough examination of these mechanisms is crucial before future potential therapeutic and preventative strategies can be unequivocally suggested.

Table 1. SCFA level alterations in brain diseases found in human studies.

Disease	SCFA		Literature	p-Values
ASD	AA	↓	f [44], f [43]	**p = 0.011, p = 0.0000003**
		↑	f [42], f [39],* u [36]	**p = 0.037, p < 0.005, p < 0.005**
		-	f [41]	p = 0.979
	BA	↓	f [44], f [43]	**p = 0.005, p = 0.005**
		↑	f [42]	**p = 0.025**
		-	f [41]	p = 0.974
	Isobutyric acid	↑	f [42]	**p = 0.022**
	Isovaleric acid	↑	f [42]	**p = 0.038**
	PA	↓	f [43]	**p = 0.002**
		↑	f [42], f [39]	**p = 0.007, p < 0.005**
		-	f [41], f [44]	p = 0.979, p = 0.243
	VA	↓	f [43]	**p = 0.005**
		↑	f [44], f [42]	**p < 0.001, p = 0.007**
MDD	AA	↓	f [67]	**p = 0.04**
		↑	f [69]	p = 0.65
	BA	-	f [67], f [69]	p = 0.68, p = 0.867
	Caproic acid	↑	f [67]	p = 0.09
	Isobutyric acid	-	f [67]	p = 0.70
		-	f [69]	p = 0.501
	Isocaproic acid	↑	f [67]	**p < 0.01**
	Isovaleric acid	-	f [67]	p = 0.4
	PA	↓	f [67]	p = 0.07
		-	f [69]	p = 0.918
	VA	↓	f [67]	p = 0.56
MS	AA	↓	f [81], s [29]	**p < 0.0001, p = 0.001**
	BA	↓	f [81], s [29]	**p < 0.05, p = 0.0001**
	Isovalerate, valerate, hexanoate, heptanoate	-	s [29]	p > 0.05
	PA	↓	f [81], s [29]	**p < 0.0001, p = 0.01**
PD	AA	↓	f [117], * p [109]	**p < 0.01, p = 0.0201**
	BA	↓	f [117]	**p < 0.01**
	Isobutyric acid	-	f [117]	p > 0.05
	Isovaleric acid	-	f [117]	p > 0.05
	PA	↓	f [117]	**p < 0.01**
	VA	-	f [117]	p > 0.05

This table shows the differences of SCFA levels of various sample materials from human patients compared to healthy controls. Significance of the data is given in the last column. ↑ symbolizes increased, ↓ decreased, whereas - symbolizes no significant change in metabolite levels found in cohorts with the specific disease. Sample material is noted as f = faecal; s = serum; p = plasma; u = urine with the associated reference as numbers in brackets; p-values < 0.05 are marked in bold letters. BA = butyric acid; AA = acetic acid; PP = propionic acid; VA = valeric acid; ASD = autism spectrum disorder; MDD = major depressive disorder; MS = multiple sclerosis; PD = Parkinson's disease. "*" marked references are sourced from reviews.

Table 2. Gut-residing bacteria found to correlate with the production of SCFAs.

SCFA	Taxa	Study
tSCFA	*Faecalibacterium, Ruminococcus, Bifidobacterium*	[39]
PA	*Bacteroides*	[39]
VA	Acidobacteria, Actinomycetaceae	[44]
BA	Streptococcaceae, Peptostreptococcaceae, Lactobacillaceae, Clostridiaceae, Family_XIII, Leuconostocaceae	[44]
PA	Desulfovibrionaceae, Streptococcaceae	[44]
AA	Desulfovibrionaceae	[44]
AA, PA	*Prevotella_9*	[81]
BA	*Clostridium, Eubacterium, Butyrivibrio*	[103]
AA	Bacteroidetes, *B.hydrogenotrophica*	[130]
BA	Lachnospiraceae, *Faecalibacterium prausnitzii, Eubacterium, Roseburia*	[130]
PA	Bacteroidetes, Proteobacteria, some Lachnospiraceae	[130]
BA	*Eubacterium ramulus*	[131]
PA	*Clostridium*	[46]
AA, PA	*Parabacteroides distasonis, Megaspheara massiliensis*	[87]
BA, VA, HA	*Parabacteroides distasonis, Megaspheara massiliensis*	[87]
PA	*Lactobacillus, Propionibacterium*	[97]
BA	*Faecalibacterium prausnitzii, Eubacterium rectale, Roserburia, Eubacterium hallii, Ruminococcus bromii*	[14]
PA	*Akkermansia municiphila*	[14]
BA	*Blautia*, Lachnospiraceae: *Coprococcus, Roseburia, Faecalibacterium, Lachnospira*	[132]
BA	Clostridia (class)	[73]
AA	*Blautia hydrogenotrophica, Clostridium, Streptococcus*	[82]
PA	*Salmonella, Roseburia inulinivorans, Ruminococcus obeum, Bacteroides, Phascolarctobacterium succinatutens, Dialister, Veillonella, Megasphaera elsdenii, Coprococcus catus*	[82]
BA	*Anaerostipes, Coprococcus catus, Eubacterium rectale, Eubacterium hallii, Faecalibacterium prausnitzii, Roseburia, Coprococcus comes, Coprococcus eutactus*	[82]

tSCFA = total SCFAs; BA = butyric acid; AA = acetic acid; PP = propionic acid; VA = valeric acid; HA = hexanoic acid. References are represented by numbers in brackets.

Table 3. Prevalence of dementia linked with various factors.

Factors	Odds Ratio	p-Value
Enterotype III	18.5 [b]	<0.001 [b]
Enterotype I	0.1 [a]	<0.001 [a]
ApoE	3.9 [a], 4.4 [b]	0.035 [a], 0.026 [b]
SLI	15.0 [a]	0.005 [a]
VSRAD	3.5 [a], 4.2 [b]	<0.001 [a,b]

Multivariable logistic regression analysis models linking the prevalence of dementia and various factors from Saji et al. [93]. [a] Model 1: inclusion of enterotype I, [b] Model 2: Inclusion of enterotype III. Abbreviations: ApoE $\varepsilon 4$ = apolipoprotein $\varepsilon 4$; SLI = silent lacunar infarct; VSRAD = voxel-based specific regional analysis system for Alzheimer's disease.

4. Non-SCFA Bacterial Metabolites

The vast majority of current studies on the GBA involve SCFAs. Our gut microbiota, however, produces metabolites far beyond the products of fibre degradation, including vitamins, polyphenol metabolites and products from amino acid metabolism (Figure 1). Each of these families of compounds are involved in various pathways and contain potential neuroactive metabolites [22]. This warrants our curiosity in exploring non-SCFA bacterial metabolites as contributors to the GBA.

4.1. Amino Acid Metabolites

Metagenomic studies suggests human gut microbes to be largely involved in amino acid metabolism [133]. Of special interest are the aromatic amino acids (AAA) tyrosine (Tyr), phenylalanine (Phe) and tryptophan (Trp). Humans are unable to produce AAA and depend on dietary sources and our gut microbiome for covering their nutritional needs. Gut bacteria are able to synthesize all three AAA de novo via the shikimate pathway [92,134]. In a first step, Trp and Phe are biosynthesized. Tyr is then synthetized from Phe. Further AAA metabolism occurs in the host as well as in gut microbes like *Lactobacillus*, Enterobacteriaceae and anaerobes of the phylum Firmicutes, that generate other metabolites. Phe and Tyr are catabolized in animals to neurotransmitters, including L-Dopa, DA, epinephrine and norepinephrine, while gut bacteria are able to produce phenolic compounds like p-cresol from Tyr and phenyl molecules from Phe. Trp is an essential precursor for the neurotransmitters serotonin and tryptamine, as well as vitamin B3 (niacin), redox cofactors NAD(P)+, plus metabolites from the kynurenine pathway [134]. On note, the kynurenine pathway in gut microbes generate metabolites associated with brain functions like indole, indole-derivatives, kynuric acid and quinolinate, which will be elaborated on in the following chapters. For a more in-depth analysis of AAA metabolism in plants, microbes as well as mammals, we refer the reader to the extensive review by Parthasarathy et al. [134].

Considering the previously described processes in AAA metabolism, it is conceivable to assume that gut microbiota might modulate neurotransmitter metabolism, synthesis, and availability in the gut, the circulatory system and the CNS. In fact, the abundance of circulating Trp can be curbed as a result of gut microbial Trp metabolization through other pathways, thereby possibly limiting the precursor for neurotransmitter synthesis in the CNS while also generating other neuroactive metabolites like indole and its derivatives [135] (Figure 3). On the other hand, gut microbes seem to elevate serotonin plasma availability after colonizing GF animals, leading to the assumption that the presence of a functioning gut microbiome contributes to physiological serotonin plasma levels [136]. More importantly, a recent study observed gut microbial involvements in Trp metabolism, providing an extensive overview of six pathways, each generating neuroactive metabolites referred to as "TRYP-6", consisting of kynurenine, quinolinate, indole, indole acetic acid (IAA), indole propionic acid (IPA) and tryptamine [135]. They identified five common gut-inhabiting phyla capable of two to six pathways. The five phyla Actinobacteria, Firmicutes, Proteobacteria, Bacteroidetes and Fusobacteria thus have been suggested to relevantly influence Trp metabolism. Investigations on a genus level revealed that *Clostridium, Burkholderia, Pseudomonas, Streptomyces* and *Bacillus* were particularly capable of generating neuroactive Trp metabolites, with the first two holding the highest potential (Table 4). Numerous pathways and metabolites in the AAA metabolism, especially Trp, show relevant effects on the CNS that seem to be intricately complex and crucial for proper brain function, thus pointing to these non-SCFAs as promising players on the GBA (Figure 3).

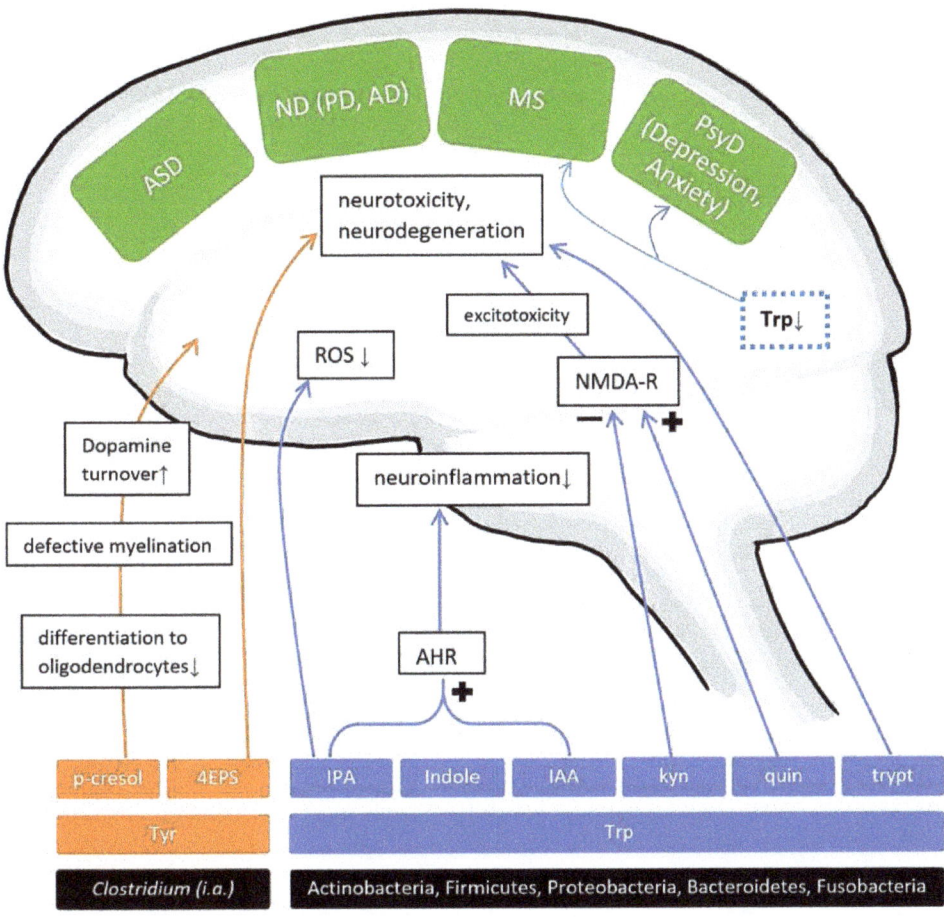

Figure 3. Hypothetical influences on brain diseases by gut bacteria-derived tyrosine and tryptophane metabolites. This figure illustrates the mechanistic effects by which gut microbial metabolites might influence brain functions related to autism spectrum disorder (ASD) and neurodegenerative disorders (NDs): Parkinson's disease (PD), Alzheimer's disease (AD), multiple sclerosis (MS) and psychiatric disorders (PsyD). Gut bacteria taking part in metabolite production are listed in black boxes situated under the orange (tyrosine metabolites) and blue boxes (tryptophane metabolites). Arrows accompanied with + or − represent an agonistic (+) or antagonistic (−) effect on a receptor, whereas unaccompanied arrows symbolize an effect described in the white boxes. ↑ = upregulated, ↓ = downregulated or lowered levels of. ROS = reactive oxygen species; NMDA-R = N-methyl-D-aspartate receptor; Trp = tryptophane; AHR = aryl hydrocarbon receptor; 4EPS = 4-ethylphenylsulfate; IPA = indole-propionic acid; IAA = indole-acetic acid; kyn = kynurenine; quin = quinolinate; trypt = tryptamine; i.a. = inter alia.

4.1.1. AAMs and Neurodevelopmental Disorders

P-cresol is a known uremic toxin, which is metabolized into p-cresol sulphate by the liver [137] and is believed to derive from Tyr fermentation in several gut bacterial species (Table 4). Significantly increased urinary and faecal levels of p-cresol were reported in autistic children, with some linking urinary levels with the clinical severity of disease [39,41,138,139]. Interestingly, p-cresol levels significantly and negatively correlate with age in ASD patients, which might suggest that younger individuals with ASD are exposed to effects from elevated p-cresol levels [41]. One study, however, did not detect significantly altered faecal levels in children with ASD [42]. As for non-human studies, p-cresol was very recently shown to dose-dependently induce and exacerbate ASD-like behaviours and significantly activate dopamine (DA) turnover in brain regions (amygdala, nucleus accumbens and striatum) in the genetically vulnerable BTBR mice model for ASD [140]. Social avoidance behaviour and increased gut levels of p-cresol were detected in GF mice, inoculated with p-cresol-producing Clostridiales (including Lachnospiraceae and Ruminococcae families), and these mice associated with defective myelination in the prefrontal cortex [141]. Additional in vitro testing showed that exposure to p-cresol interrupted the differentiation of progenitor cells into oligodendrocytes [141], suggesting that gut microbial p-cresol might impact CNS myelination through transcriptional changes. Other mechanisms by which p-cresol might negatively impact neuronal functions [140] include the inhibition of dopamine-β-hydroxylase and membrane depolarization with higher vulnerability for seizures and blunted Na^+/K^+-ATPase function. These mechanisms might demonstrate a potential for gut bacterial-derived p-cresol to play a role in disorders with disfunctions in the CNS, including ASD, MS, and neurodegenerative diseases.

In the maternal immune-activated (MIA) mouse model of autism spectrum disorder, changes in serum metabolites, showing significant elevations of two AAA bacterial metabolites 4-ethylphenylsulfate (4EPS) and indolepyruvate were found, which were completely normalized along with ASD-related behaviour, dysbiosis and impaired gut barrier after the inoculation with the probiotic *B. fragilis* [142]. Moreover, WT mice treated with the metabolite 4EPS alone manifested anxiety-like behaviour similar to MIA-mice, thus suggesting a compelling association between 4EPS and ASD. Additionally, other metabolites, two of them being serotonin and p-cresol, were elevated in the serum of MIA-mice, though not at significant levels [142]. It is essential to mention 4EPS's structural similarity to the prior mentioned p-cresol, which has links to ASD and is believed to share its producers in the gut with 4EPS, namely *Clostridia* spp. [36,140,142] (Table 4). Overall, preclinical data and some supportive human studies point towards a connection between 4EPS, indolepyruvate, p-cresol and ASD, not only as biomarkers of disease but also as putative mediators of pathogenesis.

With an extensive in silico study, Kaur et al. [135] recently detected the aforementioned "TRYP6", the six Trp metabolism pathways generating neuroactive metabolites, to be enriched in the metagenome of autistic gut microbiota. Genomes of the genera *Burkholderia* and *Pseudomonas* showed particularly large potentials for TRYP6 metabolism. *Burkholderia* holds pathways for kynurenine and quinolinate, with a lower production of IAA, indole and tryptamine, while *Pseudomonas* is a strong producer for kynurenine and a weaker one for IAA, quinolinate and tryptamine. Other enriched pathways in autistic children consisted of those generating indole and its derivative IAA by already mentioned genera *Burkholderia* and *Pseudomonas* plus *Corynebacterium*. Though microbiota from NT individuals also harboured some relatively enriched bacteria capable of producing TRYP6, namely *Alistipes* for indole and *Eggerthella* for IAA production, these genera are comparatively weak producers and thus, theorized to use indole and IAA as inter-bacterial communication tools [135]. Similarly, altered Trp metabolism in ASD has been indicated through significantly increased urinary levels of IAA, indoxyl sulphate (IS, also known as indican) and indolyl lactate in autistic children [143], though to date no data on faecal levels have been found.

In addition to Trp metabolism, altered Phe metabolism in autistic children were recently highlighted, partly based on evidence of significantly elevated Clostridia-generated Phe metabolites in the urinary profiles of ASD patients including 3-(3-hydroxyphenyl)-3-hydroxypropionic acid, 3-hydroxyphenylacetic acid and 3-hydroxyhippuric acid [36]. However, whether these metabolites might be modulated by gut bacteria remains to be elucidated.

Increased faecal levels of glutamate in children with ASD, as well as decreased GABA levels in those with pervasive developmental disorder not otherwise specified (PDD-NOS) have been previously reported [39]. Kang et al. [41] have similarly detected lower GABA faecal levels in autistic children, though these did not reach significance ($p = 0.077$). Preclinical observations in altered GABA and glutamate levels were made in a study invoking behaviours associated with ASD in GF mice through inoculation with gut microbiota derived from autistic patients. In comparison, mice receiving healthy donor FMT did not produce ASD-like behaviour [45]. Moreover, lower faecal levels of the GABA A receptor agonists 5AV and taurine were found in the first group, supporting a putative role of disturbed GABA signalling in ASD. In a further step, the exposure of an ASD mouse model to taurine or 5AV during the prenatal and weaning period produced mice with ameliorated ASD behaviour in comparison with mice treated during their juvenile stage and older mice. This suggests a critical window of vulnerability for disturbed GABA signalling during neurodevelopment [45]. Other researchers were able to uncover correlations between gut microbe genes associated with neurotransmitter metabolism and the surface area of the insula, with a focus on two microbial genes involved in GABA and glutamate metabolism, namely 4-hydroxybutyrate dehydrogenase and glutamate dehydrogenase [9]. As already mentioned, the insula is thought to be dysfunctional in many psychiatric disorders with disturbed emotion, cognition and motivation, such as affective, neurodevelopmental and neurodegenerative disorders [128]. However, it is also important to note that Kang et al. [41] were not able to detect any significant changes in gut bacterial pathways by PICRUSt database analysis between ASD and NT children. Nevertheless, these studies accumulatively show the potential involvement of gut microbial metabolites in disturbed GABA and glutamate signalling in ASD pathophysiology. Further metabolomic, metagenomic and microbial analyses of faecal amino acid metabolites (AAMs) are nonetheless highly encouraged. Compellingly, a recent study reported that GABA produced from gut bacteria (*E. coli HT115* and *P. aeruginosa PAO1*) was able to protect from neurodegeneration in the nematode C. elegans [144].

Lastly, the amplified metabolism of the amino acids Tyr, lysine, cysteine and methionine in healthy children's gut microbiomes have been found, which implies a supportive function of gut commensals during brain development, since the mentioned amino acids are not only substrates for the synthesis of structural proteins, but also neurotransmitters and biogenic amines [145].

4.1.2. AAMs and Psychiatric Disorders

No specific studies on non-SCFA faecal metabolites have been found in humans with affective disorders. However, there are a handful of reports pointing to correlations between disturbed gut microbial Trp metabolism and psychiatric disorders like anxiety and depression. Studies on acute tryptophan depletion (ATD) in humans demonstrated a correlation between the reduced levels of circulating Trp and depressive symptoms in patients, who are responsive to treatment with selective serotonin reuptake inhibitors [146,147]. ATD has also been shown to worsen depressive symptoms in patients in remission, as well as in healthy volunteers at high risk for depression [70]. Furthermore, 5-HT levels in the CNS were shown to be impacted by the amount of dietary Trp in humans [147]. This raises the question of whether a disturbed gut microbial Trp metabolism could deplete circulating Trp availability and consecutively impact 5-HT homeostasis in the CNS. The impact of gut microbiota, or the lack thereof, on the host's nervous system can be explored in GF raised animals providing the evidence for altered levels of neurotransmitters in the brain in comparison to conventionally raised control animals [148]. In support of the previous reports on humans, a recent study in GF mice showed initially higher Trp and 5-HT brain levels together with a less depressive behaviour at baseline and intriguingly, decreased Trp and 5-HT with enhanced depressive behaviour after ATD compared to the control group (specific pathogen-free mice) [149]. Additional support was obtained by findings in a rat model, which showed an induced depression to invoke gut microbial alterations as well as noticeable faecal metabolite shifts [150]. Sixteen metabolites were evaluated to be significantly distinct enough to function as depression biomarkers, including altered Trp metabolites (upregulated dextrorphan O glucuronide, 3-methyldioxyindole and down-regulated 5-methoxytryptophan) (Table 5). The others consisted of bile acid metabolites (upregulated) as well as hypoxanthine (upregulated) and fatty acid metabolites (downregulated). Additionally, the altered gut microbiota also resulted in changes of catecholamine levels in the hippocampus of depressed rats, specifically serotonin (5-HT) and DA [150].

Similarly, Clarke et al. [151] found elevated levels of 5-HT and 5-HIAA in hippocampal structures of GF male mice, as well as higher plasma levels of their precursor Trp. Considering that CNS Trp levels are to a great extent regulated by its abundance in plasma, this supports the conjecture of a humoral pathway through which gut microbes could influence serotoninergic neurotransmission by modulating Trp availability [148]. Fascinatingly, it was not possible to reinstate altered hippocampal 5-HT levels through inoculation with an intestinal microbiota in GF mice at a later stage of life, even though the serum levels of Trp were normalized. This points to a critical time window in which microbial Trp metabolism could directly impact neurodevelopment [152]. Additionally, GF animals displayed elevated stress reactivity, represented with higher corticosterone production, while also expressing lower anxiety-like behaviour that was normalized after recolonization [148]. This is intriguing, since stress hormones like cortisone shift Trp metabolism away from 5-HT production to the kynurenine pathway that generates kynurenic acid, quinolinic acid and picolinic acid [153]. While kynurenic acid invokes antagonistic effects on the α7 nicotinic acetylcholine receptor and the N-methyl-D-aspartate (NMDA) receptor, quinolinic as well as picolinic acids are agonists of the NMDA receptor with neurotoxic and depression-producing properties [152]. It is also noteworthy, that a previously mentioned study on ASD reported the induction of anxiety-like behaviour in mice following the administration of the microbial Trp metabolite 4EPS [142]. Overall, these studies might provide tangible evidence for gut microbial impact on depressive and anxious behaviour by regulating the availability of circulating Trp and consecutively, levels of Trp metabolites like 5-HT, kynurenic, quinolinic and picolinic acids. However, clear associations between gut microbial Trp metabolites and depression or anxiety seem too early to be made since studies on this subject are largely based on preclinical settings on animals.

Indole is partly produced from dietary tryptophan through the enzyme tryptophanase [154] mainly by gut bacteria *Escherichia*, *Citrobacter*, *Fusobacterium*, *Bacteroides*, *Clostridium_XIX*, *Desulfitobacterium*, *Edwardsiella*, *Providencia* and *Shigella* [135] (Table 4). Indole has also recently been shown to be associated with impaired motor activity, anxiety and depression in rats when acutely or chronically overproduced [155]. Probable pathways by which these effects occur are the activation of vagal afferences by indole and on the other hand, accumulation of oxidized indole derivatives like oxindole and isatin in the brain. Indole has been shown to activate gut mucosal L-cells to secrete glucagon-like peptide-1 (GLP-1), which then stimulates vagal afferent fibres, therefore presenting an indirect impact of indole on the CNS [156]. Oxindole is known to inhibit motor activity [155], invoke hypotension, loss of righting reflex and a reversible comatose state, while isatin is proposed an anxiogenic role by inhibiting monoamine oxidase (MAO) B and by producing antagonistic effects on benzodiazepine receptors in rodents [70]. However, Jaglin et al. [155] showed that while acute overexposure to indole in the rat gut produced depressant effects on motor activity and elevated levels of oxindole and isatin the brain, chronic exposure to indole-producing *E. coli* induced depression-associated traits (anxiety-like and helplessness behaviours) without an accumulation of oxindole and isatin in the CNS. This suggests that an indole-overproducing gut microbiome might be a risk factor for the development of anxiety and depression, while acute spikes of indole-production might profoundly decrease locomotion by the central accumulation of oxindole and isatin as well as activation of vagal afferences. Studies have further demonstrated vagal GBA connections to neurons related to reward centres, thus pointing towards a probable pathway for gut metabolites to influence the brain in neuropsychiatric disorders with disturbed reward systems [157]. A recent in silico study on microbial Trp metabolism pathways in neurological disorders called for further investigations of the gut microbiome in schizophrenia, since assumptions were too early to be made on one single available dataset, that showed altered indole, IAA and tryptamine pathways in the microbiome of schizophrenic patients [135]. The research of gut microbial influence on schizophrenia is still in its infancy, which is represented by very few analyses on microbiome compositions and no study on faecal metabolomes in schizophrenic cohorts so far. With the emerging correlations between other brain disorders and the microbiome, as well as some preclinical information on dysbiosis and probiotic studies in schizophrenia [158], further work on this particular subject remains wanting of exploration. Taking all these studies into consideration, tryptophan metabolism with its manifold metabolites seem to be intricately influenced by gut microbial metabolites and to be implicated in psychiatric disorders and brain functions.

4.1.3. AAMs and Neurodegenerative Diseases
Alzheimer's Disease

A limited number of studies have indicated adverse effects on neurons in the context of Alzheimer's disease (AD) by Trp metabolites. The decarboxylated molecule tryptamine has been associated with neurotoxicity and neurodegeneration [92,159–161] (Figure 2). Tryptamine producers commonly found in gut flora are *Holdemania*, *Desulfovibrio*, *Yersinia*, *Tyzzerella*, *Bacillus*, *Clostridium* and *Ruminococcus* [135] (Table 4). Most recent findings showed gut bacterial genomes in faecal samples of AD patients, of which one gene sequence encodes the enzyme Na-transporting NADH:Ubiquinone reductase (in *Clostridium sp.*), which produces the neuroprotectant ubiquinone. Interestingly, that enzyme is also involved in the metabolic synthesis of AAA [92]. Underlining these findings in AAA metabolism, Trp and Tyr (also GABA, taurine and valine) were found to be decreased in faecal samples of mice receiving FMT from an AD patient [97], though as noted in a previous chapter, two faecal donor samples selected out of groups of 14 healthy and 13 AD volunteers might limit the evidential impact by probable inter-individual variations.

Regarding the theory of a perturbed Trp metabolism in AD, microbial and hepatic enzymes generate kynurenine from Trp, and in succession, kynurenic acid or quinolinate. Quinolinate shows excitotoxic properties as an NMDA receptor agonist, whereas kynurenic acid ameliorates those neurotoxic effects as NMDA receptor antagonist. Therefore, this might provide a probable link between Trp metabolites and neurodegenerative processes in AD (Figure 3). In contrast to those findings, in aberrantly elevated amounts, kynurenic acid has been linked to cognitive impairments, probably caused by its antagonistic effect on the α7-nicotinic acetylcholine receptor [152]. It should be emphasized that CNS kynurenine mostly originate from the periphery and that its metabolization into kynurenic acid and quinolinate takes place in the CNS [151]. Some gut genera *Bacillus*, *Burkholderia*, *Streptomyces* and *Pseudomonas* are specially equipped for kynurenine production, while *Klebsiella*, *Bacillus* and *Burkholderia* are efficient quinolinate producers [135].

Another Trp metabolite generated from gut microbiota is indoxyl sulphate (IS), an uremic retention toxin in patients with chronic kidney disease, which has been associated with cognitive impairments [162] and various diseases of the brain such as AD, PD, MDD and MS [163]. IS was previously observed to induce nuclear factor-kappaB (NF-κB)-mediated oxidative stress in animal and in vitro studies [163,164]. Moreover, it exhibited potential neurotoxic effects in mice through perturbed microglial and astrocyte function, resulting in neuronal death [165]. This might be of interest since oxidative stress is proposed as a major process in neurodegenerative diseases [166]. Underscoring these correlations, researchers observed an elevated cerebrospinal fluid (CSF)/plasma ratio of IS in patients with PD compared to healthy counterparts [163]. This might suggest the increased crossing of IS through the BBB, a process probably facilitated by increased BBB permeability in diseases like AD and PD [167]. On the other hand, decreased IS levels in CSF, serum and faecal samples of GF and AT mice have been associated with perturbed fear extinction learning processes. These defects are common in anxiety and fear-related diseases with impaired learning and memory [168]. Considering these early preclinical and at times inconsistent findings on IS and brain disorders, future research focusing on microbiome-derived IS and its participation in neurodegenerative processes might enlighten this complicated and emerging subject. In a dementia-prone mice model, faecal metabolites seemed to differentiate from HC through higher levels of the amino acids ornithine and Tyr, which might excite further research, considering Tyr's role as precursor for several crucial neurotransmitters (norepinephrine, epinephrine and DA) as well as for the uremic toxin p-cresol. Moreover, ornithine has shown protective effects in neurotoxic ammonia [114,169], though it remains to be determined whether bacterial metabolism is involved. Nevertheless, these reports overall suggest gut microbial modulated AAA metabolites as potential components of the complex and emerging field discussing the influence of GBA in AD.

Parkinson's Disease

The analysis of gut microbial Trp metabolism in several databases of PD by Kaur et al. [135] detected enriched indole pathways and three of its producers to be differentially abundant in PD, namely *Alistipes*, *Akkermansia* and *Porphyromonas*. Concomitantly, enriched IAA production pathways in combination with increased *Lactobacillus* and *Staphylococcus* abundances were measured. Interestingly, distinct alterations of kynurenine and quinolinate pathways were undetectable, unlike in other neuropsychiatric disorders like ASD [135]. Congruously to these activated production pathways of IAA, increased IAA urinary levels were reported in patients with idiopathic PD [170,171] (Table 6). However, decreased serum IAA were observed in two cohorts of Japanese patients with idiopathic and familial PARK2-mutated PD [172,173], thus showing some inconsistencies across human studies. Some gut bacteria capable of generating IAA are *Klebsiella, Ralstonia, Staphylococcus, Bacillus, Clostridia, Bacteroides* and *Escherichia* [135,174] (Table 4). Interestingly, IAA was previously mentioned to suppress pro-inflammatory cytokine production by macrophages and act on the aryl hydrogen receptor (AHR) [109]. IAA was also able to attenuate neuroinflammation in LPS-stimulated BV2 microglia in vitro [175]. Overall, these findings point towards a probable role of altered gut microbial production of IAA in neuroinflammatory processes in PD, even if further investigations need to disentangle the complexities between gut-derived IAA and PD.

The previously mentioned metabolite and uremic toxin p-cresol (or its hepatically sulfonated form p-cresol sulphate) in ASD [142] is generated through intestinal bacterial Tyr metabolization [134], with especially strong producers within Coriobacteriaceae and Clostridium clusters XI and XIVa [137]. P-cresol sulphate has been previously associated with neurological impairments in chronic kidney disease [162]. Moreover, two recent studies reported significantly higher p-cresol sulphate levels in the CSF (yet not in plasma) from PD patients compared to samples from HC [163,176] (Table 6). Additionally, higher CSF to plasma ratios in PD was observed in one study, suggesting that individuals with PD accumulate more p-cresol sulphate in the brain than their healthy counterparts [163,176]. These findings support the relevance of a perturbed BBB allowing the increased permeation of putative neurotoxic microbial metabolites from circulation to the brain in PD [165]. Moreover, p-cresol sulphate levels in CSF associated with the presence of motor fluctuations in PD patients, suggesting a correlative connection with disease progression [163]. This is supported by the fact that p-cresol is a known inhibitor of dopamine–beta-hydroxylase [177], the enzyme facilitating the conversion from DA to norepinephrine. Therefore, alterations in the p-cresol production of the microbiome, as well as the gut bacterial impact on BBB integrity, might regulate neurotransmitter metabolism in the brain. Cirstea et al. [132] have recently provided further evidence that associates altered gut microbial metabolism, disturbed gut function (constipation and IBS) and PD. Compared to HC, PD patients harboured decreased levels of common BA-producing Clostridia, including some Lachnospiraceae genera (*Roseburia, Coprococcus*) and *Faecalibacterium*), as well as enriched bacterial clusters associated with p-cresol and phenylacetylglutamine production (*Christensenellaceae, Ruminococca, Akkermansia, Oscillospira, Mogibacteriaceae*). Moreover, increased serum levels of p-cresol and phenylacetylglutamine were measured, showing positive correlations with the presence of PD, as well as the severity of gut dysfunction. Therefore, a gut microbiome shift from BA producers to microbes generating

AAMs such as p-cresol and phenylacetylglutamine might influence symptoms of intestinal dysfunction, as well as altered circulating metabolites in patients with PD.

Manganese (Mn) has been shown to evoke neurodegenerative processes when accumulated in the brain in the context of PD [178,179]. Recent findings discovered Mn exposure to alter gut bacterial genes involved in amino acid and neurotransmitter metabolism (GABA, glycine, glutamate, Trp, Phe) in a mice model, thus giving rise to the novel proposition of gut bacterial involvement in manganese-associated neurotoxicity [180].

These findings overall suggest that members from the Clostridia class seem to be implicated in the production of AAA metabolites (phenolic and indole derivatives) associated with neurodegenerative disorders. Since Clostridia are also known as key BA producers of the human gut [73], and as the chapters above have discussed, a probable beneficial connection between BA and brain diseases, further investigations in Clostridia-derived metabolites and various brain diseases seem warranted to elucidate the relevance of these bacteria. Furthermore, our collected data on indole and indole derivatives show correlations with various brain disorders (autism, anxiety, PD) that are often accompanied with gut issues [36,110,132,181].

4.1.4. AAMs and Autoimmune Diseases of the Brain

As mentioned above, bacterial production of indole from dietary Trp might be involved in perturbed brain functions. The extensive study by Rothhammer et al. [182] has suggested, that in combination with type I interferons (IFN-Is), gut bacterial-derived metabolites might suppress neuroinflammation through agonistic effects on the aryl hydrogen receptor (AHR) on astrocytes (Figure 3). Serum levels of the AHR agonists indole, indoxyl-(3-)sulphate (IS), IPA and indole-3-aldehyde were found to be lower in patients with MS than in HC (Table 6). Furthermore, experiments conducted in EAE mice models of MS uncovered that depleted dietary Trp exacerbated disease, while the administration of the AHR agonists IS, IPA or indole-3-aldehyde reduced disease burden [182]. IS specifically was further shown to cross the BBB and to stimulate AHR on astrocytes. Not unrelatedly, another bacterial indole derivative, IAA, was able to attenuate neuroinflammation in LPS-stimulated BV2 microglia in vitro [175], which underlines the hypothesis, that bacterial-derived indoles might benefit neuroinflammatory processes by activating the AHR on brain cells. It might further be worth noting that the Trp metabolite and indole derivative IPA was shown to cross the BBB and to ameliorate harmful reactive oxygen species (ROS) in the brain as a neuroprotectant [135]. Described gut genera capable of generating IPA are few and belong to the Firmicutes phyla, namely *Clostridium*, *Peptostreptococcus*, *Escherichia* and *Proteus* [134,135] (Table 4). Therefore, the presence of these IPA-producing genera may indicate beneficial anti-oxidative properties for brain function.

Interestingly, p-cresol producing Clostridiales (including Lachnospiraceae and Ruminococcae families), appeared to be abundant in MS patients' microbiomes [79,183], which might potentially lead to similar detrimental effects on the CNS as discussed in the chapters on ASD and PD, though no reports on elevated p-cresol in MS patients exist as of now. The only MS study in humans to investigate the faecal metabolome, as far as our literature search was able to capture, provided no relevant findings on non-SCFA bacterial metabolites [29,81]. Future research is encouraged to further develop and confirm these initial findings by conducting metabolomic, gut taxonomical and metagenomic tests in the faecal samples of MS patients in order to look for correlations with bacterial metabolites beyond SCFAs.

Table 4. Gut-residing bacteria found to correlate with the production of amino acid metabolites (AAMs).

AAM	Taxa	Study
Taurine	*Alistipes HGB5, Alistipes finegoldii, Bacteroides xylanisolvens*	[45]
GABA	*Bifidobacterium, Bacteroides, Lactobacillus; Lactobacillus brevis*	[41,97]
GABA, lactate	*E. coli HT115-strain*	[144]
Serotonin	*Candida, Streptococcus, Escherichia, Enterococcus, Pseudomonas*	[135,184]
Serotonin, dopamine, norepinephrine	*Streptococcus, Enterococcus, Escherichia*	[135]
Serotonin, dopamine	*Clostridiales incertae sedis*	[150]
Norepinephrine	*Escherichia, Bacillus, Saccharomyces*	[184]
Dopamine	*Bacillus*	[184]
Acetylcholine	*Lactobacillus*	[184]
4EPS, p-cresol (sulphate)	*Clostridium*	[36,140,142]
P-cresol (sulphate)	Clostridiaceae (*Clostridium I, IV, IX, XI, XIII, XIVa, XVI*), Bacteroidaceae, Coriobacteriaceae	[109,137]
P-cresol, phenylacetylglutamine	*Oscillospira, Ruminococcus*, Mogibacteriaceae, Christensellaceae, Clostridiales, *Akkermansia*	[132]
Dextrorphan O-glucuronide, 3-methyldioxyindole(F4)	*Christensenella, Candidatus arthromitus*	[150]
"TRYP6" (Kynurenine, quinolinate, indole, IAA, IPA, tryptamine)	Actinobacteria, Firmicutes, Proteobacteria, Bacteroidetes, Fusobacteria	[135]
Quinolinate, indole, IAA, IPA, tryptamine	*Clostridium*	[135]
Kynurenine, quinolinate, indole, IAA, IPA	*Burkholderia*	[135]
Kynurenine, quinolinate, IAA, tryptamine	*Streptomyces, Pseudomonas, Bacillus*	[135]
IAA	*Bacillus, Klebsiella, Ralstonia, Staphylococcus*	[135]
Indole	*Bacteroides, Citrobacter, Clostridium_XIX, Desulfitobacterium, Edwardsiella, Escherichia, Fusobacterium, Providencia, Shigella*	[135]
	Parabacteroides distasonis, Megasphaera massiliensis *E. coli*	[87] [155]
IPA	*Clostridium, Escherichia, Proteus*	[135]
Kynurenine	*Pseudomonas, Bacillus, Burkholderia, Streptomyces*	[135]
Quinolinate	*Klebsiella, Bacillus, Burkholderia*	[135]
Tryptamine	*Holdemania, Tyzzerella, Desulfovibrio, Yersinia, Bacillus, Clostridium, Ruminococcus*	[135]
Indole, indoxyl-(3)-sulphate, IPA, indole-(3)-aldehyde	*Lactobacillus reuteri*	[182]

GABA = gamma-aminobutyric acid; TRYP6 = six Trp metabolism pathways generating the neuroactive metabolites in brackets (");
4EPS = 4-ethylphenylsulfate; IAA = indole-acetic acid; IPA = indole-propionic acid. References are listed as numbers in brackets.

Table 5. Sixteen faecal metabolites with significant correlation in rats with induced depression (adjusted from Yu et al. [150]).

Faecal Metabolites	Trend in Depressed Rats
Nicotinic acid	↑
Hypoxanthine	↑
Dextrorphan O-glucuronide	↑
3-Methoxytryptophan	↑
5-Methoxytryptophan	↓
L-Urobilin	↑
MG(0:0/20:3(5Z,8Z,11Z)/0:0)	↓
PE(14:1(9Z)/14:1(9Z))	↑
PS(18:0/22:6(4Z,7Z,10Z,13Z,16Z,19Z))	↑
Cholic acid	↑
MG(0:0/20:4(8Z,11Z,14Z,17Z)/0:0)	↓
Stearyl citrate	↓
Hyocholic acid	↑

Table 5. Cont.

Faecal Metabolites	Trend in Depressed Rats
L-Urobilinogen	↑
Deoxycholic acid	↑
Chenodeoxycholic acid	↑

Faecal levels in depressed rats compared to healthy control group: ↑ = upregulated; ↓ = downregulated. Rows marked in blue have a p-value of $p < 0.01$, whereas rows in white reached $p < 0.05$. MG = monoacylglyceride; PE = phosphatidylethanolamine; PS = phosphatidylserine

Table 6. Bacterial AAMs correlated with brain diseases or the progression of brain diseases.

Disease	Amino Acid Metabolites		Sample and Literature	p-Values
ASD	P-cresol	-	f [42]	$p = 0.884$
	P-cresol	↑	f [39], f [41], * s/p [36], u [138,139]	$p < 0.05, p = 0.04, p < 0.05, p < 0.05, p < 0.05$
	IAA, indolyl lactate	↑	u [143]	$p < 0.001$
	IS	↑	u [143]	$p < 0.05$
	Indoles (indole, 3-methylindole)	↑	f [39]	$p < 0.05$
	Serotonin, GABA	↑	* s/p [36]	$p < 0.05$
	GABA	↓	f [41]	$p = 0.077$
	3-(3-hydroxyphenyl)-3-hydroxypropionic acid, 3-hydroxyphenylacetic acid, 3-hydroxyhippuric acid	↑	* u [36]	$p < 0.05$
PD	P-cresol	↑	* c [109], c [176], s [132], cc^{a}p^a [163]	$p < 0.05, p = 0.0002, p = 0.0028, p < 0.05$
	IAA	↓	s [172,173], * s [109]	$p = 0.0083, p = 0.0258, p < 0.05$
	IAA	↑	* cp [109], u [170,171]	$p < 0.05, p$ ^{b}, $p < 0.001$
	Indole	↑	* cp [109]	$p < 0.05$
	IS	↑	c ^{a} [163]	$p < 0.05$
	Catechol sulphate, hippuric acid, 3-hydroxyhippuric acid, catechol sulphate, 3-(3-hydroxyphenyl)propionic acid, indole-3-methyl acetate, 2-furoylglycine, phenylethylamine	↓	* s [109]	$p < 0.05$
	Phenylactate, 3-(4-hydroxyphenyl)lactate	↑	* s [109]	$p < 0.05$
	3-(4-hydroxyphenyl)acetic acid, tryptamine, phenylacetic acid, aminobenzoic acid, hydroxybenzoic acid	↑	u [170,171]	$p < 0.05$
	Phenylacetylglutamine	↑	s [132]	$p = 0.004$
	Quinic acid	↑	* c [109]	$p < 0.05$
	Trimethylamine, threonate	↓	* p [109]	$p < 0.05$
	Benzoic acid, 3-(4-hydroxyphenyl)acetic acid	↓	* cp [109]	$p < 0.05$
MS	Aryl hydrocarbon receptor agonists	↓	s [182]	$p < 0.05$

This table shows the differences of AAM levels of various sample materials from human patients compared to healthy controls. p-values are listed in the last column while the significant date is written in bold letters. ↑ symbolizes increased, ↓ decreased, whereas—symbolizes no change in the metabolite levels found in cohorts with the specific disease. Sample material is noted as f = faecal; s = serum; c = cerebrospinal fluid; p = plasma; u = urine; s/p = blood samples with the associated reference as numbers in brackets. References noted with "*" are sourced from reviews. p-values < 0.05 are marked in bold letters. ^{a} correlated with progression of disease. ^{b} ($p = 0.00364$ PD in early stage of disease, $p < 0.001$ PD in mid-stage, $p = 0.056$ PD in late-stage compared to HC. (For example: cc^{a}p^a = altered cerebrospinal fluid sample, and altered cerebrospinal as well as plasma samples which correlate with disease progression). IAA = indoleacetic acid; IS = indoxyl sulphate; GABA = gamma-aminobutyric acid; IPA = indole propionic acid.

4.2. Other Metabolites

4.2.1. Trimethylamine N Oxide (TMAO)

The gut bacterial fermentation of dietary L-carnitine and phosphatidylcholine, which are abundant in red meat, produces trimethylamine (TMA). The following hepatic oxidization by flavin-containing monooxygenase 1 and 3 (FMO1 and FMO3) produces trimethylamine N oxide (TMAO), a metabolite frequently linked to increased risk of cardiovascular, metabolic and cerebrovascular disease, whether as a mediating factor, marker or bystander of disease [185–188]. Recent studies have detected TMAO in human cerebrospinal fluid (CSF), thus establishing its presence in the brain beyond the cerebrovascular system [188,189]. It is to mention that TMAO plasma levels are subject to factors besides gut microbiome composition, namely diet and liver enzyme activity. It is presently unclear how much circulating levels in the CSF depend on the de novo biosynthesis of TMAO in the brain. Recent studies have shown, however, strong correlations between CSF and plasma levels, suggesting that TMAO brain-levels largely derive from the availability in blood, thus supporting the theory of peripheral TMAO reaching the CNS [163]. Interestingly, TMAO plasma levels were found to be significantly higher in elderly humans as well as in aged mice compared to their respective younger groups [190–193]. This would be coherent with recently reported associations between shifts in gut microbiota and presence of neurodegenerative disorders [89,110,194].

By assessing TMAO CSF levels in volunteers with AD dementia, mild cognitive impairment (MCI) and healthy controls (HC), as well as correlations between TMAO CSF levels and biomarkers of AD and neurodegeneration, Vogt et al. [188] have reported the potential involvement of TMAO in AD. They found significantly higher CSF levels of TMAO in the AD and MCI groups compared to HC, with no differences between AD and MCI [195], all while controlling for age, sex and APOE ε4 genotype. Moreover, they discovered CSF TMAO levels to be significantly correlated with AD biomarkers that indicate a connection to tau pathology and axonal injury. Congruously, a different study observed plasma TMAO levels to be inversely correlated with cognitive functions (working memory, episodic memory and fluid cognition) in middle-aged to older adults [193].

Conversely, a recent study reported no differences in TMAO levels between CSF samples from PD patients and HCs. Nevertheless, significant TMAO elevations were detected in PD patients with motor fluctuations compared to those without (Table 7), thus pointing to a role of TMAO in disease progression [163].

Table 7. Other bacterial metabolites correlated with brain diseases or progression in humans.

Disease	Metabolite	Change	Literature
AD	TMAO	↑	c [188]
MCI	TMAO	↑	c [188]
PD	TMAO	↑	$c^a p p^a$ [163]
ASD	Isopropanol	↑	f [41]

AD = Alzheimer's disease; MCI = mild cognitive impairment; PD = Parkinson's disease, ASD = autism spectrum disorder; TMAO = trimethylamine N oxide, [a] correlated with the progression of disease. Significance of data is $p \leq 0.05$. ↑ symbolizes increased metabolite levels found in cohorts with the specific disease compared to healthy controls. Sample material is noted as f = faecal, c = cerebrospinal fluid, p = plasma sample with the associated reference as numbers in brackets.

Researchers have previously mentioned shared pathological arteriosclerotic and inflammatory mechanisms between cardiovascular and dementia-associated cerebrovascular diseases [93]. Literature on vascular cognitive impairment (VCI), a broad definition encompassing cognitive disorders with associations to any kind of cerebral vascular brain injury, further proposed that risk factors for VCI, including hypertension, hypercholesterolemia, diabetes mellitus, atrial fibrillation and others, might overlap the ones for AD [196]. Additionally, results in genetically modified mice previously indicated TMAO to cause the progression of atherosclerosis, a risk factor for dementia [195,197]. TMAO was further implicated with decreased reverse cholesterol transport in mice [198] and enhanced platelet hyperreactivity and thrombosis risk in mice and human subjects [199]. This might suggest a vascular aspect of the mechanism by which this bacterial metabolite might take part in the pathophysiology of AD. However, as Vogt et al. [188] found, differences in TMAO levels between healthy controls, MCI and AD groups were independent from traditional cardiovascular disease risk factors such as body mass index, blood pressure, cholesterol and fasting glucose. Positive associations between TMAO levels and biomarkers for AD and neurodegeneration were also further controlled for peripheral vascular disease risks factors, thus implying that TMAO might affect neurodegeneration by other means than vascular mechanisms. Overall, whether and to what extent TMAO might influence AD by the promotion of vascular disfunction is still to be determined at this point in time.

In studies investigating TMAO's involvement in other mechanisms of neurological diseases, this bacterial metabolite was proposed to weaken the BBB by downregulating tight junction proteins in humans [200]. After reaching the CNS, TMAO was shown to promote neuronal senescence in the hippocampus and cognitive impairment in mice by increasing oxidative stress, disturbing mitochondrial dysfunction and inhibiting the mammalian target of rapamycin (mTOR) signalling, which increased synaptic damage as well as reduced synaptic plasticity-related proteins [190]. A study with the APP/PS1 transgenic mice model of AD indicated higher TMAO-levels in plasma to be associated with cognitive and pathological deterioration, while treatment with the TMA formation inhibitor 3,3-Dimethyl-1-butanol (DMB) alleviated cognitive deterioration and defective synaptic plasticity [191]. Furthermore, DMB treatment managed to reduce hippocampal neuroinflammation and AD-associated pathologies like Aβ42, β-secretase and βCTF (β-secretase-cleaved C-terminal fragment) levels in APP/PS1 mice [191]. Similarly, a different transgenic mouse model of AD (3x Tg-AD) displayed significantly elevated plasma and brain TMAO levels in comparison to healthy controls in a recent study by Govindarajulu et al. [192]. They further incubated hippocampal brain slices of wild-type mice with TMAO and found deficits in synaptic plasticity, impaired synaptic transmission, altered presynaptic and reduced postsynaptic glutamatergic receptor units, as well as induced endoplasmatic reticulum (ER)-mediated protein kinase RNA-like endoplasmic reticulum kinase (PERK) pathway [192]. Another study has further indicated TMAO to impair cognitive function by promoting neuroinflammation and astrocyte activation in mice [193]. In addition to the association between TMAO levels and neuroinflammation and astrocyte activation in older mice, TMAO supplementation in young mice for six months exhibited a decline in memory and learning (assessed through the novel object recognition test) and indeed, elevated markers for neuroinflammation and astrocyte activation. Furthermore, human astrocyte cultures incubated with TMAO showed altered cellular morphology and markers indicating astrocyte activation, thus proposing a direct effect of TMAO on astrocytes [193]. Overall, all of these preclinical findings suggest that TMAO may provoke cognitive impairment by promoting neuroinflammation, AD-related amyloid formation, oxidative stress, as well as deficits in synaptic plasticity and function by promoting ER stress-mediated PERK signalling pathways.

Additionally, an in silico study detected significant correlations between TMAO-related genes and AD biomarkers in nine potential genetic pathways involved in both, that might underline the proposition for TMAO as a strong biomarker for AD [201]. Those nine pathways include in no specific order: the metabolism of proteins; immune system; adaptive immune system; Alzheimer's disease; axon guidance; amyotrophic lateral sclerosis (ALS); erythropoietin-producing human hepatocellular receptor A (EPHA) and B (EPHB) forward signalling and metabolism of lipids and lipoproteins. These findings might be used as groundwork for investigations of specific pathways that might elucidate a diet-microbial metabolite–brain disease axis.

Curiously, studies in mice and in vitro models reported disease-mediating as well as protective mechanisms by TMAO on processes in neurodegenerative disorders such as a reduction in amyloid aggregation in AD and PD, thus providing a new potential therapeutic target [22,200]. However, more congruous study results have been reviewed and reported on the pro-inflammatory effects of increased TMAO plasma concentrations [200]. These reports underline the need for further studies on TMAO and its combined effects on enhanced circulating pro-inflammatory mediators that can potentially cross a TMAO-induced disturbed BBB to a greater extent, and therefore promote the aforementioned neuroinflammatory and neurodegenerative effects in the brain.

Some gut bacteria found to be significantly associated with enhanced plasma TMAO were the genera *Prevotella, Mitsuokella, Fusobacterium, Desulfovibrio, Methanobrevibacter smithii*, and some from the Lachnospiraceae and Ruminococcaceae families [186] (Table 8). Three of those genera belong to the Bacteroidetes and six to the Firmicutes class, congruous with a recent study in dementia [93] that showed a significantly higher Firmicutes/Bacteroidetes ratios in demented individuals with MRI-detected silent lacunar infarctions, as well as strong correlations between dementia and low counts of *Bacteroides* along with higher counts of 'other bacteria'. Additional sources have reported the following TMA-producing genera: *Anaerococcus, Clostridium, Escherichia, Proteus, Providencia* and *Edwardsiella* [22]. Overall, future work is strongly advised to address and investigate TMAO brain levels and any correlations with the gut microbiome.

Carnitine Analogues

Given that gut metabolites related to carnitine such as TMAO affect the GBA, researchers have recently discovered two new potentially brain active metabolites, namely the carnitine analogues 3-methyl-4-(trimethylammonio)butanoate (3M4-TMAB) and 4-(trimethylammonio)pentanoate (4-TMAP) [202]. These compounds are generated by gut bacteria from the family Lachnospiraceae (*Clostridiales symbiosium* and *clostridioforme*) (Table 8) and were absent in both the gut and brain of GF mice but present in controls, thus suggesting that gut microbiota may be responsible for their presence in the brain. Importantly, these compounds were found in identical regions of white matter of the brain as carnitine and showed an inhibition of carnitine-mediated fatty acid oxidation (FAO) in a murine cell culture model of CNS white matter [202]. FAO is crucial for neuronal energy homeostasis, and inborn errors of this system may link faulty neuronal stem cell self-renewal to ASD [203,204]. Considering these findings and that increased abundance of Clostridia have been linked to ASD and other neurodevelopmental disorders [205], faulty FAO promoted by bacterial metabolites might be an important topic to explore in the future.

4.2.2. Polyphenolic Metabolites

Polyphenols derived from dietary sources are metabolized by human gut microbes to phenolic acids. Research has shown gut microbial metabolites of dietary polyphenols to accumulate in brain tissue and to modulate α-synuclein misfolding, aggregation and neurotoxicity in vitro and in an animal models [206]. Among those metabolites were 3-hydroxybenzoic acid (3-HBA), 3-(3-hydroxyphenyl)propionic acid (3-HPPA) and 3,4-dihydroxybenzoic acid (3,4-diHBA). Further investigations led to the detection of *B. ovatus* as a producer of the aforementioned metabolites that were converted from the dietary polyphenols (+)-catechin (C) and (−)-epicatechin (EC). C/EC-independent production of 3,4-diHBA, 3-HBA and dihydrocaffeic acid (DHCA), a circulating anti-inflammatory phenolic acid, also occurred through *B. ovatus, E. lenta* and *E. coli* (Table 8). In earlier studies, 3-HPPA and 3-HBA were shown to ameliorate Aβ-peptide misfolding [207], therefore underlining the potential of bacterial polyphenolic metabolites to protect from neurotoxic protein-aggregation and neurodegenerative disorders like AD and PD. Additional gut bacterial metabolism-derived polyphenols, particularly enerolactone and enterodiol, aryl-γ-valerolactone metabolites and urolithin A/B, exhibit polyphenolic neuroprotective properties [208]. Two studies have further summarized mechanisms by which brain function could be influenced by bioactive microbe-derived metabolites of polyphenols [209,210]. Direct neuroprotective impacts include modulating neuronal receptors, antioxidation, anti-inflammation and overall neuroprotective effects. Indirect mechanisms encompass the modulation of gut microbial homeostasis by supporting beneficial bacteria while decreasing pathogens, as well as improving cerebrovascular health by increased nitrogen oxide levels and vasodilatory response. Limits of the summarized findings were put by their in vitro and ex vivo-based designs.

The ability to cross the BBB is crucial for metabolites to exert neuroactive properties and ten microbe-derived polyphenolic metabolites were found to be capable of distributing in rat brains after intravenous administration [211]: 4-hydroxyhippuric acid, homovanillic acid, 4-hydroxybenzoic acid, vanillic acid, 3-HPPA, trans-ferulic acid, caffeic acid, gallic acid, 3,4-dihydroxyphenyl acetic acid and urolithin B. Taken together, the neuroactive potential of bioactive gut microbe-derived metabolites of dietary polyphenols is promising but the mode of action of these metabolites need further in depth elucidation.

Phenolic Compounds

Ferulic acid (FA), a phenolic compound, has been the focus of a handful of studies researching the GBA and has been proposed a role in cognitive development and neuroprotection. Sources of ferulic acid are plants and seeds in the human diet, as well as from gut microbial biosynthesis from dietary cyanidin, catechin and epicatechin. Some beneficial properties of FA are protection from oxidative neurological damage by ROS scavenging, neural stem cell stimulation, and the direct inhibition of Aβ aggregation [8,212–214].

Dysfunctions in Pavlovian fear extinction learning are involved in anxiety and fear-associated neuropsychiatric disorders such as PTSD [215,216]. Recently, four bacterial metabolites, of which three were phenolic compounds (phenyl sulphate, pyrocatechol sulphate and 3-(3-sulfooxyphenyl)propanoic acid), have been shown to be significantly decreased in CSF, serum and faecal samples of GF or antibiotic treated mice showing defective fear extinction learning. Further investigations discovered alterations of gene expressions in the medial prefrontal cortex, immature-like microglia, as well as perturbed structural and functional changes in neurons involved in learning processes [168].

4.2.3. Bacterial Amyloid Proteins

Amyloid proteins produced by bacteria have been an emerging subject of interest in the study of pathophysiology in PD [109]. It was reported that bacterial amyloid proteins, such as curli from *E. coli*, could induce the formation of human amyloid aggregates by cross-seeding in a prion-like fashion, as well as promote inflammatory processes by molecular mimicry [217]. The mechanism of cross-seeding was previously shown by curli-induced serum amyloid A amyloidosis in mice [218]. This was further supported by a hypothesis that the phenomenon of protein misfolding in neurodegenerative diseases might originate from the gut, possibly via bidirectional vagal fibres bypassing the circulatory system [108]. It is important to note that vagotomy has been associated with a lower risk for PD [219] and a delayed αSyn dissemination when nervous structures connecting the gut to the brain are severed [220]. Findings of αSyn aggregates in regions beyond the brain, such as the enteric nervous system and olfactory bulb, point to the phenomenon that the majority of PD patients experience gastrointestinal and olfactory dysfunctions long before their diagnosis [221]. Interestingly, hyposmia has been associated with cognitive decline, even in the context of AD [222]. A recent study observed that mice with αSyn overexpression developed PD-like pathological traits after inoculation with curli-producing *E. coli*. These mice displayed αSyn-aggregates in brain and gut tissues, as well as disturbed motor and intestinal functions [223]. Furthermore, prior research reported significantly increased amounts of αSyn aggregates in aged Fischer 344 rat brains and in *Caenorhabditis elegans* after oral inoculation with curli-producing *E. coli* in comparison with subjects colonized with identical strains lacking curli production. Moreover, exposure to curli-producing *E. coli* stimulated immune activity in rat brains, represented by enhanced neuroinflammatory markers, such as upregulated Toll-like receptor 2 (TLR2), interleukin 6, tissue necrosis factor, microgliosis and astrogliosis [224]. The similar immune response pathways to bacterial amyloids by pathogen-associated molecular pattern recognition, and the response to misfolded endogenous amyloids like αSyn and Aβ is intriguing. This illustrates the possibility that gut bacterial amyloids could prime the immune system for a neuroinflammatory response to cerebral amyloid deposits, thus leading to enhanced neuroinflammation and degeneration [217].

Species reported for curli-production are from the family *Enterobacteriaceae*, including *E. coli, Salmonella typhimurium, Citrobacter spcc., Cronobacter sakazakii* and *Proteus mirabilis*. This was recently deemed as conspicuous by researchers that observed enriched *Enterobacteriaceae spp.* in 31% of PD studies, as well as previous associations between *P. mirabilis* and a PD mouse model [109]. Other residents of the human gut were also reported to generate extracellular amyloids, namely *Streptococcus, Staphylococcus, Mycobacteria, Klebsiella* and *Bacillus spp.* [217]. Overall, these studies provide a hypothesis that bacterial amyloids could be key players in the pathogenesis of neurodegenerative diseases like PD and AD, with data pointing to their effects on amyloid aggregation and on enhanced immunoreactions in the CNS. This subject even motivated Friedland et al. [217] to propose the new term "MAPRANOSIS—the process of microbiota-associated proteopathy and neuroinflammation". However, some preclinical studies have implicated bacterial amyloids with increased clearance and decreased neuroinflammation by means of activating microglia through the receptor TREM2 [91]. Similarly, toll-like receptors 2 and 4 (TLRs) have shown contradicting effects on amyloid-related neurotoxicity and clearance through microglial activation [225]. It is difficult to draw definite conclusions regarding the effect of gut bacterial amyloids on AD and PD. Nevertheless, current data are strongly pointing to an existing connection.

Yang et al. [226] recently conducted the first study to observe implications of gut dysbiosis and faecal metabolic changes in mice with prions disease, thus providing the base for a new area of research in brain diseases with links to the gut microbiome. Of the previously mentioned metabolites, SCFAs and Trp were decreased, while Tyr increased in mice with prions disease. Furthermore, the microbiome of prion-infected mice harboured distinct compositions from HC, namely enriched Lactobacillaceae, Helicobacteraceae and decreased Prevotellaceae and Ruminococcaceae. Additionally, newly observed altered faecal metabolites consisted of various glycerophospholipids, three secondary bile acids and the toxic avermectin A2b. However, further research should investigate if these compounds are derived from gut bacterial metabolism and whether they are biomarkers or mediators of disease.

Table 8. Gut-residing bacteria found to correlate with the production of other metabolites.

Other Metabolites	Taxa	Study
TMA(O)	*Prevotella, Mitsuokella, Fusobacterium, Desulfovibrio, Methanobrevibacter smithii*; some from Lachnospiraceae and Ruminococcaceae	[186]
TMA	*Anaerococcus, Clostridium, Escherichia, Proteus, Providencia, Edwardsiella*	[22]
curli	Enterobacteriaceae (*E. coli, Salmonella typhimurium, Citrobacter freundii, Cronobacter sakazakii, Proteus mirabilis*)	[109]
curli	*E. coli*	[224]
curli	*Streptococcus, Staphylococcus, Mycobacteria, Klebsiella, Bacillus*	[217]
Nicotinamide	*Akkermansia muciniphila*	[227]
3-HBA, 3,4diHBA, DHCA	*Bacteroides ovatus*	[206]
3-methyl-4-(trimethylammonio)butanoate, 4-(trimethylammonio)pentanoate	Lachnospiraceae (Clostridiales): *C.clostridioforme, C.symbosium*	[202]

TMA(O) = trimethylamine N oxide; TMA = trimethylamine; 3-HBA = 3-hydroxybenzoic acid; 3,4-diHBA = 3,4-dihydroxybenzoic acid; DHCA = dihydrocaffeic acid. References are represented by numbers in brackets.

5. Discussion and Conclusions

Our collected data highlight the fact that research into GBA and the precise role of bacterial metabolites as key contributors is still in its infancy. The majority of studies were conducted in preclinical animal or cell models and only a limited number of human studies are contributing to the current knowledge.

Only a handful of human studies of brain diseases reported faecal SCFAs levels, making it difficult to draw definitive conclusions. Our literature search captured five studies in ASD, two in affective disorders, two in MS, one in PD and none in AD as of this point in time. Nevertheless, an overall decrease in faecal SCFA levels in ASD, affective disorders, MS and PD is apparent (Table 1). Importantly, an increase in one SCFA may be levelled out by the decrease in another SCFA in the same study. AA and PA were reported to be increased in faecal samples [39,42] in two studies, while BA was increased in one [42]. Furthermore, one study observed no significant changes across all SCFAs in ASD [41]. Therefore, it remains to be determined by in-depth studies of the human intestinal metabolome, whether distinct patterns of SCFA levels are present and relevant in different brain diseases.

Based on preclinical findings on how SCFA might impact the brain, the overall assumption points to a beneficial role. The non-exhaustive list of reported effects includes improved gut barrier and BBB integrity [19–22] and an overall shift towards anti-inflammatory processes [13,28,29,74,75,91]. As HDACI, SCFAs can epigenetically modulate the maturation of brain cells [28,84,87], enhance gene expression for enzymes relevant in catecholamine production [23] and even shift the balance of the immune system towards anti-inflammatory Treg cells and away from pro-inflammatory Th1 and Th17 cells [13,81,83]. Inflammatory processes are known to be involved in MS and to take part in neurodegenerative diseases. As SCFA levels tend to be decreased in most neurodegenerative diseases (Table 1), we might assume that a perturbed gut microbiome might lead to impaired SCFA production of gut bacteria, which might then deplete the beneficial anti-inflammatory effects on the CNS.

Regarding non-SCFA bacterial metabolites, p-cresol has yielded the most human data across studies. It is also the only metabolite with measurements in faecal samples that correlated with brain disease, namely in patients with ASD. Taken all results together (Table 6), p-cresol is significantly increased in faecal, urinary and blood samples of ASD, as well in the CSF and serum of PD patients. CSF and plasma levels of p-cresol have moreover shown to be correlated with the severity of PD [163]. This, and preclinical studies in mice models implicating p-cresol with detrimental effects on the CNS [140,141], seem to be in line with elevated levels in ASD and PD. The notion of involvements of p-cresol in ASD is supported by the finding that 4EPS, a metabolite with structural similarities to p-cresol, induces ASD-behaviour in mice.

Alterations in Trp metabolism were observed in human studies in ASD, PD and MS. Significant assessments of Trp metabolites such as indole and indole derivatives are mainly from non-faecal samples and have shown an overall increase in ASD, a decrease in MS and inconsistent results in PD (Table 6). Nevertheless, it is important to mention that two PD studies showed indole and indole derivatives to be increased in CSF [109, 163], a compartment closely connected to brain tissue. Furthermore, metagenomic tests concluded that overall Trp metabolism pathways are enriched in the gut microbiome of ASD patient cohorts, and that indole pathways are enhanced in PD microbiomes [135]. These metagenomic findings and the several reports on metabolite levels in patients seem to indicate the presence of perturbed and enriched Trp metabolism in ASD and PD. Naturally, the lack of studies testing for faecal metabolites in humans, as well as the inconsistencies within results in PD stress the limitation to unequivocally determine distinct patterns by which our gut bacteria alter Trp metabolism in various brain diseases.

Several probable mechanisms by which Trp metabolites might exert their impact were identified. Preclinical studies have indicated that indole and its derivatives (indole, IS, IPA, indole-3-aldehyde, IAA) might actually be able to limit neuroinflammation by acting as agonists on the AHR [109,182] (Figure 3). Furthermore, a shift in Trp-metabolism away from 5-HT production might partly explain the worsening of disease in individuals who are responsive to treatment with selective serotonin-reuptake inhibitors (SSRIs) [146,147]. Thus, a decrease in Trp availability might be connected to brain diseases, which is further exemplified by Trp-depletion experiments in depressed human cohorts and mice models of MS [146,147,182]. It might further be of interest that IPA was reported to ameliorate toxic ROS activity in the brain [135]. On the other hand, IS has induced oxidative stress in animal and in vitro studies [163,164], as well as displayed potential neurotoxic effects in mice through perturbed microglial and astrocyte function [165]. Moreover, an overproduction of indole was associated with anxiety and depression levels in rats [155]. Taken together, these results imply that alterations in the gut bacterial metabolism of AAA, whether it is Tyr-derived p-cresol or Trp-derived indole metabolites, could contribute to brain diseases.

The question as to whether gut bacterial amyloids like curli might contribute to or alleviate diseases with an accumulation and aggregation of misfolded proteins and neuroinflammation, cannot be unequivocally answered yet. Nevertheless, the current evidence on bacterial amyloids implies that there might be more to bacterial metabolites with connections to the brain beyond SCFAs and AAM.

The majority of evidence presented here is derived from preclinical studies, such as in vivo studies in transgenic animals, in germ-free animals or animals exposed to early-life alterations of the gut microbiota including pathogens, probiotics, or antibiotics. The validity of drawing decisive conclusions for the human physiology from animal studies is therefore conceivably limited. Moreover, the information on taxonomical alterations and associations to metabolites and diseases is non-exhaustive since this study focused on bacterial metabolites. The objective was to assess bacterial metabolites independently as probable determinants of disease, thus shifting the focus away from their producers. The need for further work in deciphering the vast and intricate correlations between gut microbial communities, faecal metabolites and the presence of brain dysfunction, is definitely acknowledged and deemed as necessary.

Results regarding the potential protective or aggravating role of bacterial metabolite groups on brain diseases are still few and require additional confirmation. A final assessment of the importance of faecal metabolomic changes in brain diseases, however, is problematic as of now. The difficulties lie in the heterogeneity of disease manifestations and varying technological methods to assess varying sample sources. Furthermore, confounders like gender, genetics, dietary factors, medication and lifestyle, as well as subtypes of bacterial species, might contribute to insignificant or falsified results. Therefore, additional independent research applying methodical standardization is essential to ensure comparable and reproducible data. Determining not only taxonomical data, but also conducting functional analyses through metagenomic and metabolomic testing of faecal samples would crucially increase the robustness of discovered associations. This might further develop, confirm or refute today's initial findings on correlations between bacterial metabolites and brain diseases. Interests lie in the discovery and unravelment of GBA mechanisms, as well as the study of bacterial metabolites as promising key contributors to brain diseases. Successful findings of such might be crucial in identifying aetiological and pathophysiological processes, thus efficaciously supporting future research in novel treatments and the prevention strategies of brain diseases.

Author Contributions: Conceptualization, S.M.-S.T. and M.H.M.; methodology, S.M.-S.T. and M.H.M.; validation, M.H.M.; formal analysis, S.M.-S.T. and M.H.M.; investigation, S.M.-S.T.; resources, S.M.-S.T.; data curation, S.M.-S.T.; writing—original draft preparation, S.M.-S.T.; writing—review and editing, S.M.-S.T. and M.H.M.; visualization, S.M.-S.T.; supervision, M.H.M.; project administration, M.H.M. and S.M.-S.T. All authors have read and agreed to the published version of the manuscript.

Funding: This research received no external funding.

Institutional Review Board Statement: Not applicable.

Informed Consent Statement: Not applicable.

Data Availability Statement: Data sharing not applicable. No new data were created or analyzed in this study. Data sharing is not applicable to this article.

Acknowledgments: The authors thank David P. Wolfer for valuable comments.

Conflicts of Interest: The authors declare no conflict of interest.

Abbreviations

CNS	central nervous system
SCFA	short-chain fatty acids
AAM	amino acid metabolites
ASD	autism spectrum disorder
MS	multiple sclerosis
PD	Parkinson's disease
AD	Alzheimer's disease
GIT	gastrointestinal tract
GBA	gut–brain axis
BBB	blood–brain barrier
BA	butyric acid
PA	propionic acid
AA	acetic acid
VA	valeric acid
TMAO	trimethylamine N-oxide
IS	indoxyl sulphate
4EPS	4-ethylphenylsulfate
IAA	indole acetic acid
IPA	indole propionic acid
IBS	irritable bowel syndrome
GF	germ free
WT	wild type
HDACI	histone deacetylase inhibition/inhibitor
NT	neurotypical
FMT	faecal microbiome transplants
HC	healthy controls
DBH	dopamine beta-hydroxylase
MDD	major depressive disorder
HAB	high anxiety-like behaviour
NaB	sodium butyrate
αSyn	alpha-synuclein protein
AAA	aromatic amino acids
Tyr	tyrosine
Phe	phenylalanine
Trp	tryptophan
5-HT	serotonin
ATD	acute tryptophan depletion
DA	dopamine
AHR	aryl hydrogen receptor

References

1. Martin, R.; Makino, H.; Cetinyurek Yavuz, A.; Ben-Amor, K.; Roelofs, M.; Ishikawa, E.; Kubota, H.; Swinkels, S.; Sakai, T.; Oishi, K.; et al. Early-Life Events, Including Mode of Delivery and Type of Feeding, Siblings and Gender, Shape the Developing Gut Microbiota. *PLoS ONE* **2016**, *11*, e0158498. [CrossRef]
2. Jasarevic, E.; Rodgers, A.B.; Bale, T.L. A novel role for maternal stress and microbial transmission in early life programming and neurodevelopment. *Neurobiol. Stress* **2015**, *1*, 81–88. [CrossRef]
3. Rybnikova, E. Brain, antibiotics, and microbiota—How do they interplay? An Editorial for 'Antibiotics-induced modulation of large intestinal microbiota altered aromatic amino acid profile and expression of neurotransmitters in the hypothalamus of piglets' on page 219. *J. Neurochem.* **2018**, *146*, 208–210. [CrossRef]
4. Mehrian-Shai, R.; Reichardt, J.K.V.; Harris, C.C.; Toren, A. The Gut-Brain Axis, Paving the Way to Brain Cancer. *Trends Cancer* **2019**, *5*, 200–207. [CrossRef] [PubMed]
5. Moher, D.; Liberati, A.; Tetzlaff, J.; Altman, D.G. Preferred reporting items for systematic reviews and meta-analyses: The PRISMA statement. *PLoS Med.* **2009**, *6*, e1000097. [CrossRef]

6. Miller, T.L.; Wolin, M.J. Pathways of acetate, propionate, and butyrate formation by the human fecal microbial flora. *Appl. Environ. Microbiol.* **1996**, *62*, 1589–1592. [CrossRef] [PubMed]
7. Rooks, M.G.; Garrett, W.S. Gut microbiota, metabolites and host immunity. *Nat. Rev. Immunol.* **2016**, *16*, 341–352. [CrossRef]
8. Westfall, S.; Lomis, N.; Kahouli, I.; Dia, S.Y.; Singh, S.P.; Prakash, S. Microbiome, probiotics and neurodegenerative diseases: Deciphering the gut brain axis. *Cell. Mol. Life Sci.* **2017**, *74*, 3769–3787. [CrossRef]
9. Labus, J.S.; Hollister, E.B.; Jacobs, J.; Kirbach, K.; Oezguen, N.; Gupta, A.; Acosta, J.; Luna, R.A.; Aagaard, K.; Versalovic, J.; et al. Differences in gut microbial composition correlate with regional brain volumes in irritable bowel syndrome. *Microbiome* **2017**, *5*, 49. [CrossRef]
10. Mayer, E.A.; Savidge, T.; Shulman, R.J. Brain-gut microbiome interactions and functional bowel disorders. *Gastroenterology* **2014**, *146*, 1500–1512. [CrossRef]
11. Theodorou, V.; Ait Belgnaoui, A.; Agostini, S.; Eutamene, H. Effect of commensals and probiotics on visceral sensitivity and pain in irritable bowel syndrome. *Gut Microbes* **2014**, *5*, 430–436. [CrossRef] [PubMed]
12. Lin, L.; Zhang, J. Role of intestinal microbiota and metabolites on gut homeostasis and human diseases. *BMC Immunol.* **2017**, *18*, 2. [CrossRef]
13. Haghikia, A.; Jorg, S.; Duscha, A.; Berg, J.; Manzel, A.; Waschbisch, A.; Hammer, A.; Lee, D.H.; May, C.; Wilck, N.; et al. Dietary Fatty Acids Directly Impact Central Nervous System Autoimmunity via the Small Intestine. *Immunity* **2015**, *43*, 817–829. [CrossRef] [PubMed]
14. Hijova, E. Gut bacterial metabolites of indigestible polysaccharides in intestinal fermentation as mediators of public health. *Bratisl. Lek. Listy* **2019**, *120*, 807–812. [CrossRef] [PubMed]
15. Dalile, B.; Van Oudenhove, L.; Vervliet, B.; Verbeke, K. The role of short-chain fatty acids in microbiota-gut-brain communication. *Nat. Rev. Gastroenterol. Hepatol.* **2019**, *16*, 461–478. [CrossRef]
16. Lewis, K.; Lutgendorff, F.; Phan, V.; Söderholm, J.D.; Sherman, P.M.; McKay, D.M. Enhanced translocation of bacteria across metabolically stressed epithelia is reduced by butyrate. *Inflamm. Bowel Dis.* **2010**, *16*, 1138–1148. [CrossRef]
17. Peng, L.; Li, Z.R.; Green, R.S.; Holzman, I.R.; Lin, J. Butyrate enhances the intestinal barrier by facilitating tight junction assembly via activation of AMP-activated protein kinase in Caco-2 cell monolayers. *J. Nutr.* **2009**, *139*, 1619–1625. [CrossRef]
18. Obrenovich, M.E.M. Leaky Gut, Leaky Brain? *Microorganisms* **2018**, *6*, 107. [CrossRef]
19. Sampson, T.R.; Mazmanian, S.K. Control of brain development, function, and behavior by the microbiome. *Cell Host Microbe* **2015**, *17*, 565–576. [CrossRef]
20. Braniste, V.; Al-Asmakh, M.; Kowal, C.; Anuar, F.; Abbaspour, A.; Tóth, M.; Korecka, A.; Bakocevic, N.; Ng, L.G.; Kundu, P.; et al. The gut microbiota influences blood-brain barrier permeability in mice. *Sci. Transl. Med.* **2014**, *6*, 263ra158. [CrossRef]
21. Hoyles, L.; Snelling, T.; Umlai, U.K.; Nicholson, J.K.; Carding, S.R.; Glen, R.C.; McArthur, S. Microbiome-host systems interactions: Protective effects of propionate upon the blood-brain barrier. *Microbiome* **2018**, *6*, 55. [CrossRef]
22. Parker, A.; Fonseca, S.; Carding, S.R. Gut microbes and metabolites as modulators of blood-brain barrier integrity and brain health. *Gut Microbes* **2020**, *11*, 135–157. [CrossRef]
23. Nankova, B.B.; Agarwal, R.; MacFabe, D.F.; La Gamma, E.F. Enteric bacterial metabolites propionic and butyric acid modulate gene expression, including CREB-dependent catecholaminergic neurotransmission, in PC12 cells—Possible relevance to autism spectrum disorders. *PLoS ONE* **2014**, *9*, e103740. [CrossRef] [PubMed]
24. Stilling, R.M.; van de Wouw, M.; Clarke, G.; Stanton, C.; Dinan, T.G.; Cryan, J.F. The neuropharmacology of butyrate: The bread and butter of the microbiota-gut-brain axis? *Neurochem. Int.* **2016**, *99*, 110–132. [CrossRef] [PubMed]
25. Fernandes, M.F.; de Oliveira, S.; Portovedo, M.; Rodrigues, P.B.; Vinolo, M.A.R. Effect of Short Chain Fatty Acids on Age-Related Disorders. *Adv. Exp. Med. Biol.* **2020**, *1260*, 85–105. [CrossRef] [PubMed]
26. Silva, Y.P.; Bernardi, A.; Frozza, R.L. The Role of Short-Chain Fatty Acids from Gut Microbiota in Gut-Brain Communication. *Front. Endocrinol.* **2020**, *11*, 25. [CrossRef] [PubMed]
27. Bachem, A.; Makhlouf, C.; Binger, K.J.; de Souza, D.P.; Tull, D.; Hochheiser, K.; Whitney, P.G.; Fernandez-Ruiz, D.; Dähling, S.; Kastenmüller, W.; et al. Microbiota-Derived Short-Chain Fatty Acids Promote the Memory Potential of Antigen-Activated CD8+ T Cells. *Immunity* **2019**, *51*, 285–297.e5. [CrossRef]
28. Erny, D.; Hrabě de Angelis, A.L.; Jaitin, D.; Wieghofer, P.; Staszewski, O.; David, E.; Keren-Shaul, H.; Mahlakoiv, T.; Jakobshagen, K.; Buch, T.; et al. Host microbiota constantly control maturation and function of microglia in the CNS. *Nat. Neurosci.* **2015**, *18*, 965–977. [CrossRef] [PubMed]
29. Park, J.; Wang, Q.; Wu, Q.; Mao-Draayer, Y.; Kim, C.H. Bidirectional regulatory potentials of short-chain fatty acids and their G-protein-coupled receptors in autoimmune neuroinflammation. *Sci. Rep.* **2019**, *9*, 8837. [CrossRef] [PubMed]
30. Hug, H.; Mohajeri, M.H.; La Fata, G. Toll-Like Receptors: Regulators of the Immune Response in the Human Gut. *Nutrients* **2018**, *10*, 203. [CrossRef]
31. Oleskin, A.V.; Shenderov, B.A. Neuromodulatory effects and targets of the SCFAs and gasotransmitters produced by the human symbiotic microbiota. *Microb. Ecol. Health Dis.* **2016**, *27*, 30971. [CrossRef] [PubMed]
32. Varela, R.B.; Valvassori, S.S.; Lopes-Borges, J.; Mariot, E.; Dal-Pont, G.C.; Amboni, R.T.; Bianchini, G.; Quevedo, J. Sodium butyrate and mood stabilizers block ouabain-induced hyperlocomotion and increase BDNF, NGF and GDNF levels in brain of Wistar rats. *J. Psychiatr. Res.* **2015**, *61*, 114–121. [CrossRef] [PubMed]

33. Barichello, T.; Generoso, J.S.; Simões, L.R.; Faller, C.J.; Ceretta, R.A.; Petronilho, F.; Lopes-Borges, J.; Valvassori, S.S.; Quevedo, J. Sodium Butyrate Prevents Memory Impairment by Re-establishing BDNF and GDNF Expression in Experimental Pneumococcal Meningitis. *Mol. Neurobiol.* **2015**, *52*, 734–740. [CrossRef] [PubMed]
34. Costa-Mattioli, M.; Sonenberg, N.; Richter, J.D. Translational regulatory mechanisms in synaptic plasticity and memory storage. *Prog. Mol. Biol. Transl. Sci.* **2009**, *90*, 293–311. [CrossRef] [PubMed]
35. Buffington, S.A.; Huang, W.; Costa-Mattioli, M. Translational control in synaptic plasticity and cognitive dysfunction. *Annu. Rev. Neurosci.* **2014**, *37*, 17–38. [CrossRef]
36. Srikantha, P.; Mohajeri, M.H. The Possible Role of the Microbiota-Gut-Brain-Axis in Autism Spectrum Disorder. *Int. J. Mol. Sci.* **2019**, *20*, 2115. [CrossRef]
37. Nitschke, A.; Deonandan, R.; Konkle, A.T. The link between autism spectrum disorder and gut microbiota: A scoping review. *Autism* **2020**, *24*, 1328–1344. [CrossRef] [PubMed]
38. Averina, O.V.; Kovtun, A.S.; Polyakova, S.I.; Savilova, A.M.; Rebrikov, D.V.; Danilenko, V.N. The bacterial neurometabolic signature of the gut microbiota of young children with autism spectrum disorders. *J. Med. Microbiol.* **2020**, *69*, 558–571. [CrossRef] [PubMed]
39. De Angelis, M.; Piccolo, M.; Vannini, L.; Siragusa, S.; De Giacomo, A.; Serrazzanetti, D.I.; Cristofori, F.; Guerzoni, M.E.; Gobbetti, M.; Francavilla, R. Fecal microbiota and metabolome of children with autism and pervasive developmental disorder not otherwise specified. *PLoS ONE* **2013**, *8*, e76993. [CrossRef]
40. Carlson, A.L.; Xia, K.; Azcarate-Peril, M.A.; Goldman, B.D.; Ahn, M.; Styner, M.A.; Thompson, A.L.; Geng, X.; Gilmore, J.H.; Knickmeyer, R.C. Infant Gut Microbiome Associated with Cognitive Development. *Biol. Psychiatry* **2018**, *83*, 148–159. [CrossRef]
41. Kang, D.W.; Ilhan, Z.E.; Isern, N.G.; Hoyt, D.W.; Howsmon, D.P.; Shaffer, M.; Lozupone, C.A.; Hahn, J.; Adams, J.B.; Krajmalnik-Brown, R. Differences in fecal microbial metabolites and microbiota of children with autism spectrum disorders. *Anaerobe* **2018**, *49*, 121–131. [CrossRef]
42. Wang, L.; Christophersen, C.T.; Sorich, M.J.; Gerber, J.P.; Angley, M.T.; Conlon, M.A. Elevated fecal short chain fatty acid and ammonia concentrations in children with autism spectrum disorder. *Dig. Dis. Sci.* **2012**, *57*, 2096–2102. [CrossRef] [PubMed]
43. Adams, J.B.; Johansen, L.J.; Powell, L.D.; Quig, D.; Rubin, R.A. Gastrointestinal flora and gastrointestinal status in children with autism—Comparisons to typical children and correlation with autism severity. *BMC Gastroenterol.* **2011**, *11*, 22. [CrossRef]
44. Liu, S.; Li, E.; Sun, Z.; Fu, D.; Duan, G.; Jiang, M.; Yu, Y.; Mei, L.; Yang, P.; Tang, Y.; et al. Altered gut microbiota and short chain fatty acids in Chinese children with autism spectrum disorder. *Sci. Rep.* **2019**, *9*, 287. [CrossRef]
45. Sharon, G.; Cruz, N.J.; Kang, D.W.; Gandal, M.J.; Wang, B.; Kim, Y.M.; Zink, E.M.; Casey, C.P.; Taylor, B.C.; Lane, C.J.; et al. Human Gut Microbiota from Autism Spectrum Disorder Promote Behavioral Symptoms in Mice. *Cell* **2019**, *177*, 1600–1618.e17. [CrossRef]
46. El-Ansary, A.; Shaker, G.H.; El-Gezeery, A.R.; Al-Ayadhi, L. The neurotoxic effect of clindamycin-induced gut bacterial imbalance and orally administered propionic acid on DNA damage assessed by the comet assay: Protective potency of carnosine and carnitine. *Gut Pathog.* **2013**, *5*, 9. [CrossRef]
47. Al-Mosalem, O.A.; El-Ansary, A.; Attas, O.; Al-Ayadhi, L. Metabolic biomarkers related to energy metabolism in Saudi autistic children. *Clin. Biochem.* **2009**, *42*, 949–957. [CrossRef]
48. MacFabe, D.F.; Cain, D.P.; Rodriguez-Capote, K.; Franklin, A.E.; Hoffman, J.E.; Boon, F.; Taylor, A.R.; Kavaliers, M.; Ossenkopp, K.P. Neurobiological effects of intraventricular propionic acid in rats: Possible role of short chain fatty acids on the pathogenesis and characteristics of autism spectrum disorders. *Behav. Brain Res.* **2007**, *176*, 149–169. [CrossRef]
49. Alfawaz, H.; Al-Onazi, M.; Bukhari, S.I.; Binobead, M.; Othman, N.; Algahtani, N.; Bhat, R.S.; Moubayed, N.M.S.; Alzeer, H.S.; El-Ansary, A. The Independent and Combined Effects of Omega-3 and Vitamin B12 in Ameliorating Propionic Acid Induced Biochemical Features in Juvenile Rats as Rodent Model of Autism. *J. Mol. Neurosci.* **2018**, *66*, 403–413. [CrossRef] [PubMed]
50. Choi, J.; Lee, S.; Won, J.; Jin, Y.; Hong, Y.; Hur, T.Y.; Kim, J.H.; Lee, S.R. Pathophysiological and neurobehavioral characteristics of a propionic acid-mediated autism-like rat model. *PLoS ONE* **2018**, *13*, e0192925. [CrossRef] [PubMed]
51. Kratsman, N.; Getselter, D.; Elliott, E. Sodium butyrate attenuates social behavior deficits and modifies the transcription of inhibitory/excitatory genes in the frontal cortex of an autism model. *Neuropharmacology* **2016**, *102*, 136–145. [CrossRef]
52. Harrington, R.A.; Lee, L.C.; Crum, R.M.; Zimmerman, A.W.; Hertz-Picciotto, I. Serotonin hypothesis of autism: Implications for selective serotonin reuptake inhibitor use during pregnancy. *Autism Res.* **2013**, *6*, 149–168. [CrossRef]
53. Ching, M.S.; Shen, Y.; Tan, W.H.; Jeste, S.S.; Morrow, E.M.; Chen, X.; Mukaddes, N.M.; Yoo, S.Y.; Hanson, E.; Hundley, R.; et al. Deletions of NRXN1 (neurexin-1) predispose to a wide spectrum of developmental disorders. *Am. J. Med. Genet. B Neuropsychiatr. Genet.* **2010**, *153*, 937–947. [CrossRef] [PubMed]
54. Kim, H.G.; Kishikawa, S.; Higgins, A.W.; Seong, I.S.; Donovan, D.J.; Shen, Y.; Lally, E.; Weiss, L.A.; Najm, J.; Kutsche, K.; et al. Disruption of neurexin 1 associated with autism spectrum disorder. *Am. J. Hum. Genet.* **2008**, *82*, 199–207. [CrossRef]
55. Szatmari, P.; Paterson, A.D.; Zwaigenbaum, L.; Roberts, W.; Brian, J.; Liu, X.Q.; Vincent, J.B.; Skaug, J.L.; Thompson, A.P.; Senman, L.; et al. Mapping autism risk loci using genetic linkage and chromosomal rearrangements. *Nat. Genet.* **2007**, *39*, 319–328. [CrossRef]
56. Boccuto, L.; Lauri, M.; Sarasua, S.M.; Skinner, C.D.; Buccella, D.; Dwivedi, A.; Orteschi, D.; Collins, J.S.; Zollino, M.; Visconti, P.; et al. Prevalence of SHANK3 variants in patients with different subtypes of autism spectrum disorders. *Eur. J. Hum. Genet.* **2013**, *21*, 310–316. [CrossRef] [PubMed]

57. Mohajeri, M.H.; La Fata, G.; Steinert, R.E.; Weber, P. Relationship between the gut microbiome and brain function. *Nutr. Rev.* **2018**, *76*, 481–496. [CrossRef] [PubMed]
58. Liu, F.; Horton-Sparks, K.; Hull, V.; Li, R.W.; Martínez-Cerdeño, V. The valproic acid rat model of autism presents with gut bacterial dysbiosis similar to that in human autism. *Mol. Autism* **2018**, *9*, 61. [CrossRef] [PubMed]
59. Christensen, J.; Grønborg, T.K.; Sørensen, M.J.; Schendel, D.; Parner, E.T.; Pedersen, L.H.; Vestergaard, M. Prenatal valproate exposure and risk of autism spectrum disorders and childhood autism. *Jama* **2013**, *309*, 1696–1703. [CrossRef]
60. Ingram, J.L.; Peckham, S.M.; Tisdale, B.; Rodier, P.M. Prenatal exposure of rats to valproic acid reproduces the cerebellar anomalies associated with autism. *Neurotoxicol. Teratol.* **2000**, *22*, 319–324. [CrossRef]
61. Cohen, O.S.; Varlinskaya, E.I.; Wilson, C.A.; Glatt, S.J.; Mooney, S.M. Acute prenatal exposure to a moderate dose of valproic acid increases social behavior and alters gene expression in rats. *Int. J. Dev. Neurosci.* **2013**, *31*, 740–750. [CrossRef]
62. D'Souza, A.; Onem, E.; Patel, P.; La Gamma, E.F.; Nankova, B.B. Valproic acid regulates catecholaminergic pathways by concentration-dependent threshold effects on TH mRNA synthesis and degradation. *Brain Res.* **2009**, *1247*, 1–10. [CrossRef]
63. Fukuchi, M.; Nii, T.; Ishimaru, N.; Minamino, A.; Hara, D.; Takasaki, I.; Tabuchi, A.; Tsuda, M. Valproic acid induces up- or down-regulation of gene expression responsible for the neuronal excitation and inhibition in rat cortical neurons through its epigenetic actions. *Neurosci. Res.* **2009**, *65*, 35–43. [CrossRef] [PubMed]
64. Stilling, R.M.; Ryan, F.J.; Hoban, A.E.; Shanahan, F.; Clarke, G.; Claesson, M.J.; Dinan, T.G.; Cryan, J.F. Microbes & neurodevelopment—Absence of microbiota during early life increases activity-related transcriptional pathways in the amygdala. *Brain Behav. Immun.* **2015**, *50*, 209–220. [CrossRef] [PubMed]
65. AbuHasan, Q.; Reddy, V.; Siddiqui, W. Neuroanatomy, Amygdala. In *StatPearls*; StatPearls Publishing LLC.: Treasure Island, FL, USA, 2020.
66. Lu, J.; Lu, L.; Yu, Y.; Cluette-Brown, J.; Martin, C.R.; Claud, E.C. Effects of Intestinal Microbiota on Brain Development in Humanized Gnotobiotic Mice. *Sci. Rep.* **2018**, *8*, 5443. [CrossRef] [PubMed]
67. Skonieczna-Żydecka, K.; Grochans, E.; Maciejewska, D.; Szkup, M.; Schneider-Matyka, D.; Jurczak, A.; Łoniewski, I.; Kaczmarczyk, M.; Marlicz, W.; Czerwińska-Rogowska, M.; et al. Faecal Short Chain Fatty Acids Profile is Changed in Polish Depressive Women. *Nutrients* **2018**, *10*, 1939. [CrossRef] [PubMed]
68. Deng, F.L.; Pan, J.X.; Zheng, P.; Xia, J.J.; Yin, B.M.; Liang, W.W.; Li, Y.F.; Wu, J.; Xu, F.; Wu, Q.Y.; et al. Metabonomics reveals peripheral and central short-chain fatty acid and amino acid dysfunction in a naturally occurring depressive model of macaques. *Neuropsychiatr. Dis. Treat.* **2019**, *15*, 1077–1088. [CrossRef] [PubMed]
69. Kelly, J.R.; Borre, Y.; O'Brien, C.; Patterson, E.; El Aidy, S.; Deane, J.; Kennedy, P.J.; Beers, S.; Scott, K.; Moloney, G.; et al. Transferring the blues: Depression-associated gut microbiota induces neurobehavioural changes in the rat. *J. Psychiatr. Res.* **2016**, *82*, 109–118. [CrossRef] [PubMed]
70. Caspani, G.; Kennedy, S.; Foster, J.A.; Swann, J. Gut microbial metabolites in depression: Understanding the biochemical mechanisms. *Microb. Cell* **2019**, *6*, 454–481. [CrossRef] [PubMed]
71. Fond, G.; Loundou, A.; Hamdani, N.; Boukouaci, W.; Dargel, A.; Oliveira, J.; Roger, M.; Tamouza, R.; Leboyer, M.; Boyer, L. Anxiety and depression comorbidities in irritable bowel syndrome (IBS): A systematic review and meta-analysis. *Eur. Arch. Psychiatry Clin. Neurosci.* **2014**, *264*, 651–660. [CrossRef]
72. Schmidtner, A.K.; Slattery, D.A.; Gläsner, J.; Hiergeist, A.; Gryksa, K.; Malik, V.A.; Hellmann-Regen, J.; Heuser, I.; Baghai, T.C.; Gessner, A.; et al. Minocycline alters behavior, microglia and the gut microbiome in a trait-anxiety-dependent manner. *Transl. Psychiatry* **2019**, *9*, 223. [CrossRef] [PubMed]
73. Pryde, S.E.; Duncan, S.H.; Hold, G.L.; Stewart, C.S.; Flint, H.J. The microbiology of butyrate formation in the human colon. *FEMS Microbiol. Lett.* **2002**, *217*, 133–139. [CrossRef]
74. Haase, S.; Haghikia, A.; Wilck, N.; Muller, D.N.; Linker, R.A. Impacts of microbiome metabolites on immune regulation and autoimmunity. *Immunology* **2018**, *154*, 230–238. [CrossRef] [PubMed]
75. Kim, C.H.; Park, J.; Kim, M. Gut microbiota-derived short-chain Fatty acids, T cells, and inflammation. *Immune Netw.* **2014**, *14*, 277–288. [CrossRef] [PubMed]
76. Miller, A.H.; Raison, C.L. The role of inflammation in depression: From evolutionary imperative to modern treatment target. *Nat. Rev. Immunol.* **2016**, *16*, 22–34. [CrossRef] [PubMed]
77. Van de Wouw, M.; Boehme, M.; Lyte, J.M.; Wiley, N.; Strain, C.; O'Sullivan, O.; Clarke, G.; Stanton, C.; Dinan, T.G.; Cryan, J.F. Short-chain fatty acids: Microbial metabolites that alleviate stress-induced brain-gut axis alterations. *J. Physiol.* **2018**, *596*, 4923–4944. [CrossRef]
78. Jamshidian, A.; Shaygannejad, V.; Pourazar, A.; Zarkesh-Esfahani, S.H.; Gharagozloo, M. Biased Treg/Th17 balance away from regulatory toward inflammatory phenotype in relapsed multiple sclerosis and its correlation with severity of symptoms. *J. Neuroimmunol.* **2013**, *262*, 106–112. [CrossRef]
79. Jangi, S.; Gandhi, R.; Cox, L.M.; Li, N.; von Glehn, F.; Yan, R.; Patel, B.; Mazzola, M.A.; Liu, S.; Glanz, B.L.; et al. Alterations of the human gut microbiome in multiple sclerosis. *Nat. Commun.* **2016**, *7*, 12015. [CrossRef] [PubMed]
80. Chen, J.; Chia, N.; Kalari, K.R.; Yao, J.Z.; Novotna, M.; Paz Soldan, M.M.; Luckey, D.H.; Marietta, E.V.; Jeraldo, P.R.; Chen, X.; et al. Multiple sclerosis patients have a distinct gut microbiota compared to healthy controls. *Sci. Rep.* **2016**, *6*, 28484. [CrossRef] [PubMed]

81. Zeng, Q.; Junli, G.; Liu, X.; Chen, C.; Sun, X.; Li, H.; Zhou, Y.; Cui, C.; Wang, Y.; Yang, Y.; et al. Gut dysbiosis and lack of short chain fatty acids in a Chinese cohort of patients with multiple sclerosis. *Neurochem. Int.* **2019**, *129*, 104468. [CrossRef]
82. Xiao, S.; Jiang, S.; Qian, D.; Duan, J. Modulation of microbially derived short-chain fatty acids on intestinal homeostasis, metabolism, and neuropsychiatric disorder. *Appl. Microbiol. Biotechnol.* **2020**, *104*, 589–601. [CrossRef] [PubMed]
83. Melbye, P.; Olsson, A.; Hansen, T.H.; Sondergaard, H.B.; Bang Oturai, A. Short-chain fatty acids and gut microbiota in multiple sclerosis. *Acta Neurol. Scand.* **2019**, *139*, 208–219. [CrossRef] [PubMed]
84. Chen, T.; Noto, D.; Hoshino, Y.; Mizuno, M.; Miyake, S. Butyrate suppresses demyelination and enhances remyelination. *J. Neuroinflamm.* **2019**, *16*, 165. [CrossRef] [PubMed]
85. Dopkins, N.; Nagarkatti, P.S.; Nagarkatti, M. The role of gut microbiome and associated metabolome in the regulation of neuroinflammation in multiple sclerosis and its implications in attenuating chronic inflammation in other inflammatory and autoimmune disorders. *Immunology* **2018**, *154*, 178–185. [CrossRef] [PubMed]
86. Erkkinen, M.G.; Kim, M.O.; Geschwind, M.D. Clinical Neurology and Epidemiology of the Major Neurodegenerative Diseases. *Cold Spring Harb. Perspect. Biol.* **2018**, *10*. [CrossRef]
87. Ahmed, S.; Busetti, A.; Fotiadou, P.; Vincy Jose, N.; Reid, S.; Georgieva, M.; Brown, S.; Dunbar, H.; Beurket-Ascencio, G.; Delday, M.I.; et al. In vitro Characterization of Gut Microbiota-Derived Bacterial Strains with Neuroprotective Properties. *Front. Cell. Neurosci.* **2019**, *13*, 402. [CrossRef]
88. Li, J.M.; Yu, R.; Zhang, L.P.; Wen, S.Y.; Wang, S.J.; Zhang, X.Y.; Xu, Q.; Kong, L.D. Dietary fructose-induced gut dysbiosis promotes mouse hippocampal neuroinflammation: A benefit of short-chain fatty acids. *Microbiome* **2019**, *7*. [CrossRef]
89. Vogt, N.M.; Kerby, R.L.; Dill-McFarland, K.A.; Harding, S.J.; Merluzzi, A.P.; Johnson, S.C.; Carlsson, C.M.; Asthana, S.; Zetterberg, H.; Blennow, K.; et al. Gut microbiome alterations in Alzheimer's disease. *Sci. Rep.* **2017**, *7*, 13537. [CrossRef] [PubMed]
90. Zhuang, Z.Q.; Shen, L.L.; Li, W.W.; Fu, X.; Zeng, F.; Gui, L.; Lü, Y.; Cai, M.; Zhu, C.; Tan, Y.L.; et al. Gut Microbiota is Altered in Patients with Alzheimer's Disease. *J. Alzheimers Dis.* **2018**, *63*, 1337–1346. [CrossRef]
91. Bostancıklıoğlu, M. The role of gut microbiota in pathogenesis of Alzheimer's disease. *J. Appl. Microbiol.* **2019**, *127*, 954–967. [CrossRef]
92. Paley, E.L.; Merkulova-Rainon, T.; Faynboym, A.; Shestopalov, V.I.; Aksenoff, I. Geographical Distribution and Diversity of Gut Microbial NADH:Ubiquinone Oxidoreductase Sequence Associated with Alzheimer's Disease. *J. Alzheimers Dis.* **2018**, *61*, 1531–1540. [CrossRef]
93. Saji, N.; Niida, S.; Murotani, K.; Hisada, T.; Tsuduki, T.; Sugimoto, T.; Kimura, A.; Toba, K.; Sakurai, T. Analysis of the relationship between the gut microbiome and dementia: A cross-sectional study conducted in Japan. *Sci. Rep.* **2019**, *9*, 1008. [CrossRef]
94. Nie, P.; Li, Z.; Wang, Y.; Zhang, Y.; Zhao, M.; Luo, J.; Du, S.; Deng, Z.; Chen, J.; Chen, S.; et al. Gut microbiome interventions in human health and diseases. *Med. Res. Rev.* **2019**, *39*, 2286–2313. [CrossRef] [PubMed]
95. Zhang, L.; Wang, Y.; Xiayu, X.; Shi, C.; Chen, W.; Song, N.; Fu, X.; Zhou, R.; Xu, Y.F.; Huang, L.; et al. Altered Gut Microbiota in a Mouse Model of Alzheimer's Disease. *J. Alzheimers Dis.* **2017**, *60*, 1241–1257. [CrossRef]
96. Zheng, J.; Zheng, S.J.; Cai, W.J.; Yu, L.; Yuan, B.F.; Feng, Y.Q. Stable isotope labeling combined with liquid chromatography-tandem mass spectrometry for comprehensive analysis of short-chain fatty acids. *Anal. Chim. Acta* **2019**, *1070*, 51–59. [CrossRef]
97. Fujii, Y.; Nguyen, T.T.T.; Fujimura, Y.; Kameya, N.; Nakamura, S.; Arakawa, K.; Morita, H. Fecal metabolite of a gnotobiotic mouse transplanted with gut microbiota from a patient with Alzheimer's disease. *Biosci. Biotechnol. Biochem.* **2019**, *83*, 2144–2152. [CrossRef] [PubMed]
98. Mohajeri, M.H.; Leuba, G. Prevention of age-associated dementia. *Brain Res. Bull.* **2009**, *80*, 315–325. [CrossRef]
99. Ho, L.; Ono, K.; Tsuji, M.; Mazzola, P.; Singh, R.; Pasinetti, G.M. Protective roles of intestinal microbiota derived short chain fatty acids in Alzheimer's disease-type beta-amyloid neuropathological mechanisms. *Expert Rev. Neurother.* **2018**, *18*, 83–90. [CrossRef]
100. Sun, J.; Xu, J.; Ling, Y.; Wang, F.; Gong, T.; Yang, C.; Ye, S.; Ye, K.; Wei, D.; Song, Z.; et al. Fecal microbiota transplantation alleviated Alzheimer's disease-like pathogenesis in APP/PS1 transgenic mice. *Transl. Psychiatry* **2019**, *9*, 189. [CrossRef]
101. Peleg, S.; Sananbenesi, F.; Zovoilis, A.; Burkhardt, S.; Bahari-Javan, S.; Agis-Balboa, R.C.; Cota, P.; Wittnam, J.L.; Gogol-Doering, A.; Opitz, L.; et al. Altered histone acetylation is associated with age-dependent memory impairment in mice. *Science* **2010**, *328*, 753–756. [CrossRef]
102. Govindarajan, N.; Agis-Balboa, R.C.; Walter, J.; Sananbenesi, F.; Fischer, A. Sodium butyrate improves memory function in an Alzheimer's disease mouse model when administered at an advanced stage of disease progression. *J. Alzheimers Dis.* **2011**, *26*, 187–197. [CrossRef]
103. Bourassa, M.W.; Alim, I.; Bultman, S.J.; Ratan, R.R. Butyrate, neuroepigenetics and the gut microbiome: Can a high fiber diet improve brain health? *Neurosci. Lett.* **2016**, *625*, 56–63. [CrossRef] [PubMed]
104. Nguyen, T.D.; Prykhodko, O.; Fak Hallenius, F.; Nyman, M. Monovalerin and trivalerin increase brain acetic acid, decrease liver succinic acid, and alter gut microbiota in rats fed high-fat diets. *Eur. J. Nutr.* **2019**, *58*, 1545–1560. [CrossRef]
105. Soliman, M.L.; Combs, C.K.; Rosenberger, T.A. Modulation of inflammatory cytokines and mitogen-activated protein kinases by acetate in primary astrocytes. *J. Neuroimmune Pharm.* **2013**, *8*, 287–300. [CrossRef] [PubMed]
106. Marino, B.L.B.; de Souza, L.R.; Sousa, K.P.A.; Ferreira, J.V.; Padilha, E.C.; da Silva, C.H.T.P.; Taft, C.A.; Hage-Melim, L.I.S. Parkinson's Disease: A Review from Pathophysiology to Treatment. *Mini-Rev. Med. Chem.* **2020**, *20*, 754–767. [CrossRef]
107. Brettschneider, J.; Del Tredici, K.; Lee, V.M.; Trojanowski, J.Q. Spreading of pathology in neurodegenerative diseases: A focus on human studies. *Nat. Rev. Neurosci.* **2015**, *16*, 109–120. [CrossRef] [PubMed]

108. Braak, H.; Del Tredici, K.; Rüb, U.; de Vos, R.A.; Jansen Steur, E.N.; Braak, E. Staging of brain pathology related to sporadic Parkinson's disease. *Neurobiol. Aging* **2003**, *24*, 197–211. [CrossRef]
109. Van Kessel, S.P.; El Aidy, S. Bacterial Metabolites Mirror Altered Gut Microbiota Composition in Patients with Parkinson's Disease. *J. Parkinsons Dis.* **2019**, *9*, S359–S370. [CrossRef]
110. Gerhardt, S.; Mohajeri, M.H. Changes of Colonic Bacterial Composition in Parkinson's Disease and Other Neurodegenerative Diseases. *Nutrients* **2018**, *10*, 708. [CrossRef]
111. Hasegawa, S.; Goto, S.; Tsuji, H.; Okuno, T.; Asahara, T.; Nomoto, K.; Shibata, A.; Fujisawa, Y.; Minato, T.; Okamoto, A.; et al. Intestinal Dysbiosis and Lowered Serum Lipopolysaccharide-Binding Protein in Parkinson's Disease. *PLoS ONE* **2015**, *10*, e0142164. [CrossRef] [PubMed]
112. Scheperjans, F.; Aho, V.; Pereira, P.A.B.; Koskinen, K.; Paulin, L.; Pekkonen, E.; Haapaniemi, E.; Kaakkola, S.; Eerola-Rautio, J.; Pohja, M.; et al. Gut microbiota are related to Parkinson's disease and clinical phenotype. *Mov. Disord.* **2015**, *30*, 350–358. [CrossRef] [PubMed]
113. Boertien, J.M.; Pereira, P.A.B.; Aho, V.T.E.; Scheperjans, F. Increasing Comparability and Utility of Gut Microbiome Studies in Parkinson's Disease: A Systematic Review. *J. Parkinsons Dis.* **2019**, *9*, S297–S312. [CrossRef] [PubMed]
114. Sanguinetti, E.; Collado, M.C.; Marrachelli, V.G.; Monleon, D.; Selma-Royo, M.; Pardo-Tendero, M.M.; Burchielli, S.; Iozzo, P. Microbiome-metabolome signatures in mice genetically prone to develop dementia, fed a normal or fatty diet. *Sci. Rep.* **2018**, *8*, 4907. [CrossRef]
115. Kim, S.; Kwon, S.H.; Kam, T.I.; Panicker, N.; Karuppagounder, S.S.; Lee, S.; Lee, J.H.; Kim, W.R.; Kook, M.; Foss, C.A.; et al. Transneuronal Propagation of Pathologic α-Synuclein from the Gut to the Brain Models Parkinson's Disease. *Neuron* **2019**, *103*, 627–641.e7. [CrossRef]
116. Houser, M.C.; Tansey, M.G. The gut-brain axis: Is intestinal inflammation a silent driver of Parkinson's disease pathogenesis? *Npj Parkinsons Dis.* **2017**, *3*, 1–9. [CrossRef] [PubMed]
117. Unger, M.M.; Spiegel, J.; Dillmann, K.U.; Grundmann, D.; Philippeit, H.; Bürmann, J.; Faßbender, K.; Schwiertz, A.; Schäfer, K.H. Short chain fatty acids and gut microbiota differ between patients with Parkinson's disease and age-matched controls. *Parkinsonism Relat. Disord.* **2016**, *32*, 66–72. [CrossRef]
118. Sampson, T.R.; Debelius, J.W.; Thron, T.; Janssen, S.; Shastri, G.G.; Ilhan, Z.E.; Challis, C.; Schretter, C.E.; Rocha, S.; Gradinaru, V.; et al. Gut Microbiota Regulate Motor Deficits and Neuroinflammation in a Model of Parkinson's Disease. *Cell* **2016**, *167*, 1469–1480.e12. [CrossRef] [PubMed]
119. Sun, M.F.; Zhu, Y.L.; Zhou, Z.L.; Jia, X.B.; Xu, Y.D.; Yang, Q.; Cui, C.; Shen, Y.Q. Neuroprotective effects of fecal microbiota transplantation on MPTP-induced Parkinson's disease mice: Gut microbiota, glial reaction and TLR4/TNF-α signaling pathway. *Brain Behav. Immun.* **2018**, *70*, 48–60. [CrossRef] [PubMed]
120. Wakade, C.; Chong, R. A novel treatment target for Parkinson's disease. *J. Neurol. Sci.* **2014**, *347*, 34–38. [CrossRef]
121. Donohoe, D.R.; Garge, N.; Zhang, X.; Sun, W.; O'Connell, T.M.; Bunger, M.K.; Bultman, S.J. The microbiome and butyrate regulate energy metabolism and autophagy in the mammalian colon. *Cell Metab.* **2011**, *13*, 517–526. [CrossRef]
122. Stefanko, D.P.; Barrett, R.M.; Ly, A.R.; Reolon, G.K.; Wood, M.A. Modulation of long-term memory for object recognition via HDAC inhibition. *Proc. Natl. Acad. Sci. USA* **2009**, *106*, 9447–9452. [CrossRef]
123. Vecsey, C.G.; Hawk, J.D.; Lattal, K.M.; Stein, J.M.; Fabian, S.A.; Attner, M.A.; Cabrera, S.M.; McDonough, C.B.; Brindle, P.K.; Abel, T.; et al. Histone deacetylase inhibitors enhance memory and synaptic plasticity via CREB:CBP-dependent transcriptional activation. *J. Neurosci.* **2007**, *27*, 6128–6140. [CrossRef]
124. Sherwin, E.; Sandhu, K.V.; Dinan, T.G.; Cryan, J.F. May the Force Be With You: The Light and Dark Sides of the Microbiota-Gut-Brain Axis in Neuropsychiatry. *CNS Drugs* **2016**, *30*, 1019–1041. [CrossRef] [PubMed]
125. Paiva, I.; Pinho, R.; Pavlou, M.A.; Hennion, M.; Wales, P.; Schütz, A.L.; Rajput, A.; Szego, M.É.; Kerimoglu, C.; Gerhardt, E.; et al. Sodium butyrate rescues dopaminergic cells from alpha-synuclein-induced transcriptional deregulation and DNA damage. *Hum. Mol. Genet.* **2017**, *26*, 2231–2246. [CrossRef]
126. Kidd, S.K.; Schneider, J.S. Protection of dopaminergic cells from MPP+-mediated toxicity by histone deacetylase inhibition. *Brain Res.* **2010**, *1354*, 172–178. [CrossRef] [PubMed]
127. St. Laurent, R.; O'Brien, L.M.; Ahmad, S.T. Sodium butyrate improves locomotor impairment and early mortality in a rotenone-induced Drosophila model of Parkinson's disease. *Neuroscience* **2013**, *246*, 382–390. [CrossRef] [PubMed]
128. Namkung, H.; Kim, S.H.; Sawa, A. The Insula: An Underestimated Brain Area in Clinical Neuroscience, Psychiatry, and Neurology: (Trends in Neuroscience 40, 200–207, 2017). *Trends Neurosci.* **2018**, *41*, 551–554. [CrossRef]
129. Van Kessel, S.P.; Frye, A.K.; El-Gendy, A.O.; Castejon, M.; Keshavarzian, A.; van Dijk, G.; El Aidy, S. Gut bacterial tyrosine decarboxylases restrict levels of levodopa in the treatment of Parkinson's disease. *Nat. Commun.* **2019**, *10*, 310. [CrossRef]
130. Marietta, E.; Horwath, I.; Taneja, V. Microbiome, Immunomodulation, and the Neuronal System. *Neurotherapeutics* **2018**, *15*, 23–30. [CrossRef]
131. Rodriguez-Castano, G.P.; Dorris, M.R.; Liu, X.; Bolling, B.W.; Acosta-Gonzalez, A.; Rey, F.E. Bacteroides thetaiotaomicron Starch Utilization Promotes Quercetin Degradation and Butyrate Production by Eubacterium ramulus. *Front. Microbiol.* **2019**, *10*, 1145. [CrossRef]

132. Cirstea, M.S.; Yu, A.C.; Golz, E.; Sundvick, K.; Kliger, D.; Radisavljevic, N.; Foulger, L.H.; Mackenzie, M.; Huan, T.; Finlay, B.B.; et al. Microbiota Composition and Metabolism Are Associated with Gut Function in Parkinson's Disease. *Mov. Disord.* **2020**. [CrossRef]
133. Gill, S.R.; Pop, M.; Deboy, R.T.; Eckburg, P.B.; Turnbaugh, P.J.; Samuel, B.S.; Gordon, J.I.; Relman, D.A.; Fraser-Liggett, C.M.; Nelson, K.E. Metagenomic analysis of the human distal gut microbiome. *Science* **2006**, *312*, 1355–1359. [CrossRef]
134. Parthasarathy, A.; Cross, P.J.; Dobson, R.C.J.; Adams, L.E.; Savka, M.A.; Hudson, A.O. A Three-Ring Circus: Metabolism of the Three Proteogenic Aromatic Amino Acids and Their Role in the Health of Plants and Animals. *Front. Mol. Biosci.* **2018**, *5*, 29. [CrossRef]
135. Kaur, H.; Bose, C.; Mande, S.S. Tryptophan Metabolism by Gut Microbiome and Gut-Brain-Axis: An in silico Analysis. *Front. Neurosci.* **2019**, *13*, 1365. [CrossRef] [PubMed]
136. Wikoff, W.R.; Anfora, A.T.; Liu, J.; Schultz, P.G.; Lesley, S.A.; Peters, E.C.; Siuzdak, G. Metabolomics analysis reveals large effects of gut microflora on mammalian blood metabolites. *Proc. Natl. Acad. Sci. USA* **2009**, *106*, 3698–3703. [CrossRef] [PubMed]
137. Saito, Y.; Sato, T.; Nomoto, K.; Tsuji, H. Identification of phenol- and p-cresol-producing intestinal bacteria by using media supplemented with tyrosine and its metabolites. *FEMS Microbiol. Ecol.* **2018**, *94*. [CrossRef]
138. Gabriele, S.; Sacco, R.; Cerullo, S.; Neri, C.; Urbani, A.; Tripi, G.; Malvy, J.; Barthelemy, C.; Bonnet-Brihault, F.; Persico, A.M. Urinary p-cresol is elevated in young French children with autism spectrum disorder: A replication study. *Biomarkers* **2014**, *19*, 463–470. [CrossRef] [PubMed]
139. Altieri, L.; Neri, C.; Sacco, R.; Curatolo, P.; Benvenuto, A.; Muratori, F.; Santocchi, E.; Bravaccio, C.; Lenti, C.; Saccani, M.; et al. Urinary p-cresol is elevated in small children with severe autism spectrum disorder. *Biomarkers* **2011**, *16*, 252–260. [CrossRef]
140. Pascucci, T.; Colamartino, M.; Fiori, E.; Sacco, R.; Coviello, A.; Ventura, R.; Puglisi-Allegra, S.; Turriziani, L.; Persico, A.M. P-cresol Alters Brain Dopamine Metabolism and Exacerbates Autism-Like Behaviors in the BTBR Mouse. *Brain Sci.* **2020**, *10*, 233. [CrossRef]
141. Gacias, M.; Gaspari, S.; Santos, P.M.; Tamburini, S.; Andrade, M.; Zhang, F.; Shen, N.; Tolstikov, V.; Kiebish, M.A.; Dupree, J.L.; et al. Microbiota-driven transcriptional changes in prefrontal cortex override genetic differences in social behavior. *Elife* **2016**, *5*. [CrossRef]
142. Hsiao, E.Y.; McBride, S.W.; Hsien, S.; Sharon, G.; Hyde, E.R.; McCue, T.; Codelli, J.A.; Chow, J.; Reisman, S.E.; Petrosino, J.F.; et al. Microbiota modulate behavioral and physiological abnormalities associated with neurodevelopmental disorders. *Cell* **2013**, *155*, 1451–1463. [CrossRef]
143. Gevi, F.; Zolla, L.; Gabriele, S.; Persico, A.M. Urinary metabolomics of young Italian autistic children supports abnormal tryptophan and purine metabolism. *Mol. Autism* **2016**, *7*, 47. [CrossRef]
144. Urrutia, A.; García-Angulo, V.A.; Fuentes, A.; Caneo, M.; Legüe, M.; Urquiza, P.; Delgado, S.E.; Ugalde, J.; Burdisso, P.; Calixto, A. Bacterially produced metabolites protect C. elegans neurons from degeneration. *PLoS Biol.* **2020**, *18*, e3000638. [CrossRef] [PubMed]
145. Hollister, E.B.; Riehle, K.; Luna, R.A.; Weidler, E.M.; Rubio-Gonzales, M.; Mistretta, T.A.; Raza, S.; Doddapaneni, H.V.; Metcalf, G.A.; Muzny, D.M.; et al. Structure and function of the healthy pre-adolescent pediatric gut microbiome. *Microbiome* **2015**, *3*, 36. [CrossRef]
146. Delgado, P.L.; Charney, D.S.; Price, L.H.; Aghajanian, G.K.; Landis, H.; Heninger, G.R. Serotonin function and the mechanism of antidepressant action. Reversal of antidepressant-induced remission by rapid depletion of plasma tryptophan. *Arch. Gen. Psychiatry* **1990**, *47*, 411–418. [CrossRef] [PubMed]
147. Young, S.N. Acute tryptophan depletion in humans: A review of theoretical, practical and ethical aspects. *J. Psychiatry Neurosci.* **2013**, *38*, 294–305. [CrossRef]
148. Clarke, G.; Grenham, S.; Scully, P.; Fitzgerald, P.; Moloney, R.D.; Shanahan, F.; Dinan, T.G.; Cryan, J.F. The microbiome-gut-brain axis during early life regulates the hippocampal serotonergic system in a sex-dependent manner. *Mol. Psychiatry* **2013**, *18*, 666–673. [CrossRef] [PubMed]
149. Lukić, I.; Getselter, D.; Koren, O.; Elliott, E. Role of Tryptophan in Microbiota-Induced Depressive-Like Behavior: Evidence from Tryptophan Depletion Study. *Front. Behav. Neurosci.* **2019**, *13*, 123. [CrossRef]
150. Yu, M.; Jia, H.; Zhou, C.; Yang, Y.; Zhao, Y.; Yang, M.; Zou, Z. Variations in gut microbiota and fecal metabolic phenotype associated with depression by 16S rRNA gene sequencing and LC/MS-based metabolomics. *J. Pharm. Biomed. Anal.* **2017**, *138*, 231–239. [CrossRef]
151. Ruddick, J.P.; Evans, A.K.; Nutt, D.J.; Lightman, S.L.; Rook, G.A.; Lowry, C.A. Tryptophan metabolism in the central nervous system: Medical implications. *Expert Rev. Mol. Med.* **2006**, *8*, 1–27. [CrossRef] [PubMed]
152. O'Mahony, S.M.; Clarke, G.; Borre, Y.E.; Dinan, T.G.; Cryan, J.F. Serotonin, tryptophan metabolism and the brain-gut-microbiome axis. *Behav. Brain Res.* **2015**, *277*, 32–48. [CrossRef] [PubMed]
153. Lapin, I.P.; Oxenkrug, G.F. Intensification of the central serotoninergic processes as a possible determinant of the thymoleptic effect. *Lancet* **1969**, *1*, 132–136. [CrossRef]
154. Abramowitz, M.K.; Meyer, T.W.; Hostetter, T.H. Chapter 18—The Pathophysiology of Uremia. In *Chronic Kidney Disease, Dialysis, and Transplantation*, 3rd ed.; Himmelfarb, J., Sayegh, M.H., Eds.; W.B. Saunders: Philadelphia, PA, USA, 2010; pp. 251–264.

155. Jaglin, M.; Rhimi, M.; Philippe, C.; Pons, N.; Bruneau, A.; Goustard, B.; Dauge, V.; Maguin, E.; Naudon, L.; Rabot, S. Indole, a Signaling Molecule Produced by the Gut Microbiota, Negatively Impacts Emotional Behaviors in Rats. *Front. Neurosci.* **2018**, *12*, 216. [CrossRef] [PubMed]
156. Buckley, M.M.; O'Brien, R.; Brosnan, E.; Ross, R.P.; Stanton, C.; Buckley, J.M.; O'Malley, D. Glucagon-Like Peptide-1 Secreting L-Cells Coupled to Sensory Nerves Translate Microbial Signals to the Host Rat Nervous System. *Front. Cell. Neurosci.* **2020**, *14*, 95. [CrossRef] [PubMed]
157. Han, W.; Tellez, L.A.; Perkins, M.H.; Perez, I.O.; Qu, T.; Ferreira, J.; Ferreira, T.L.; Quinn, D.; Liu, Z.W.; Gao, X.B.; et al. A Neural Circuit for Gut-Induced Reward. *Cell* **2018**, *175*, 665–678.e23. [CrossRef]
158. Cuomo, A.; Maina, G.; Rosso, G.; Beccarini Crescenzi, B.; Bolognesi, S.; Di Muro, A.; Giordano, N.; Goracci, A.; Neal, S.M.; Nitti, M.; et al. The Microbiome: A New Target for Research and Treatment of Schizophrenia and its Resistant Presentations? A Systematic Literature Search and Review. *Front. Pharm.* **2018**, *9*, 1040. [CrossRef] [PubMed]
159. Paley, E.L.; Denisova, G.; Sokolova, O.; Posternak, N.; Wang, X.; Brownell, A.L. Tryptamine induces tryptophanyl-tRNA synthetase-mediated neurodegeneration with neurofibrillary tangles in human cell and mouse models. *Neuromol. Med.* **2007**, *9*, 55–82. [CrossRef]
160. Paley, E.L. Tryptamine-induced tryptophanyl-tRNAtrp deficiency in neurodifferentiation and neurodegeneration interplay: Progenitor activation with neurite growth terminated in Alzheimer's disease neuronal vesicularization and fragmentation. *J. Alzheimers Dis.* **2011**, *26*, 263–298. [CrossRef]
161. Paley, E.L.; Perry, G.; Sokolova, O. Tryptamine induces axonopathy and mitochondriopathy mimicking neurodegenerative diseases via tryptophanyl-tRNA deficiency. *Curr. Alzheimer Res.* **2013**, *10*, 987–1004. [CrossRef] [PubMed]
162. Yeh, Y.C.; Huang, M.F.; Liang, S.S.; Hwang, S.J.; Tsai, J.C.; Liu, T.L.; Wu, P.H.; Yang, Y.H.; Kuo, K.C.; Kuo, M.C.; et al. Indoxyl sulfate, not p-cresyl sulfate, is associated with cognitive impairment in early-stage chronic kidney disease. *Neurotoxicology* **2016**, *53*, 148–152. [CrossRef] [PubMed]
163. Sankowski, B.; Księżarczyk, K.; Raćkowska, E.; Szlufik, S.; Koziorowski, D.; Giebułtowicz, J. Higher cerebrospinal fluid to plasma ratio of p-cresol sulfate and indoxyl sulfate in patients with Parkinson's disease. *Clin. Chim. Acta* **2020**, *501*, 165–173. [CrossRef] [PubMed]
164. Dou, L.; Jourde-Chiche, N.; Faure, V.; Cerini, C.; Berland, Y.; Dignat-George, F.; Brunet, P. The uremic solute indoxyl sulfate induces oxidative stress in endothelial cells. *J. Thromb. Haemost.* **2007**, *5*, 1302–1308. [CrossRef] [PubMed]
165. Adesso, S.; Magnus, T.; Cuzzocrea, S.; Campolo, M.; Rissiek, B.; Paciello, O.; Autore, G.; Pinto, A.; Marzocco, S. Indoxyl Sulfate Affects Glial Function Increasing Oxidative Stress and Neuroinflammation in Chronic Kidney Disease: Interaction between Astrocytes and Microglia. *Front. Pharm.* **2017**, *8*, 370. [CrossRef]
166. Singh, A.; Kukreti, R.; Saso, L.; Kukreti, S. Oxidative Stress: A Key Modulator in Neurodegenerative Diseases. *Molecules* **2019**, *24*, 1583. [CrossRef]
167. Gray, M.T.; Woulfe, J.M. Striatal blood-brain barrier permeability in Parkinson's disease. *J. Cereb. Blood Flow Metab.* **2015**, *35*, 747–750. [CrossRef] [PubMed]
168. Chu, C.; Murdock, M.H.; Jing, D.; Won, T.H.; Chung, H.; Kressel, A.M.; Tsaava, T.; Addorisio, M.E.; Putzel, G.G.; Zhou, L.; et al. The microbiota regulate neuronal function and fear extinction learning. *Nature* **2019**, *574*, 543–548. [CrossRef] [PubMed]
169. Zieve, L.; Lyftogt, C.; Raphael, D. Ammonia toxicity: Comparative protective effect of various arginine and ornithine derivatives, aspartate, benzoate, and carbamyl glutamate. *Metab. Brain Dis.* **1986**, *1*, 25–35. [CrossRef]
170. Luan, H.; Liu, L.F.; Tang, Z.; Zhang, M.; Chua, K.K.; Song, J.X.; Mok, V.C.; Li, M.; Cai, Z. Comprehensive urinary metabolomic profiling and identification of potential noninvasive marker for idiopathic Parkinson's disease. *Sci. Rep.* **2015**, *5*, 13888. [CrossRef] [PubMed]
171. Luan, H.; Liu, L.F.; Meng, N.; Tang, Z.; Chua, K.K.; Chen, L.L.; Song, J.X.; Mok, V.C.; Xie, L.X.; Li, M.; et al. LC-MS-based urinary metabolite signatures in idiopathic Parkinson's disease. *J. Proteome Res.* **2015**, *14*, 467–478. [CrossRef]
172. Hatano, T.; Saiki, S.; Okuzumi, A.; Mohney, R.P.; Hattori, N. Identification of novel biomarkers for Parkinson's disease by metabolomic technologies. *J. Neurol. Neurosurg. Psychiatry* **2016**, *87*, 295–301. [CrossRef]
173. Okuzumi, A.; Hatano, T.; Ueno, S.I.; Ogawa, T.; Saiki, S.; Mori, A.; Koinuma, T.; Oji, Y.; Ishikawa, K.I.; Fujimaki, M.; et al. Metabolomics-based identification of metabolic alterations in PARK2. *Ann. Clin. Transl. Neurol.* **2019**, *6*, 525–536. [CrossRef]
174. Gao, J.; Xu, K.; Liu, H.; Liu, G.; Bai, M.; Peng, C.; Li, T.; Yin, Y. Impact of the Gut Microbiota on Intestinal Immunity Mediated by Tryptophan Metabolism. *Front. Cell. Infect. Microbiol.* **2018**, *8*, 13. [CrossRef]
175. Kim, D.-C.; Quang, T.H.; Yoon, C.-S.; Ngan, N.T.T.; Lim, S.-I.; Lee, S.-Y.; Kim, Y.-C.; Oh, H. Anti-neuroinflammatory activities of indole alkaloids from kanjang (Korean fermented soy source) in lipopolysaccharide-induced BV2 microglial cells. *Food Chem.* **2016**, *213*, 69–75. [CrossRef] [PubMed]
176. Willkommen, D.; Lucio, M.; Moritz, F.; Forcisi, S.; Kanawati, B.; Smirnov, K.S.; Schroeter, M.; Sigaroudi, A.; Schmitt-Kopplin, P.; Michalke, B. Metabolomic investigations in cerebrospinal fluid of Parkinson's disease. *PLoS ONE* **2018**, *13*, e0208752. [CrossRef]
177. Southan, C.; DeWolf, W.E., Jr.; Kruse, L.I. Inactivation of dopamine beta-hydroxylase by p-cresol: Evidence for a second, minor site of covalent modification at tyrosine 357. *Biochim. Biophys. Acta* **1990**, *1037*, 256–258. [CrossRef]
178. Crossgrove, J.; Zheng, W. Manganese toxicity upon overexposure. *NMR Biomed.* **2004**, *17*, 544–553. [CrossRef] [PubMed]
179. Reaney, S.H.; Bench, G.; Smith, D.R. Brain accumulation and toxicity of Mn(II) and Mn(III) exposures. *Toxicol. Sci.* **2006**, *93*, 114–124. [CrossRef] [PubMed]

180. Chi, L.; Gao, B.; Bian, X.; Tu, P.; Ru, H.; Lu, K. Manganese-induced sex-specific gut microbiome perturbations in C57BL/6 mice. *Toxicol. Appl. Pharm.* **2017**, *331*, 142–153. [CrossRef] [PubMed]
181. Fowlie, G.; Cohen, N.; Ming, X. The Perturbance of Microbiome and Gut-Brain Axis in Autism Spectrum Disorders. *Int. J. Mol. Sci.* **2018**, *19*, 2251. [CrossRef]
182. Rothhammer, V.; Mascanfroni, I.D.; Bunse, L.; Takenaka, M.C.; Kenison, J.E.; Mayo, L.; Chao, C.C.; Patel, B.; Yan, R.; Blain, M.; et al. Type I interferons and microbial metabolites of tryptophan modulate astrocyte activity and central nervous system inflammation via the aryl hydrocarbon receptor. *Nat. Med.* **2016**, *22*, 586–597. [CrossRef]
183. Cekanaviciute, E.; Yoo, B.B.; Runia, T.F.; Debelius, J.W.; Singh, S.; Nelson, C.A.; Kanner, R.; Bencosme, Y.; Lee, Y.K.; Hauser, S.L.; et al. Gut bacteria from multiple sclerosis patients modulate human T cells and exacerbate symptoms in mouse models. *Proc. Natl. Acad. Sci. USA* **2017**, *114*, 10713–10718. [CrossRef]
184. Mohanta, L.; Das, B.C.; Patri, M. Microbial communities modulating brain functioning and behaviors in zebrafish: A mechanistic approach. *Microb. Pathog.* **2020**, *145*, 104251. [CrossRef]
185. Chong-Nguyen, C.; Duboc, H.; Sokol, H. The gut microbiota, a new cardiovascular risk factor? *Presse Med.* **2017**, *46*, 708–713. [CrossRef]
186. Fu, B.C.; Hullar, M.A.J.; Randolph, T.W.; Franke, A.A.; Monroe, K.R.; Cheng, I.; Wilkens, L.R.; Shepherd, J.A.; Madeleine, M.M.; Le Marchand, L.; et al. Associations of plasma trimethylamine N-oxide, choline, carnitine, and betaine with inflammatory and cardiometabolic risk biomarkers and the fecal microbiome in the Multiethnic Cohort Adiposity Phenotype Study. *Am. J. Clin. Nutr.* **2020**, *111*, 1226–1234. [CrossRef]
187. Velasquez, M.T.; Ramezani, A.; Manal, A.; Raj, D.S. Trimethylamine N-Oxide: The Good, the Bad and the Unknown. *Toxins* **2016**, *8*, 326. [CrossRef]
188. Vogt, N.M.; Romano, K.A.; Darst, B.F.; Engelman, C.D.; Johnson, S.C.; Carlsson, C.M.; Asthana, S.; Blennow, K.; Zetterberg, H.; Bendlin, B.B.; et al. The gut microbiota-derived metabolite trimethylamine N-oxide is elevated in Alzheimer's disease. *Alzheimers Res. Ther.* **2018**, *10*, 124. [CrossRef]
189. Del Rio, D.; Zimetti, F.; Caffarra, P.; Tassotti, M.; Bernini, F.; Brighenti, F.; Zini, A.; Zanotti, I. The Gut Microbial Metabolite Trimethylamine-N-Oxide Is Present in Human Cerebrospinal Fluid. *Nutrients* **2017**, *9*, 1053. [CrossRef]
190. Li, D.; Ke, Y.; Zhan, R.; Liu, C.; Zhao, M.; Zeng, A.; Shi, X.; Ji, L.; Cheng, S.; Pan, B.; et al. Trimethylamine-N-oxide promotes brain aging and cognitive impairment in mice. *Aging Cell* **2018**, *17*, e12768. [CrossRef] [PubMed]
191. Gao, Q.; Wang, Y.; Wang, X.; Fu, S.; Zhang, X.; Wang, R.T. Decreased levels of circulating trimethylamine N-oxide alleviate cognitive and pathological deterioration in transgenic mice: A potential therapeutic approach for Alzheimer's disease. *Aging* **2019**, *11*, 8642–8663. [CrossRef]
192. Govindarajulu, M.; Pinky, P.D.; Steinke, I.; Bloemer, J.; Ramesh, S.; Kariharan, T.; Rella, R.T.; Bhattacharya, S.; Dhanasekaran, M.; Suppiramaniam, V.; et al. Gut Metabolite TMAO Induces Synaptic Plasticity Deficits by Promoting Endoplasmic Reticulum Stress. *Front. Mol. Neurosci.* **2020**, *13*, 138. [CrossRef]
193. Brunt, V.E.; LaRocca, T.J.; Bazzoni, A.E.; Sapinsley, Z.J.; Miyamoto-Ditmon, J.; Gioscia-Ryan, R.A.; Neilson, A.P.; Link, C.D.; Seals, D.R. The gut microbiome-derived metabolite trimethylamine N-oxide modulates neuroinflammation and cognitive function with aging. *Geroscience* **2020**. [CrossRef] [PubMed]
194. Alkasir, R.; Li, J.; Li, X.; Jin, M.; Zhu, B. Human gut microbiota: The links with dementia development. *Protein Cell* **2017**, *8*, 90–102. [CrossRef]
195. Wang, Z.; Klipfell, E.; Bennett, B.J.; Koeth, R.; Levison, B.S.; Dugar, B.; Feldstein, A.E.; Britt, E.B.; Fu, X.; Chung, Y.M.; et al. Gut flora metabolism of phosphatidylcholine promotes cardiovascular disease. *Nature* **2011**, *472*, 57–63. [CrossRef] [PubMed]
196. Gorelick, P.B.; Scuteri, A.; Black, S.E.; Decarli, C.; Greenberg, S.M.; Iadecola, C.; Launer, L.J.; Laurent, S.; Lopez, O.L.; Nyenhuis, D.; et al. Vascular contributions to cognitive impairment and dementia: A statement for healthcare professionals from the american heart association/american stroke association. *Stroke* **2011**, *42*, 2672–2713. [CrossRef]
197. Wu, P.; Chen, J.; Tao, J.; Wu, S.; Xu, G.; Wang, Z.; Wei, D.; Yin, W. Trimethylamine N-oxide promotes apoE(-/-) mice atherosclerosis by inducing vascular endothelial cell pyroptosis via the SDHB/ROS pathway. *J. Cell Physiol.* **2020**, *235*, 6582–6591. [CrossRef] [PubMed]
198. Koeth, R.A.; Wang, Z.; Levison, B.S.; Buffa, J.A.; Org, E.; Sheehy, B.T.; Britt, E.B.; Fu, X.; Wu, Y.; Li, L.; et al. Intestinal microbiota metabolism of L-carnitine, a nutrient in red meat, promotes atherosclerosis. *Nat. Med.* **2013**, *19*, 576–585. [CrossRef] [PubMed]
199. Zhu, W.; Gregory, J.C.; Org, E.; Buffa, J.A.; Gupta, N.; Wang, Z.; Li, L.; Fu, X.; Wu, Y.; Mehrabian, M.; et al. Gut Microbial Metabolite TMAO Enhances Platelet Hyperreactivity and Thrombosis Risk. *Cell* **2016**, *165*, 111–124. [CrossRef] [PubMed]
200. Janeiro, M.H.; Ramírez, M.J.; Milagro, F.I.; Martínez, J.A.; Solas, M. Implication of Trimethylamine N-Oxide (TMAO) in Disease: Potential Biomarker or New Therapeutic Target. *Nutrients* **2018**, *10*, 1398. [CrossRef] [PubMed]
201. Xu, R.; Wang, Q. Towards understanding brain-gut-microbiome connections in Alzheimer's disease. *BMC Syst. Biol.* **2016**, *10* (Suppl. S3), 63. [CrossRef]
202. Hulme, H.; Meikle, L.M.; Strittmatter, N.; van der Hooft, J.J.J.; Swales, J.; Bragg, R.A.; Villar, V.H.; Ormsby, M.J.; Barnes, S.; Brown, S.L.; et al. Microbiome-derived carnitine mimics as previously unknown mediators of gut-brain axis communication. *Sci. Adv.* **2020**, *6*, eaax6328. [CrossRef] [PubMed]

203. Knobloch, M.; Pilz, G.A.; Ghesquière, B.; Kovacs, W.J.; Wegleiter, T.; Moore, D.L.; Hruzova, M.; Zamboni, N.; Carmeliet, P.; Jessberger, S. A Fatty Acid Oxidation-Dependent Metabolic Shift Regulates Adult Neural Stem Cell Activity. *Cell Rep.* **2017**, *20*, 2144–2155. [CrossRef] [PubMed]
204. Xie, Z.; Jones, A.; Deeney, J.T.; Hur, S.K.; Bankaitis, V.A. Inborn Errors of Long-Chain Fatty Acid β-Oxidation Link Neural Stem Cell Self-Renewal to Autism. *Cell Rep.* **2016**, *14*, 991–999. [CrossRef]
205. Argou-Cardozo, I.; Zeidán-Chuliá, F. Clostridium Bacteria and Autism Spectrum Conditions: A Systematic Review and Hypothetical Contribution of Environmental Glyphosate Levels. *Med. Sci.* **2018**, *6*, 29. [CrossRef]
206. Ho, L.; Zhao, D.; Ono, K.; Ruan, K.; Mogno, I.; Tsuji, M.; Carry, E.; Brathwaite, J.; Sims, S.; Frolinger, T.; et al. Heterogeneity in gut microbiota drive polyphenol metabolism that influences α-synuclein misfolding and toxicity. *J. Nutr. Biochem.* **2019**, *64*, 170–181. [CrossRef] [PubMed]
207. Wang, D.; Ho, L.; Faith, J.; Ono, K.; Janle, E.M.; Lachcik, P.J.; Cooper, B.R.; Jannasch, A.H.; D'Arcy, B.R.; Williams, B.A.; et al. Role of intestinal microbiota in the generation of polyphenol-derived phenolic acid mediated attenuation of Alzheimer's disease β-amyloid oligomerization. *Mol. Nutr. Food Res.* **2015**, *59*, 1025–1040. [CrossRef]
208. Reddy, V.P.; Aryal, P.; Robinson, S.; Rafiu, R.; Obrenovich, M.; Perry, G. Polyphenols in Alzheimer's Disease and in the Gut-Brain Axis. *Microorganisms* **2020**, *8*, 199. [CrossRef] [PubMed]
209. Filosa, S.; Di Meo, F.; Crispi, S. Polyphenols-gut microbiota interplay and brain neuromodulation. *Neural Regen. Res.* **2018**, *13*, 2055–2059. [CrossRef] [PubMed]
210. Feng, X.; Li, Y.; Brobbey Oppong, M.; Qiu, F. Insights into the intestinal bacterial metabolism of flavonoids and the bioactivities of their microbe-derived ring cleavage metabolites. *Drug Metab. Rev.* **2018**, *50*, 343–356. [CrossRef]
211. Gasperotti, M.; Passamonti, S.; Tramer, F.; Masuero, D.; Guella, G.; Mattivi, F.; Vrhovsek, U. Fate of microbial metabolites of dietary polyphenols in rats: Is the brain their target destination? *ACS Chem. Neurosci.* **2015**, *6*, 1341–1352. [CrossRef]
212. Cheng, C.Y.; Su, S.Y.; Tang, N.Y.; Ho, T.Y.; Chiang, S.Y.; Hsieh, C.L. Ferulic acid provides neuroprotection against oxidative stress-related apoptosis after cerebral ischemia/reperfusion injury by inhibiting ICAM-1 mRNA expression in rats. *Brain Res.* **2008**, *1209*, 136–150. [CrossRef] [PubMed]
213. Yabe, T.; Hirahara, H.; Harada, N.; Ito, N.; Nagai, T.; Sanagi, T.; Yamada, H. Ferulic acid induces neural progenitor cell proliferation in vitro and in vivo. *Neuroscience* **2010**, *165*, 515–524. [CrossRef]
214. Fuertes, A.; Perez-Burillo, S.; Apaolaza, I.; Valles, Y.; Francino, M.P.; Rufian-Henares, J.A.; Planes, F.J. Adaptation of the Human Gut Microbiota Metabolic Network During the First Year After Birth. *Front. Microbiol.* **2019**, *10*, 848. [CrossRef] [PubMed]
215. Fullana, M.A.; Albajes-Eizagirre, A.; Soriano-Mas, C.; Vervliet, B.; Cardoner, N.; Benet, O.; Radua, J.; Harrison, B.J. Fear extinction in the human brain: A meta-analysis of fMRI studies in healthy participants. *Neurosci. Biobehav. Rev.* **2018**, *88*, 16–25. [CrossRef] [PubMed]
216. Singewald, N.; Holmes, A. Rodent models of impaired fear extinction. *Psychopharmacology* **2019**, *236*, 21–32. [CrossRef] [PubMed]
217. Friedland, R.P.; Chapman, M.R. The role of microbial amyloid in neurodegeneration. *PLoS Pathog.* **2017**, *13*, e1006654. [CrossRef]
218. Lundmark, K.; Westermark, G.T.; Olsén, A.; Westermark, P. Protein fibrils in nature can enhance amyloid protein A amyloidosis in mice: Cross-seeding as a disease mechanism. *Proc. Natl. Acad. Sci. USA* **2005**, *102*, 6098–6102. [CrossRef]
219. Svensson, E.; Horváth-Puhó, E.; Thomsen, R.W.; Djurhuus, J.C.; Pedersen, L.; Borghammer, P.; Sørensen, H.T. Vagotomy and subsequent risk of Parkinson's disease. *Ann. Neurol.* **2015**, *78*, 522–529. [CrossRef]
220. Pan-Montojo, F.; Schwarz, M.; Winkler, C.; Arnhold, M.; O'Sullivan, G.A.; Pal, A.; Said, J.; Marsico, G.; Verbavatz, J.M.; Rodrigo-Angulo, M.; et al. Environmental toxins trigger PD-like progression via increased alpha-synuclein release from enteric neurons in mice. *Sci. Rep.* **2012**, *2*, 898. [CrossRef]
221. Miraglia, F.; Colla, E. Microbiome, Parkinson's Disease and Molecular Mimicry. *Cells* **2019**, *8*, 222. [CrossRef] [PubMed]
222. Bienenstock, J.; Kunze, W.A.; Forsythe, P. Disruptive physiology: Olfaction and the microbiome-gut-brain axis. *Biol. Rev. Camb. Philos. Soc.* **2018**, *93*, 390–403. [CrossRef] [PubMed]
223. Sampson, T.R.; Challis, C.; Jain, N.; Moiseyenko, A.; Ladinsky, M.S.; Shastri, G.G.; Thron, T.; Needham, B.D.; Horvath, I.; Debelius, J.W.; et al. A gut bacterial amyloid promotes α-synuclein aggregation and motor impairment in mice. *Elife* **2020**, *9*. [CrossRef] [PubMed]
224. Chen, S.G.; Stribinskis, V.; Rane, M.J.; Demuth, D.R.; Gozal, E.; Roberts, A.M.; Jagadapillai, R.; Liu, R.; Choe, K.; Shivakumar, B.; et al. Exposure to the Functional Bacterial Amyloid Protein Curli Enhances Alpha-Synuclein Aggregation in Aged Fischer 344 Rats and Caenorhabditis elegans. *Sci. Rep.* **2016**, *6*, 34477. [CrossRef]
225. Caputi, V.; Giron, M.C. Microbiome-Gut-Brain Axis and Toll-Like Receptors in Parkinson's Disease. *Int. J. Mol. Sci.* **2018**, *19*, 1689. [CrossRef] [PubMed]
226. Yang, D.; Zhao, D.; Shah, S.Z.A.; Wu, W.; Lai, M.; Zhang, X.; Li, J.; Guan, Z.; Zhao, H.; Li, W.; et al. Implications of gut microbiota dysbiosis and metabolic changes in prion disease. *Neurobiol. Dis.* **2020**, *135*, 104704. [CrossRef]
227. Blacher, E.; Bashiardes, S.; Shapiro, H.; Rothschild, D.; Mor, U.; Dori-Bachash, M.; Kleimeyer, C.; Moresi, C.; Harnik, Y.; Zur, M.; et al. Potential roles of gut microbiome and metabolites in modulating ALS in mice. *Nature* **2019**, *572*, 474–480. [CrossRef]

MDPI
St. Alban-Anlage 66
4052 Basel
Switzerland
Tel. +41 61 683 77 34
Fax +41 61 302 89 18
www.mdpi.com

Nutrients Editorial Office
E-mail: nutrients@mdpi.com
www.mdpi.com/journal/nutrients

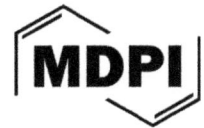

www.ingramcontent.com/pod-product-compliance
Lightning Source LLC
LaVergne TN
LVHW070458100526
838202LV00014B/1745